PRINCIPLES OF CLINICAL BIOCHEMISTRY

Principles of Clinical Biochemistry

Scientific Foundations

SECOND EDITION

Edited by

David L. Williams
MA MB PhD FRSC MRCPath
Consultant Chemical Pathologist, Royal Berkshire Hospital, Reading; Visiting Reader in Clinical Biochemistry, University of Surrey, Guildford

and

Vincent Marks
DM FRCP(Ed) FRCP FRCPath
Professor of Clinical Biochemistry, University of Surrey, Guildford; Consultant Chemical Pathologist, St Luke's Hospital, Guildford, Surrey

Heinemann Medical Books

Heinemann Medical Books

An imprint of Heinemann Professional Publishing Ltd
Halley Court, Jordan Hill, Oxford   OX2 8EJ

OXFORD   LONDON   SINGAPORE   NAIROBI   IBADAN   KINGSTON

First published
as *Scientific Foundations of Clinical Biochemistry*
   Vol 1: Analytical Aspects 1978
   Vol 2: Clinical Practice 1983

Second edition 1988

British Library Cataloguing in Publication Data

Principles of clinical biochemistry
   scientific foundations.—2nd ed.
   1. Medicine. Biochemistry
   I. Williams, David L. (David Llewelyn)
   II. Marks, Vincent   III. Williams, David L.
   (David Llewelyn). Scientific foundations
   of clinical biochemistry
   612′.015

ISBN 0 433 36389 4

Typeset and printed in Great Britain at The Bath Press, Avon

PREFACE TO THE FIRST EDITION

The application of analytical chemistry to the furtherance of medical knowledge began in earnest during the late nineteenth century with the work of such pioneers as Thudicum. These workers looked upon themselves as chemical pathologists whose determination it was to elucidate the chemistry of disease and by doing so to increase their understanding. It was only much later that the results of chemical analyses on biological fluids, initially especially on urine, began to be applied to the recognition and differentiation of disease in individual patients and this heralded the beginning of the era of clinical chemistry. Organizationally, these two branches of what can now best be described as clinical biochemistry remained separate; the elucidation and extension of knowledge of the biochemical basis of disease remaining firmly in the hands of clinicians, medical investigators and academic biochemists and the application of that knowledge to individual patients developing as a branch of clinical pathology. The artificiality of this division and its detriment to the growth and proper utilization of chemical and biological knowledge for the general benefit of mankind has not prevented its perpetuation in many parts of the world. Recognition is long overdue that clinical biochemistry, which can be defined as the application of analytical chemistry and a knowledge of biochemistry to the improvement in understanding, diagnosis, treatment and prevention of disease in man, is a single unified scientific discipline. It encompasses a number of subdivisions which have for many years masqueraded as separate academic disciplines such as metabolic medicine, chemical pathology, clinical chemistry and analytical chemistry and biochemistry. All seek to achieve the same objective, namely, the improvement of the health of individuals and of the community.

It was with this view of clinical biochemistry in mind that the editors embarked upon the preparation of this textbook on the Scientific Basis of Clinical Biochemistry. For the sake of convenience the work has been divided into two volumes. The first, here presented, is concerned with the analytical principles and techniques used to obtain the data which are the bed rock of medical knowledge and understanding. They are the same regardless of whether the data are used for the benefit of individual patients or as a contribution to the general corpus of scientific knowledge.

Volume II is concerned with the interpretive aspects and, therefore, more concerned with practicalities than the present one in which no attempt has been made, except by way of illustration, to describe particular analytical methods of managerial procedures in detail. These are usually best obtained from the original publications.

The subject matter chosen for inclusion in the two volumes is similar to that taught to MSc students in Clinical Biochemistry at the University of Surrey and to students on other advanced courses in clinical biochemistry.

PREFACE TO THE SECOND EDITION

Progress in the technology of clinical biochemistry has made a second edition of the *Scientific Foundations of Clinical Biochemistry* essential if it is to continue to fulfil its aim of providing, in readable form, a text on the scientific basis upon which that technology is based. Almost without exception the chapters retained from the first edition have been rewritten or pruned and updated, whilst some have been dropped because they have outgrown their usefulness. New developments, not foreseen in the earlier edition, have been given chapters of their own.

Increasingly, manufacturers of laboratory reagents and equipment are assuming responsibility for supplying clinical biochemists with the tools necessary for them to produce analytical data. But, without an understanding of the way that the reagents and equipment work and operate, the clinical biochemist is reduced to little more than an automaton dependent on the 'black box' he feigns to control. It is to provide that understanding that this volume is dedicated.

The many helpful comments we received following publication of the first edition have enabled us to produce a textbook that we believe will meet the requirements of all of those aspiring to pursue a career in clinical biochemistry, whether as a practitioner or manufacturer of equipment and reagents.

As in the first edition, the subject matter chosen for inclusion is similar to that taught to MSc students in Clinical Biochemistry at the University of Surrey, and to students on other advanced courses of clinical biochemistry.

We regret that Ronald F. Nunn, our co-editor of the first edition and a founder of the course on which this book is based, died in September, 1988.

David L. Williams
Vincent Marks

September, 1988

CONTENTS

SECTION 1

GENERAL TOPICS

SECTION 2

PHYSICAL MEASUREMENTS

SECTION 3

CHROMATOGRAPHY AND ELECTROPHORESIS

SECTION 4

BIOLOGICAL MEASUREMENTS

SECTION 5

AUTOMATION AND COMPUTING

* Deceased

LIST OF CONTRIBUTORS

G. Wynne Aherne, BSc PhD
   Experimental Officer and Research Fellow,
   University of Surrey, Guildford.

Josephine Arendt, BSc PhD
   Reader in Clinical Biochemistry, University of
   Surrey, Guildford.

Lucille Bitensky, MB BCh PhD DSc MRCP
   FRCPath
   Deputy Head of the Division of Cellular Biology,
   Kennedy Institute of Rheumatology, London.

R. C. Boguslaski, PhD
   Executive Vice President, Environmental Test
   Systems, Elkhart, Indiana, USA.

Alan M. Bold, MA BM BCh DCC MCB CChem
   FRSC FRCPath
   Consultant Chemical Pathologist, King Faisal
   Specialist Hospital and Research Centre, Riyadh,
   Kingdom of Saudi Arabia.

J. W. Bridges, BSc PhD CChem CBiol FRSC FIBiol
   MRCPath MInstEnvSci
   Director of the Robens Institute of Industrial and
   Environmental Health and Safety, and Professor
   of Toxicology, University of Surrey, Guildford.

Peter M. G. Broughton, BSc MCB FRSC FRCPath
   Deputy Director, Wolfson Research
   Laboratories, Queen Elizabeth Medical Centre,
   Birmingham.

Brendan M. Buckley MB MSc DPhil FRCPI
   Consultant Chemical Pathologist, Sandwell
   District Hospital, West Bromwich; Senior Clinical
   Lecturer, University of Birmingham.

David Burnett, PhD
   Consultant Clinical Biochemist, North-West
   Hertfordshire Health Authority

J. Chakraborty, MSc PhD CChem MRSC
   MRCPath.
   Senior Lecturer in Clinical Biochemistry,
   University of Surrey, Guildford.

G. S. Challand, PhD MCB FRSC
   Top Grade Biochemist, Royal Berkshire
   Hospital, Reading, Berkshire.

J. Chayen, PhD DSc MInstP FIBiol
   Head of the Division of Cellular Biology and the
   WHO Collaborative Centre for Cytochemical
   Bioassays, Kennedy Institute of Rheumatology,
   London.

Yannis Clonis, MSc PhD
   Senior Research Associate, Institute of
   Biotechnology, University of Cambridge.

J. G. H. Cook BSc PhD
   Top Grade Biochemist, Royal Sussex County
   Hospital, Brighton.

Martin Crowder, BSc DIC PhD
   Senior Lecturer in Mathematics, University of
   Surrey, Guildford.

J. B. Dawson, BSc PhD FInstP CPhys MIPSM
   Reader in Medical Physics and Acting Head of
   Department of Medical Physics, University of Leeds.

André De Bats, PhD
   Public Relations Consultant, Medical, Scientific
   and Technical Public Relations, Ascot, Berkshire.

Callum G. Fraser, BSc PhD FAACB
   Top Grade Biochemist and Honorary Senior
   Lecturer, Ninewells Hospital and Medical School,
   Dundee.

P. Garcia-Webb, MB BS MD FRCPA FAACB
   Clinical Biochemist, Sir Charles Gairdner
   Hospital and Consulting Biochemist to the King
   Edward Memorial Hospital, Nedlands, Western
   Australia.

R. Goodburn, BSc PhD
   Senior Biochemist, Ashford District Hospital,
   Ashford, Middlesex.

Barry J. Gould, MSc PhD
   Senior Lecturer in Biochemistry, University of
   Surrey, Guildford.

Julia B. Green, BSc
   Research Officer, Physics Department and
   Robens Institute of Industrial and Environmental
   Health and Safety, University of Surrey,
   Guildford.

D. W. Hill, MSc PhD DSc FInstP FIEE
   Regional Scientific Officer, North-East Thames
   Regional Health Authority.

Richard H. Hinton, BA PhD MRCPath
   Reader in Cell Pathology and Acting Head,
   Toxicology Unit, Robens Institute of Industrial
   and Environmental Heath and Safety, University
   of Surrey, Guildford.

R. Hubbard, BSc PhD CChem MRSC
   Lecturer in Immunology and Biochemistry,
   University of Surrey, Guildford.

Daphne F. Jackson, OBE DSc FInstP CPhys FIEE
   CEng
   Professor of Physics and Dean of the Faculty of
   Science, University of Surrey, Guildford.

R. U. Koenigsberger, PhD CChem FRSC
   Lecturer in Chemistry (retired), University of
   Surrey, Guildford.

C. R. Lowe, BSc PhD
   Director, Institute of Biotechnology, University
   of Cambridge.

Norman Lynaugh, BSc PhD
   Division Manager, VG Instruments Group
   (North), Manchester.

D. V. Mabbs, PhD MInstP
   Physicist to the Royal Berkshire Hospital,
   Reading, Berkshire (retired)

Vincent Marks, DM FRCP FRCPath
Professor of Clinical Biochemistry and Head of
Department of Biochemistry, University of
Surrey; Consultant Chemical Pathologist, St
Lukes Hospital, Guildford.

Donald W. Moss, MA PhD DSc
Professor of Clinical Enzymology and Honorary
Biochemist, Hammersmith Hospital, London.

Graham R. Parlett, BSc PhD
Lecturer, University of Surrey, Guildford.

C. P. Price, BSc MA PhD MCB CChem FRSC
Professor of Chemical Pathology, The London
Hospital Medical School.

Bernard F. Rocks, MSc PhD CBiol CChem MIBiol
FRSC
Top Grade Biochemist, Royal Sussex County
Hospital, Brighton Sussex.

Leslie J. Russell, BSc PhD CChem MRSC
Director of Technical Development, Cambridge
Life Sciences plc, Cambridge.

A. M. Stokes, BSc PhD
Commercial Development Manager, Monsanto
Chemical Company, St Louis, Missouri, USA.

David G. Taylor, PhD CPhys MInstP
Senior Lecturer in Physics, University of Surrey,
Guildford.

J. D. Teale, BSc PhD
Principal Biochemist, St Lukes Hospital, Guildford.

P. M. Timms, BSc. Dip CB
Acting Head of Clinical Biochemistry Department,
National Guard, King Khaled Hospital, Jeddah,
Saudi Arabia.

P. Vadgama, MB BS BSc PhD MRCPath
Professor of Clinical Biochemistry, University of
Manchester; Honorary Consultant Chemical
Pathologist, Hope Hospital, Salford.

Arthur W. Walker, BSc PhD MCB FRCPath
Top Grade Biochemist, St Lukes Hospital,
Guildford.

Bert Walter, PhD
Manager, Diabetes R & D Department, Miles
Diagnostics, Elkhart, Illinois, USA.

J. T. Whicher, MA MB BChir MSc MRCPath
Professor of Chemical Pathology, University of
Leeds.

D. L. Williams, MA MB CChem PhD MRCPath
FRSC
Consultant Chemical Pathologist and Head of
Clinical Biochemistry Department, Royal
Berkshire Hospital, Reading; Visiting Reader in
Clinical Biochemistry, University of Surrey,
Guildford.

Alan G. E. Wilson, BSc PhD
Senior Research Specialist and Head of the
Biochemical Toxicology and Metabolism Section,
Environmental Health Laboratory, Monsanto
Company, St Louis, Missouri, USA.

1. Laboratory Tests
Vincent Marks

INTRODUCTION

All clinical biochemistry tests have two essential components, (1) an analytical result and (2) its interpretation. Factors that influence the reliability of analytical results are discussed elsewhere in this volume, and in this chapter we are concerned exclusively with interpretation. It cannot be stressed too often, or too strongly, that analytically perfect results can, if wrongly interpreted, be just as harmful as incorrect data properly interpreted, especially as the latter will usually prompt further investigation—whereas the former are unlikely to do so.

PURPOSE OF LABORATORY TESTS

Laboratory tests are carried out for a variety of reasons. One of the commonest is to help the clinician establish a diagnosis upon which a rational approach to treatment and prognosis can be based. They are, however, used increasingly in treatment, to monitor the concentration of body constituents or drugs as a guide to further action. This is particularly important in those cases where too little treatment is ineffective but too much is harmful, such as in the chemotherapy of cancer and in haemodialysis therapy for renal failure.

Laboratory tests can, when carried out in a logical and orderly manner, be uniquely useful in elucidating the mechanism of disease not only in individual patients but generally. This was indeed the original reason for performing biochemical tests on patients and accounts for the term chemical pathology which means literally the study of the chemical basis of disease.

Less worthy reasons for performing, or requesting, laboratory tests are (1) as a substitute for thought or as a delaying tactic until the patient's illness either declares itself more clearly or resolves itself spontaneously; (2) as a real or supposed safeguard against a subsequent, possibly totally unwarranted, charge of criminal medical negligence; (3) as a prop to morale, especially in young and relatively insecure doctors entrusted with more responsibility than their clinical experience and knowledge justifies; (4) serendipitomania; which is the term used to describe the common habit of ordering all the laboratory tests one can think of in the hope of 'falling onto' a disease. Between them these less worthy reasons account for 20–80% of the tests carried out in clinical laboratories, the exact figure depending upon the standard and type of clinical medicine practised in the locality and the attitude of the laboratory director.

The reason for, and the purpose of, a laboratory test may profoundly effect the way it is performed. It is clearly more important, for example, to have a prompt, if only approximately correct analysis on a patient suspected of suffering from a potentially curable, but rapidly progressive and permanently damaging, condition—such as hypoglycaemia—than a delayed but accurate result, if this is the only alternative. Likewise, a method that may be insufficiently specific to distinguish one drug from another closely related to it under some circumstances may, nevertheless, be ideal for monitoring treatment with either drug alone.

As pointed out elsewhere in this volume it is an important function of clinical biochemists, by and large, to advise clinicians about which tests are best suited to solving their particular patients' problems. Few doctors, for example, really want to know what a patient's 24-h urinary 17-oxosteroid excretion is, although they may request it rather than lose face by asking for help in elucidating the role of the adrenal cortex in their patient's illness. The reason why a laboratory request is made is, therefore, an important part of the process whereby an analytical result becomes a clinically useful piece of information.

GENERAL CLASSIFICATION OF BIOCHEMICAL TESTS IN CLINICAL MEDICINE

Clinical biochemistry tests usually involve measuring the concentration of one or more substances in the blood, plasma, serum, saliva or urine of a patient and relating the result, so obtained, to a series of reference values obtained from healthy subjects, or other individuals who resemble the propositus as closely as possible in all respects except their freedom from the disease under suspicion. From time to time it is both necessary and desirable to examine other fluids such as CSF; peritoneal and pleural exudates; transudates; synovial and cystic fluids; duodenal aspirates and faeces; or to determine the rate of production (or utilization) of a substance in unit time rather than merely its concentration in one of the biological fluids.

Meaningful interpretation of clinical biochemistry tests requires consideration of both the intra- and extra-laboratory factors that are capable of influencing the result; where intralaboratory factors are those that relate exclusively to the analysis—such as its sensitivity, specificity, precision and accuracy—and extralaboratory factors are those that relate the analytical result to the individual patient from whom the specimen originated.

There has been an understandable tendency, in the past, for clinicians and clinical biochemists to emphasize the importance of intralaboratory factors—to the neglect of extralaboratory ones—partly because the latter are more difficult to control but mainly because their true significance is not fully appreciated. This lack of appreciation has its origins in history when clinical biochemistry tests were more concerned with gross or qualitative deviations from the norm than to subtle changes in quantity.

EXTRALABORATORY FACTORS

Extralaboratory factors capable of influencing the result and/or meaning of clinical laboratory tests are summarized in Table 1. They can, for convenience, be considered under two headings, namely those that relate (1) to the patient as an individual, (2) to the specimen collected from him.

In the section that follows it will not be possible to do more than give one or two examples of the way each extralaboratory factor can influence the result or interpretation of clinical biochemistry tests. The reader will doubtless think of numerous additional examples for himself.

Age and Sex

Many of the commonly measured constituents of the blood and plasma vary according to the subject's age and sex. Changes with age are especially profound during the first few years of life, particularly in the neonatal period. Many substances which have long been considered to change very little in concentration with increasing age are now known, largely as a result of massive population screening, to change quite markedly. Examples of this include plasma urea and glucose concentrations both of which increase with advancing years.

TABLE 1

EXTRALABORATORY FACTORS CAPABLE OF INFLUENCING THE RESULT AND/OR MEANING OF CLINICAL LABORATORY ANALYSES

'Patient determined' variables	Technical considerations
(1) Age	(a) Site of collection of specimen, e.g. venous or capillary
(2) Sex	
(3) Pregnancy	
(4) Stage of menstrual cycle	(b) Temporal relationship of specimen collection to physical examination or 'treatment'
(5) Body size	
(6) Ethnic group	
(7) Genetic variant	
(8) Place of domicile	(c) Cleanliness and composition of equipment used to collect and transport specimens to laboratory
(9) Normal diet	
(10) Interval since last meal	
(11) Time of day	
(12) Posture during test	
(13) Recent exercise	(d) Interval between collection of the specimen and its receipt in the laboratory
(14) Mental state during test	
(15) Non-specific illness	
(16) Medication	
	(e) Conditions of storage of specimen
	(f) Method of measurement

Plasma uric acid is possibly the best-known example of a substance, apart from the obviously sex-related steroid hormones, whose concentration in plasma is markedly different in men and women, but there are many others including various plasma proteins and certain enzymes, e.g. CK.

Stage of Menstrual Cycle

Measured values for sex hormones, and possibly many other constituents of the blood and urine, must be related to reference values appropriate to the stage of the patient's menstrual cycle for their full clinical significance to be appreciated.

Pregnancy

This not only profoundly affects the plasma concentration and amount excreted in the urine of virtually every hormone it is possible to measure, but also the concentration of many other substances ranging from plasma proteins and enzymes to electrolytes and vitamins.

Body Size

Body size alone appears to have little effect upon the *concentration* of different substances in blood and plasma. It does, however, have a profound bearing upon *total quantities*, such as blood volume, total body water, renal blood flow and glomerular filtration rate. Body size is especially important in determining the total amount of a substance excreted (or produced) in unit time whether it be a minute, an hour or a day.

The bigger an individual the more of a substance is usually produced, but what should be the standard or reference unit of bigness is still unsettled. It has, for example, long been customary to relate measurements of metabolic rate to body surface area, but this is arbitrary and an equally strong case could be made for standardizing it against either lean body weight or height. Doing so, however, appears to reduce the discriminatory function of the investigation, even though the measurement of weight or height is much more reliable than the calculation of body surface area from tables. Most other clinical biochemistry measurements in which the total amount of a substance, rather than just its concentration, is determined are either related to body weight, e.g. ml of blood per kg body weight, or to nothing at all as though the absolute value has clinical significance in its own right, e.g. mmol/24 h.

Ethnic Group; Habitat and Diet

There are large differences in the mean plasma cholesterol concentration of inhabitants in different parts of the world. This is due partly to ethnic differences but also to differences in their diet and way of life.

A striking example of the effect of geography, alone, on the biochemistry of healthy human beings is the difference in thyroidal ^{131}I uptake according to whether the subject lives in a high or low iodine-providing habitat. The thyroid glands of normal healthy residents of low iodine-providing, goitrous areas of the world, for example, take up radio-iodine rapidly and avidly giving them a 'neck-uptake' which would readily qualify them for a diagnosis of thyrotoxicosis if the results obtained were to be compared with reference values derived from inhabitants of fish-eating, iodine-rich communities such as the UK.

Time Elapsed Since Last Meal

It is well recognized that blood glucose concentration normally rises after a meal and then gradually falls to, or below, preprandial levels before finally returning to what is quaintly referred to as the 'fasting level' but which itself decreases still further if fasting is continued beyond the customary 12–14 h.

Probably most of the commonly measured constituents of plasma also vary in concentration according to the time elapsed since the last meal but scant attention has been paid to this possibility in the past apart from plasma lipids and, to a lesser extent, inorganic phosphate. Nevertheless whilst it would seem desirable always to collect specimens for analysis from patients after an overnight fast in order to minimize variations due to meals this is not always practicable and might itself obscure important and diagnostically significant differences between individuals. It must be remembered that the terms 'postprandial' and 'fasting' are, to a large extent, arbitrary and have different meanings in different parts of the world. In Britain a 'fasting' specimen is generally one collected after a 12–16 h fast; elsewhere it may be one collected after only 6–8 h without food depending upon local custom.

Time of Day

The rate of production of many endogenous compounds and/or their concentration in plasma, varies according to time of day. Probably the best-known example of this is the plasma cortisol concentration; peak plasma levels normally being observed about 8–9 a.m. and minimum levels about midnight. Other commonly measured substances which show similar, though less well marked diurnal fluctuations are plasma total iron and inorganic phosphate concentrations, both of which tend to be lower in the afternoon than in the morning.

Posture

The assumption of the upright posture after a moderate period of recumbency leads to haemoconcentration in the order of 10–20% within the space of 15 minutes or so and as a result of increased seepage of crystalloid rich ultrafiltrate of blood from the intra- to extravascular compartment of the extracellular fluid. When specimens collected from standing or sitting subjects are compared with those from recumbent subjects, this haemoconcentration effect increases by up to 20% the plasma concentration of most proteins and of those small molecular weight substances, such as cortisol, thyroxine, copper and iron, which are largely or completely bound or complexed to them. This important source of difference between clinical biochemistry measurements made on hospital inpatients—who are usually recumbent—and 'reference' populations who are usually ambulant, is often overlooked as is its ability to account for many of the apparently inexplicable fluctuations in plasma constituents often observed during serial measurements on individuals.

The use of a tourniquet to obtain blood from 'difficult' veins merely exaggerates the effects of haemoconcentration observed with changes in posture. These effects may become so great that serious errors of interpretation may occur, especially in relation to calcium, whose concentration in blood is normally controlled within very fine limits and is also modified by the plasma albumin concentration.

The effect of posture on the rate of gastric emptying, and consequently on the rate of absorption, of say a glucose load given in the course of a glucose tolerance test, is usually totally ignored both by clinical biochemists and clinicians even though it may profoundly affect the whole future of an individual patient's life. Results obtained from recumbent subjects are not strictly speaking comparable with those obtained in sitting or ambulant ones who, when given a large glucose load to drink, for example, are much more likely to exhibit reactive hypoglycaemia than are recumbent subjects. Yet how often is the posture of a subject during a test procedure controlled, still less recorded, except in research publications?

Physical Exercise and Mental State

Both physical exercise and mental state are capable of affecting bodily functions including the secretion and/or production of various hormones and intermediate metabolites which eventually pass into the blood and urine where they can be measured. Both fear and exercise are potent stimuli to growth hormone secretion, for example, and must be taken into account when attempting to interpret a plasma growth hormone measurement made on a nervous patient.

Prolonged inactivity, such as that produced by confinement to bed, can also profoundly affect metabolic responses—such as the ability to dispose of large oral glucose loads—and can in this way lead to erroneous conclusions when comparisons are made between the test data and reference values obtained from ordinary mobile individuals.

Non-specific Illness

Since one of the main purposes of clinical biochemistry testing is to aid (specific) diagnosis it is important to recognize that many biochemical parameters are altered non-specifically by all sorts of diseases. Changes as a result of moderate to severe illness in the concentration of the so-called acute phase proteins are probably the best recognized examples of this type of non-specific response; the fall in plasma iron concentration, the appearance of a glucose intolerance and the drop in plasma sodium concentration as a consequence of sick-cell-syndrome are others.

Drugs

Recognition that all sorts of drugs and other xenobiotics, whether prescribed or self-administered, can profoundly interfere with clinical biochemistry analyses or drastically alter their significance is surprisingly recent and still insufficiently appreciated by most clinicians.

The problem of drug interference with laboratory tests first came to the fore in the course of making measurements of plasma protein bound iodine when contamination of specimens received in the laboratory with iodine-containing x-ray contrast media not only invalidated the test on that particular specimen but that of all other specimens in the same and possibly several ensuing batches.

Some of the problems caused by drugs in clinical biochemistry are purely technical and can be overcome by using more specific analytical procedures *providing the problem is recognized*. In other cases the drug may induce a genuine physiological change in the individual to whom it has been administered which is reflected in a genuine alteration in the concentration or amount of substance measured in the laboratory. Since the reference population will not have been receiving the same drugs as the propositus intelligent interpretation of even regular clinical biochemistry results obtained from patients receiving drug therapy may be very difficult or impossible. This has not prevented practitioners from doing it, sometimes with unfortunate consequences for the patients. The list of recognized drug effects on clinical biochemistry tests is already so large that it can only be encompassed by a massive and constantly updated computer-based data storage and retrieval system such as that operated by Dr J. Salway at the University of Surrey. Since no single medical practitioner can be expected to carry even a small fraction of such a list around in his head it is encumbant upon him to let the analyst know, by recording it on the request form, what drugs the patient is receiving—or recently has received—in order that misinterpretation of the result from this cause can be minimized.

Technical Considerations

Timing of Specimen Collection. The temporal relationship between specimen collection and physical examination of the patient or administration of a drug can occasionally influence the interpretation of a clinical biochemistry test result. Errors have arisen for example, because a raised plasma CK concentration caused by an intramuscular injection given for relief of pain has been wrongly attributed to a myocardial infarct. At a more prosaic level I am amazed how often the first specimen sent to the laboratory for blood glucose analysis in a patient suspected of having hypoglycaemia, was collected *after* the patient had already been given intravenous glucose!

Many clinical biochemists and pharmacologists are concerned lest the enormous potential value to patients of blood drug measurements in the monitoring and regulation of drug therapy is vitiated by the seeming inability of a small minority of doctors and nurses to comprehend the importance of timing the collection of specimens correctly in relation to the last dose of drug. The data obtained if such care is taken can be clinically useful instead of being merely accurate results of a totally uninterpretable analysis.

Collection Site. Most blood specimens submitted for analysis are collected from a peripheral vein but occasionally they are obtained from an artery or nest of capillaries. The difference in source of the specimen can have either a trivial or major effect upon the analytical result and its significance, depending on the substance measured and the circumstances of its collection. Blood gas measurements are clearly more meaningful when made on arterial or, failing that, on arterialized capillary or venous blood, than when performed on an 'ordinary' venous sample. Different criteria must also be employed, for example, in interpreting blood glucose data obtained during oral glucose tolerance tests according to whether capillary or venous blood is analysed.

It is sometimes overlooked that venous, unlike arterial blood, is not homogeneous throughout the body, but reflects the anatomy, physiology and biochemistry of the tissues from which it comes. The difference between blood derived from different parts of the body, and from superficial versus deep veins, is most clearly seen with regard to substances such as glucose and lactate which are utilized or produced at different rates by different tissues.

Failure to take anatomy into account is responsible for the far from rare occasion when blood for analysis is collected from a vein into which an infusion is being given more peripherally. Unless spotted as the cause of error and depending on the substance being measured, this practice can lead to catastrophic misinterpretation of the analytical data with serious consequences for the patient. At best it leads to troublesome investigation into the cause of a clearly anomalous result.

Errors of interpretation have occurred because urine, obtained by percutaneous puncture, has been submitted to the laboratory for analysis in the mistaken belief that it was amniotic fluid; and bronchial secretions obtained through a misplaced Ryle's tube have been analysed in the mistaken belief that they were gastric juice. These are not isolated examples but merely illustrative of the necessity to take all factors into account when interpreting analytical data.

Equipment Used to Collect and Transport Specimens to the Laboratory. Swabs, needles and syringes used to collect, and containers used to transport specimens from the patient to the laboratory, for analysis, may need to be specially treated in order to prevent interference with subsequent chemical analyses and their interpretation. The use of an iodine swab to clean the skin before collecting blood for a protein-bound iodine test used, in the days when this was a popular test, to be as important a source of error as is the use of either ethyl alcohol or propanol impregnated swabs prior to the collection of blood for ethanol determinations today.

Failure to clean the skin properly before blood is collected may introduce large and potentially serious errors of interpretation. So may the use of syringes from which metals, or other materials, either leach out or adsorb causing erroneously high or low results respectively. The pots into which specimens are collected may occasionally contain, unbeknownst to the collector or analyst, either through ignorance or accident, the very substance it is intended to measure. Plasma lithium determinations, for example, may be increased—but not by so large an amount as immediately to arouse suspicion—by collecting blood into pots containing lithium heparin; and factitious elevation of plasma potassium levels because of contamination of the heparin pots with potassium instead of lithium or ammonium heparin is a well-recognized cause of error in clinical biochemistry practice.

The addition of more, or less, of a blood sample to a pot containing a preservative than the amount for which the pot was designed may also cause errors, either by failing to preserve adequately the constituents being measured, or by interfering with the analysis. Too high a concentration of sodium fluoride resulting from the addition of too little blood to the pot may, by interfering with the analytical procedure, produce a factitiously low blood glucose level; alternatively too low a concentration of fluoride may fail to prevent glycolysis and so also produce a falsely low value.

The use of syringes and/or pots made of glass instead of plastic, and onto which the hormone adsorbs both rapidly and irreversibly, is an important source of error in plasma ACTH and other hormone assays. Some assays are affected by one or more of the commonly used anticoagulants whilst yet others are invalidated by the use of serum instead of plasma. There are no rigid rules; experimentation, observation and constant vigilance are the only safeguards in this difficult area of clinical laboratory practice.

Storage of Specimens

Interval Between Collection and Analysis. The passage of time affects the concentration of many blood constituents once it has been shed from the body; some are destroyed and others are generated in the interval between the collection of the specimen and its analysis in the laboratory. The situation is further complicated by the fact that many substances of clinical importance are present in vastly different concentrations in the plasma and red cells. The best known example of confusion arising because of this is the elevation of plasma potassium levels that occurs whenever blood is allowed to stand overnight or for even shorter periods especially at refrigeration temperatures, before separation of the red cells from the plasma. Fortunately most clinical biochemists recognize a high 'plasma' potassium concentration resulting from this cause as an artifact and so prevent its misinterpretation but this is not always the case. Less seem to be aware that prolonged contact between red cells and plasma once they have been shed from the body may produce high plasma aminotransferase and lactic dehydrogenase values.

Some enzymes 'deteriorate' rapidly *in vitro* no matter how well the specimen is preserved. The clinical usefulness of red cell ALA dehydratase measurements as a test for chronic alcoholism or lead poisoning, for example, is greatly reduced by its instability which *in vitro* leads to a halving of its activity within 30 minutes of its collection no matter what treatment is employed.

Many of the more commonly measured red-cell and plasma enzymes are also unstable *in vitro* and are profoundly influenced by conditions of storage such as temperature and light.

Rapidly metabolized intermediate metabolites, such as pyruvate and lactate can be formed or utilized by red and white cells present in the specimen between the time of its collection and its analysis unless special precautions are taken to prevent it. Some compounds may be liberated from platelets or other organized constituents of the blood during clotting and a further group of substances such as fibrinogen and other coagulation factors, are either utilized or converted into other compounds. The 5-hydroxytryptamine in blood is contained almost exclusively within the platelets and is liberated into the serum during clotting.

Conditions of Storage. Some of the low molecular weight polypeptide hormones, such as ACTH, glucagon and PTH, are rapidly destroyed by enzymes present in plasma and must, therefore, be protected by the addition of suitable antiproteolytic agents to the blood immediately it is collected. Chilling of the specimen before and during centrifugation may also be required to ensure maximum stability. But whilst chilling—both during preparation and storage—usually increases stability, some plasma constituents such as aldolase, alanine aminotransferase and pre-β-lipoprotein (VLDL) are damaged by it. Alternate freezing and thawing is particularly damaging to proteins including those that are relatively stable at either temperature alone.

Ultra-violet irradiation or daylight destroys bilirubin remarkably quickly, and the mere standing of a blood or plasma specimen on a bench in direct sunlight can convert an abnormal icteric serum into a 'normal' one very rapidly and without anyone being the wiser.

Preservatives are often added to urine to prevent bacterial growth and/or prevent autodestruction of certain labile constituents such as adrenaline. Unfortunately there is no single all-purpose preservative; instead the correct one must be chosen according to the substance to be measured and the analytical method employed. Consequently the preservative used may vary from one laboratory to another, even for the same constituent, a fact that is insufficiently appreciated by laboratory users to whom methodology is often merely a tiresome detail!

Conclusion. It is axiomatic that an analysis is only as reliable as the specimen it is done on. As so many extralaboratory factors are capable of influencing the analytical result, its interpretation and clinical significance, it is perhaps more surprising that clinical biochemistry determinations are clinically useful than that they have limitations.

Proper documentation of the patient and the specimens obtained from him, including the conditions of collection, will undoubtedly help reduce the risk of misinterpreting the results of analytical tests. But whilst knowledge of the preventable sources of interpretive error is a step in the direction of their total elimination, constant vigilance is also required if previously unknown or unforeseen causes of interference are to be avoided completely.

TYPES OF LABORATORY TESTS

Most clinical biochemistry tests are performed on blood, plasma or serum as:

1. 'discretionary' or 'one-off' tests designed or intended to answer specific questions;
2. an admission profile;
3. part of a dynamic function test; or
4. an integral part of a metabolic work-up.

or on cells obtained by biopsy, aspiration or amniocentesis.

Strictly speaking *all* clinical biochemistry tests are urgent as their purpose is to help the clinician relieve the patient from suffering as quickly as possible. In practice, however, it is customary to divide tests, arbitrarily, into those which are urgent and those which are less urgent. The basis of this classification will be discussed later.

The Discretionary or 'One-off' Test

Discretionary tests were the original and are still the commonest type of clinical biochemistry investigation. They can be looked upon as being designed to answer a specific question such as 'does this patient have a high blood urea concentration? (which would lend weight to my tentative diagnosis of kidney disease)' or 'does this patient have an increased amount of blood in his faeces? (which might account for his anaemia)'. If the result of a discretionary test conforms to that postulated by the hypothesis (which in practice is usually unformulated), it is generally described as 'consistent with' or 'supporting' the putative diagnosis. An analytical result cannot, as some would like to believe, confirm or establish a diagnosis; it can only help strengthen (or weaken) it. The only exception to this rule is when the 'diagnosis' is itself a chemical definition, e.g. uraemia, hypercalcaemia or hypoglycaemia, in which case it is more properly termed a description, like lameness, and is an invitation to further investigation and elucidation.

Analyses performed on blood and plasma are

almost invariably quantitative, but those performed on urine and faeces are often qualitative or only semi-quantitative. This is not altogether bad since quantitative measurements performed on excreta are usually clinically meaningless unless expressed in terms of mass of substance excreted per unit time and not merely as concentration per unit volume. In order to express results in terms of mass per unit time, it is necessary either to collect an accurately timed specimen, which is usually extremely difficult, or to use an internal standard. The best-known example of an endogenous internal standard is creatinine, whose excretion in the urine is usually more or less constant, both throughout the day and from day to day in the same individual, and is related, in general, to muscle bulk rather than to variations in diet, activity and the subject's current state of health. In the faeces non-absorbable substances such as chromium sesquioxide and copper thiocyanate taken in known amounts at regular intervals throughout the day for a period of at least three days, have been used as internal standards. This manoeuvre enables the investigator to express the substance in which he is interested in terms of mass excreted per g of reference material and hence—by calculation—per unit time; without having to depend upon the notoriously unreliable 'timed' faecal collection.

Discretionary tests have a number of practical advantages. They may tell the clinician all he wants to know in order to make or dismiss a diagnosis or alter his treatment and because they require only a single specimen—which can often be collected at the patient's first attendance—are generally convenient for doctor, patient and laboratory alike. Their major disadvantage is that they are generally insensitive and non-specific. Quite serious kidney disease can be present, for example, before the blood urea concentration becomes diagnostically high and conversely a high blood urea concentration does not—by itself—indicate renal damage.

Discretionary tests, as ordinarily performed, are often uninterpretable because the conditions under which the specimen was collected were uncontrolled, or unrecorded, or both. For many substances, as we have already seen, it is important to know the time of day when the specimen was collected and the patient's mental and physical state at the time, when he last ate, and the nature and quantity of any drugs he might have been taking. All these factors, and many others, are capable of affecting the clinical significance of an analytical result but are often ignored because their proper control and documentation takes medical time as well as 'inconveniencing' the patient. Nevertheless, whilst most doctors and clinical biochemists know of cases in which the condition of a patient has been wrongly diagnosed and consequently wrongly treated, because laboratory results were misinterpreted, either through ignorance or oversight, almost all of the information relating to this topic is merely anecdotal.

The main reason 'one-off' tests are requested is to gain additional information to support a tentative diagnosis—often referred to, incorrectly, as 'confirming' it—or to monitor treatment. Because analyses are usually carried out by a third person and can be expressed numerically, they may carry more weight with junior and inexperienced doctors than is clinically justified. Clinical biochemists recognizing this and wishing to minimize the consequences of analytical errors, sometimes advocate double checking all abnormal results for analytical errors. A genuinely 'abnormal' result which is wrongly reported (or interpreted) as 'normal' may, however, be equally damaging, since it may be thought wrongly to have 'excluded' the original tentative diagnosis of a potentially curable illness. As an example of this one can quote the early dismissal of a tentative clinical diagnosis of spontaneous hypoglycaemia due to insulinoma on the basis of a single 'normal' blood glucose concentration. Another is hypothyroidism which, once suspected and dismissed by the finding of a 'normal' plasma thyroxine concentration, is unlikely to be reconsidered by the same clinician for many years. During this time the patient will have continued to suffer unnecessarily from a completely curable disease.

An insurmountable disadvantage of 'one-off' tests is that they represent the conditions prevailing in the patient's body at a single moment in time, whereas many diseases tend to be episodic both in their nature and manifestations. The timing of specimen collection may be absolutely crucial, therefore, if it is to provide useful clinical information. For example, a positive 'diagnosis' of hypoglycaemia can be made only by the demonstration of a low blood glucose concentration. This is much more likely if blood is collected from the patient whilst he is symptomatic than when he is in remission, which is most of the time.

'One-off' tests provide the investigator with no information about the biochemical flux or metabolic turnover rate of the substances he is measuring. Nor are they usually very helpful in elucidating the pathophysiological mechanism of a particular disease, although they may suggest lines of further investigation. The discovery of a high blood urea concentration may indicate excessive urea production, decreased elimination, dehydration or a combination of the three. Further investigative steps must be taken to find out which is correct.

Biochemical Profile

The concept of the 'biochemical profile' stems from the fact that sometimes more clinically useful information can be obtained by measuring the concentration of two or more interdependent substances and considering the results collectively than by considering them individually. Amongst the better known examples of 'biochemical profiles' are 'plasma electrolytes' (i.e. sodium, potassium, chloride, bicarbonate and urea); the so-called 'liver function tests' (more accurately referred to as differential diagnosis of jaundice tests), e.g. plasma bilirubin, aspartate aminotransferase, alkaline phosphatase and plasma proteins; and the 'calcium screen', e.g. plasma calcium, inorganic phosphate and alkaline phosphatase.

It is important to distinguish 'biochemical profiling', which is carried out on patients, i.e. people who have symptoms and are, therefore, dis-eased, from the seemingly similar process of 'biochemical screening' which is performed on uncomplaining asymptomatic individuals. Although the constituents of the two types of test are the same, their purpose (and function) is different. Neither type is clinically very useful.

The main advantages of 'biochemical profiles' are that they are (a) convenient for the doctor, patient and laboratory alike, especially if a multi-channel analyser is available to carry out all of the analyses on a single sample without further subdivision within the laboratory; (b) generally much cheaper to perform than the sum of their constituent parts; (c) sometimes all that is required to establish or substantiate the tentative clinical diagnosis; (d) very occasionally able to provide information, especially after computer-assisted multivariate analysis, which cannot otherwise be readily obtained.

With the large multi-channel analysers now available from many manufacturers, it often costs very little more, and sometimes less, to perform six, twelve or even twenty different analyses on a single specimen 'on-line' than to perform two or three discretionary tests using single-channel equipment. The true cost-benefit of this approach to analytical biochemistry has still to be established, however. The evidence available lends no support to the argument that indiscriminate profiling using such equipment either reduces overall intralaboratory costs or cuts down in-patient time in hospital.

An important disadvantage of the 'biochemical profile' is that, like 'one-off' discretionary tests, it provides information about the chemistry of the blood at only a single point in time. Profiles tend to be insensitive and unhelpful clinically unless at least one of their constituents is grossly abnormal. Clinicians receiving the data may actually overlook clinically important information in the welter of unrequested and uninterpretable information, a condition well recognized as data fatigue.

A further practical disadvantage of the 'biochemical profile' is that biochemical anomalies may be uncovered that are of no particular clinical relevance and possibly totally innocent. Their discovery may cause alarm and meddlesome medical interference or, at best, additional unwarranted investigation. It is difficult, at the present time, to see how this inherent disadvantage of indiscriminate biochemical testing can be overcome except by suppressing unrequested information or better, by abandoning it.

Dynamic Function Tests

One of the main attributes of living things is their ability to react, in a characteristic and quantifiable manner, to external stimulation. The loss or alteration of this facility is sometimes the cause of a patient's disease; more often, however, it occurs as an associated epiphenomenon which can be used clinically as an indicator of incipient pathology—sometimes long before permanent anatomical damage has developed.

Comparison of a patient's response to a standardized stimulus with that obtained in a suitable reference group, is referred to as a dynamic function test and it bears the same relation to the 'one-off' discretionary test as a movie film does to a photographic 'still'. Dynamic function tests are not confined to clinical biochemistry, indeed virtually all 'physiological tests' employed in medicine fall into this category.

The conventional oral glucose tolerance test is probably the best known example of a dynamic function test. So important has it become that many notable authorities use the glucose tolerance test, not merely as an aid to the diagnosis of diabetes mellitus, but to define it. This practice is both illogical and clinically unsound and is responsible for much of the confusion that surrounds the definition, diagnosis, understanding and treatment of the diabetic syndrome. It is so firmly entrenched, however, that it will be extremely difficult to dispel until some better and more specific definition can be produced.

Examples of other dynamic function tests employed in clinical biochemistry are given in Table 2. They vary in complexity, both in their performance and in their interpretation, from such simple procedures as the synacthen test for adrenocortical reserve to the pancreozymin-secretin test, with duodenal intubation, for pancreatic exocrine function.

In the main, dynamic function tests have greater sensitivity and are more organ and/or disease specific than 'one-off' tests or 'biochemical profiles'. Moreover, unlike the latter, dynamic function tests can provide information about the nature and mechanism of a patient's illness, especially when this is primarily due to a biochemical lesion.

Most dynamic function tests can be performed on out-patients if suitable accommodation is available. Ideally, these tests should be carried out in special investigation units where all the necessary equipment, staff and facilities are immediately available but failing this, ordinary out-patient facilities can be used.

Dynamic function tests are necessarily time-consuming for both the patient and the investigator, whether he be a doctor, biochemist, technician or nurse. Some patient preparation, such as overnight fasting and the withholding or administration of drugs; limitation of exercise and maintenance of the recumbent posture, is generally necessary before the test can be carried out, and a varying amount of technical clinical expertise is usually also required. This may be very little, as in the case of the urine concentration test for renal tubular function which can be carried out by an intelligent patient on himself after only a few minutes instruction. On the other hand, the collection of bile from the duodenum as part of the secretin-pancreozymin test for chronic pancreatic disease, requires considerable skill in addition to the services of a radiology department with fluoroscopic facilities.

The greatest difficulty with this type of test is undoubtedly in obtaining reliable and applicable reference values, especially since many of the investigations are not only time consuming and to a greater or lesser extent unpleasant, but also potentially hazardous.

upon a metabolic work-up, to have some idea of the possible causes of the patient's illness and to know roughly what investigations are most likely to reveal it. It must never be forgotten that in the course of a metabolic work-up the patient is often grossly inconvenienced and suffers a variable amount of additional discomfort but has no guarantee that he will necessarily benefit from it. For this reason the vainglorious hope that mere initiation of a series of undirected investigations will reveal the cause of a patient's problems should be strongly discouraged except as part of an ethically acceptable experiment to which the patient has given his informed consent.

In the past the metabolic work-up was used extensively to investigate disorders of energy and mineral metabolism, which generally involved accurately

TABLE 2

SELECTION OF DYNAMIC FUNCTION TESTS EMPLOYED IN CLINICAL BIOCHEMISTRY

Name of test	Duration (hours)	System tested	Degree of 'medical' expertise
Dexamethasone	–	Adrenal cortex	0
Synacthen	0·75	Adrenal cortex	±
Bromsulphthalein	1–2	Liver	+ +
Intravenous fructose	1–2	Fructose metabolism	+ +
Oral glucose	2–3	Glucose homeostasis	±
Insulin stress	2–3	Hypothalamic-pituitary	+ + +
2-deoxyglucose	2–3	Adrenomedullary	+ + +
Creatinine clearance	2–4	Glomerular filtration	+
Secretin pancreozymin	2–4	Exocrine pancreas	+ + +
Pentagastrin	12–14 (overnight)	Gastric mucosa	+ +
Urine concentration	>24	Renal tubules	±

Programmed Intensive Investigation or 'Metabolic Work-Up'

A definitive diagnosis, sufficiently strong to serve as the basis for treatment, can usually be made on the patient's history and physical examination with or without the aid of a small number of laboratory investigations. In some cases, however, the cause of a patient's ill health remains obscure and more intensive investigation than can easily be performed on an out-patient basis becomes necessary. In cases where the underlying abnormality is wholly or predominantly biochemical, rather than anatomic, psychogenic or infective, such an intensive investigation can properly be referred to as a metabolic (or endocrinological) work-up which may either be unique to the individual patient or follow a well-defined protocol.

The details of a metabolic work-up naturally varies according to the nature of the patient's illness and the investigator's understanding of it. Often some measure of dietary or other control is required in order to produce as nearly standardized conditions as possible so as to facilitate comparison with reference populations. It is essential, before embarking

timed collections of urine and faeces. Because of historical development it is still widely believed that all metabolic work-ups require urine and faecal collections and the performance of balance studies. This is not so. Elucidation of the pathogenesis of hypoglycaemia, for example, from amongst the hundred or more possible causes, may require a metabolic work-up but virtually never involves the making of measurements on either urine or faeces. Such measurements may be required, however, for elucidation of other types of inherited and acquired metabolic disorder.

The chemical and immunochemical analysis of tissue biopsies, collected under a variety of different but standardized conditions, may constitute part of a metabolic work-up. Such analyses may be limited to a single static measurement, e.g. the amount of iron per gram of liver tissue in a biopsy specimen from a patient believed to be suffering from haemochromatosis, or alternatively may involve detailed dynamic examination of complex intracellular metabolic pathways such as those involved in glycolysis in a piece of muscle obtained from a patient with suspected glycogen storage disease type V (McArdle's syndrome).

Despite their drawbacks, metabolic work-ups can be looked upon as the epitome of clinical biochemistry bringing, as they do, the concerted skills of analytical biochemists, molecular biologists and practising clinicians, to the help of individual patients. Time alone will tell how far expenditure on this type of investigation is financially justified on the basis of the number of individuals who are converted from chronic invalids, as a result of metabolic and/or endocrine disease, into fit and gainfully employed members of the community.

'Emergency' Assays

In theory all clinical laboratory investigations are urgent since, ostensibly, the sole reason for performing them is either to hasten diagnosis—and hence the inauguration of effective treatment—or to monitor and possibly adjust treatment already under way. In practice, however, many of the biochemical tests requested on patients contribute only a small, and non-essential, component to the overall clinical picture, which usually depends much more heavily on information derived from other sources, notably the clinical history and physical examination. Nevertheless, in an important minority of cases, biochemical data are vital to the correct management of the case and may indeed be required urgently if the patient is not to suffer irremedial harm. Tests performed under these circumstances can conveniently be described as 'emergency' assays to distinguish them from those with lesser degrees of urgency.

A convenient definition of an emergency assay is that it arises when a physician requires a result in order to establish *immediately* what treatment is appropriate and not merely to satisfy his curiosity. It must be recognized that this definition accepts the essential arbitrariness of the term 'emergency' since it depends, in part, upon individual value judgements.

A distinction is sometimes made between emergency work arising during normal working or office hours and that arising at other times. Such a distinction is unfortunate. It tends to blur the real distinction between urgent and non-urgent tests which is dictated solely by clinical and not by administrative or financial considerations although it must be recognized that these factors cannot be ignored completely.

Some laboratories are organized on a 24 h a day, seven days a week basis, but evidence that this is either cost-effective or beneficial to individual patients has not so far been produced. The majority of laboratories, therefore, continue to distinguish between 'regular' and out-of-hours work. Many laboratories have a special section devoted exclusively to the performance of emergency investigations, which is manned, equipped and located separately from the rest of the department. It must be recognized, however, that whilst emergency laboratories may be practicable in large institutions they may not be in small or impoverished ones and compromise solutions must be applied.

There is convincing evidence that, in the absence of a special laboratory devoted to them, analyses carried out on an emergency basis are seldom as accurate or precise as similar tests carried out under ordinary conditions. There are many reasons for this unfortunate state of affairs, chief amongst them being the necessity to employ relatively junior, and/or inexperienced staff —who normally work in other sections of the pathology laboratory—to perform out-of-hours analyses. Some of these organizational difficulties can be overcome by utilizing 'dedicated equipment' and prepacked reagents which are ideal for emergencies and well within the budget of even the most impoverished laboratory.

The decision about the biochemical investigations that could or should be made available on an emergency basis is influenced by many factors; some of them technical and clinical; others, of necessity, financial and administrative. Some biochemical analyses cannot, for purely technical reasons, be made available to clinicians sufficiently quickly to influence the decision to treat. It might, for example, be desirable to know the plasma thyroid hormone levels in a patient suspected of suffering from thyrotoxic crisis (thyroid-storm) but the danger to the patient's health—including the risk of death—of delaying treatment until the result of the test became available, is so much greater than the risk of causing damage by instituting treatment solely on clinical evidence, that no experienced clinician would consider doing so.

Authorities differ in their views on the tests that should be available on an emergency basis; most would accept those listed in Table 3 as a minimum.

TABLE 3
EMERGENCY CLINICAL BIOCHEMISTRY TESTS

Generally available		Under special circumstances	
Plasma:	Sodium	*Plasma:*	AST
	Potassium		Osmolality
	Bicarbonate		Lithium
	Urea		Iron
	Calcium		Barbiturate
	Amylase		Carbon
	CK		monoxide
	Bilirubin		Digoxin
	Salicylate	*Blood:*	Lead
	Paracetamol		
	Fibrinogen		
Blood:	pH, $P\text{CO}_2$, $P\text{O}_2$		
CSF:	Glucose		
	Protein		
Urine:	Porphobilinogen (qualitative)		

Analytical procedures which might reasonably be expected to be available on an emergency basis in all but the smallest clinical biochemistry laboratory.

There are, however, no hard and fast rules. Every case must be considered on its merits. The general rule that only tests, the result of which will influence *immediate* treatment, should be considered as genuine emergencies, provides a useful yardstick.

Side-room Tests

Several, usually semi-quantitative, clinical biochemistry tests have traditionally been performed either at the bedside or in the practitioner's own office. These tests which include urinalysis for sugar, blood glucose measurement and protein and faecal tests for occult blood, are amongst the most important 'routine' analytical procedures used in clinical medicine. In hospitals they are usually assigned to the most junior and inexperienced person on the ward to perform. This accounts for the very high percentage of erroneous results produced under these circumstances and of which the majority of clinicians, and administrators (and clinical biochemists) are unaware. The high percentage of erroneous results obtained under average working conditions should not be allowed to detract from the very real advantage of side-room testing which is growing in importance rapidly and inexorably. Instead, clinical biochemists should ensure, by careful monitoring of the results of such tests, that full advantage is taken of technological advances, which enable biochemical analyses to be performed where and when they are required rather than after transportation of the specimen to a remote laboratory.

Screening

The concept of well-person screening is based on the unproven belief that presymptomatic diagnosis of real or potential disease is always both possible and advantageous. The undoubted success of mass x-ray screening for detecting pulmonary tuberculosis at a stage when symptoms were still trivial, infectivity high and irreversible destruction of the lungs minimal, encouraged belief in the general validity of the concept. It was further fortified when curative therapy with streptomycin and other tuberculocidal drugs led to virtual eradication of the disease in the endogenous population of the UK and other developed countries.

Extension of the philosophy of 'well-person' screening to other clinical areas has, unfortunately, not been accompanied by such clear-cut evidence of benefit to individual subjects or to the community. The advantages accruing to asymptomatic individuals screened for so-called early diabetes, for example, and other currently incurable diseases are so dubious that many people doubt the wisdom of this exercise either on economic or clinical grounds. There is currently no convincing evidence that detection of conditions, like atherosclerosis and osteoporosis, of such 'minimal' degree as to be symptomless alters the patient's ultimate prognosis. There is, on the other hand, reason to believe that the disastrous consequences of inducing hypochondriasis and/or non-disease in previously healthy individuals, by the imprudent handling of results of laboratory screening tests has been insufficiently appreciated by enthusiasts.

From a clinical or patient-orientated point of view, there is no particular virtue in being able to diagnose asymptomatic disease unless some action can be taken which has been *proved*, beyond doubt, to produce more benefit than harm. Mere belief—however, fervent—that this or that 'treatment' will produce benefit is not enough. It would be just as absurd however, to say that biochemical screening has absolutely no value: its place in preventing the mental and physical damage that can result from the uncontrolled ravages of certain inborn errors of metabolism, such as phenylketonuria, is so well established as to be unshakeable: but these are conditions for which there is an effective preventive treatment. These diseases differ too from certain other conditions revealed by some mass-screening programmes in that they are clinical entities—not merely biochemical anomalies or markers of dubious or unknown significance.

There is so much still to be learned about biochemical individuality that the inauguration, in healthy subjects, of large-scale programmes to detect minor or even major deviations from what is arbitrarily called the norm is premature. Two exceptions to this general rule are (1) the use of biochemical screening techniques to detect, especially in the neonatal period, inborn errors of metabolism and other diseases which are amenable to correction *before* irreparable physical damage has occurred and (2) the use of regular screening or 'check-ups' on people working, or habitually coming into contact with cumulative toxic agents such as lead, mercury and pesticides. Here the detection of the toxic agent in the body fluid either by direct analysis or by its biochemical effects can lead to correction before irreparable damage has developed.

A further place where screening has an important role to play is the detection of carriers of genetic disease using gene probes and in fetuses at risk of genetic or acquired disease, by means of amniocentesis.

EVALUATION OF TESTS

It is amazing, in view of the fact that one of the main purposes of clinical biochemistry testing is to benefit individual patients, how little attention has been given, in the past, to assessing the true clinical usefulness of a biochemical test before introducing it into regular use.

In this, as in other areas of medicine, there are no hard and fast rules and each new test procedure must be evaluated on its own individual merits. Consideration must, however, be given to its precision and accuracy; sensitivity and specificity; discrimination, predictive value and patient acceptability, as well as to its effectiveness and cost. It will be readily appreciated, from this list of conditions, that a specific analytical procedure may be wholly justified as a biochemical test in one clinical situation but not in another. It emphasizes the conceptual difference between a simple analysis and a clinical biochemistry test which, as was pointed out at the beginning of this chapter, always contains an interpretive as well as an analytical component.

Many of the clinical biochemistry tests currently carried out in clinical laboratories would probably not be requested or undertaken if their true contribution to the patient's overall wellbeing could be properly evaluated. This evaluation is however difficult to carry out and few investigators have even attempted to do so. What evidence there is suggests that whilst clinical biochemistry (and other laboratory) tests are invaluable or indispensable in a small but important group of subjects they are in the majority of patients at best only moderately or slightly helpful. Sometimes they may be frankly misleading and counterproductive.

Evaluation of the clinical usefulness of analyses as ordinarily carried out in hospital laboratories has led some clinical biochemists, including the author of this chapter, to advocate greater use of the resources available to them for the investigation of patients for whom clinical biochemistry has a unique role to play—either in the diagnosis or management of their disease—rather than on the provision of a more or less uniformly thin blanket of routine investigations on every patient regardless. Adoption of such a philosophy will undoubtedly require radical rethinking by many clinicians and clinical biochemists, but will in the long run assuredly be to their advantage as well as to that of their patients.

FURTHER READING

Asher R. (1954). Straight and crooked thinking in medicine. *Br. Med. J*; **2**: 460.
(*Witty and pithy comments by a superior clinician who was also a master of the written word.*)

Barnett R. N. (1967). Profile admission data. *Clin. Chem*; **13**: 81.
(*A short letter to the editor putting the arguments against producing clinical biochemistry profiles on everyone.*)

Bold A. M. (1976). Clinical chemistry reporting: problem and proposals. *Lancet*; **i**: 951.
(*A clear exposition of the necessity for the integration of extra- and intralaboratory information in order to obtain an interpretable result.*)

Bradwell A. P., Carmalt M. H. B., Whitehead T. P. (1974). Explaining the unexpected abnormal results of biochemical profile investigations. *Lancet*; **ii**: 1071.
(*The title is self-explanatory.*)

Caraway W. T. (1962). Chemical and diagnostic specificity of laboratory tests: effect of hemolysis, lipemia, anticoagulants, medications, contaminants, and other variables. *Am. J. Clin. Pathol*; **37**: 445.

(*One of the first detailed descriptions of the role of extralaboratory factors in the production and interpretation of clinical biochemistry data.*)

Caraway W. T. (1971). Accuracy in clinical chemistry. *Clin. Chem*; **17**: 63.
(*An updating of his earlier paper.*)

Carter P. M., Davison A. J., Wickings H. V. I., Zilva J. F. (1974). Quality and quantity in chemical pathology. *Lancet*; **ii**: 1555.
(*A worthwhile discussion of priorities in clinical biochemistry.*)

Galen R. S., Gambino S. R. (1975). *Beyond Normality: The Predictive Value and Efficiency of Medical Diagnosis*. New York: Wiley.
(*The seminal work on the predictive value of tests.*)

Hampton J. R., Harrison M. J. G., Mitchell J. R. A., Prichard J. S., Seymour C. (1975). Relative contributions of history-taking, physical examination, and laboratory investigation to diagnosis and management of medical outpatients. *Br. Med. J*; **2**: 486.
(*The title is self-explanatory.*)

Holland W. W., Whitehead T. P. (1974). Value of new laboratory tests in diagnosis and treatment. *Lancet*; **ii**: 391.
(*The title is self-explanatory.*)

Lancet (1967). Interpretation of laboratory tests. *Lancet*; **i**: 1091.
(*A leading article in* The Lancet *which was amongst the first critically to examine this problem—deals virtually exclusively with clinical biochemistry.*)

Lancet (1973). Is more really better?; *Lancet*; **i**: 977.
(*Also deals virtually exclusively with clinical biochemistry.*)

Lancet (1975). Mass screening for cretinism. *Lancet*; **ii**: 356.
(*Is this one of the few disorders worth screening for despite the apparent technical difficulties?.*)

Landon J., Sanders P., Peppiatt R., Clayton B., Jenkins P., Cotgrove I. (1971). Emergency chemical pathology service in central London. *Lancet*; **ii**: 480.
(*The title is self-explanatory.*)

Marks V., Alberti K. G. M. M., eds (1985). *Clinical Biochemistry Nearer the Patient*. Edinburgh: Churchill Livingstone.

Marks V., Alberti, K. G. M. M., eds (1986). *Clinical Biochemistry Nearer the Patient II*. Eastbourne: Transmedica.
(*Two books describing modern trends.*)

Meador C. K. (1965). The art and science of non-disease. *New Engl. J. Med*; **272**: 92.
(*The first quasi-humorous and satirical delineation of 'non-disease'.*)

Office of Health Economics. The health care dilemma 1975, Office of Health Economics, No. 53.
(*A short and very readable booklet on the dilemmas produced by well-person screening.*)

Sackett D. L. (1973). The usefulness of laboratory tests in health-screening programs. *Clin. Chem*; **19**: 366.
(*Well worth reading.*)

Sackett D. L., Holland W. W. (1975). Controversy in the detection of disease. *Lancet*; **ii**: 357.
(*The title is self-explanatory.*)

Sunderman F. W. (1975). Current concepts of 'normal values',: 'reference values', and 'discrimination values' in clinical chemistry. *Clin. Chem*; **21**: 1873.
(*The title is self-explanatory.*)

Todd J. W. (1968). Cost and complexity of medicine. *Lancet*; **ii**: 823.
(*A clinician's view of some overvalued activities including laboratory investigations.*)

Whitby L. G. (1974). Screening for disease: definitions and criteria. *Lancet*; **ii**: 819.
(*The first, and in some ways the most useful, of a series of articles on the value of screening.*)

Wirth W. A., Thompson R. L. (1965). The effect of various conditions and substances on the results of laboratory procedures. *Am. J. Clin. Pathol*; **43**: 579.
(*The title is self-explanatory.*)

Zilva J. F. (1970). Collection and preservation of specimens for chemical pathology. *Br. J. Hosp. Med*; December, 845.
(*The title is self-explanatory.*)

2. Evaluation and Introduction of New Tests into the Laboratory

Alan M. Bold and Peter Timms

Introduction
Analytical robustness, accuracy and precision
Clinical value
    Sensitivity
    Specificity
    Decision limits
Predictive values
Patient selection
Site for test performance
Cost
Feasibility
The Clinical Biochemical report of the future

INTRODUCTION

The literature on evaluating new tests has grown steadily over the last decade or so (see bibliography of selected key references at the end of the chapter). This demonstrates amongst both clinical biochemists and clinicians an increasing awareness of the importance of rigorous and objective study of new investigations before their introduction into the routine repertoire. Before a new test is introduced by a laboratory, several questions should be answered. These will vary with circumstances (for an American view, see the article by Barnett[1]). For all laboratories, the following is a minimum check list for consideration.

1. Under local conditions, what will be the analytical robustness, accuracy and precision?
2. Under local conditions, what is the clinical value of the test?
3. What strategy is to be adopted for selection of patients to be investigated?
4. Where is the most appropriate site for the test to be performed?

5. How much will the test cost? Will it be an additional test, or does it replace an existing test? How much is demand likely to increase?
6. How feasible is it to introduce the test? Are there adequate facilities of space, instrumentation, spare time and ability of staff, and revenue costs? Can the test be adequately standardized, and quality assurance procedures established?

Too frequently, a test is introduced for no clearly defined reason, and with inadequate consideration of possible future problems. In general, a new test may be introduced for one of three reasons.

1. Because a test is required for statutory purposes, such as obligatory tests to be carried out on potential blood donors.
2. To keep Dr X happy, where Dr X can be anyone from a green junior doctor to the Professor of Medicine.
3. Because someone in the laboratory has read or heard of a new test, and 'it seems it might be useful'.

Statutory requirements are usually based on a great deal of information. In each of the latter cases, the idea may be impulsive, planted by an interesting article, lecture, or even a plausible salesman. In both cases, where laboratory work is reimbursed, profit may be an additional motive. Increasingly, however, world-wide pressure is mounting to cut the costs of laboratory services, to meet demand for other aspects of health care.

If there is to be scope to introduce new tests of genuine value, there is a need to break the vicious circle, in which long-established tests are requested far more often than is justified. Confusion and muddled thinking are rife, with both pathology staff and clinicians assuming uncritically that because a service is provided, it must be of established value. This was eloquently described by Morgan,[2] referring to electrolytes, but in principle applicable to all investigations '...the situation is perpetuated, and even allowed to worsen, because clinicians believe that if we in the laboratory make these measurements freely available—as we do, day and night—then they must be useful; whereas in the laboratories we believe that if the clinicians request these measurements in large numbers—as they do, day and night—then they must be useful'.

In this chapter, we seek to provide guidance on evaluating new tests. We draw on our own experience, supplemented by the published work of many colleagues, as indicated in the bibliography.

First, since any evaluation is time consuming, we address the question, why evaluate? Where a test has already been thoroughly evaluated and the work published, there is no need for each laboratory to carry out a full-scale evaluation. Frequently, unfortunately, either the evaluation is incomplete, or the results are not directly transferable to the local laboratory. Available instrumentation may differ from that on which the test was originally evaluated. The required analytical skill may be lacking. The population of local patients to be studied may be very different from that studied in a published evaluation. In practice therefore, some evaluation is needed to verify that the test is valuable and reliable in the local population, and in the hands of local staff. Senior laboratory staff must judge how short or extensive the evaluation should be. Where important data are lacking, work may need to be put in hand to rectify the deficiencies. We seek below to discuss and suggest possible approaches to the questions posed above.

ANALYTICAL ROBUSTNESS, ACCURACY AND PRECISION

These are analytical problems dealt with in detail elsewhere in this book. Here, only a few short points will be made, relevant to evaluating the suitability of the proposed test for local use. By robust we mean, 'How will the test perform in day-to-day work?' Is the analyte labile? Are the reagents used stable? Do the instruments function reliably under routine conditions? Can the test be carried out by staff after brief training, or will it require staff dedicated to it, because of the long training required? What will be its 'routine conditions variance', to use Whitehead's term?[3] And, not least, does the patient require special preparation, such as fasting, or the cancellation of various drugs, before the specimen can be collected? Accuracy and precision, or to use the currently preferred terms, inaccuracy and imprecision, are the measures of the closeness with which the analytical results approach the true results and of their reproducibility. Accuracy is a theoretical concept, and for relatively few tests is a definitive method available with which other analytical procedures can be compared. More frequently, but still not widely available, there is a reference method, with a detailed protocol. Test results on a new method can be compared with the reference method. In their absence, one can only compare the proposed method with the best available local method. In practice, therefore, one needs to know how inaccurate and imprecise the test is not only when carried out under ideal conditions, but also under prevailing conditions.

It is highly desirable that analytical methods are as accurate, precise and robust in routine practice as possible. Poor performance impairs interpretation of data, particularly when comparing results from different centres. But analytical performance is not an end in itself, however desirable. It should be subservient to a defined clinical need. Technological progress may one day make it possible to determine an analyte concentration to say three, four or five significant figures. But such an aim to achieve the 'state of the art' should proceed only when it is cost effective, and contributes to serving a definite clinical need.

Selection of which new test methodologies to evaluate is no academic exercise. Every new issue of the major journals devoted to clinical biochemistry includes several new or improved analytical procedures. The clinical biochemist is presented with an ever lengthening list of analytes which, thanks to new technology, can be determined in biological material. Sometimes a method becomes available for the first time. More frequently, a new method is presented, that is allegedly better than its predecessor. It is a professional responsibility, requiring experience and judgement, to select those methods that are a genuine advance. Several authors[4,5,6] have attempted to define what are goals for analytical performance, in a clinical setting. In practice, however, there remain wide divergences of opinion between clinical biochemists and clinicians about just how precise and accurate analytical methods need to be. This is not surprising, as there is a relative paucity of convincing data on the amount of contribution that improvement of analytical standards makes to improving clinical decisions. So recommendations of desirable accuracy are based on different criteria, such as biological (intra-individual) variation, achievable analytical accuracy, or the subjective views of clinicians. Too little attention is paid to the fact that the *desirable* goals may not be cost effective, and that they may vary with the clinical situation, such as making an important diagnosis, or screening or monitoring therapy. The need for co-ordinating analytical accuracy with interpretation in individual diagnostic problems cannot be over stressed.

Let us consider examples. It has been stated that the analytical imprecision of routine plasma calcium measurement is unsatisfactory for clinical purposes. It is true that the intra-individual variation is small, and also that the range for plasma calcium in a reference population is narrow. It is obvious that a precise method for determining calcium is desirable, for example to diagnose primary hyperparathyroidism. It is less clear how precise this should be. On the one hand, factors such as diet, venous stasis, and whether the patient is ambulant or recumbent can affect the result by at least 5%, a much bigger source of error than the imprecision with reputable routine methods of analysis. On the other hand, in borderline hypercalcaemia, interpretation of so-called definitive investigations such as plasma parathyroid hormone concentration can be difficult. Furthermore, many patients with borderline hypercalcaemia have few or no symptoms; thus surgery to explore the neck for a parathyroid adenoma or hyperplasia is dubiously justifiable. We await a study that shows how much benefit there would be for patients in reducing analytical imprecision for plasma calcium from, say, a coeffient of variation of 2% to 0·5%.

Most routine methods can determine urate in plasma with precision and accuracy more than adequate for diagnosing the hyperuricaemia of gout; but are inaccurate at low urate concentrations, which might for example alert to the possibility of deficiency of xanthine oxidase or purine nucleotide phosphorylase. In such circumstances, a more specific technique such as by HPLC might be needed.

These are but two examples of the need to link the clinical problem to be solved and the analytical method used. Even commoner is the analysis of sodium and potassium. Here with good modern instruments, results can confidently be reported to respectively plus or minus 1 and 0·1 mmol/l respectively, or close to these figures. But clinically, no action would be taken unless changes were much greater than those due to analytical error.

CLINICAL VALUE

There is a large measure of professional consensus on how tests should be evaluated for analytical imprecision and inaccuracy. Detailed protocols have been produced, and many excellent evaluations of analytical procedures have been published. But evaluation of the clinical usefulness of a test is much more difficult. A test must offer more than a number or report to be inserted in the case notes. It must provide information that can assist in some way, in isolation or in combination with other tests or clinical data, in the management of a patient. It may help positively, by supporting a provisional diagnosis, or negatively by helping to exclude a diagnosis. It may help in monitoring therapy, or in assessing prognosis. It must always be remembered that in addition to the direct cost of the test, there can be unpredictable indirect costs. A test may suggest an unsuspected diagnosis. If, because of non-specificity of the test this is a false trail, needless distress may be caused, or treatment or discharge of the patient may be delayed while further tests are carried out to disprove the false diagnosis. The responsibility for requesting the test in the first place rests with the clinician. But laboratory staff who provide a service for any test need to ensure that it has value and that its limitations are known and publicized.

Tests should therefore be carefully evaluated to assess their clinical value, including those clinical conditions in which the test is helpful. It is also highly desirable to study those clinical conditions in which the test may mislead. Galen[7] and Sheps and Schechter[8] are amongst authors who have drawn attention to the inadequacy of many such evaluations.

There are five major problems in evaluating the clinical value of tests:

1. An accurate clinical diagnosis is required in all patients in whom the test is to be evaluated. Furthermore, this diagnosis should be established independently of the test under evaluation. This is sometimes difficult or impossible to achieve. It is particularly difficult in the very patients where the test has most potential use, namely clinically borderline cases.

2. To provide data suitable for rigorous statistical treatment, large numbers of such cases need to be studied. For uncommon diseases this could involve a lengthy, or multi-centre study.

3. Critical evaluation shows that most tests are not as helpful as their advocates would like. It is natural to want to publish work demonstrating how useful a test is, or how much better it is than a previously used test. It requires uncommon determination to document the limitations of a new test. Morgan's critical study of the large number of requests for plasma electrolytes[2] is one of the few that advocate a drastically reduced number of requests for well-established, allegedly cheap and simple tests.

4. Investigations are increasingly being scrutinized for their cost effectiveness. Any evaluation of the clinical usefulness of a test should ideally include a study of costs and benefits. In fact such studies are virtually non-existent. It is difficult enough accurately to cost a test, though some proposals have been published (see below, and papers by Broughton and colleagues[9,10]). There are no agreed ways of putting a financial value on a test result, even when this can be shown to lead to a diagnosis, or improve treatment. The cost effectiveness of screening surveys for congenital hypothyroidism and phenylketonuria has been established. The cost here is life-long institutional care, which can be prevented by early diagnosis and treatment. But it is much less easy to measure the economic value, for example, of improved control of epilepsy through monitoring levels of anticonvulsants in blood, or early, possibly pre-symptomatic, diagnosis of a curable condition such as hyperparathyroidism through routine calcium measurement in hospital patients.

5. It is difficult enough to assess the value of a single diagnostic test. In practice, many tests are requested repeatedly, perhaps to assist in monitoring treatment, or to demonstrate the progress of a disease such as chronic renal failure. In hospital, repeat tests may account for a high proportion of the workload. To our knowledge, there has been no critical survey

of the value of a test in relation to frequency of requesting. Plasma glucose and potassium measurements are two common examples of valuable tests, often requested many times for one patient during a hospital admission. Where repeats are needed, clinical judgement determines whether they are requested weekly or hourly. It is our impression that the timing of requests has more to do with convenience and routine, e.g. every day or every Monday morning, than with any scientific data on optimal frequency.

There will remain tricky problems. However, progress has been made, and some statistical tools for studying the clinical value of a test have been described, notably by Galen and Gambino[11] and Statland.[12] Their work is based on the theorem 'An essay toward solving a problem in the doctrine of chance' by the Reverend Thomas Bayes, published in 1763. If data are available about the sensitivity and specificity of a test in a given population, in which the prevalence of the disease tested for is known, the probability of an abnormal test result confirming the disease, or of a normal result excluding the disease, can be calculated.

The terms used are:
True positive: a test result adjudged abnormal in a patient with the suspected disease.
False positive: a test result adjudged abnormal in a patient who does not have the suspected disease.
True negative: a test result adjudged normal in a patient who does not have the suspected disease.
False negative: a test result adjudged normal in a patient who does have the suspected disease.

The decision whether the patient does or does not have the suspected disease is usually made retrospectively, after consideration of all factors, including the natural history of the patient's condition and possibly response to treatment. Ideally precise criteria for diagnosis should be described. The test result is adjudged normal or abnormal either by comparison with a defined reference interval, or with a decision level (*see* below).

Sensitivity

This is a measure of the likelihood of a test being abnormal in a given disease. If the test is abnormal in a high proportion of patients with the disease, its sensitivity is high. Sensitivity is assessed by determining the proportion of patients with the disease that are correctly identified by the test. Thus if 100 patients have a given disease of whom 95 show an abnormal test result, the remaining five who have the disease but have normal test results are false negatives. The sensitivity would be 95%. In more general terms,

Sensitivity =

$$\frac{\text{Number of true positives} \times 100}{\text{Number of true positives} + \text{false negatives}}$$

Specificity

This is a measure of the likelihood of a test being normal in patients who after full investigation turn out not to have the suspected disease. So for a test to have good specificity, it should give normal results (true negatives) in a high proportion of those tested in whom the suspected diagnosis is eventually ruled out. A non-specific test will mislead by having a high proportion of false positives. In general terms,

Specificity =

$$\frac{\text{Number of true negatives} \times 100}{\text{Number of true negatives} + \text{number of false positives}}$$

Decision Limits

Conventionally, a test result is interpreted as 'normal' or 'abnormal' relative to the range found in a suitable reference population. A great deal of work has gone into collecting data and defining reference populations. Wherever possible, the reference population studied should be similar to that of the patients to be studied, except free from disease. Wherever possible allowance is made for significant differences with age or between the sexes. Ideally allowance should be made also for race, diet, time of day and the differences between ambulant and recumbent patients.

Statland[12] has drawn attention to the need for decision levels in place of reference intervals. The ideal test, which is both 100% specific and sensitive, does not exist. The ideal and 'real-life' situations are depicted graphically in Figs 1 and 2.

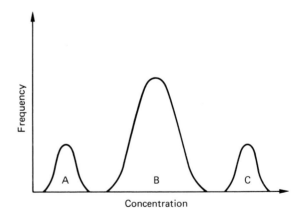

Fig. 1 Hypothetical distribution of test values in health and disease for an ideal test. *A* represents a disease with low test values, *B* the normal population and *C* a population with a disease with high values.

Figure 2 would be typical of many tests of endocrine function. Most cases of severe hypo- or hyperfunction are clearly distinguished by the test. Less severe cases unfortunately have test values overlapping with those in apparently healthy individuals.

Decision levels 1 and 6 maximize specificity, but some sensitivity is lost. Decision levels 3 and 4 maximize sensitivity but at the expense of specificity. Decision levels 2 and 5 would represent a typical compromise, and is the easiest solution in practice provided the limitations are appreciated. For specific diagnostic problems, a different approach may need to be used.

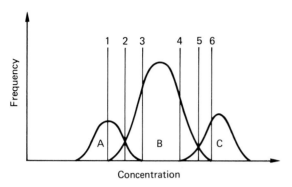

Fig. 2 The real life situation for the conditions in Fig. 1. Lines 1 to 6 are possible decision levels.

For example, a lowish level of hypercalcaemia (e.g. at the 95 or 97·5 percentile of the reference population) may be chosen when screening for possible primary hyperparathyroidism. This ensures that few cases are missed. But false positives would have to be excluded at some cost, e.g. by more specialized tests such as measuring the parathyroid hormone concentration. For diseases which are difficult or impossible to treat, it is undesirable for a test to give *any* false positives. In such a circumstance, a decision level should be chosen to maximize specificity.

PREDICTIVE VALUE

This provides a statistical probability of an 'abnormal' result being diagnostic for a suspected disease. Since tests are generally far from perfect, even when analytically reliable, it is important for the purpose of interpretation to know how likely it is that a given result will provide the correct diagnosis. It is a truism that test results need to be interpreted in the light of all clinical data available. But when clinical history and examination are ambiguous and other investigations unhelpful, a clinician may turn to a clinical biochemist with the question 'Has my patient got such and such a disease?' The question cannot be answered 'Yes' or 'No'; but 'probably' or 'probably not'. An experienced clinician or clinical biochemist can answer intuitively. Where data on sensitivity and specificity at a given decision level are known, and where the prevalence of the suspected disease in the population studied is known, the probability can be quantitated. It has to be admitted that too frequently these data are not known, or at best are incomplete and imperfect. But progress, and computer technology, are increasing the occasions where the predictive value of tests can be given. The calculation can be simpli-

fied as follows. For a positive result, the predictive value =

$$\frac{\text{The number of true positives in the population studied} \times 100}{\text{The total number of positives (true and false)}}$$

For a negative result, the same principle would apply, negative replacing positive in the equation. Worked examples illustrate the principles.

1. Let us take a favourable situation. A test for myocardial infarction, for a given decision level, has a sensitivity of 95%, specificity of 95%, and in the population studied (let us say those patients with chest pain and a possible diagnosis of myocardial infarction) a prevalence of 1 in 5. If 1000 patients were studied, the following statistics would apply.

	No. of patients	True positives	True negatives	False positives	False negatives
Chest pain with myocardial infarction	200	190			10
Chest pain without myocardial infarction	800		760	40	

Thus for a positive result, 190 are true positives, 40 false positives. The predictive value is therefore

$$\frac{190}{190 + 40} \times 100 = 82·6\%$$

Tests with 95% specificity and sensitivity would be considered good tests. Yet a positive result is only correct just over 8 times out of ten. Conversely, a doctor might want to know how confidently he can exclude a diagnosis. For the situation described above, a true negative occurs in 760 patients, a false negative in 10. The predictive value for a negative result is therefore

$$\frac{760}{760 + 10} \times 100 = 98·7\%$$

This is much more satisfactory. It illustrates the importance of the prevalence of the suspected disease in the population studied.

2. Let us now consider the situation for a test again with 95% sensitivity and specificity, but now used as a screening test. Suppose in these circumstances the disease prevalence is 1:100. Thus in 10 000 patients,

	No. of patients	True positives	False positives	True negatives	False negatives
Patients with suspected disease	100	95			5
Patients without suspected disease	9900		495	9405	

The predictive result for a positive result is

$$\frac{95}{95 + 495} \times 100 = 16 \cdot 1\%$$

Similarly, the predictive value of a negative result is

$$\frac{9405}{9405 + 5} \times 100 = 99 \cdot 95\%$$

With such a test, a doctor is happy when the result is negative; but the odds against a positive being diagnostic are worse than 1 in 6.

3. The decision levels in the above test could be adjusted to improve the predictive value for a positive result, i.e. to improve specificity and reduce false positives.

Thus by changing the decision level, specificity can be increased to say 99%. There will be a corresponding loss of sensitivity which in our hypothetical example may fall to say 90%.

Recalculation of predictive values for the above population would now give:

	No. of patients	True positive	False positive	True negative	False negative
Patients with suspected disease	100	90			10
Patients without suspected disease	9900		99	9801	

The predictive value for a positive result would now be

$$\frac{90}{90 + 99} \times 100 = 47 \cdot 6\%$$

in other words much better than previously, but not quite as helpful as tossing a coin!

The predictive value for a negative result would be 9801 (9801 + 10) or 99·9%.

In routine practice, it is common for more than a single test to be requested. If it is required that both tests be positive for a disease to be diagnosed, specificity is improved, but sensitivity reduced. Conversely, if abnormality of either one of the tests is used for diagnosis, then sensitivity is improved, specificity reduced.

Further examples are given by Galen and Gambino,[11] and Galen.[7] The review by Griner and colleagues[13] describes predictive value data in relation to a wide range of investigations other than clinical biochemical tests.

We now consider examples of recent studies of test evaluation.

McKenna and colleagues[14] have carried out a careful evaluation of a series of tests to distinguish osteoporosis from osteomalacia. Theirs is one of a handful of published studies which use predictive value data. An invasive technique, bone biopsy, was used to determine diagnosis, based on quantifying osteoid volume. This does beg the question, but is a good example of authors precisely defining their diagnostic criteria: osteomalacia was diagnosed if the osteoid volume was greater than 2·4%. No one feature, clinical, radiological or biochemical, accurately diagnosed all cases. The presence of proximal myopathy and low serum 25-hydroxy-vitamin D concentration were 100% specific, but had sensitivity of 31% and 70% respectively using the authors' criteria. By constructing an index, with features allocated a numerical score, they were able to define a range, 15–35%, where a biopsy was needed for diagnosis, thus reducing, if the retrospective survey were confirmed prospectively, the need for invasive biopsy by about 75%. However, the serum 25-hydroxy-vitamin D concentration and alkaline phosphatase activity, though unfortunately not measured in all cases, would have predicted virtually 100% of cases as published, *if optimal decision levels had been selected.*

Steinberg and colleagues[15] carried out various tests including plasma amylase activity in a study to distinguish acute pancreatitis from other causes of abdominal pain. They studied 39 patients with acute pancreatitis and 127 controls with abdominal pain due to a variety of conditions such as acute appendicitis, biliary tract disease and acute cholecystitis. Sonography, computed tomography and laparotomy were used to provide the 'definitive' diagnosis. The authors demonstrate how, by using an optimal cut-off as the decision level rather than the upper limit of normal, specificity can be improved from 88·9 to 98·5%, without any loss of sensitivity. This significantly improves the predictive value of a positive test. The authors themselves admit, however, that there are problems inherent in such an evaluation. Thus, how accurate was their 'gold standard' for diagnosis, of sonography, computed tomography and laparotomy? How much was the series biased by referral of patients suspected of having acute pancreatitis by physicians who already knew that the patient's plasma amylase activity was raised?

These examples illustrate the problems involved in interpretation, when the odds are changed by the way in which the test is used; in other words used as a screening test, or used as a confirmatory test when there is a reasonable likelihood on clinical grounds of the suspected disease being present. Some screening programmes are clearly here to stay. But unselective requests for investigations, including a large biochemical profile in the absence of a reasonable clinical suspicion, can cause problems. Increased understanding of such problems, and economic constraints, are changing the atmosphere for introducing new tests. There is a great need for highly specific tests. Screening tests that are highly sensitive, but lack specificity, may be needed to avoid missing an important diagnosis, but they should not be introduced without first answering the question 'How do we confirm positive results?'

PATIENT SELECTION

The study of this problem is inextricably linked with the previous section. Both common sense and the worked examples indicate that the diagnostic value of a test is very largely determined by appropriate selection of patients. A test is requested for:

1. Diagnosis—this may be to confirm a suspected clinical diagnosis (discretionary investigation) or may be a screening test or profile requested without clinical indication.
2. Monitoring—to assess the general or specific response to treatment (e.g. therapeutic drug monitoring).
3. Prognosis—to assess the severity of a disease (e.g. assessing myocardial infarct size by measuring the magnitude of rise in serum activity of a 'cardiac' enzyme such as creatine kinase over a period of time; or assessing natural progression of a disease, such as chronic glomerulonephritis by serial measurements of creatinine).

In each situation, custom and practice affect the tests selected, and the patients in whom the test is requested. It is fascinating to observe the inter-hospital and intra-hospital variation in test requesting practice, even by clinicians in the same specialty. Some doctors seem to manage with minimal laboratory investigation; others request an extensive battery of tests for even straightforward cases. It is undeniable that the possibility of medico-legal liability on the one hand, and documentation for a careful prospective research survey on the other, affect test requesting practice. Aside from that, differences are often illogical. Kaplan and colleagues[16] recently reported a survey of preoperative screening in 2785 cases admitted for routine surgery. They concluded that roughly 60% of tests requested were not clinically indicated; of these, only 0·22% uncovered abnormalities of potential significance, *none of which, according to the clinical record, altered the management of the patients.* Their conclusion, though still to be tested in the courts, is interesting '... a complication traceable to an overlooked result more readily suggests legal liability than does a complication possibly related to the absence of a test that neither hospital policy nor the medical literature considers appropriate'. This represents, we believe, a note of sanity. This is not the place for an extended treatise on indications for requesting tests. We do recommend the following guidelines:

1. Follow hospital policy, and the general consensus of medical and scientific practice. It is unwise for anyone to risk omitting an investigation that is available if it is standard practice to request it. This admittedly cautious policy needs to be complemented by many more detailed studies of the clinical value of tests. Only by hard evidence can the scientific climate be changed so that it is normal *not* to request certain non-specific tests in given clinical conditions.
2. Apart from the medico-legal aspect, it is fundamental to investigation to ask the question 'What problem am I seeking to solve with this test?' And more specifically, 'What will I do in managing this patient that will be different if a test result is high (or low) compared with the management if it is normal?' Measurement of plasma glucose, calcium, potassium levels, blood gases, and various hormone concentrations, are some of the tests which when abnormal can lead to different treatment, depending on the result. Plasma cholesterol measurement is an example of a test which when abnormal *could* lead to treatment. But a doctor ought to ask himself what treatment he would institute in an 85-year-old man suffering from hypertension if he discovered the patient's plasma cholesterol to be say, 9·0 mmol/l. In a 15 year old patient, a vigorous attempt at treatment would be indicated. But in the elderly . . .? Similarly, serum creatine kinase or other 'cardiac enzyme' activity is frequently requested when, in our experience, the diagnosis of myocardial infarction has been established with virtually 100% certainty on clinical and electrocardiographic grounds. If in such a case the request is queried, the clinician is frequently defensive. The argument that 'We always do the cardiac enzymes on our cases with chest pain' seems to die hard. Yet since the diagnosis of myocardial infarction has already been established, a normal creatine kinase result would hardly change the management.
3. Where tests are done routinely for screening, there should be a clear policy for action when results are abnormal. If no decision level can be defined that would change action, then the rationale for requesting the test is non-existent.
4. This may be summed up as: think, discriminate.

Unfortunately, habits die hard, and busy clinicians will claim that there is no time for such discriminating requesting of laboratory tests. The senior staff of the clinical biochemistry laboratory can play a vital role by encouraging discrimination in the use of tests, and where necessary querying or even refusing certain requests which cannot be rationally justified. There is a need for day-to-day clinical liaison, and easy approachability of laboratory staff by clinicians. Aside from this, the following steps can help.

1. New investigations should only be introduced into the laboratory repertoire when their clinical value has been established. This means ideally that sensitivity, specificity and predictive values should be known for likely clinical problems before the habit of requesting the new test becomes ingrained.
2. Pathology request forms, wherever practicable,

should contain the minimum of 'boxes', thus reducing 'tick' requests to a few common and well-established tests. All other tests would have to be requested by hand.

3. Clinical biochemists should play an on-going role through attendance at clinical meetings, etc., to educate other staff in discriminating investigation. This invariably means that the clinical biochemist must first be fully conversant with all the facts about tests which are abused.

SITE FOR TEST PERFORMANCE

There is much to be said for the modern trend for tests being performed nearer the patient. Home measurement of blood glucose, for example, introduces a level of monitoring, and hence education and motivation of the patient, that is unattainable by other means. Whether this necessarily improves the life expectancy of diabetics is another matter.

In hospital, whether in ICU, ward or clinic, or in a clinic outside the hospital, there are advantages and disadvantages to siting analytical instruments outside the laboratory. Advantages include: speed of availability of results; instant opportunity to check unexpected results; rapid opportunity to institute or amend treatment. Disadvantages include: limited training of staff in analysis, and consequent problems in recognizing and solving malfunctions of the instrument; problems in storage of results, particularly if these are normally input on-line to a computer system; discrepancies between local and pathology laboratory results; and the cost of carrying out analyses in small batches.

Improvements in technology have changed the situation dramatically over the last few years. The disadvantages are rapidly getting less. When the decision on where a test should be performed lies with senior laboratory staff, the pros and cons should be weighed carefully. In our view, the great majority of tests, in most situations, are best carried out by trained personnel in a proper laboratory. Where it is essential for clinical management for results to be available more rapidly or more frequently than can be achieved by the hospital laboratory, as for blood gases in ICUs, or blood glucose in wards where there are many diabetics, on-site analysis may be required. Close liaison between clinical, ward and laboratory staff is essential. By selecting appropriate instrumentation, training *a limited* number of users and explaining any consistent differences between methods, everyone gains.

COST

A detailed description of costing of laboratory tests is outside the scope of this chapter. Those interested should refer to the article by Broughton and Woodford.[10] Here we would simply point out that anyone contemplating the evaluation of a new test with a view to adding it to the laboratory repertoire must make an attempt to assess the cost. Costs will be:

1. Direct. These are the capital cost of any instrument required, plus that of any installation or services, an allowance for maintenance and capital depreciation, the cost of reagents and other consumables, and of staff time directly devoted to the analysis.

2. Indirect. This includes indirect consumables, such as laboratory computer, centrifuges, rates, heating, lighting, transport and a large number of miscellaneous items which are part and parcel of running a laboratory. Also allowance must be made for indirect labour such as specimen collection, separation and storage, clerical work. A major cost, but one that is difficult to allocate accurately to any test, is that of the salaries of staff engaged in supervision, administration, research and development.

Costing is complicated by the variability of batch size. The unit cost is much more expensive for the analysis of one or two specimens than a batch of 100 or so specimens. Where the anticipated workload is uneconomically low, it may be preferable to arrange for a referral laboratory to carry out the test, at least until local demand makes a local service cost effective. Where detailed costing is not feasible, a useful rule of thumb is that *in general* about 80 to 85% of laboratory costs are for labour. Thus for a typical analysis, if the total consumables cost per request can be calculated, under local conditions and for batch sizes anticipated, this cost multiplied by a factor of 4 to 6 will give an estimate of cost that is at least reasonably realistic.

FEASIBILITY

Depending on the nature of the test and numbers of requests anticipated, the decision whether or not to introduce a new test may be easy or difficult. Before time is spent on any of the evaluation stages described above, a brief feasibility study should be carried out. The following questions should be considered.

1. Is space available? The requirement for space must include space for any new instrument, storage of specimens and consumables.

2. Can the staff cope? One must consider whether there is spare time for the new test, or whether additional staff will be required. Also training needs and the skills and experience required must be assessed.

3. Are there any safety problems? Problems could arise if explosive gases or solvents are needed, or toxic or potentially carcinogenic reagents essential.

4. Are there problems associated with standardization and quality assurance? Many new tests are developed in research laboratories. Mater-

ial for standardization may have been prepared locally, and not be widely available. Even where standardization is not a problem, quality assurance material may not be available.

5. Can the data be computerized? In many laboratories, work is reported via a computer. Entry of new data to a laboratory computer is usually no problem; but it is important to check in advance that new tests can be accommodated without extensive programming, particularly if large numbers of tests on a multi-channel analyser are planned.

6. Will the budget stand the new test? Unless the new test is specially funded, this is a topical problem. Wherever possible, an old test should be excised from the repertoire, particularly if the new test supersedes it. When the new test is particularly helpful, possible rapid growth in requests should be anticipated. This happened for example, when it became feasible to determine prolactin. Possible methods of controlling unreasonable requests should be planned.

THE CLINICAL BIOCHEMICAL REPORT OF THE FUTURE

All reports should include, in addition to necessary patient-identifying data, analytical result, units, biological fluid. Date and time are desirable, as well as conditions, e.g. fasting, for lipid analyses, or inspired oxygen for blood gases. Reference intervals, relevant for the patient's age and sex, should be added. For Government laboratories, in cost-conscious times, the cost might be added. Computerized, potentially interactive, data banks could enable any interfering drug therapy to be indicated. The ideal would include also the analytical confidence limits of the method used; and perhaps, one fine day, a predictive value for a positive or negative result, using decision levels relevant to the clinical problem to be solved. The possibilities released by technology, and the pressures produced by financial constraints, could combine to bring such a dream at least a little nearer reality.

REFERENCES

1. Barnett R. N. (1983). Planning and instituting new tests in the clinical laboratory. In *Clinics in Laboratory Medicine: Symposium on Laboratory Management* (Tiersten D., ed.) **3**: 413.
2. Morgan D. B. (1981). Why plasma electrolytes? *Ann. Clin. Biochem*; **18**: 275.
3. Whitehead T. P. (1977). *Quality Control in Clinical Chemistry*. New York: Wiley.
4. Barnett R. N. (1968). Medical significance of laboratory results. *Am. J. Clin. Pathol*; **50**: 671.
5. Cotlove E., Harris E. K., Williams G. Z. (1970). Biological and analytic components of variation in long-term studies of serum constituents in normal subjects. III. Physiological and medical implications. *Clin. Chem*; **16**: 1028.
6. Fraser C. G. (1983). Desirable performance standards for clinical chemistry tests. *Adv. Clin. Chem*; **23**: 299.
7. Galen R. S. (1981). Evaluating published data. In *Laboratory Diagnosis and Patient Monitoring: Clinical Chemistry* (Galen R. S., Brennan L., eds) p. 39. Oradell, New Jersey: Medical Electronics Co.
8. Sheps S. B., Schechter M. T. (1984). The assessment of diagnostic tests. A survey of current medical research. *J. Am. Med. Assoc*; **252**: 2418.
9. Broughton P. M. G., Hogan T. C. (1981). A new approach to the costing of clinical laboratory tests. *Ann. Clin. Biochem*; **18**: 330.
10. Broughton P. M. G., Woodford F. P. (1983). Benefits of costing in the clinical laboratory. *J. Clin. Pathol*; **36**: 1028.
11. Galen R. S., Gambino S. R. (1975). *Beyond Normality: The Predictive Value and Efficiency of Medical Diagnoses*. New York: Wiley.
12. Statland B. E. (1981). Decision levels. In *Laboratory Diagnosis and Patient Monitoring: Clinical Chemistry* (Galen R. S., Brennan L., eds) p. 53. Oradell, New Jersey: Medical Electronics Co.
13. Griner P. F., Mayewski J., Mushlin A. I., Greenland P. (1981). Selection and interpretation of diagnostic tests and procedures. *Ann. Int. Med*; **94**: 553.
14. McKenna M. J., Freaney R., Casey O. M., Towers R. P., Muldowney F. P. (1983). Osteomalacia and osteoporosis: evaluation of a diagnostic index. *J. Clin. Pathol*; **36**: 245.
15. Steinberg W. M., Goldstein S. S., Davis N. D., Shamma'a J., Anderson K. (1985). Diagnostic assays in acute pancreatitis. A study of sensitivity and specificity. *Ann. Int. Med*; **102**: 576.
16. Kaplan E. B., Sheiner L. B., Boeckmann A. J., Roizen M. F., Beal S. L., Cohen S. N., Nicoll D. (1985). The usefulness of preoperative laboratory screening. *J. Am. Med. Assoc*; **253**: 3576.

FURTHER READING

Berwick D. M. (1985). Screening in health fairs. A criticial review of benefits, risks and costs. *J. Am. Med. Assoc*; **254**: 1492.
Burke D. M. (1982). Test strategies in selected clinical problems. In *Clinics in Laboratory Medicine: Test Selection Strategies* (Benson E. S., Connolly D. P., Burke D. M., eds) **2**: 789. Philadelphia: Saunders.
Gräsbeck R., Alström T. (eds) (1981). *Reference Values in Laboratory Medicine*. Chichester: Wiley.
Robertson E. A., Zweig M. H., Steirteghem C. Van (1983). Evaluating the clinical efficacy of laboratory tests. *Am. J. Clin. Pathol*; **79**: 78.

3. Laboratory Management
David Burnett

INTRODUCTION

It is the intention of the author in this chapter to provide an introductory framework on which the reader can develop an interest in laboratory management rather than to deal comprehensively with every aspect of the topic.

Laboratory management involves the need to organize, a verb that can be defined as 'to arrange or dispose things or a body of people in order to carry out some purpose effectively'. This definition summarizes the structure of this chapter. Clearly 'to carry out some purpose' is the *objective* or *goal* of a clinical laboratory and 'to arrange or dispose' concerns the *organizational structure*. The 'things or body of people' are the *resources* available and the final word in the definition 'effectively' indicates the need for *monitoring* and *assessment of performance* to confirm that the set objectives have been achieved.

OBJECTIVES OR GOALS

The overall goal of a clinical laboratory is to provide results that are relevant to the care of patients. The immediate implications of this goal are that the results produced should be (a) reliable, (b) timely, and (c) interpretable. Furthermore a laboratory should be actively and constantly involved in (d) research and the development of new techniques and (e) assessing the clinical value of new tests and the continuing usefulness of current procedures. As resources available for health care are not infinite there is also a responsibility to achieve the goal cost-effectively in order not to detract from the provision of other aspects of patient care.

Consideration of whether a result is reliable or not involves the general aspects of quality assurance and the more specific areas of quality control and quality assessment. The general aspects are the most easily overlooked; for example, was the sample collected from the correct patient?, was the patient properly prepared?, was the specimen properly collected, transported and separated for analysis? When the analysis itself is completed there are further management responsibilities to ensure that the results despatched to the requesting clinician actually arrive. When the result arrives it should be legible; in other words has the printer ribbon been replaced or the photocopier serviced regularly?

A quality control system requires that acceptable limits of performance should be defined for the precision, bias, sensitivity and specificity of each assay. A valuable review has been published summarizing the different approaches to defining acceptable limits of performance.[1] Once the acceptable limits of performance have been set then monitoring the quality of the analytical process is possible.

The quality of the results will in large part be determined by the choice of equipment and methodology. Automated techniques are generally more precise than manual ones; the specificity of an immunoassay may avoid interference that is known to be a problem with a particular colorimetric or fluorimetric assay. Choice of equipment or method will be determined by the clinical requirement and the limits of performance defined accordingly. Seeking greater precision for an assay when the clinical situation does not demand it may not be cost effective. The use of quality control implies that if a problem is detected in a certain analytical batch then action can be taken to avoid erroneous patient results being sent from the laboratory.

A further check to the reliability of results is obtained by participation in quality assessment schemes in which the assay of an analyte by a particular laboratory is compared with results obtained by many laboratories. As there is a time interval between the return of results and the final assessment there is not the opportunity for immediate action. However, the opportunity for long-term evaluation of a laboratory's performance and the information to be obtained about other methods makes participation in such schemes essential.

Meaningful results must be reliable but they must also be timely and the users of the service and their needs must be identified. The provision of all services in a central location is being increasingly questioned. In units such as intensive care and coronary care the results may be needed urgently and with such frequency that local provision is necessary. The volume and range of assays required from a laboratory needs to be established together with a prediction of future needs if the correct resources are to be allocated and timeliness maintained.

Once reliable and timely results are available then

a further role of the clinical laboratory is to participate in their interpretation. To ensure that results are interpretable means the report must provide sufficient information to enable the result to be used in a meaningful way. In an ideal world some estimate of the imprecision of the results would be provided together with a reference range appropriate to the age, sex and ethnic origin of the patient. Some reporting systems include an indication, graphical or otherwise, as to whether the particular result is abnormal. Advice on further appropriate investigations should be considered part of an interpretation. The way in which results are interpreted and reported should be determined in consultation with clinicians in order that failures of communication are minimized.

Involvement in the research and development of new techniques is essential for any clinical laboratory, and will have a major impact on the laboratory's ability to continue to provide meaningful results. The recruitment of good staff and their motivation, together with the effective use of all other resources are related to an active research and development programme. Budgetary provision must be made for attendance at appropriate scientific and medical meetings, and for library and information services.

If new lamps were readily exchanged for old then the importance of assessing the clinical value of new tests and the continuing usefulness of current procedures would not be so important. The need to make value judgements as to which tests should be introduced and which phased out has until recently been avoided by a continuing growth in the resource allocation for health care. There are, however, now clear indications that the honeymoon is over and the introduction of a new test should not take place without some attempt to make a prospective evaluation of its role in patient care.

ORGANIZATIONAL STRUCTURE

Conventional Approaches

A typical organizational chart of a business is shown in Fig. 1, with at its head the Director/General Manager to whom are answerable the various functional managers. It is possible to recognize in a large clinical laboratory that all these functions exist even if the names are unfamiliar and even if there are no specifically designated managers of these functions.

Production can be regarded as analysing the specimens received, marketing—finding out what the client (patient/doctor) wants or needs, research and development—new tests and clinical applications, personnel—recruiting, training, appraisal and rewarding personnel etc. Such a structure would not be necessary for a smaller or satellite laboratory which might conveniently be regarded as an isolated production unit, the head of which was answerable to the Production Manager of the main organization.

It is more important, however, to consider whether the structure or culture represented by Fig. 1 is the correct one for the jobs or goal which the clinical laboratory has to perform. Perhaps there is no one correct structure or culture for an organization. A mix of different cultures may be necessary, both to accommodate the different groups of staff who work in the organization and the different types of job. This mix of organizational approaches or cultures have been termed[2] 'The theory of cultural propriety'.

Greek Gods and Laboratories

In his book *Gods of Management—who they are, how they will work, and why they will fail* Handy[2] develops the theme that it is useful to recognize 'four gods of management', each giving its name to a cult or philosophy of management and thus to an organizational culture. Each of these cultures is given a formal name and picture which is represented in Fig. 2.

Zeus, the head of the gods in Greek mythology was famed for his impulses and the power of his presence. Apollo is characterized as being fond of rules and order. Athena is a goddess, protectress of problem solvers, and Dionysus, the supreme individualist.

Only a brief summary of each type of culture can be given here. The Club Culture (Zeus) is represented pictorially by a spiders web in which the radiating lines represent divisions based on function or perhaps product. These lines are those of the traditional organization chart (Fig. 1) but the crucial lines are the encircling lines near the centre, lines of power and influence. The spider, Zeus represents the patriachal tradition, irrational but often benevo-

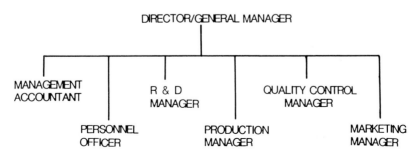

Fig. 1 Organization of a typical business.

THE GOD	THE PICTURE	THE CULTURE
ZEUS		CLUB
APOLLO		ROLE
ATHENA		TASK
DIONYSUS		EXISTENTIAL

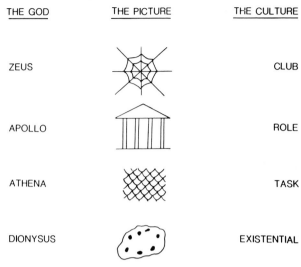

Fig. 2 The 'four gods of management'.

lent power, impulsiveness and charisma—it is a good culture for speed of decision but the quality of decision will depend upon the calibre of Zeus.

The Role Culture (Apollo) is one we think of as an 'organization'. It is based on definitions of the role or the job to be done not on personalities. It assumes that man is rational and everything can be analysed in a logical fashion. The picture is a Greek Temple, drawing its beauty from its pillars which represent the functions and divisions in a role organization. The pediment at the top is where the functional heads join to form a board of management. It is a good culture if tomorrow is like yesterday and stability and predictability are assumed and encouraged. It works very efficiently if this is so, but is not good at responding to change.

The Task Culture (Athena) see management as basically concerned with the continuous and successful solution of problems. Performance is judged in terms of solved problems. The picture is of a net, it draws its resources from various parts of the organizational system in order to tackle the problem in hand. Power lies at the interstices of the net, not at the top as in the role culture or at the centre as in the club culture. The organization is a network of loosely linked task forces, each largely self-contained but with a specific responsibility within an overall strategy. Expertise is the base of power and influence. It is a useful culture for situations of challenge and change, its leadership comes from the common purpose of the group.

Finally the Existential Culture (Dionysus). Existentialism starts from the assumption that the world is not part of some higher purpose, and we are not simply instruments of some higher power, but that if anyone is responsible for us and our world then it is ourselves. As Professor Handy says 'we are in charge of our own destinies but that is not a recipe for self-indulgent selfishness, for Kant's categorical imperative applies, that whatever we ordain or wish

for ourselves must be equally applicable to the rest of mankind'.[2] In this culture, the individual does not exist for the organization, the organization exists to help the individual achieve his purpose. It is an excellent culture where the talent or skill of the individual is the crucial asset, think of barristers in chambers or doctors in a group practice. However, when the effectiveness say of a particular doctor increasingly depends on the skills of other professions, this culture becomes less appropriate.

Jobs in this thesis are divided into three broad types; steady-state jobs are best suited to Apollonian culture and represented by a square □. They are programmable because they are predictable, handled by systems and routines, rules and procedures. Development jobs which deal with new situations or problems are for Athenian cultures and represented by a creative cell ⊙. Not all problems however are developmental, some may be described as asterisk (*) situations, where the rule book has failed and instinct and speed are likely to be better than logical analysis or creative problem-solving. A supervisor comes to the head of the department and says 'Tom's refusing to do any more blood glucose measurements to-day because the new houseman has been rude to him on the phone'. These situations require personal intervention, a role for Zeus or Dionysus?

Evolution and New Challenges

Professor Handy's analysis* is particularly valuable because as one reads it, one can see individuals in an organization as being, say, more Athenian than Apollonian, and see parts of the organization, a situation, or a job as being more suited to a particular type of organizational culture. Is it not that at the dawn of time clinical laboratories were directed by a general pathologist, a Zeus-like person, famed for his impulses and the power of his presence, originally able to operate in a Dionysian culture of one because it was his talents and skills which were the sole asset of the organization.

Then as the clinical laboratory developed, specialties emerged, heads of haematology, biochemistry, microbiology and histopathology either separated their departments or formed uneasy Dionysian cultures. The range and scope of work done in the clinical laboratory increased and the introduction of scientific and technical personnel meant that the assets of the organization were more widespread and an Apollonian or role culture started to emerge, co-existing uneasily with its Dionysian sometimes Zeus-like directorship. As the technology increased, workloads increased, created in the case of non-selective multichannel analysers by the technology itself, and those who controlled the technology had more

* This section of the chapter owes almost everything to the ideas developed by Professor Charles Handy which is hereby acknowledged with the proviso that any misinterpretation of his ideas is the author's responsibility.

power. While the resource available for health care could be guaranteed to keep pace with the demand then a stable environment existed which favoured the Apollonian culture. Of course there would be pockets where the Goddess Athena, protectress of problem solvers held sway with, at best, clinicians and medical, scientific and technical personnel working together to evaluate the clinical importance of some new test or procedure.

At the present time, however, the clinical laboratory faces two new challenges, particularly in the so-called advanced countries. First, the resources available for health care are no longer infinite, and as people live longer the cost of their social and medical care increases and serious questions of priorities in the use of resources emerge. How much should be spent on the clinical laboratory services as against, for example, the care of the elderly? Secondly, technologies are appearing, particularly the so-called dry chemistry systems, that allow analysis which could only previously be carried out in sophisticated laboratories by highly trained technicians and scientists, to be performed by relatively unskilled staff in the clinic or in the ward without significant loss of precision and accuracy. Apollonian culture is faced with change, Athena and her problem solvers may establish a new system that will work but who will maintain it twenty-four hours a day, three hundred and sixty-five days a year, or is this the opportunity for the Dionysian physician to take back to himself the asset, uncontrolled and unsupervised? A better awareness of how we work and behave in clinical laboratories is essential if the different professional groups with their tendencies to cultural preference are to work together constructively to face the changes and challenges outlined.

RESOURCES AND THEIR MANAGEMENT

The resources of a clinical laboratory comprise the people who work for it, directly or indirectly, the place in which the work is done and the equipment and reagents etc. which are used to run the equipment and to accomplish the work. All these resources require financing and therefore financial acumen is an increasingly important aspect of laboratory management.

People

It is often said that people are the greatest asset of any organization but perhaps one to which the least detailed attention is given. In large organizations the personnel aspects of a laboratory are often handled by a personnel department, separate from the laboratory. Whilst it is important to have expert advice available for placement of advertisements, preparation and formulation of contracts and the legal aspects of job descriptions, it is important that recruitment, selection, career development and apprai-

sals should firmly be in the hands of the appropriate level of management within the laboratory itself.

Job descriptions are seen to be particularly important in the Apollo culture of our large laboratories. Exponents of job descriptions require the job title and place of work to be stated, the overall scope and purpose of the job to be described, relationships above, below and lateral to be defined etc. and thus a box is created which defines the role and places the person clearly within a particular part of the temple. Furthermore it is seen as a joint contract between manager and managed. Annual review of job content and of performance are expected, career development is discussed and perhaps corrective training. The system will work in an Apollo culture, providing the managers' appraisals are fair and job requirement is reasonably static and does not demand too much initiative. Dionysian directors of laboratories may see job descriptions as necessary for others but not for themselves, Athenians feel they are restricted by their prescriptive nature and Zeusians would not have time to read them. All this is not to deny that individuals in an organization need to understand their role and responsibilities but simply to indicate that in a rapidly changing world inflexible job descriptions are not the be all and end all of an effective organization.

Within any organization good communication is important, if a laboratory is small enough then no formal system is necessary. Many large laboratories develop regular formal meetings to discuss at different organizational levels aspects of budget control, quality control and customer complaints, etc., all of which may give an individual a sense of being part of and contributing to the organization. On the other hand meetings may be held simply because they are scheduled and their mere existence should not be seen as evidence of good communication.

Blanchard and Johnson[3] in a deceptively simple book called 'The One-Minute Manager' have taken what they have learned in their studies of medicine and in behavioural sciences about how people work best with each other, and created an allegory which introduces the three secrets of a One-Minute Manager. By 'best' they mean how people produce valuable results, and feel good about themselves, the organization and the other people with whom they work.

The One-Minute Manager feels that a one-minute goal and its performance standard should take no more than 250 words to express, be on no more than a single page and be able to be read in one minute. It involves people understanding not only their responsibilities but what will be regarded as a good performance. The second and third secrets of the One-Minute Manager also concern communication but are also to do with motivation, one minute praisings involve helping people to reach their full potential by catching them doing something right, telling them so, making them see that you feel good about what they did right and how it helps the organization and the other people who work there. One-minute reprimands are in two parts and an essential prerequisite is that you tell people beforehand that you are going to let them know how they are doing and in no uncertain terms. The first half of the reprimand must take place immediately and be specific and express the reprimand in no uncertain terms. After four seconds uncomfortable silence to let them feel how you feel, the second half of the reprimand should show them by shaking their hands or indicating that you are on their side, that you value them in spite of their particular performance in this situation. When a reprimand is over it is over. If this all sounds too simple, give it a chance, it only takes a few minutes to read!

Where are future managers of clinical laboratories to come from, what qualities and what type of training should they receive? The November 1984 issue of the Laboratory Accreditation Newsletter of the College of American Pathologists contains a statement concerning the knowledge and performance criteria for a clinical laboratory director. It states that to function effectively in fulfilling the duties and responsibilities as director of a clinical laboratory, a person should possess broad knowledge of clinical medicine, sciences basic to medicine, and the clinical laboratory sciences. It then lists certain abilities which are deemed to be required (Table 1). The aspect that seems to be rather poorly defined concerns the skills of interpersonal relationships. Perhaps the 'One-Minute Manager' should be added to the list.

TABLE 1

ABILITIES REQUIRED FOR A CLINICAL LABORATORY DIRECTOR

— Function as a peer member of the medical community.

— Define, implement and monitor standards of performance concerning the utility and value of laboratory services.

— Use and correlate laboratory data for diagnosis and patient management.

— Perform strategic planning for setting goals and developing and allocating resources appropriate to the medical environment.

— Relate and function effectively with accrediting, regulatory, local and administrative groups; the medical community; and the population serviced.

— Provide effective and efficient administration of laboratory services, including budget planning and control, with responsible financial management.

— Communicate effectively to relate correlations and interpretation of laboratory data to clinicians.

— Provide educational direction for the medical, laboratory, and lay communities.

— Perform or direct research and development appropriate to the institution.

The training of general managers in the National Health Service is a major concern at the present time, and a recent report[4] emphasized the shifting views on the nature of the adult learning process, away from the didactic to the 'experiential'. Management training involves changing attitudes. Stewart[5] comments that many 'commercial companies are worried about how to develop an understanding of, and sensitivity to, people. How to change a good scientist or technician who has been primarily concerned with things, into a manager who is sufficiently interested and aware of people to be sensitive to their reactions and to be able to adjust his behaviour accordingly'. It is sometimes assumed that doctors with their experience of dealing with patients should be well-prepared to be good managers. However, the patient/doctor relationship is different in nature, and medical education with its increasing burden of facts to assimilate leaves little time to develop skills of communication. A great deal must be learned by all groups in the clinical laboratory if good management is to be achieved.

Workplace

Laboratory Design. The opportunity to participate in designing a new laboratory may only come once, or not at all to the professionals who work in laboratories. Until recently laboratory designs have tended to be rather static in nature, to have rooms with designated functions and fixed services. Changes are difficult to accomplish without major disruption or lengthy planning procedures which result in the accommodation once again being out of date before it can be occupied.

Different jobs in a clinical laboratory will require a different environment. Work involving radioisotopes may require an area of containment and restricted access. Cervical cytology screening will require a quiet area for concentration but open enough to enable some communication to offset the tedium of such routine work. A large multichannel analyser may be placed in an open area with ease of access to facilitate the arrival of samples. What is required is design with a high degree of flexibility, where benches can be changed or totally removed for the introduction of floor-standing equipment and services provided and altered without involving the specialized skills of electricians, plumbers etc. Walls need not be permanent but present-day partitions give the illusion of permanence and the benefit of flexibility. Good design gives the people who have to work in the laboratory the ability to control and alter their own environment.

Such designs are becoming available all over the world and in the United Kingdom are manufactured on design work done by the Laboratory Investigation Unit of the Department of Education and Science.[6] Benches are free standing tables (see Fig. 3 [1]), clamped together to enhance stability. Services for

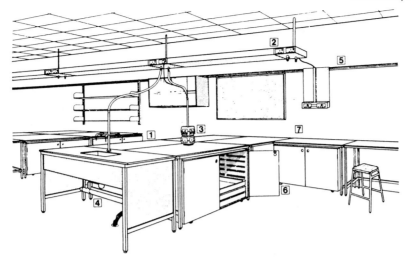

Fig. 3 Ideal laboratory design.

the benches are provided by overhead booms [2], natural gas, air, hydrogen, etc. Electricity, water and purified water can all be provided by this system. Gases and electricity can be received on a particular bench from above through service bollards [3] which can bolt to a number of different parts of a bench. Water is provided by appropriate pressure tubing to sinks as required; drainage from these sinks can be collected in a glass or appropriate plastic drainage system emptying via any of a number of outlets in a drainage grid [4]. Changing the configuration of the laboratory is a matter of disconnecting services from overhead booms and from the drainage grid, moving the tables as required and reconnecting. Flexibility of wall-mounted furnishings, shelves and noticeboards is achieved by using a top track system [5] upon which these items hang. Underbench units [6] mounted on castors provide flexibility and having 'safe' laminated tops [7] can be used as extra work surfaces.

Health and Safety. The safety of all staff who work in clinical laboratories must be a cause for constant concern and surveillance. In many countries through government agencies, trades unions and professional groups, codes of practice are introduced to safeguard the health and safety of laboratory personnel. Regulations in the UK concerning the manner in which to deal with potentially infected specimens and the design of safety cabinets are contained in the 'Code of Practice for the Prevention of Infection in Clinical Laboratories and Post-mortem Rooms',[7] and other codes cover such topics as AIDS and the use of radioactive isotopes. Translating these codes into local rules which can be understood, implemented and sustained in practice over long periods of time is a most important and difficult part of management. The employer's responsibilities may be clear but if the code of practice is provisional and advisory rather than mandatory, the resources are not always readily

made available. The responsibility of the employee towards his own health and safety, to those he works with, and to those entering the clinical laboratory as patients, visitors, representatives or as cleaning and maintenance staff, needs to be stressed in any local rules concerning health and safety. The interrelated effects of stress at work, job dissatisfaction, and physical and mental ill-health are not often very fully discussed and Cooper[8] provides a useful introduction.

Equipment and Reagents

As with the opportunity to design a new laboratory, the opportunity to purchase large items of equipment only occurs at infrequent (7–10 year) intervals. A Head of Department appointed at the age of 35 might make his first decision two years later and further decisions when aged 44, 51, 58 and finally in the year he retires. This last decision might be his best if his age was a reflection of his wisdom and he had consulted with his staff, or his worst if he had lost touch and talked to nobody. In clinical biochemistry one large analyser might well represent 50–75% of the total capital equipment in the laboratory. The followers of Apollo will take delight in the many national and international protocols available for equipment evaluation. Athenians will certainly have a problem to solve but one cannot help a sneaking feeling that it will be Zeus who makes the final decision by ringing up other members of his club and asking them what they feel about instrument x.

A major problem of coming to a rational decision in this area is the dichotomy of finance, the capital often coming from a different source from that which provides revenue with which to run and maintain the equipment. Thus if capital is easy and revenue tight, it predisposes the decision towards instruments with laundry systems rather than disposable cuvettes, towards low cost reagents which require more quality control within the laboratory as compared with dry chemistry systems which have inherent in their price the manufacturers' contribution to reliability and quality control.

When instrumentation and reagents are equal in terms of precision, accuracy, sensitivity and specificity, it is ease of use, stability and reliability that one will look for and pay for if a busy laboratory is to avoid hassle and continue to provide meaningful results cost effectively. Seven or ten years after purchase the final validation of choice will be known! Purchase of instruments and reagents are a major management role.

Financial Management

There is in health care increasing emphasis on the proper financial management of laboratories. Accounting procedures are required which not only record the total costs incurred in running the laboratory but also analyse these costs, to identify the specific costs of different work done by the laboratory. It is relatively easy to identify the direct costs associated with the laboratory such as the salaries and other direct staff costs; the cost of consumables, reagents, and quality control materials; the maintenance of equipment; and the cost of depreciation of capital equipment used in the laboratory: but the assessment of other costs such as buildings, heating, lighting, laundry and library services, is more difficult and will have to be obtained from the departments that provide these services.

The accounting procedures must be designed so that figures produced will relate to the purpose for which such figures are to be used. For instance, most financial accounting systems will allow the current expenditure on assay kits to be compared to a budget target for the current month and also to the cumulative expenditure to date against an annual budget figure. They do not usually make it possible to examine the cost of materials actually used for e.g., TSH assays in order that the cost per test may be identified. Information regarding costs may be used in different ways; for instance, it is important to know the cost of running a certain instrument, particularly when it is becoming unreliable, as this will affect a decision about its replacement. The cost of doing say 30 glucose assays on a 'stat' instrument in contrast to doing the same number on a batch analyser would affect the choice of the replacement equipment.

In a profit-making environment the charge made to the patient will reflect the cost of a test and in this respect we might need to know the cost of doing one test at night as compared to a test which was one of a daytime batch. In a non-profit making environment, a major benefit of an accurate costing of a test would be the ability to compare the cost of a test in one laboratory to the cost of the same test in another laboratory. It would also be possible in a clinical costing exercise to allocate the cost of tests to a clinical department, a particular clinician, or a patient's stay in hospital, and thereby assist in a comparison of costs of similar clinical departments, clinicians, or patients in different hospitals.

Another area in which accurate costing becomes a vital ingredient is clinical budgeting. In this a clinician or clinical specialty will be given a pre-agreed workload for the year and an appropriate budget to cover the cost of that workload. To arrive at the costs of achieving the workload it will be necessary for the clinician or clinical specialty to accept a charge from the laboratory for the number of tests he has requested, and this charge becomes revenue for the laboratory and expenditure from the clinical budget. The clinician will then, it is hoped, clearly understand the cost of what he does and utilize his resources to maximize his efficiency. Unnecessary requests to the laboratory should be eliminated.

It follows that if the clinicians reduce their demands on the laboratory, and the charge for a test has been fixed at an average cost when the laboratory had a high output, then since it is suggested that salaries represent 75% of total costs a fall in revenue will necessitate a reduction of staff. However, since there is a minimum staffing level for certain jobs irrespective of throughput, care should be taken to include consideration of this when fixing the unit charge.

MONITORING OR ASSESSMENT OF PERFORMANCE

The ultimate in monitoring and assessing performance would be to determine whether the goal of the clinical laboratory which has been previously defined as producing 'meaningful results for patient care' has been achieved. Such an overall assessment is very complex and the best we can do is to examine performance in the separate parts of the process. We can with certain limitations, assess the reliability of our results and also attempt to evaluate the continuing usefulness of current techniques and the clinical value of new ones. Finally it is possible to establish performance indicators to see if we produce our results cost effectively.

The issue for most laboratories is not, should monitoring and assessment be done, for quality control and assessment procedures are already a part of laboratory culture. The concern is that the performance indicators devised should be reliable and robust, and if they are that they should be used intelligently and constructively, not simplistically and without consultation.

Quality Control and Assessment

The area of monitoring the reliability of results has already been discussed in this chapter under objectives or goals and is dealt with elsewhere in this volume (Chapter 6). Only two aspects will be dealt with here because of their management implications.

First, it is important to be aware that things are not always as they seem to be. Good quality control results for pH using ampoules of tonometered aqueous buffer solutions do not exclude the possibility that deposits of protein have affected the measuring electrode and that patients results are wrong, neither do bad results for Po_2 mean the Po_2 electrode is malfunctioning, unless care has been taken to control the ambient temperature at which an ampoule is reconstituted. Results from an external assessment scheme which suggest poor performance may result from a matrix effect from the control material when used in a particular assay or equally a performance being compared to an inappropriate method mean.

Secondly, quality control and assessment is required for tests done in side rooms on wards, in intensive care units and ultimately for patients analysing their own blood glucoses. A standard of performance which is a statutory requirement in one country for tests done in a laboratory cannot be ignored just because it happens to be in a diabetic clinic.

Clinical Value or Usefulness

Holland and Whitehead[10] gave a good, clear account of the evaluation that should be undertaken before any new investigation is introduced as routine. They suggested two main criteria, the efficiency of the test and the method of measurement and the effectiveness of the test in improving the diagnosis and treatment. Monitoring and assessment of precision and accuracy are fundamental to measuring the efficiency of a new test. The use of reference values produced from a carefully defined reference population are an essential part of the interpretability of a test and therefore affect its efficiency. Techniques for the evaluation of a test, in terms of sensitivity, are described by Galen and Gambino.[11] Sensitivity and specificity are independent of the prevalence of a particular disease in the population tested. The predictive value of a test (the proportion of true positive results in relation to the total number of positives given by the test) is related to prevalence and this markedly affects a test's value in diagnosis. To determine the true effectiveness of a test, a firm end-point of patient benefit, such as reduced morbidity or mortality is necessary, rather than a simple conversion of a physiological variable such as blood glucose to a 'normal level'.

Economic aspects cannot be ignored and are often quoted to support the case for pre- and post-natal screening for diseases such as spina bifida, phenylketonuria and hypothyroidism, the cost of the screening being offset against the cost of hospitalization and social care. It is an essential part of laboratory management to be involved in such cost-benefit analyses.

Performance Indicators

As previously mentioned the difficulty with performance indicators is being certain that they are reliable and robust and if used in comparisons, that like is measured against like. In the section on financial management, mention was made of limitations in present accounting procedures, but a further problem for performance indicators in pathology concerns the method of recording workload. Certain performance indicators recently promulgated by the DHSS in the United Kingdom try to evaluate requests (which are not uniformly measured from hospital to hospital) against the number of technical staff employed in the laboratory and take no account of scientific, medical or ancillary staffing levels.[12]

More sophisticated methods of measurement workload take into account not only the number of tests performed but time taken in different situations.[13] These systems produce information invaluable to the management process but require time and money to implement. While costing and accounting practices vary and workload recording is primitive, the prospect of valid comparisons between laboratories remains remote.

MANAGING

The task of managing a clinical laboratory means tackling many different types of jobs. As Professor Handy says 'the "manager" therefore has to embrace within himself all the four cultures. He has to emulate each god in the appropriate circumstances. If you want an explanation for the lure of management, this is it—the simultaneous call of four gods'. The problem is that this may be for some people impossible and they will revert when tired or stressed to their favourite culture. Cultural tolerance will reduce this pressure and there are many opportunities within a laboratory service to create for people 'meaningful jobs'. If this is accomplished then 'meaningful results' for patient care will not be far behind.

REFERENCES

1. Fraser C. G. (1983). Desirable performance standards for clinical chemistry tests. *Adv. Clin. Chem*; **23**: 299.
2. Handy C. (1985). *Gods of Management.* London: Pan Books.
3. Blanchard K., Johnson S. (1983). *The One Minute Manager.* Fontana Paperbacks.
4. Eastel M., Thomas M. (1984). *The Development of the General Manager.* Nuffield Provincial Hospital Trust.
5. Stewart R. (1967). *The Reality of Management.* London: Pan Books.
6. Raby A. H. (1985). Laboratory design—traditional or flexible. *Inst. Med. Lab. Sci. Gazette*; **29**: 557.
7. Dept. of Health and Social Services (1978). *Code of Practice for the Prevention of Infection in Clinical Laboratories and Post-mortem Rooms.* London: HMSO.
8. Cooper C. L. (1985). The stress of work: An overview. *Aviat. Space Environ. Med*; **56**: 627.
9. Fraser C. G., Sanger R. (1985). Better laboratory

evaluations of instruments and kits are required. *Clin. Chem*; **31**(5): 667.

10. Holland W. W., Whitehead T. P. (1974). Value of new laboratory tests in diagnosis and treatment. *Lancet*; **ii**: 391.

11. Galen R. S., Gambino S. R. (1975). *Beyond Nor-mality*. Chichester: Wiley.

12. Stenton P. (1985). Performance Indicators in Pathology. *Inst. Med. Lab. Sci. Gazette*; **29**: 316.

13. Penner D. W. (1982). The workload recording method. A management tool for the Clinical Laboratory. *Human Pathol*; **13**: 393.

4. The Collection, Transportation and Storage of Specimens

C. G. Fraser

Introduction
Subject preparation
  Documentation
  Controllable factors
Specimen collection
  Blood specimens
  Urine specimens
  Cerebrospinal fluid specimens
  Faeces specimens
Transportation
Storage

INTRODUCTION

The primary purpose of the clinical chemistry laboratory is to provide test results early enough to influence clinical decision-making. To achieve this laudable objective, it is necessary for the analytical performance characteristics of the tests to reach or surpass certain standards.[1] However, even an excellent analytical method cannot provide a valid result unless the subject is carefully prepared and the specimen correctly collected, transported to the laboratory, handled, and stored prior to analysis. This chapter delineates the problems associated with these crucial steps in the cycle of obtaining a test result, and suggests strategies for minimizing the potential difficulties.

SUBJECT PREPARATION

Many pre-analytical factors affect clinical chemistry test results. These may be divided into two groups. First, there are factors which cannot be modified by either clinical or laboratory staff: these require careful *documentation* prior to or at the time of specimen collection in order to facilitate later interpretation of test results. Secondly, there are variable factors which influence test results and these must not only be documented but must be *controlled* as far as possible. These factors are discussed below; they have been reviewed in detail by Young.[2]

Documentation

Age. Many quantities of interest are affected by age and therefore this must be documented in order for the laboratory to report appropriate reference values. There are conflicting reports in the literature concerning the changes that occur with age but it is certain that plasma concentrations of phosphate, urea and creatinine rise in an almost linear fashion and alkaline phosphatase activity falls after the pubertal growth period and then rises in the elderly; some data have been provided on such changes.[3] During the neonatal period and childhood, many quantities change markedly and the compendium of Meites[4] provides an excellent reference source.

Sex. Prior to puberty, the sex of the patient has little influence on clinical chemistry quantities. During the reproductive phase of life, there are many differences between men and women. Due to the influence of oestrogens, the activities of alanine and aspartate aminotransferases, and the concentrations or activities of albumin, alkaline phosphatase, proteins, calcium and magnesium are higher in the plasma of women than of men, whilst iron, ferritin and bilirubin levels are lower.

Body Mass. The plasma concentrations or activities of certain quantities including creatinine, creatine kinase, cholesterol, triglycerides, urate and triiodothyronine are positively correlated with body mass.

Pregnancy. The many changes in clinical chemistry quantities during pregnancy have been reviewed by Lind.[5] Because the plasma volume increases during pregnancy and the erythrocyte volume increases, but to a lesser degree, the changes seen are often considered to be due to dilution. This is an oversimplification and, while the levels of plasma proteins, albumin, urea, creatinine, iron, sodium, potassium, calcium and magnesium do fall, certain quantities do not change including phosphate and alanine and aspartate aminotransferase activities and others, including caeruloplasmin, transferrin and lipoproteins, rise. Many hormonal changes also occur as a consequence of pregnancy.

Food and Drink Intake. Habitual diet can influence clinical chemistry quantities. Moreover, intake of particular foods can pose difficulties; for example, ingestion of foods containing serotonin or vanillin may lead to elevated levels of urinary 5-hydroxyindoleacetic acid and hydroxymethoxymandelic acid respectively. Alcohol intake has many effects which are dependent on a number of factors including whether the individual is an abuser or non-abuser, the amount of alcohol consumed and the time of specimen collection after ingestion. Serum enzyme activities, including alkaline phosphatase, aspartate aminotransferase and lactate dehydrogenase, are elevated after even a single intake of alcohol and gamma-glutamyl transferase activity is also elevated in this situation in addition to being elevated in the majority of habitual drinkers.

Stress. Mental or physical stress leads to increased plasma concentrations of many hormones including cortisol, growth hormone and prolactin. One to two days after a stressful event, for example, myocardial infarction, a reduction in the plasma concentrations of iron, transferrin and cholesterol are sometimes noticed. In general, specimens should not be collected when the patient is stressed by illness or surgical procedures unless the test result is required for immediate patient care.

Exercise. After exercise, plasma activities of creatine kinase, aspartate aminotransferase and lactate dehydrogenase are increased as are the concentrations of many hormones including cortisol, growth hormone, prolactin and plasma renin activity. The magnitude of these effects is dependent on the amount of exercise undertaken and on whether the individual is physically trained or not.

Previous Clinical Care. The effects of previous clinical care on clinical chemistry quantities should not be forgotten. Surgery usually causes increased aspartate aminotransferase activity, blood transfusion can lead to transient hyperbilirubinaemia, intramuscular injection results in increased serum creatine kinase activity, and prostatectomy causes increased serum acid phosphatase activity although palpation of the prostate usually does not lead to this effect. Immobilization itself has some interesting metabolic effects but plasma concentrations do not generally show significant effects unless illness such as Paget's disease or fractures lead to increased plasma calcium and phosphate concentrations due to increased bone turnover.

Drug Effects. There are more than 25 000 references in the literature on the effects of drugs on clinical laboratory investigations and detailed coverage in this chapter is therefore impossible. There are comprehensive documents enumerating such effects.[6,7]

Drugs can cause difficulties in interpretation through their effects on physiological and biochemical mechanisms and these *in vivo* effects account for 80% of drug–test interactions. Important effects are those due to oral contraceptives which, through their oestrogenic activity, lead to increased concentrations of many binding proteins including thyroxine-binding globulin, transcortin, sex hormone-binding globulin and transferrin and can lead to changes in those test results of value in assessment of liver function in some women. Thiazide diuretics often cause hyperuricaemia and hypercalcaemia. Phenytoin, barbiturates and other anti-epileptic drugs can cause elevated gamma-glutamyl transferase activity because of hepatic microsomal enzyme induction. Narcotics can result in hyperamylasaemia, hyperamylasuria and hyperlipasaemia due to their effect of contracting the sphincter of Oddi. Drugs may also interfere with the analytical methodology used but these *in vitro* effects are becoming less important as newer, more specific, analytical techniques are introduced.

Controllable Factors

Posture. When an individual rises from a recumbent position, water shifts out of the vascular compartment and large molecules and the small molecules bound to large molecules become relatively more concentrated. Plasma concentrations of proteins, albumin, cholesterol, triglycerides, iron, thyroxine, cortisol and activities of enzymes rise by 8 to 10%. Plasma calcium concentrations rise by 4–5% because only about half the total calcium is protein bound. The concentrations of drugs change in a similar manner depending on how much is protein bound. The changes seen when rising from a sitting position are of the order of 60–70% of those that occur in changing from recumbent to standing positions.

Time. Many clinical chemistry quantities show biological rhythms. These may be of a daily nature, as shown in Fig. 1 for cortisol, growth hormone and prolactin. During the reproductive phase of life, monthly rhythms are seen for many blood and urinary quantities, for example, in serum luteotrophin, oestradiol and progesterone (Fig. 2). An awareness of such rhythms is vital because it is necessary to collect specimens at times at which reference values are well documented. Moreover, demonstration of absence of a biological rhythm may provide valuable diagnostic information.

It is important to consider the time of specimen collection most carefully before performing analyses for therapeutic drugs. Generally, specimens should be taken before the patient receives further drugs. Specimens should certainly not be taken within seven hours of taking digoxin, lithium or valproate. It is also relevant to remember that adequate time should be allowed for a new steady state to be reached following change in drug dosage.

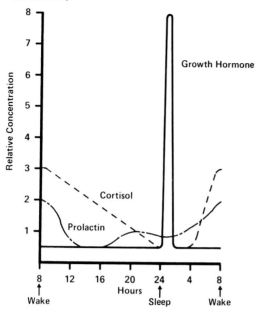

Fig. 1 Daily rhythms seen in plasma levels of cortisol, growth hormone and prolactin.

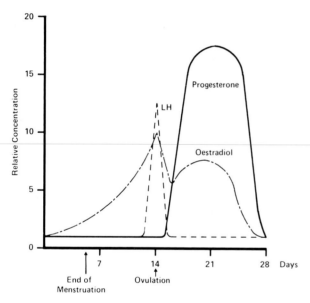

Fig. 2 Monthly rhythms in luteotrophin (LH), oestradiol and progesterone in plasma during the reproductive phase of life.

Dietary State. Recent intake of food can considerably influence many clinical chemistry quantities because of the lipaemia that can occur which interferes with certain analytical techniques. As a general rule, it is preferable that all specimens be collected when the patient is in the fasting state.

SPECIMEN COLLECTION

Blood Specimens

Containers. Few laboratories now prepare containers for blood specimens; in most countries either dispos-

able glass or plastic tubes are used to contain specimens collected by conventional venepuncture or by evacuated tube systems.

The containers may contain no anticoagulant or preservative and subsequent analyses are performed on the serum obtained by centrifugation after formation of a clot. In some respects, serum is the preferred matrix since a clearer specimen is obtained.

Anticoagulants and preservatives widely used in clinical chemistry are shown in Table 1. Lithium heparinized plasma is often used but it should be noted that lithium analyses, electrophoretic studies and certain immunoassays cannot be performed on

TABLE 1
COMMONLY USED ANTICOAGULANTS

Anticoagulant	Concentration
Lithium heparin	12 Units per ml blood
K₂EDTA	2·0 mg per ml blood
Fluoride/oxalate	1·0 mg sodium fluoride plus 3·0 mg potassium oxalate per ml blood

such specimens. It is undoubtedly quicker to obtain plasma specimens for analysis than to wait for clot formation and retraction but it should be recognized that, if the specimen is not centrifuged with sufficient force (3000 g) for long enough (15 min), platelets will not be removed[8] and subsequent analysis will lead to artefactually high lactate dehydrogenase activity if methods which cause platelet lysis are used. Ladenson *et al.*[9] have reviewed the small differences between serum and plasma. These should be borne in mind when clinical laboratories receive both types of specimen. Because the clotting process presumably releases some erythrocyte contents, reference intervals for plasma potassium and phosphate concentrations, and aspartate aminotransferase and lactate dehydrogenase activities are lower than the corresponding intervals for serum.

When multiple specimens are being withdrawn using vacuum tube systems, the order of draw is important to prevent cross-contamination. Serum should be collected first and then the order recommended[10] is citrate, heparin, K₂EDTA and oxalate/fluoride.

Contamination of specimens with anticoagulant can cause difficulties. K₂EDTA invalidates potassium, calcium, magnesium and alkaline phosphatase activity assays. Fluoride/oxalate causes artefactual hypernatraemia, hyperkalaemia and hypocalcaemia. Excess heparin, when used for anticoagulation of specimens for arterial blood pH and gas analyses, causes decreased pH and increased $P\text{CO}_2$; this problem can be avoided by use of syringes containing lyophilized heparin.

Contamination. Blood specimens should be collected from carefully prepared collection sites which are clean, sterile and not contaminated. Specimens should not be contaminated with extraneous materials. Air bubbles, for example, cause Po_2 levels to rise in arterial blood specimens in as little as 3 minutes.

Collection Site. Capillary blood is often collected from neonates and children and from adults either in out-patient clinics or when venepuncture has proved traumatic. Capillary and venous blood do differ, the concentration of glucose being higher and those of potassium, proteins and calcium being lower.

Often individuals from whom specimens are collected are being given intravenous therapy. Blood taken proximal to the infusion site will be contaminated with the intravenous fluid being given. This will be simple to detect when glucose is being administered because a dilution of all quantities will be seen. Contamination with physiological saline may be more difficult to observe but hyperchloraemia in the presence of eunatraemia and low levels of other quantities is detected in most cases.

Tourniquet Application. A tourniquet is often applied to aid venepuncture but, should venous occlusion be prolonged, water and small molecules and ions will pass out of the vascular space. As a result, large molecules (such as proteins, albumin and enzymes) and small moieties bound in whole or in part to proteins (such as calcium, cholesterol, triglycerides, bilirubin, some drugs and many hormones) can be raised to high or equivocal levels. Moreover, prolonged stasis is said to lead to local hypoxia and quantities present in erythrocytes, including potassium, phosphate, aspartate aminotransferase and lactate dehydrogenase, can diffuse out and cause raised plasma levels. As a general rule, therefore, the use of minimum venous occlusion is advised.

Haemolysis. Haemolysis can be caused by a number of factors including traumatic venepuncture, forcing blood through the needle and use of wet or dirty tubes. Freezing and thawing of blood specimens causes massive haemolysis.

The compositions of plasma and erythrocytes are very different as is shown in Table 2. When haemolysis is present, two effects may be seen. First, those quantities which are present at high concentrations or activities, including potassium, phosphate, magnesium, aspartate aminotransferase and lactate dehydrogenase, will be elevated. Secondly, spectrophotometric interference can introduce errors which are very method dependent and cannot, therefore, be dealt with in depth in this chapter.

Urine Specimens

The analysis of a random or spot urine specimen may provide valuable clinical information; urinalysis using commercial reagent dipsticks and assays of sodium, potassium and osmolality are usually performed on such specimens.

It is more usual to collect timed specimens of urine and the two important considerations are, first, that the patient is given clear instructions which leave no room for ambiguity and, secondly, that the correct preservative and/or stabilizer is used.

Simple instructions for the collection of urine are shown in Table 3. Although urinary creatinine output

TABLE 3
THE COLLECTION OF URINE SPECIMENS

1. Use the collection bottle provided.
2. At the start of the 24 hour collection, empty the bladder and DISCARD THIS SPECIMEN OF URINE. Note the exact time on the bottle label.
3. All the urine passed during the next 24 hours must be collected in the bottle which should be kept in a cool place or preferably in a refrigerator at 4°C.
4. On the following day, at EXACTLY the time noted on the label on the previous day, empty the bladder and add this urine to the collection bottle. Note the EXACT time on the bottle label.
5. If any urine is discarded in error, a new collection should be started.
6. If a bowel movement is anticipated during the collection period, collect the urine first and add it to the collection bottle. If the urine is contaminated, a new collection should be started.

is not absolutely constant, analyses in serial specimens from an individual is thought by some to provide a useful check on the adequacy of timed collections.

Urine collections may require preservation to prevent bacterial growth or may require a stabilizer to prevent degradation of constituents. There is a paucity of publications dealing with this subject but a recent review[11] has suggested use of the preservatives and stabilizers shown in Table 4. Merthiolate is used as sodium merthiolate 150 mg per container, boric acid as 27 g per container and thymol as one crystal per container.

Correct stabilization is important because, for example, calcium and phosphate will precipitate out

TABLE 2
AVERAGE COMPOSITION OF PLASMA AND ERYTHROCYTES

Quantity	Units	Plasma	Erythrocytes
Glucose	mmol/l	5·0	4·1
Calcium	mmol/l	2·50	0·25
Phosphate	mmol/l	1·20	4·20
Sodium	mmol/l	140	16
Potassium	mmol/l	4	100
Chloride	mmol/l	104	52
Bicarbonate	mmol/l	25	10
Urea	mmol/l	5·5	4·0
Aspartate aminotransferase	U/l	25	500
Lactate dehydrogenase	U/l	180	30 000

TABLE 4
PRESERVATIVES AND STABILIZERS FOR URINE COLLECTIONS

Quantity	Preservative	Stabilizer
Sodium	4°C or merthiolate, boric acid or thymol	Nil
Potassium	4°C or merthiolate, boric acid or thymol	Nil
Osmolality	4°C or merthiolate, boric acid or thymol	Nil
Urea	4°C or merthiolate, boric acid or thymol	Nil
Creatinine	4°C or merthiolate, or thymol	Nil
Calcium	Nil	50 ml of 3 mol/l HCl
Phosphate	Nil	50 ml of 3 mol/l HCl
Urate	Nil	15 ml of 2 mol/l NaOH
Proteins	4°C or merthiolate or thymol	Nil
Glucose	4°C or merthiolate	Nil
Chloride	4°C or merthiolate, boric acid or thymol	Nil
Oxalate	Nil	50 ml of 3 mol/l HCl
Hydroxymethoxymandelic acid	Nil	50 ml of 3 mol/l HCl
5-Hydroxyindoleacetic acid	Nil	50 ml of 3 mol/l HCl
Amylase	4°C or merthiolate or thymol	Nil

of solution if the pH is not acidic and urate will precipitate if the pH is not alkaline. While these situations can be retrieved in the laboratory by thorough mixing of the entire collection after appropriate adjustment of pH, this strategy cannot be successful for quantities which degrade on standing at inappropriate pH; for example, 5-hydroxyindoleacetic acid and hydroxymethoxymandelic acid must be collected into acid.

Certain widely advocated stabilizers do cause analytical difficulties. For example, glacial acetic acid causes significant negative interference in methods for 5-hydroxyindoleacetic acid which use nitrosonaphthol with extraction.

Cerebrospinal Fluid Specimens

Cerebrospinal fluid, obtained by lumbar puncture, is analysed for few clinical chemistry quantities. It is important to note that specimens which are contaminated with blood cannot be analysed for proteins because the cerebrospinal fluid contains very much less protein than blood. Moreover, cells may be present in the fluid and specimens for glucose analyses must be collected into fluoride/oxalate containers.

Faeces Specimens

Analysis of faeces is largely confined nowadays to electrolyte balance and fat excretion studies. Irregularities in bowel habits make the timing of any collection difficult. Carmine red and charcoal faecal markers, given orally every few days, have been used for this purpose but, at best, are only a crude index of the collection period.

Considerable improvement in the accuracy of faecal collections has been achieved by the use of continuous chromium sesquioxide markers. Details of this method, together with its evaluation, can be found in the study by Rose.[12]

TRANSPORTATION

It is generally advisable to transport all specimens to the clinical laboratory without delay. This is particularly necessary for those quantities present in erythrocytes which will leak out when the plasma glucose has been metabolized.

Specimens for blood pH and gas analyses must be transported to the laboratory on ice. Delay of more than 20 minutes causes Po_2 levels to change significantly if the specimen is at 4°C or room temperature. These changes also take place even at 0°C in 30 minutes. pH and Pco_2 levels are rather more stable and do not change significantly for at least 30 minutes, even at room temperature.

Many laboratories analyse glucose in non-preserved specimens. This is to be deprecated because, as shown in Fig. 3, glucose is unstable, the degrada-

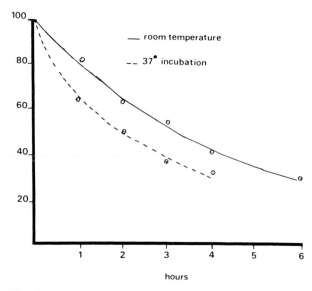

Fig. 3 Loss in plasma glucose in a specimen collected in lithium heparin without preservative.

tion seen depending on a number of factors. Iodoacetate has been used as an antiglycolytic agent but is now rarely used because it is relatively unstable and fluoride/oxalate does not interfere in most modern analytical methods. It should be noted that the rate of glucose metabolism is very high in premature neonates and no preservative may be truly effective; rapid transportation on ice is probably the best approach.

Transportation of specimens from outside the clinical laboratory is the subject of legislation in many countries. Polystyrene packs provide a robust and economical way of transport. Specimens which must arrive in the laboratory in a frozen state create a problem. Wide-necked vacuum flasks with dry ice in the base provide the best means for transportation but are not suitable for posting. They must therefore be transported by road or rail and arrangements must be made for timely pickup and delivery.

This subject and UK regulations have been dealt with in detail by Wilding et al.[13]

STORAGE

Clinical laboratories may not be able to analyse all specimens as soon as they have been received and therefore it is necessary to have knowledge of the stability of clinical chemistry quantities. Information[13] on the stability of commonly analysed quantities in serum or plasma is shown in Table 5. Urine, as well as plasma, should be analysed as soon as possible, although a delay of 2–3 days will not significantly alter most investigations. For long-term storage, lyophilization is the most satisfactory procedure although storage at $-70°C$ is likely to be adequate.

REFERENCES

1. Fraser G. C. (1983). Desirable performance standards for clinical chemistry tests. *Adv. Clin. Chem*; **23**: 299–339.
2. Young D. S. (1979). Biological variability. In *Clinical Diagnosis of Disease*. (Brown S. S., Mitchell F. L., Young D. S., eds) pp. 1–113. Amsterdam: Elsevier.
3. Gräsbeck R., Alström T., eds (1981). *Reference Values in Laboratory Medicine*. Chichester: Wiley.
4. Meites S., ed. (1981). *Paediatric Clinical Chemistry*, 2nd edn. Washington: Am. Assoc. of Clinical Chemists.
5. Lind T. (1980). Clinical chemistry of pregnancy. *Adv. Clin. Chem*; **21**: 1–24.
6. Young D. S., Pestaner L., Gibberman V. (1975). Effects of drugs on clinical tests. *Clin. Chem*; **21**: 1D–432D.
7. Tryding N., Lindblad C. G., eds (1983). *Drug Effects in Clinical Chemistry*, 3rd edn. Stockholm: Apoteksbolaget.
8. Duggan P. F., Hurley T., Martin N. (1985). Centrifugation speeds and removal of platelets from heparinised plasma. *Clin. Chem*; **31**: 1082.
9. Ladenson J. H., Tsai L. B., Michawl J. M., Kessler G., Joist J. H. (1974). Serum versus heparinised plasma for eighteen common chemistry tests. *Am. J. Clin. Pathol*; **62**: 545–552.
10. Calam R. R., Cooper M. H. (1982). Recommended order of draw for collecting blood samples into additive containing tubes. *Clin. Chem*; **28**: 1399.
11. Shephard M. D. S., Mazzachi R. D. (1983). The collection, preservation, storage and stability of urine specimens for routine clinical biochemical analysis. *Clin. Biochem. Rev*; **4**: 61.
12. Rose G. A. (1964). Experiences with the use of interrupted carmine red and continuous chromium sesquioxide marking of human faeces. *Gut*; **5**: 274.
13. Wilding P., Zilva J. F., Wilde C. E. (1977). Transport of specimens for clinical chemistry analysis. *Ann. Clin. Biochem*; **14**: 301–6.

FURTHER READING

Fraser C. G. (1986). *Interpretation of Clinical Chemistry Laboratory Data*. Edinburgh: Blackwell Scientific.
Slockbower J. M., Blumenfeld T. A. (1983). *Collection and Handling of Laboratory Specimens: A Practical Guide*. Philadelphia: Lipincott.

TABLE 5
STABILITY OF SERUM OR PLASMA QUANTITIES WITHOUT PRESERVATIVES

Quantity	Room Temperature	4°C	Frozen
Acid phosphatase	15 min	3 h	7 days
Alanine aminotransferase	3 days	7 days	Stable
Albumin	7 days	1 month	Stable
Alkaline phosphatase	7 days	7 days	Stable
Amylase	Stable	Stable	Stable
Aspartate aminotransferase	3 days	7 days	Stable
Bilirubin	2 days	6 days	Stable
Calcium	7 days	10 days	Stable
Cholesterol	7 days	7 days	Stable
Cortisol	1 day	7 days	Stable
Creatine kinase	2 days	7 days	1 month
Creatinine	1 day	2 days	Stable
Gamma-glutamyl transferase	7 days	7 days	Stable
Glucose	45 min	1 day	Stable
Iron	4 days	7 days	Stable
Lactate dehydrogenase	7 days	Unstable	Unstable
Magnesium	7 days	7 days	Stable
Phosphate	4 days	7 days	Stable
Potassium	14 days	14 days	Stable
Proteins	7 days	1 month	Stable
Sodium	14 days	14 days	Stable
Thyroxine	2 days	4 days	Stable
Triglycerides	5 days	7 days	Stable
Urate	3 days	7 days	Stable
Urea	4 days	7 days	Stable

5. The Statistical Treatment of Biological Data
Martin Crowder

INTRODUCTION

As the aim of this chapter is to present a useful range of basic techniques in a limited number of pages, many details and extensions are omitted. The books listed at the end are suggested for further reading.

There are two major movements under way in contemporary statistical practice. The first, now well established, is the increasing use of computer packages by scientists to process their data. Unfortunately, there is a natural tendency among such clients to accord the computer output too much respect and place too much weight on what it tells them. It is worth remembering that statistical packages are usually written by computer programmers who, though experts in their field, are probably neither practising statisticians nor familiar with the user's particular problem. In my view the answer to this problem is that the client should know exactly what the computer is doing to his data. If he has performed the same computations by hand, even if only on small training data sets, he should have acquired some feeling for what the result means in practice rather than in theory. Of course, the more complex statistical techniques often require far too much computational effort for this, but the principle stands: one can gain vital insight from the simpler calculations which is applicable across the board. This chapter therefore concentrates on the basic pen and paper (plus calculator, perhaps) techniques.

The second movement is more fundamental. It stems from a growing dissatisfaction over the past decade or so with traditional statistical wisdom. Lack of space precludes discussion of the issues in general here, but the essential points will be brought out in context below.

DATA PRESENTATION AND SUMMARY

Before the development of formal methods of examining data, statistics simply meant records of a numerical character such as may be found in certain government reports. However, when records are examined it is usually with a view to drawing general conclusions about the situation giving rise to the data rather than because of a fascination for staring at columns of figures.

Suppose that a fairly large amount of data is under scrutiny. We now describe methods for extracting from it features of possible interest; this is essentially a process of reduction from a mass of figures to a few summarizing characteristics. In subsequent sections other situations are discussed and appropriate statistical methods are demonstrated.

Frequency Distributions and Histograms

The data in Table 1 are measurements of potassium level taken on 83 patients in routine hospital screening.

Visual inspection of the observations in this sample reveals that they vary from 2·8 at the lower end to 5·6 at the upper. One might also detect that the spacing of the values is wider towards the extremes of the data than nearer the middle, in other words the density of points is not constant along the scale. These

TABLE 1
POTASSIUM LEVELS FOR 83 SUBJECTS

3·5	4·6	4·4	3·6	4·2	5·6	2·8	3·0	3·9	3·4	3·9	4·3	4·2	4·2	3·8
4·6	4·1	4·9	4·4	4·0	3·5	4·6	4·3	3·8	3·7	4·0	4·1	3·7	4·0	3·7
4·1	4·0	4·2	3·7	3·8	4·0	3·5	3·6	4·2	3·9	3·2	3·2	3·3	3·9	3·2
5·2	4·3	3·6	4·1	3·8	4·4	3·8	3·9	4·2	4·2	3·9	4·9	4·0	4·0	4·0
4·3	4·9	4·8	4·2	4·0	4·1	4·5	4·5	3·5	3·8	2·9	4·2	3·6	4·0	4·6
4·2	3·7	3·6	4·3	4·4	4·4	3·3	3·8							

TABLE 2
FREQUENCY DISTRIBUTION FOR THE DATA IN TABLE 1

Class	Frequency	Relative frequency (%)	Cumulative frequency	Relative cumulative frequency (%)
2·8 to	3	3·6	3	3·6
3·1 to	5	6·0	8	9·6
3·4 to	10	12·0	18	21·6
3·7 to	18	21·7	36	43·3
4·0 to	25	30·2	61	73·5
4·3 to	12	14·5	73	88·0
4·6 to	5	6·0	78	94·0
4·9 to	3	3·6	81	97·6
5·2 to	1	1·2	82	98·8
5·5	1	1·2	83	100·0

two characteristics, the range of values and their density distribution, can be demonstrated more clearly as follows. We construct a grid on the scale by taking a convenient number of intervals (say ten) starting at 2·8 at equal spacings of 0·3. Then we examine the data and count the number of values falling in each of our constructed intervals. This process of *grouping* the data into *classes* produces the *frequency distribution* in Table 2.

In the first two columns of the table, the first class (2·8 up to, but not including, 3·1) is seen to contain three of the original measurements, i.e. the *frequency* in this class is 3, the points 2·8, 2·9 and 3·0 being *grouped* together. Thus we can now learn at a glance from the frequency distribution the range of values and the distribution of frequencies among the classes. It is often preferable to present information pictorially, and in this case a graphical display of the frequency distribution is called a *histogram* (Fig. 1). The varying density of points along the scale can then be appreciated visually. For many purposes *relative frequencies* are preferable to the absolute frequencies we have been using. These are obtained by dividing the latter by the total number of observations in the sample. For instance, the first class contains 3 observations out of 83 so its relative frequency is 3/83 = 0·036, or 3·6%; these percentages are given in the third column of Table 2. Similarly, by adding relative frequencies, the proportion of sample values between 3·1 and 4·0 is 0·397 or 39·7%. Sometimes we may wish to discuss how many of the points fall below (or above) some given value, rather than how many lie between given limits. For this purpose *cumulative frequencies* are used; in Table 2 they are given in the fourth column. In the fifth column the corresponding *relative cumulative frequencies* are expressed as percentages; for example 94% of the observations fall below the value 4·9. Fig. 2 is a *cumulative frequence plot* (or *ogive*).

This summarizing process is now discussed in more detail in order to bring out certain problems which need to be resolved in practice.

1. Ten classes were taken as convenient for the data. Had fewer been taken, less detail would

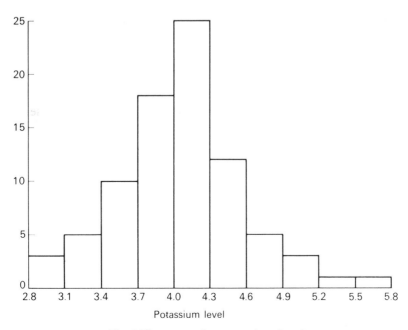

Fig. 1 Histogram for potassium levels.

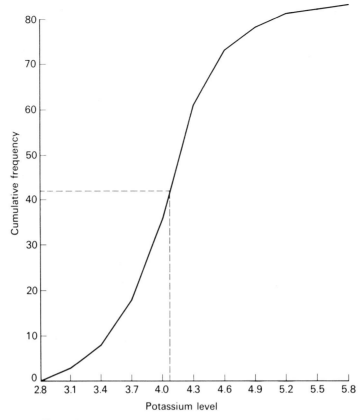

Fig. 2 Cumulative frequency plot for potassium levels.

have been evident in the histogram; this may be appreciated by pooling adjacent pairs of classes, thus obtaining only five groups. On the other hand, if the number of classes had been 25, say, the histogram would have taken on an irregular appearance, most of the classes containing very few observations. Clearly, a compromise is called for, and this will depend on the data available, although about ten classes will usually convey the required information adequately.

2. The grid values were taken to be equi-spaced. This is not always necessary. Occasionally it is argued that because of the different densities of points at different parts of the measurement scale higher resolution (obtained by narrowing the classes) is required in some places but not in others. However, the practice of having unequal class intervals introduces some minor and troublesome details, for which the reader is referred to the more extensive accounts in the reference list.

3. Having decided on the grid points, a rule for borderline values must be operated. For instance if the heights of a group of people were recorded to the nearest inch, it is an arbitrary decision whether 68 in. is to be included in a class 67–68 in. or the adjacent 68–69 in. Consistency being the determining virtue, one might allocate each observation to the corresponding left-hand class, so that 68 in. goes into 67–68 in., 69 in. goes into 68–69 in., etc. But this has the effect of making everyone half an inch shorter. Clearly in this example the difficulty can be avoided by choosing classes which begin and end on half inches, e.g. 68·5–69·5 in. Equivalently, the horizontal scale on the histogram can be shifted by half an inch and any subsequent computations corrected by the same amount. With the data on potassium levels this bias is 0·05 since the values are recorded to the nearest tenth, e.g. 3·7 representing any value between 3·65 and 3·75.

4. A point related to the previous one concerns the type of measurements being treated. It has been assumed implicitly in the above description that these are *continuous*, i.e. there is a range along the scale within which an observation can take any value, at least as far as the limits of accuracy of the recording device permit. But there are also *discrete* measurements, the possible values for an observation being a sequence of isolated points; examples are the number of bacterial colonies on a slide (in general, counts), or the stage of a disease (scores or grades). In drawing up a frequency distribution for discrete data, points similar to those discussed in (3) will have to be considered;

in fact the histogram is often given in the form of a sequence of vertical bars, based on the possible observation values, instead of adjacent rectangles.

Measures of Location and Dispersion

In addition to purely descriptive presentation of the data certain numerical indices can be computed which summarize particular aspects of the sample. Also, such values are often needed as input for further calculations.

Location. Central values can be located in an informal way by inspecting the histogram. But how may a definite figure be assigned for this purpose?

1. Suppose that the original raw data are available, and denoted by $x_1, x_2, \ldots, x_n$; this general notation indicates that there are n measurements of a variable x, the subscripts $1, 2, \ldots$ merely distinguishing the different observations, and not necessarily implying that they have been, for instance, put in increasing order of size. Thus, if our observations are 5·3, 7·4, 6·6, 6·2, 8·0 then n is 5, x_1 is 5·3, x_2 is 7·4, etc. The *mean* of these data is

$$\bar{x} = \Sigma x_i / n;$$

the $\bar{x}$ notation is standard and Σx_i means $(x_1 + x_2 + \ldots + x_n)$, i.e. Σx_i is an instruction to add together the x values, the dummy subscript i running from 1 to n. Thus,

$$\Sigma x_i = 5 \cdot 3 + 7 \cdot 4 + \ldots + 8 \cdot 0 = 33 \cdot 5$$

and $\bar{x}$ is $33 \cdot 5 / 5 = 6 \cdot 7$; the mean, 6·7, is just the (arithmetic) average, and so provides a value which is 'central' for the data. The same feat is accomplished in a different way by the *median* which is just the half-way point. Ordering the data according to increasing size gives (5·3, 6·2, 6·6, 7·4, 8·0). The median is 6·6, the middle one. If n had been even instead of odd, there would be two middle values, and it is a convention to average these two in obtaining the median, e.g. if the 8·0 is deleted from our sample, the median becomes $\frac{1}{2}(6 \cdot 2 + 6 \cdot 6) = 6 \cdot 4$.

2. Now suppose that the raw data are not available, and we have to work from a frequency distribution—this is often the case in published reports of large amounts of data. In Fig. 1 we see only that three of the original figures were between 2·8 and 3·1 (exclusive of the higher figure), whereas to compute $\bar{x}$ we apparently require their exact values. As a first approximation let us select the value 2·9 as representative of data points falling in the first class; 2·9 is in fact the mid-point of measurements allocated to the first class, and is called the *class mark*. Thus the contribution of the three in question

to the overall sum of values is $(2 \cdot 9 + 2 \cdot 9 + 2 \cdot 9)$ or $3 \times 2 \cdot 9$. Denoting the j-th class mark (j runs from 1 to 10) by x and the corresponding frequency by f (where $x_1 = 2 \cdot 9$ and $f_1 = 3$), the contribution by the j-th class to the overall sum is $f_j x_j$, and so the Σx_i occurring above is now replaced by

$$\Sigma f_j x_j = (3 \times 2 \cdot 9) + (5 \times 3 \cdot 2) + \ldots \\ + (1 \times 5 \cdot 6) = 332 \cdot 8.$$

Thus $\bar{x} = \Sigma f_j x_j / n = 332 \cdot 8 / 83 = 4 \cdot 01$. This is an approximation to the value that would have been obtained using the exact measurements and seems crude because of the initial assumption that all the values within a class are clustered at one point. However, the same formula is obtained on the more credible hypothesis that values within classes are uniformly distributed about the class mark; this becomes obvious when one realizes that $\bar{x}$ is the 'point of balance' or 'centre of gravity' of the observations along the x-scale, and is unchanged by shifting them from their uniformly spaced positions to their class marks. The determination of sensible class marks depends on the situation since some knowledge of the data, and the method of construction of the frequency distribution, is used. In this case we took account of the fact that the figures were continuous measurements originally recorded to one decimal place and that a 'left-hand class' rule was used for allocating borderline cases.

For the *median* we argue as follows. Since the sample size n is 83 we are looking for the 42nd observation. Inspection of the cumulative frequencies in Table 2 shows that this occurs somewhere in the class 4·0–4·3. If such a statement is not adequate, it may be refined as follows. Assuming that the 25 observations in this class are uniformly distributed between 3·95 and 4·25, the sixth one along is at $3 \cdot 95 + (6/25)(4 \cdot 25 - 3 \cdot 95) = 4 \cdot 02$, which value may be taken as the median. An alternative quicker determination can be made if the cumulative frequency plot is available; in Fig. 2 the horizontal dotted line is drawn first, starting at 42 on the cumulative frequency axis, then the x-value corresponding to the point where this horizontal line meets the curve is taken as the median.

In the case of grouped data there is a third commonly used method of quoting a central value. This is the *mode*, the point of highest density of the distribution; inspection of Table 2 shows that the mode belongs to the class 4·0–4·3 and may be taken as 4·1 (the class mark). The *mode* is really a different type of index from the *mean* and *median* in that it locates the region of highest density. If, as is common, this occurs near the centre of the data, the three indices will be fairly close. However, for certain types of measurement the values cluster more towards one end, and tail off gradually at the other, in which case the essential differences between the three indices become apparent. Occasionally the mode is used for raw, ungrouped data, but it is not ideally suited to this case since, for instance, observations may coincide by chance far from the true region of highest density, especially in fairly small samples. If the frequency distribution has two (or more), separated, high-scoring classes there are two (or more) modes and the distribution is *bimodal* (or *multimodal*) instead of *unimodal*.

There are refinements of the median. We may specify a fraction other than one half and look for a point on the x-scale below which this fraction of the distribution lies. Such points are called *quantiles* in general. In the case of the fractions $\frac{1}{4}$, $\frac{1}{2}$ and $\frac{3}{4}$, the three corresponding quantiles are given the special name *quartiles*, the middle one being the median; thus the quartiles cut the distribution into quarters. Other special cases are *deciles* (tenths) and *percentiles* (hundredths). A convenient method for finding quantiles is that described above for the median using the cumulative frequency plot. Referring to Fig. 2, and taking the $\frac{1}{3}$ quantile as an example, the horizontal dotted line should be drawn one-third of the way up the vertical scale, corresponding to a frequency 83/3. (In fact the exact $\frac{1}{3}$ and $\frac{2}{3}$ cuts occur at frequencies 28 and 56 for this set of data.) It may be verified that the $\frac{1}{3}$ quantile obtained by this method is 3·86.

With regard to the relative merits of the mean, median and mode, we note that the mean is useful because it can be combined and compared easily between different sets of data. It is also much more tractable theoretically, so that most formal statistical methods use the mean rather than the median or the mode. The median is unaffected by the extreme values or by the shape of the distribution in the *tails* far from the centre; the mode really indicates the position of the 'high point(s)' of the distribution.

Dispersion. We now turn to a second feature of the data which can be expressed quantitatively, namely the spread, or dispersion, of values. There are many ways of measuring it, but we consider only the most important one. The sample *variance* s^2 is computed (for raw data) as

$$s^2 = \Sigma(x_i - \bar{x})^2/(n - 1)$$

this means that first $\bar{x}$ is subtracted from each x (thus forming $x_i - \bar{x}$), the n resulting differences are each squared, then added, and finally divided by $(n - 1)$. Intuitively, to measure the spread, we are considering the distances of the points x_i from the central value $\bar{x}$; in fact we are averaging the squared distances, $(x_i - \bar{x})^2$. If the distances are not squared, zero is always obtained as the average, because the mean is so positioned that the negative deviations $(x_i - \bar{x})$ balance exactly the positive ones. The use of $(n - 1)$ instead of n in this average is a technical convenience. The following variants of s^2 are commonly quoted:

s, the sample *standard deviation*, is the square root of the variance, and has the same units as the original data; $s/\bar{x}$, the sample *coefficient of variation*, expresses s as a fraction (or often as a percentage) of $\bar{x}$. The computations are illustrated using the above sample of five observations: the differences $(x_i - \bar{x})$ are $(-1·4, 0·7, -0·1, -0·5, 1·3)$; these have squares $(1·96, 0·49, 0·01, 0·25, 1·69)$ which sum to 4·40; thus the sample variance $s^2 = 4·40/4 = 1·1$, the standard deviation $s = 1·1^{1/2} = 1·05$, and the coefficient of variation $s/\bar{x} = 1·05/6·7 = 0·16$ (or 16%). For grouped data, the formula for s^2 is modified in a similar fashion to that for $\bar{x}$, and becomes

$$s^2 = \Sigma f_j(x_j - \bar{x})^2/(n - 1)$$

In the case of the potassium levels data

$$s^2 = (1/82)\{3(2·9 - 4·01)^2 + \ldots \\ + 1(5·6 - 4·01)^2\} = 0.26,$$

$s = 0·51$ and $100s/\bar{x} = 12·8\%$. Note: for ease of calculation (but not for interpretation) we may use the following:

$$\Sigma(x_i - \bar{x})^2 = \Sigma x_i^2 - n\bar{x}^2$$
$$\Sigma f_j(x_j - \bar{x})^2 = \Sigma f_j x_j^2 - n\bar{x}^2$$

When different sets of data are combined a pooled mean and a pooled variance can be computed without recourse to the original figures. For two independent samples:

$$\text{pooled sample mean } \bar{x} = \frac{n_1\bar{x}_1 + n_2\bar{x}_2}{n_1 + n_2},$$

$$\text{pooled sample variance } s^2 = \frac{(n_1 - 1)s_1^2 + (n_2 - 1)s_2^2}{(n_1 - 1) + (n_2 - 1)}.$$

These are both weighted averages of the separate quantities with more weight being given to the larger sample. The pooled mean $\bar{x}$ is just that which would be obtained by throwing the samples together (since the numerator is the total sum of both sets of values, and the denominator is the total size of the two samples); its use carries the implication that the corresponding populations have equal mean values (the term 'population' is explained below). The use of a pooled variance similarly relies upon an assumption of equal population variances, but not necessarily of equal means; s^2 is not the value which would be obtained by amalgamating the samples unless by chance $\bar{x}_1 = \bar{x}_2$.

Theoretical Distributions

So far we have been dealing with a sample of observations. But these are drawn from a *population* of values, that is, the collection of all possible measurements of that type. In the example, the population measurements could be thought of as the complete set of potassium levels which could possibly have resulted from the screening exercise in that week, or perhaps that month or year. The population will almost invariably be regarded as infinite, or at least as consisting of a sufficiently large number of members for any finite-population adjustments to be unnecessary.

Consider now the effect on a histogram like Fig. 1 if we could carry on increasing our sample size n indefinitely. As n grows, the class widths could be

Two further characteristics of the distributions are the so-called *skewness* and *kurtosis*, usually denoted by γ_1 and γ_2 respectively. The former, γ_1, describes the degree of asymmetry, i.e. whether the distribution is lopsided and leans in one direction or the other, and the latter, γ_2, is affected by the nature of the peak and tails of the distribution. Fig. 4 illustrates positive, negative and zero values of skewness and kurtosis.

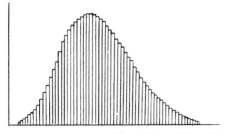 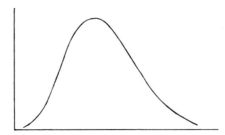

Fig. 3 Transition of histogram to density curve.

made smaller without introducing an irregular appearance until eventually a smooth curve is obtained. The process is illustrated in Fig. 3. In order to prevent the size of the graph becoming unmanageable as the class frequencies become large, a conventional standardization is made that the total area enclosed is unity. The smooth limiting curve illustrates the relative density of points along the x-scale in the whole population; it is called a *density curve*.

Relative frequencies were used to obtain the proportion of sample values between two given points on the x-scale; the same is possible with the density curve. For instance the area beneath the curve between the points 3·0 and 4·0 represents the proportion of the population values in that range. Another interpretation of this is that, if an observation is taken at random from the population, the probability that it will be between 3·0 and 4·0 is equal to the area in question. If instead of 3·0 and 4·0 we take the two points closer and closer together, the area, and hence the probability, tends to zero, representing virtual impossibility; if the two points are taken successively further apart so that eventually the whole population will be enclosed, and hence an area tending to 1, we have a representation of virtual certainty. Thus a scale for probability is developed, ranging from 0 to 1.

The numerical characteristics considered above for samples have their analogues in the population. For instance, the sample mean $\bar{x}$ and sample variance s^2 will in general take different values for different samples from a given population, but the population mean μ and population variance σ^2 are fixed constants. Usually, population characteristics such as μ and σ^2 (generally called *parameters*) are unknown and the purpose of computing $\bar{x}$ and s^2 is to estimate them. It is vital to keep clear the distinction between $\bar{x}$ and μ, and between s^2 and σ^2.

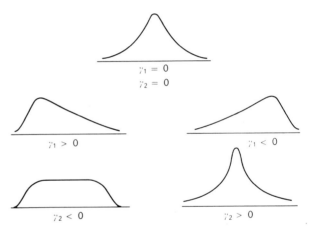

Fig. 4 Illustration of skewness and kurtosis coefficients.

STATISTICAL INFERENCE AND THE NORMAL DISTRIBUTION

We have looked at some ways of boiling down the data and presenting it in more easily digested summary form, either graphically or numerically. This is the *descriptive* side of statistics. The other side is *inferential*, i.e. using the sample to draw conclusions about the population. In this there is no particular interest in the sample *per se*, only as a means of gaining information about the underlying mechanisms generating it. The logical basis of many conventional statistical methods is *repeated sampling* which is now discussed.

Repeated Samples

Recall the sample of observations used above for illustration: 5·3, 7·4, 6·6, 6·2, 8·0. We saw that, for this sample, $n = 5$, $\bar{x} = 6·7$ and $s^2 = 1·1$. Let us suppose that this is one typical member of a continuing series, e.g. resulting from routine daily calibration checks on some system. Thus our sample here is viewed in the context of similar, repeated samples each yielding its own particular mean $\bar{x}$ and variance s^2. Concentrating on the set of $\bar{x}$-values so produced, we have a 'sample' of them in effect. Correspondingly there is an underlying 'population' of $\bar{x}$-values generated from repeated samples in the above manner. This theoretical $\bar{x}$-distribution will have all the characteristics that any distribution has, in particular a mean and a variance. It does not come as a complete surprise that this mean is μ (the same as the underlying mean of the raw observations) and this variance is σ^2/n (n^{-1} times the raw data variance, reflecting the increased precision of averages over raw data). To summarize, over repeated samples $\bar{x}$ has a distribution with mean μ and variance σ^2/n.

The above considerations are mathematically correct (as can be proved), but are they practically useful? One thing that they do yield is a scale of accuracy for $\bar{x}$ as an estimate of μ. Because $\bar{x}$ has variance σ^2/n, its standard deviation is $\sigma/n^{1/2}$ and this is a measure of dispersion of the $\bar{x}$-distribution, i.e. it gives a qualitative assessment of how close $\bar{x}$-values are to their mean μ on average. Now σ^2 is usually unknown—if we are trying to estimate μ then presumably we do not know its value (otherwise the exercise is pointless), and then probably the same goes for σ^2. Hence, the measure used in practice is $s/n^{1/2}$ (replacing σ by its sample estimate s), which is called the *standard error of the mean* (sem for short). Thus the sem, $s/n^{1/2}$, is usually quoted along with $\bar{x}$ to convey a measure of precision. But this precision, remember, is an average value over repeated samples. For one thing the repeated sample setting is often only hypothetical, i.e. our sample is really one-off. For another, this average precision tells us nothing definite about our particular $\bar{x}$, only about such $\bar{x}$'s in general. We will return to this defect below when we discuss confidence intervals; in order to do this we make a slight digression first to investigate a particular distribution.

Normal Distribution

The variety of possible shapes of density curve for continuous variables is enormous, all that is required is that the total area be 1 and that the curve never dip below the x-scale. However, there is one which frequently occurs in statistical theory and practice. This is the Normal (or Gaussian) curve. A Normal distribution with mean μ and variance σ^2 is referred to briefly as $N(\mu,\sigma^2)$; if the distribution of values in the population of measurements of a variable x is described by this curve we say simply that x is $N(\mu,\sigma^2)$. The form of the curve is given by

$$f(x) = \frac{1}{\sigma\sqrt{(2\pi)}} \exp\{-(x-\mu)^2/2\sigma^2\} \text{ for } -\infty < x < \infty,$$

where $f(x)$ denotes the density at the point x, and this is illustrated in Fig. 5. The bell-shaped curve is symmetric about μ and has points of inflexion at $\mu \pm \sigma$; the range of values is the whole line, $-\infty$ to $+\infty$, but the density tends very strongly towards zero in the tails of the distribution.

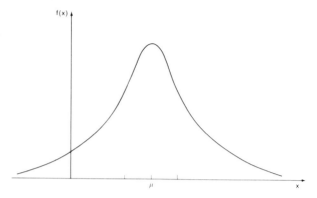

Fig. 5 Normal density curve.

Normal distributions are used extensively in statistics and so we have to gain some working knowledge of them. In particular we will need to be able to find areas under the curve between specified points. Clearly, there are many different Normal distributions, one for each pair (μ,σ^2). In fact, only one of them need be studied since, as will be explained below, they are all closely related.

We choose $N(0,1)$, known as the *standard* Normal distribution, for the discussion of areas. There are many different sets of tables which give such information in various forms, e.g. the *Cambridge Elementary Statistical Tables*.[1] We introduce the conventional notation $\Phi(x)$ for the area beneath the $N(0,1)$ density curve to the left of the point x; thus as x moves from $-\infty$ to 0 and then to $+\infty$, $\Phi(x)$ increases from 0 to $\frac{1}{2}$ and then to 1. Figure 6 illustrates the quantity $\Phi(x)$

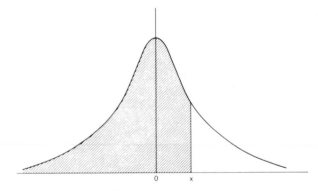

Fig. 6 The shaded area is $\Phi(x)$.

and some selected values are given in Table 3. For instance, we can find that the area

1. to the left of $x = 1\cdot50$ is $0\cdot933$,
2. between points $x = 1\cdot00$ and $x = 3\cdot10$ is $0\cdot999 - 0\cdot841 = 0\cdot158$,

TABLE 3
SELECTED VALUES OF $\Phi(x)$

x	$\Phi(x)$	x	$\Phi(x)$
0·00	0·500	1·96	0·975
0·50	0·692	2·00	0·977
0·67	0·750	2·50	0·994
1·00	0·841	2·58	0·995
1·50	0·933	3·10	0·999
1·64	0·950	3·29	0·9995

3. to the right of $x = 2\cdot50$ is $1 - 0\cdot994 = 0\cdot006$ (since the total area is 1),
4. to the left of $x = -2\cdot5$ is $0\cdot006$ (using the symmetry of $N(0,1)$ about 0),
5. between $x = -1\cdot0$ and $x = 0\cdot5$ is $(0\cdot841 - 0\cdot5) + (0\cdot692 - 0\cdot5) = 0\cdot533$.

A sketch along the lines of Fig. 6 will help in such computations.

There are many properties possessed by Normal distributions among which the following are especially useful for our purposes.

1. If x is $N(\mu,\sigma^2)$, then for any constants b and c, $x + b$ is $N(\mu + b, \sigma^2)$ and cx is $N(c\mu,c^2\sigma^2)$.
2. If x is $N(\mu_x,\sigma_x^2)$ and y is $N(\mu_y,\sigma_y^2)$ then $x + y$ is $N(\mu_x + \mu_y, \sigma_x^2 + \sigma_y^2)$, provided x and y are statistically *independent*.

In (1) the assertion is that if the variable x, which originally has population distribution $N(\mu,\sigma^2)$, is 'corrected' by a constant amount b, then the distribution of 'corrected' values is $N(\mu + b, \sigma^2)$. That the new mean is $\mu + b$ is not surprising, nor is the fact that the variance σ^2 is unchanged, since we have merely shifted the x-values along the scale by an amount b (this holds for any initial distribution, not just Normal); it might even be assumed that the new distribution is a Normal one without question, since the curve has been moved along without change of shape, and this assumption is justified. Similar considerations apply for a 'correction factor' c in (1); attention is drawn to the new variance, c^2 times the old one since variance has the units of x-squared. A special case of (1) is when we take $b = -\mu$, so that $x - \mu$ is $N(0,\sigma^2)$. If we now take $c = 1/\sigma$, we obtain $(x - \mu)/\sigma$ is $N(0,1)$. This process, of first subtracting the mean μ, and then dividing by the standard deviation σ, is called *standardizing*; the result is a standard Normal variable. In this way any Normal distribution can be reduced to $N(0,1)$. As an example of standardizing, suppose that y is $N(2\cdot7, 4\cdot0)$ and we wish to find the probability that a randomly chosen y-observation lies below $3\cdot42$; we shall write this probability as $P[y \leqslant 3\cdot42]$. Using (1), $z = (y - 2\cdot7)/2$ is $N(0,1)$ and the required probability is equal to

$$P[z \leqslant (3\cdot42 - 2\cdot7)/2];$$

this is in turn equal to $\Phi((3\cdot42 - 2\cdot7)/2) = \Phi(0\cdot36)$ which lies between $0\cdot500$ and $0\cdot692$ (see Table 3—it is in fact $0\cdot641$). Similarly $P[y \leqslant 0\cdot0] = \Phi(-1\cdot35)$ which lies between $0\cdot067$ and $0\cdot159$ ($0\cdot088$ in fact), and

$$\begin{aligned}
&P[1\cdot7 \leqslant y \leqslant 4\cdot7] \\
&= P[-0\cdot5 \leqslant z \leqslant 1\cdot0] \\
&= \Phi(1\cdot0) - \Phi(-0\cdot5) \\
&= 0\cdot841 - (1 - 0\cdot692) = 0\cdot533.
\end{aligned}$$

In (2) we start with two different Normal variables x and y and (as can be proved) find that their sum is again Normal with the indicated mean and variance. The meaning of statistical independence in this context is probably most easily illustrated by an example. Considering married couples, suppose x is the husband's height and y that of his wife. Over the set of husbands x will have a distribution of values, and the likely size of an x chosen at random can be inferred from the corresponding density curve. However, suppose that of the pair (x,y), y is already known. Does this lead to a modified estimate of x? If not, that is if the wife's height gives no information about the likely value of her husband's height (or, more precisely, if the x-distributions for different y-values are the same), they are independent.

We can make the following deductions from (1) and (2); in (2), $(x - y)$ is $N(\mu_x - \mu_y, \sigma_x^2 + \sigma_y^2)$ (the variances are *added*); if $\bar{x}$ is the sample mean of n independent observations $(x_1, \ldots, x_n)$ all from $N(\mu,\sigma^2)$, then $\bar{x}$ is $N(\mu,\sigma^2/n)$. The second of these is used many times in what follows. There are powerful results in the theory of probability to the effect that, under certain conditions, the assumptions (i) that $x_1, \ldots, x_n$, have the same distribution, (ii) that this distribution is Normal, and (iii) that they are independent, may be weakened, and yet the result that $\bar{x}$ is Normal still holds, but in a limiting form, i.e., the distribution of $\bar{x}$ becomes arbitrarily close to Normal as n increases. Thus the statistical methods presented below, which apparently depend on assuming independence and Normality for the observations, are more widely applicable.

Confidence Interval for the Mean

We return now to the problem left hanging before our digression on the Normal distribution. That is, given a sample of observations and hence $\bar{x}$ as an estimate of μ, how can we quantify the quality of this estimate? Recall that the sem, $s/n^{1/2}$, gave a guide to the width of the $\bar{x}$-distribution over repeated samples. What we do now is to pursue the same route a little further to give a more definite result.

As n increases (i.e., as the sample becomes larger), the $\bar{x}$-distribution tends towards the Normal. If the raw data x-distribution is Normal to start with, then the $\bar{x}$-distribution is precisely Normal for any n. The more the x-distribution differs in shape from the Normal, the larger we should expect n will have to be before the $\bar{x}$-distribution becomes near-Normal, speaking loosely. (On a technicality, there are x-distributions so badly behaved that $\bar{x}$ never approaches

Normality for any n, but these are of little practical importance in the present context.) Let us suppose then that the $\bar{x}$-distribution *is* Normal, or, at least, close enough to Normal for the following argument to give useful results in practice.

Since $\bar{x}$ is $N(\mu,\sigma^2/n)$, the standardized version $z = (\bar{x} - \mu)/(\sigma/n^{1/2})$ is $N(0,1)$.

Thus $P[-1{\cdot}96 \leqslant z \leqslant 1{\cdot}96] = 0{\cdot}95$ (referring to Table 3) which, by elementary algebra, is equivalent to $P[\bar{x} - 1{\cdot}96\ \sigma/n^{1/2} \leqslant \mu \leqslant \bar{x} + 1{\cdot}96\sigma/n^{1/2}] = 0{\cdot}95$. In words, there is 95% probability (or confidence) that the computed range, $\bar{x} - 1{\cdot}96\sigma/n^{1/2}$ to $\bar{x} + 1{\cdot}96\sigma/n^{1/2}$, will cover μ; the range $\bar{x} \pm 1{\cdot}96\sigma/n^{1/2}$ is called a 95% *confidence interval* for μ. If the $1{\cdot}96$ is replaced by $2{\cdot}58$, a 99% confidence interval results—the greater the confidence, the wider the interval.

A complication is that the value of σ, the population standard deviation, is probably unknown, so the interval cannot be found explicitly. However, we might attempt to retrieve the situation by inserting s, the sample standard deviation, in place of σ as an estimate of it. This approximation has the effect that instead of using $N(0,1)$ for the distribution of $(x - \mu)/(s/n^{1/2})$, we use a slightly different distribution known as Student's t. A further point is that, whereas in the former case the single distribution $N(0,1)$ served for any sample size n, now we have to take account of n in deciding which version of the t-distribution to use. The different versions are conveniently indexed by a quantity called the *degrees of freedom* denoted by ν, so it is just a question of deciding which value of ν to take—in the present case ν is equal to $(n-1)$. Some values of t are given in Table 4. The formula then becomes $\bar{x} \pm ts/n^{1/2}$ and, recalling $s/n^{1/2}$ as the standard error of the mean, is sometimes approximated by the rule '$\bar{x}$ plus or minus two standard errors' since the 95% t-values are near 2.

TABLE 4
SELECTED VALUES FOR STUDENT'S t

	95%	99%
$\nu =$ 3	3·18	5·84
6	2·45	3·71
10	2·23	3·17
20	2·09	2·85
40	2·02	2·70

Example. For simplicity let us take the first seven observations in Table 1; these data on potassium levels are (3·5. 4·6, 4·4, 3·6, 4·2, 5·6, 2·8). We find $\bar{x} = 28{\cdot}7/7 = 4{\cdot}1$ and $s^2 = 4{\cdot}90/6 = 0{\cdot}8167$. The quantity ν is 6 here so, for a 95% confidence interval, the tabulated t-value is 2·45 (*see* Table 4). Thus the interval is $4{\cdot}1 \pm 2{\cdot}45\ (0{\cdot}8167/7)^{1/2}$, i.e., $4{\cdot}1 \pm 0{\cdot}8$. This means that our estimate of μ, the mean potassium level in the population from which the sample is drawn, is 4·1 and, further, there is 95% confidence

that the interval, $4{\cdot}1 \pm 0{\cdot}8$ on this occasion, includes μ.

Having examined the computations involved in a confidence interval let us now examine the logical basis. The interval $4{\cdot}1 \pm 0{\cdot}8$ in the example results from a particular sample of seven observations. The fundamental argument is that over repeated similar samples of size seven, the same calculation will yield intervals (one per sample) of which 95% will span μ. As a long-run frequency statement this is perfectly correct. As an *informative* statement about μ it is, at best, evasive. Even if the repeated sampling framework were real, and not just hypothetical as it often is, we do not know whether the particular interval $4{\cdot}1 \pm 0{\cdot}8$ covers μ or not. All we know is that it is either one of those 95% that do cover μ, or one of those 5% which do not. It is very tempting to infer that it covers μ with *probability* 95%, which is the way in which most users tend to interpret it and which would be a useful informative statement. But, unfortunately, that is not what we have got. Probability statements in the sense used here cannot be made about μ, 4·1 or 0·8 since these are not random quantities varying over repeated trials. In the confidence interval argument the probability statement applies to $\bar{x}$ and s, the only random quantities. There is not space here to discuss the various attempts to resolve these logical difficulties. One justification for retaining the traditional statistical approach is that it is familiar and usually gives the 'right' answers, but perhaps for the 'wrong' reasons. Another, rather pragmatic, consideration is that most of the scientific literature which one has to read uses traditional statistics and this is only very gradually changing.

Estimation of Normal Ranges

When a test is made on a patient a judgement has then to be made whether the result is 'normal' or not. (Note the distinction between 'normal' and 'Normal' in this section; 'normal' refers to a result expected in a healthy subject; 'Normal' refers to a distribution of results.) For continuous measurements, to specify what is normal and what is abnormal, a range is usually taken which contains the values for most healthy individuals in the relevant population. There are inherent difficulties in establishing this range: (1) a clinically healthy individual may happen to have an 'abnormal' value for the test, or *vice-versa*; (2) borderline cases need further investigation; (3) the test might lack discriminatory power because the variation in levels between individuals swamps the comparatively small average difference between normals and abnormals; (4) there may be large within-individual variation due to diurnal cycles, time of last meal, etc.; (5) the normal range may have been determined for an inappropriate population (e.g. a range for human subjects in general may not be the most appropriate one for male children).

We consider here only the statistical question of how normal ranges may be determined. We will suppose that for this purpose there is available a large number n of measurements $(x_1, \ldots, x_n)$ on 'normal' individuals, and that this sample is truly representative of the target population of normal values, i.e., our sample is not contaminated by values from unhealthy individuals, and represents a 'fair selection' of the possible measurements. Let us suppose that the normal range is to be defined by an upper limit such that 2·5% of values lie above it, and a lower limit such that 2·5% lie below it; we thus include 95% of normal values. In other circumstances different definitions may be more suitable, such as having a single upper limit. The percentage included is also subject to such considerations as the risk of misclassification. With 95% limits, we will wrongly classify, on average, 5% of normal individuals as being abnormal; this error is usually, but not always, less serious than the complementary one of missing genuinely abnormal cases because the limits are too wide.

The problem then is to estimate from the sample the values $q_{2.5}$ and $q_{97.5}$ below which lies 2·5% and 97·5% respectively of the population. Probably the most straightforward way is to use for estimates the 2·5% and 97·5% sample quantiles; for instance, for the data on potassium levels we see from a construction similar to that for the sample median that these points are at 2·96 and 5·42. However, it is more customary to base the procedure on the assumption that the population of measurements is Normal, say $N(\mu, \sigma^2)$. Then the 2·5% and 97·5% points are respectively $\mu - 1.96\sigma$ and $\mu + 1.96\sigma$ (see Table 3), the obvious estimates being $\bar{x} - 1.96s$ and $\bar{x} + 1.96s$. Since $\bar{x}$ and s^2 are unlikely to be exactly equal to μ and σ^2, the estimated range will not contain exactly 95% of the population. In practice it may be important not to leave this imprecision to chance, but to try to ensure (with a high degree of confidence) that the estimated range has at least 95% content. The problem comes under the heading 'tolerance intervals' and, in brief, its solution is to increase the above factor 1·96; to include at least 95% of the population with a confidence of 90% the factor to be used is 2·28 when $n = 50$ and 2·17 when $n = 100$. Such factors have been tabulated. Unlike the methods based on $\bar{x}$, to be described below, this determination of normal ranges relies quite heavily on the assumed Normality of the distribution, a question discussed in the next subsection.

In practice normal ranges are usually found by referring to published work, though often the statistical technique of deriving them described above has not been applied and the sets of data on which they are based are quite small.

Assessing Normality

Many techniques have been developed for judging whether a given sample may reasonably be assumed to have been drawn from a Normal population. Two are described here:

1. *Normal plotting*. A useful graphical method is based on the simple question 'If the population is Normal what spacings would be expected between observations in a sample of size n?'. If we can calculate these then their degree of correspondence with the observed values will give an assessment of Normality. It turns out that, on average, the observations will be so positioned that the $(n + 1)$ intervals between adjacent pairs (the first interval stretching from $-\infty$ to the smallest, the next interval from the smallest to the second smallest, ..., the last interval from the largest to $+\infty$) contain equal amounts of probability, $(n + 1)^{-1}$. For instance, if $n = 3$ we can deduce from Table 3 that the 'expected observations' (e's say) for $N(0,1)$ are roughly $(-0.67, 0.0, 0.67)$—four intervals each containing probability 0·25. In general, supposing that the x's in the sample have been put in increasing order, the standardized values $(x - \mu)/\sigma$ should be roughly equal to these e's. Thus a plot of the ordered x's against the e's should be roughly a straight line, with slope and intercept near σ and μ respectively. The laborious aspect of converting the probability intervals $(n + 1)^{-1}$ into e's, with $N(0,1)$ tables, is circumvented by the use of Normal *probability plotting paper* which does the job automatically on one scale. On such graph paper, where the conversion is on the horizontal scale, one merely plots the points $(k/(n + 1), x_{(k)})$, where $x_{(k)}$ denotes the k-th smallest observation. If the points appear to lie near a straight line the Normality hypothesis is accepted: concavity upwards (downwards) indicates positive (negative) skewness. In Fig. 7 the potassium data exhibit slight positive skewness.

2. *Goodness-of-fit test*. If the underlying distribution is Normal the histogram should exhibit a similar shape to that shown in Fig. 5. In other words, for some values of μ and σ^2, there is a Normal curve which will fit the outline of the histogram fairly closely. A formal test for Normality based on this idea is the chi-square goodness-of-fit test (*see below*).

There remains the question of what to do when it is judged that the population is not Normal. One answer is that for methods based on $\bar{x}$ it does not matter very much provided the sample size n is reasonably large, say 50 or more; if n is not large it is difficult to assess non-Normality from the sample anyway. However, there are circumstances, such as those encountered in making inferences about σ^2 (using s^2) and deriving normal ranges, in which Normality is important. In such cases, one may either seek methods which do not rely on assumptions about the form of the population density curve (so-called

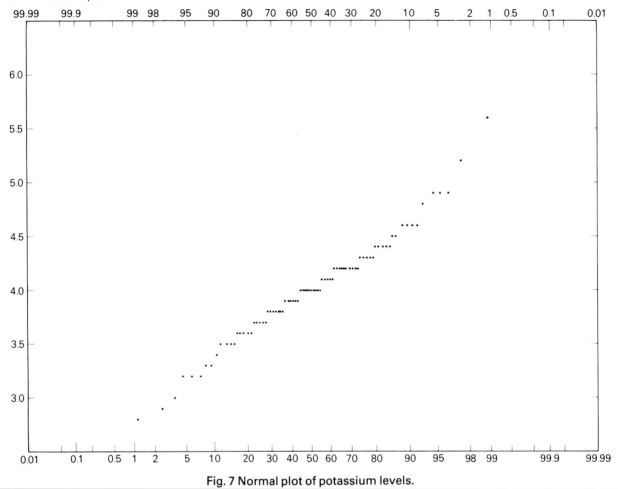

Fig. 7 Normal plot of potassium levels.

distribution-free methods), or just seek a transformation of the data until the Normality assumption is acceptable. For instance, if the distribution exhibits positive skewness, as many do in practice, replacing each observation by its square root (assuming all the values are positive) may remove this feature since the larger values in the right-hand tails of the distribution are pulled in towards zero by a larger distance; a similar, greater effect is achieved by taking logarithms. If the values are not all positive the preliminary addition of a suitable constant will make them so. The variety of possible transformations is vast and for most common types of data it should not be too hard to find one with the desired effect. Some further discussion of these points is given by Sokal and Rohlf.[2]

METHODS FOR MEANS AND VARIANCES

Test for a Specified Mean

As before, suppose we have a sample of x's, but we wish to use it not to estimate μ from first principles but to assess the plausibility of some conjectured value of μ. For instance, a certain theory might predict that μ should be equal to μ_0 and the observations are made to judge whether they lend support to the theory or not. It is the convention to say that we have a *null hypothesis*, H_0, that μ has the value μ_0; this is usually written $H_0: \mu = \mu_0$. Various kinds of *alternative hypothesis* H_1 may be appropriate depending on the situation. Very often H_1 is vague, merely stating that μ has some unspecified value other than μ_0, in this case we write $H_1: \mu \neq \mu_0$. We shall consider only this type of alternative but remark that methods for certain other types are similar to that given here.

Let us then derive a rule for deciding between $H_0: \mu = \mu_0$ and $H_1: \mu \neq \mu_0$ on the basis of a sample $(x_1, \ldots, x_n)$ from $N(\mu, \sigma^2)$. If H_0 is true, $\bar{x}$ can be standardized using

$$\mu_0: z = (\bar{x} - \mu_0)/(\sigma/n^{1/2}).$$

Thus, under H_0, the probability that z will be between -1.96 and $+1.96$ is 0.95, and so if this is in fact observed we can say that the data do not strongly contradict H_0. On the other hand, if the computed z is greater than 1.96 in absolute size then, if H_0 is to be believed, an event with the rather low probability of 0.05 (1 in 20) has occurred; alternatively, this occurrence throws suspicion on H_0.

More precisely, suppose that the total probability in the tails of the Normal distribution, outside the range between $-z$ and $+z$, is p; for instance, if $z = 1.50$ (or -1.50), $p = 2(1 - 0.933) = 0.134$ from Table 3. Then p is the probability, under H_0, of obtaining a value as extreme as or more extreme than z. The smaller p, the less likely is z under H_0, roughly speaking. Formal statements such as 'H_0 is rejected at the 5% level of significance' were used to convey that $p < 0.05$, but nowadays more attention is focused on the actual p-value obtained as a measure of conflict between data and hypothesis. A common label for p is 'the observed significance level'. However, use of the word significance can be misleading for what is statistically significant (p very small) may be of no practically important significance at all, and *vice-versa*. For this reason perhaps routine use of the jargon 'p-value' is excusable since it eliminates the ambiguity.

When σ is unknown, as is usual, it is replaced by the sample value s and the t-distribution with $\nu = n - 1$ degrees of freedom is used. We have then the so-called *t-test* based on the quantity $t_{n-1} = (\bar{x} - \mu_0)/(s/n^{1/2})$, which is just the ratio of $(\bar{x} - \mu_0)$ to its standard error.

Example. Taking the seven potassium levels again, suppose $H_0: \mu = 4.2$. We calculate $t_6 = (\bar{x} - \mu_0)/(s/n^{1/2}) = (4.1 - 4.2)/(0.816/7)^{1/2} = -0.29$ and see, from Table 4, that $p > 0.05$ (since -0.29 is within the tabulated value 2.45): a p-value such as this, greater than 5%, is not generally regarded as implying strong conflict between the data and H_0.

Test Between Two Means

Consider now the situation where two independent samples are available, summarized as $(n_1, \bar{x}_1, s_1^2)$ and $(n_2, \bar{x}_2, s_2^2)$, and we wish to compare the underlying means μ_1 and μ_2. Let us assume that, after transformation if necessary, the first sample consists of observations from a population $N(\mu_1, \sigma_1^2)$ and the second is from $N(\mu_2, \sigma_2^2)$. Also, we will only examine the procedure appropriate for the very commonly occurring null hypothesis $H_0: \mu_1 = \mu_2$, other hypotheses involving μ_1 and μ_2 being dealt with on broadly similar lines. The alternative is taken as $H_1: \mu_1 \neq \mu_2$, again, a special but illustrative case. It is natural to base a test of H_0 on the sample difference of means, $\bar{x}_1 - \bar{x}_2$, small (or large) values indicating support for (or against) H_0. What is needed is a scale for assessment of $\bar{x}_1 - \bar{x}_2$, and this is provided as before by its standard error. Without going into too much detail, it turns out that the extension of the formula $s/n^{1/2}$, the standard error of $\bar{x}$ in a single sample, to the case of $\bar{x}_1 - \bar{x}_2$ is $(s_1^2/n_1 + s_2^2/n_2)^{1/2}$. Further, to avoid difficulties not germane to our purpose, we will assume that $\sigma_1^2 = \sigma_2^2$; this means that the two populations to be compared, presumably of similar types of measurement, may differ in their mean levels (μ_1 and μ_2) but have the same spread of values as measured by the variances σ_1^2 and σ_2^2. This assump-

tion can be tested (*see below*). In this case, s_1^2 and s_2^2, which estimate σ_1^2 and σ_2^2 respectively, can be pooled to provide a single estimate of the common value: the formula for this pooled s^2 has been given above (p. 40). Thus the standard error of $\bar{x}_1 - \bar{x}_2$ becomes $(s^2/n_1 + s^2/n_2)^{1/2}$ or, equivalently, $s(n_1^{-1} + n_2^{-1})^{1/2}$ and our standardized test statistic is $t_\nu = (\bar{x}_1 - \bar{x}_2)/s(n_1^{-1} + n_2^{-1})^{1/2}$. The degrees of freedom for this *two-sample t-test* are $\nu = (n_1 - 1) + (n_2 - 1)$, an obvious extension of the single sample $n - 1$ rule.

Example. The data are muscle tissue mercury levels in monkeys to whom a drug has been administered.

low dose: 165, 123, 138, 126, 218.
medium dose: 205, 163, 90, 88, 158, 129, 147.

The summary figures are

$(n_1, \bar{x}_1, s_1^2) = (5, 152.0, 1554.5)$ and
$(n_2, \bar{x}_2, s_2^2) = (7, 140.0, 1742.0)$,
and the pooled variance $s^2 = 1667.0$. Thus,
$t_{10} = 12.0/\{1667.0(5^{-1} + 7^{-1})\}^{1/2} = 12.0/23.91 = 0.50 \, (p > 0.05)$

the p-value exceeds 5% (since 0.50 is within ± 2.23, from Table 4) and so the data do not conflict strongly with H_0. Had t been large (and, correspondingly, p small) we should probably have wished to give an estimate of the size of the difference between μ_1 and μ_2, instead of leaving it at the rather bald statement that there does seem to be one. This estimate here is $\bar{x}_1 - \bar{x}_2 = 12.0$, with standard error 23.91. The corresponding 95% confidence interval for $\mu_1 - \mu_2$ is $12.0 \pm (2.23 \times 23.91) = 12.0 \pm 53.3$, computed in the same way as that for a single mean value on p. 39.

Finally, we return to the assumption $\sigma_1^2 = \sigma_2^2$ made for the t-test here. This can be tested from the data as follows. If it is true, then $F = s_1^2/s_2^2$ should not differ too greatly from unity, since $\sigma_1^2/\sigma_2^2 = 1$. Thus we need a scale for assessing the departure of the observed value F from 1. As in the case of testing means, the distribution of F over repeated samples yields a p-value for F to measure conflict between the data and the assumption $\sigma_1^2 = \sigma_2^2$. Such values are tabulated[1] and for details of the procedure the reader is referred to Snedecor and Cochran.[3] For illustration, when $n_1 = n_2 = 10$, the range of F corresponding to $p > 0.05$ is $(0.336, 2.98)$, i.e., F-values within this range are close enough to 1 for us to conclude that there is not strong evidence in the sample against the hypothesis $\sigma_1^2 = \sigma_2^2$.

Matched Pairs

Sometimes the observations in the two samples are matched in pairs consisting of one from each sample. For instance, suppose it is suggested that a certain clinical treatment can affect a particular enzyme level, thus effecting a desired improvement in a body function. The plasma enzyme activities before treatment (x_1) and those after treatment (x_2) are recorded on n patients, resulting in n pairs of measurements. To treat these observations as before, that is, as a sample of x_1's and an independent sample of x_2's whose means are to be compared, is inappropriate. There will be substantial variation amongst the x_1's and amongst the x_2's, so the sample variances s_1^2 and s_2^2, and hence the pooled variance s^2, will not be small, thus in computing the two-sample t-test, the denominator will not be small, assuming the sample size n is not enormous. The numerator is $(\bar{x}_1 - \bar{x}_2)$ (presumably H_0 will specify a zero treatment effect, i.e., that $\mu_1 = \mu_2$). If there is a consistent but small difference between levels before and after treatment, then $(\bar{x}_1 - \bar{x}_2)$ will be small and so the computed t-value will be small, resulting in a non-significant test result. (Statistically, the assumption of independence is violated; a consistent difference would imply that the distribution of x_1 or of x_2 varies according to the value of the other.) The correct procedure is suggested by examination of the initial conjecture—it is the individual differences $d = x_1 - x_2$ which are important. A one-sample t-test is applied to the d's, assuming that they constitute a random sample from $N(\mu_d, \sigma_d^2)$.

Example. For arithmetic convenience we illustrate the test using just five sets of enzyme levels.

Patient	1	2	3	4	5
x_1	10	16	5	12	4
x_2	12	20	6	14	5
d	2	4	1	2	1

We have $n = 4$, $\bar{d} = 10/5 = 2.0$, $s_d^2 = 6/4 = 1.5$, so that

$$t_3 = (\bar{d} - 0)/(s_d/n^{1/2}) = 3.65$$

From Table 4, $0.05 > p > 0.01$ indicating a moderate conflict between data and null hypothesis.

In this particular example, on closer inspection of the data, it seems that the percentage difference between x_1 and x_2 rather than the absolute difference, is fairly consistent. These percentages are $D_1 = (2/10) \times 100 = 20$, $D_2 = (4/16) \times 100 = 25$, $D_3 = 20$, $D_4 = 16.67$, and $D_5 = 25$. If we make the distributional assumption, alternative to that above, that the D's are independent $N(\mu_D, \sigma_D^2)$, we may base our test on percentage differences: $t = (\bar{D} - 0)/(s_D/n^{1/2}) = 13.2$, which is clearly significant. A 95% confidence interval for μ_D is $21.3 \pm 3.18(0.1298/5)^{1/2}$, i.e., 21.3 ± 5.1.

We stress again the difference between the test statistics for the paired and unpaired cases. The numerators are the same, that is $\bar{d} = \bar{x}_1 - \bar{x}_2$, but the denominator $s_d/n^{1/2}$ in the paired case may well be much smaller than the unpaired one, thus resulting in greater sensitivity in detecting a real difference.

Discussion

At this point we pause to examine more critically the test procedures described above.

1. There seems to be confusion in some quarters over the use of the t-distribution as opposed to the Normal distribution in assessing these test statistics. For example, in testing for a specified mean some students have the impression that for $n \leq 30$ one refers the test statistic $(\bar{x} - \mu_0)/(s/n^{1/2})$ to Table 4 whereas for $n > 30$ one refers to Table 3, i.e., the test statistic is regarded as undergoing a magic transformation from a t-distribution to a Normal one at $n = 30$. Although the numerical values in the two tables are similar for $n > 30$, the recommendation of a sudden change of rule for $n > 30$ is puzzling, has no obvious logical foundation, and is unnecessary.

2. Consider the example on the two-sample t-test (*see* p. 47). Is the null hypothesis $H_0: \mu_1 = \mu_2$ tenable? In other words, is it possible that different levels of the drug should have precisely the same effect? Note the word 'precisely', not 'almost equal' or 'differing little', but 'precisely', for this is what the t-test tests. If the answer is no then, surely, the test is pointless. Such 'sharp' hypotheses are often used, not because there is any prior belief in their possible truth, but as an approximation to a more sensible hypothesis like $|\mu_1 - \mu_2| \leq 0.1$. Unfortunately, though, the t-test is only appropriate for the sharp version $|\mu_1 - \mu_2| = 0$. In fact, it can be proved that, as one might suspect, if μ_1 and μ_2 are not equal, however close, then p can be made as small as required by taking n large enough. In other words, any such sharp hypothesis, if not precisely true, will always conflict with a sufficiently large data set (under some mild technical provisos). The practical resolution of this is not to perform a significance test but to estimate $\mu_1 - \mu_2$. Then, besides avoiding the logical objection, one conveys more information, i.e., how large is $\mu_1 - \mu_2$, by quoting $\bar{x}_1 - \bar{x}_2$, and how precisely it is estimated (by quoting the associated standard error).

3. Our third point is just to emphasize again, as was done on p. 43 in connection with confidence intervals, the repeated-sampling foundation of these tests. An attempt has been made to avoid the more extreme concomitants of the traditional approach by emphasizing the p-value as a measure in its own right, rather than as determining a decision on whether H_0 is true or false.

CHI-SQUARE TESTS

This section is concerned with discrete data in the form of counts, or frequencies. The reader is reminded of the distinction between discrete and continuous data as mentioned in p. 38.

The statistical methods to be described are approximate. In the previous section if the x's were precisely Normally distributed then the derived t-values have exactly the t-distribution (over repeated samples). However, it is understood that even if the x-distribution is not Normal the answers obtained should not be too seriously affected provided n is not too small. It is in this sense that the following methods are approximate.

Goodness-of-fit

The procedure is best explained by examples.

Example 1. It is predicted that the four main varieties of a particular disorder should be equally common in a particular human subpopulation. Of 1200 cases diagnosed, the numbers of cases of the different types are 334, 316, 257 and 293. (We must be satisfied first that the sample is representative of the target population, e.g. that the four types have equal likelihoods of being recorded.) To test the prediction, regarded as a null hypothesis H_0, we compare the *observed* frequencies (334, 316, 257, 293) with those which would be *expected* (300, 300, 300, 300). The differences between observed and expected frequencies $(o - e)$, are (34, 16, −43, −7). We wish to obtain a single overall measure of discrepancy between the o's and e's. A straight addition of the differences is useless since their sum is zero; by construction the e's sum to 1200, the same as the o's, therefore the $(o - e)$'s sum to zero. The sum of square differences, $34^2 + 16^2 + (-43)^2 + (-7)^2 = 3310$ avoids the problem of cancellation of positive and negative contributions, by making them all positive. However, this is still not quite right. A difference of 34, for instance, should carry more weight if it were associated with an expected frequency e of 30 than when $e = 3000$, say. This could be taken into account by using a weighted sum of squared $(o - e)$'s, such that $(o - e)^2$ would be divided by 30 or 3000 as appropriate. In the present example this differential weighting does not occur since the e's are all equal, but nevertheless the overall discrepancy measure is generally calculated as $X^2 = \Sigma (o - e)^2/e$, with divisors e for the individual contributions. Thus $X^2 = (34^2/300) + (16^2/300) + (43^2/300) + (7^2/300) = 110\cdot33$. Next, we need to know whether this is an unusually large value or not in the general run of things, i.e., we need a p-value to tell us how often an X^2 of this size or more would occur in repeated samples with H_0 true. This is obtained by referring to the chi-square distribution (hence the name of the test) in Table 5. Accepting, for a moment, that the second row ($\nu = 3$) of the table is appropriate, we see that $p < 0\cdot01$ because $110\cdot33 > 11\cdot34$, i.e., our observed X^2 value lands beyond the 1% column of the table. (The table tells us that X^2 value $11\cdot34$ or greater will occur with probability $0\cdot01$ over repeated samples under H_0.)

Notes

1. The rule for degrees of freedom ν (i.e., which

TABLE 5
SELECTED χ^2 VALUES

	0·95	0·10	0·05	0·01
$\nu = 1$	0·004	2·71	3·84	6·63
3	0·35	6·25	7·81	11·34
6	1·64	10·64	12·59	16·81
10	3·94	15·99	18·31	23·21
20	10·85	28·41	31·41	37·57
40	26·51	51·81	55·76	63·69

row of Table 5 to enter) is $\nu = k - 1 - $ (no. of parameters estimated) where k is the number of categories ($k = 4$ in Example 1) and the adjustment for parameters estimated will be explained below (it does not occur in Examples 1 and 2).

2. As the e's increase (strictly, towards ∞) the distribution of X^2 (over repeated samples under H_0) tends to the so-called chi-square (χ^2) distribution. For finite e-values the distribution of X^2 is only approximately χ^2, and if any e is below about 2 or 3 the approximation may be too inaccurate. In such cases it is usual to pool the offending categories (*see* Example 3).

3. For this test it is large values of X^2 which correspond to small p, i.e., conflict with H_0. The usual caveat applies: if H_0 is not *precisely* true then the larger the sample, the smaller p.

4. If an unusually small value of X^2 is observed (i.e., very near zero) one cannot regard it as conflicting with H_0, but other things should be checked such as the arithmetic and the fidelity of the observations.

5. Suppose that data gathered from different areas of the country are to be used to test the same basic hypothesis. However, for one reason or another (e.g. the use of differently defined categories in different areas), the sets of data cannot be directly pooled. In such a case, a χ^2 test may be performed on each separate set, and then the X^2 values added to produce an overall X^2, also adding the individual degrees of freedom. For example, if the separate data sets produce $X_3^2 = 7\cdot11$, $X_5^2 = 11\cdot04$ and $X_2^2 = 7\cdot49$, then, overall, $X_{10}^2 = 25\cdot64$ and $p < 0\cdot01$ from Table 5. (The degrees of freedom here appear as subscripts to X^2, as is usual.)

Example 2. Patients with cirrhosis of the liver are asked to complete a questionnaire on their admission to hospital concerning their eating habits. The object is to assess possible nutritional deficiencies. The collection of such data might also be compared with the established general population pattern. Suppose that the national figure for a certain deficiency is 10%, and 15 out of 100 cirrhosis patients exhibit it. The categories are 'deficient' and 'not deficient', with $k = 2$, the observed frequencies are (15, 85), and the expected frequencies are (10, 90). Thus

$X_1^2 = \Sigma(o-e)^2/e = (15-10)^2/10 + (85-90)^2/90 = 2.78$ and $0.10 > p > 0.05$ from Table 5 since $2.71 < 2.78 < 3.84$: the conflict between the data and H_0 (that the cirrhosis patients follow the national pattern) is not strong. We can give the estimate 0.15 (or 15%) for the proportion q of cirrhosis patients exhibiting the deficiency. A corresponding 95% confidence interval consists of those values q for which the corresponding X^2 does not exceed 3.84, i.e., for which

$$(15 - 100q)^2/100q + (85 - 100\bar{q})^2/100\bar{q} \leqslant 3.84,$$

where $\bar{q} = 1 - q$: after some algebraic manipulation, the interval is 0.15 ± 0.07.

Example 3. Let us see whether the distribution of potassium levels in p. 36 can be considered Normal. Since the Normal distribution has two parameters, μ and σ^2, and the null hypothesis of Normality does not specify values for them, they must be estimated. For this purpose $\bar{x} = 4.01$ and $s^2 = 0.26$ are used. In the frequency distribution there are $k = 10$ classes, the observed frequencies (o's) being (3, 5, 10, 18, 25, 12, 5, 3, 1, 1). The e's are obtained as follows, using Normal tables[1] more extensive than Table 3: the proportion of $N(4.01, 0.26)$ below the point 3.05 (i.e., in the first class) is

$$\Phi((3.05 - 4.01)/0.26^{1/2}) = \Phi(-1.88) = 0.0301,$$

so the expected frequency is $83 \times 0.0301 = 2.50$; the proportion of $N(4.01, 0.26)$ between 3.05 and 3.35 (i.e., in the second class) is

$$\Phi((3.35 - 4.01)/0.26^{1/2}) - 0.0301$$
$$= \Phi(-1.29) - 0.301$$
$$= 0.0985 - 0.0301$$
$$= 0.0684,$$

so the expected frequency is $83 \times 0.0684 = 5.68$. In this way the e's are found as (2.50, 5.68, 11.65, 17.70, 18.97, 14.49, 7.89, 3.07, 0.85, 0.20). Since the last three e's are rather small (see Note (2) above) they are pooled so that k becomes 8 and the last $o - e$ is $5 - 4.12$. Now

$$\chi_5^2 = \Sigma(o-e)^2/e = (3 - 2.50)^2/2.50 + \ldots = 4.01.$$

(The degrees of freedom are $\nu = 8 - 1 - 2 = 5$ since two parameters were estimated.) From Table 5, interpolating between $\nu = 3$ and 6, we see that $p > 0.10$ indicating no strong conflict between the data and the Normality hypothesis.

Contingency Tables

The preceding analysis can be applied to two-way (and higher-way) classifications in which an object is categorized according to both attributes A and B. When a sample of n objects is examined a frequency is obtained for each combination of A and B and it is usual to present the data as a two-way con-tingency table. The statistical analysis is most easily shown by examples.

Example 1. Consider an immunological investigation in which 120 rats are examined to determine the status of a particular substance A in the blood—each rat is classified as A_1 or A_2. After exposure to a bacterial infection the rat may be affected (B_1) or not (B_2). The interest lies in any possible association between A and B, in particular, whether an A_1-rat is more, or less likely to succumb than an A_2-rat. The observed frequencies are given in the 2×2 table (Table 6A); we see that of the 70 A_1-rats, 15 were affected whereas of the 30 A_2-rats, 20 were affected.

TABLE 6A
OBSERVED FREQUENCIES

	B_1	B_2	Total
A_1	15	55	70
A_2	20	10	30
Total	35	65	100

The null hypothesis H_0 to be tested is one of no association between A and B. If H_0 is true, the proportion of A_1-rats affected, $15/70$, should be about the same as that for A_2-rats, $20/30$; hence both proportions should be roughly equal to the overall proportion affected, $35/100$. In other words, under H_0, the expected frequency in the A_1B_1-cell of Table 6B

TABLE 6B
EXPECTED FREQUENCIES

	B_1	B_2	Total
A_1	24.5	45.5	70
A_2	10.5	19.5	30
Total	35	65	100

is $35/100$ths of 70, i.e., $35 \times 70/100 = 24.5$, and that in A_2B_1 is $35 \times 30/100 = 10.5$; similarly the e's for cells A_1B_2, A_2B_2 are respectively $65 \times 70/100 = 45.5$ and $65 \times 30/100 = 19.5$. Thus we have o's in the right hand table, and e's in the left, and can therefore compute

$$X^2 = \Sigma(o-e)^2/e$$
$$= (15 - 24.5)^2/24.5 + (55 - 45.5)^2/45.5$$
$$\quad + (20 - 10.5)^2/10.5 + (10 - 19.5)^2/19.5$$
$$= 18.9$$

We refer X^2 to the χ_1^2 distribution: from Table 5, $p < 0.01$ since $18.9 > 6.63$, and so the data indicate an association between A and B—in fact it appears that A_1-rats have a smaller chance of being affected than A_2-rats. The reason that the number of degrees of freedom is 1 for a 2×2 table is as follows. Using the rule $\nu = k - 1 -$ (number of estimated parameters) we have $k = 4$ and two estimated parameters. These are the proportions of A_1-rats (estimated as $70/100$) and of B_1-rats ($35/100$); these figures (or their equivalents) were used in the computation of expected frequencies under H_0.

Example 2. We look at a larger two-way contingency table now with $r = 3$ rows and $s = 4$ columns (Table 7A); the observed frequencies are shown unbracketed. Let us test the null hypothesis H_0 of no association between A and B. Looking first at

TABLE 7A

	B_1	B_2	B_3	B_4	Total
A_1	22	43	15	36	116
	(21·7)	(40·3)	(16·0)	(38·1)	
A_2	41	87	32	66	226
	(42·3)	(78·3)	(31·2)	(74·1)	
A_3	59	96	43	112	310
	(58·0)	(107·4)	(42·8)	(101·8)	
Total	122	226	90	214	652

the marginal totals in the right-hand column we see that the overall distribution of relative frequencies between the A-classes is ($116/652$, $226/652$, $310/652$). Under H_0, this 3-way division should be roughly the same in each B-class, that is, in each column. In the first column then, the expected frequencies under H_0 (shown bracketed in the table) are obtained by sharing out the total 122 among the three rows in the proportions $116/652:226/652:310/652$. Thus the e for the A_1B_1-cell of the table is $116 \times 122/652 = 21·7$, and that for A_2B_1 is $226 \times 122/652 = 42·3$. The general rule for computing e's is, symbolically,

$$e(A_iB_j) = (i\text{-th row sum}) \times (j\text{-th column sum})/n,$$

n being the total number of objects classified (652 here). For A_3B_1 we may either compute $310 \times 122/652 = 58·0$, or notice that the three expected frequencies must sum to 122, and therefore that the last member of the column is easily obtained by subtraction, $122 - (21·7 + 42·3) = 58·0$. Amplifying this last remark, once the e's for the first three columns have been found, those for the B_4 column may be obtained also by subtraction (e.g. $116 - (21·7 + 40·3 + 16·0) = 38·1$). Thus in general only $(r-1)(s-1)$ e's have to be computed laboriously; alternatively it may be preferable to compute all rs e's using the formula, reserving the agreement of marginal totals of o's and e's for a check on the arithmetic.

We can now calculate X^2

$$\begin{aligned}
&= \Sigma(o - e)^2/e \\
&= (22 - 21·7)^2/21·7 + \dots \text{(12 summands)} \\
&= 4·53.
\end{aligned}$$

To find $\nu = k - 1 - $ (number of parameters estimated) we note that $k = rs = 3 \times 4 = 12$, and that

we need the marginal distributions in the table to compute the e's; the latter information is supplied by any $2(= r - 1)$ row totals and any $3 (= s - 1)$ column totals, since $n = 652$ is given, and thus the number of parameters estimated (i.e. $(r-1) + (s-1)$) is $2 + 3 = 5$. Thus $\nu = 12 - 1 - 5 = 6$; in general

$$\nu = rs - 1 - (r-1) - (s-1) = (r-1)(s-1).$$

From Table 5 $p > 0·10$, since $4·53 < 10·64$, and we conclude that the data show no strong evidence of A–B association.

TABLE 7B

	B_1	B_2	B_3	B_4
A_1	0·004	0·182	0·062	0·116
A_2	0·040	0·967	0·021	0·885
A_3	0·017	1·210	0·001	1·022

If the result had been significant we would normally wish to be more specific about the form of the association indicated by the data. There are various methods for this, among which is an examination of the individual contributions to X^2. These are shown in Table 7B with the largest underlined. It appears that, as far as H_0 is concerned, these four cells are most aberrant, and an inspection of the original table of observed and expected frequencies indicates the directions of the departures.

A general point is that the marginal totals (apart from n) are supposed to be random, not fixed. In the first example the total number of A_1-rats (70) was not known in advance; all four totals (70, 30, 35, 65) were observed, not fixed, although of course $n = 100$ was predetermined. It is under these circumstances that the large-sample approximation used above, of the X^2 distribution as χ_ν^2 with $\nu = (r-1)(s-1)$, is appropriate. However, often one set of marginal totals is fixed; we might have deliberately chosen 70 A_1-rats and 30 A_2-rats for the experiment. It is perhaps slightly unfortunate that exactly the same approximation as before turns out to be appropriate, thus obscuring the logical differences.

LEAST SQUARES, REGRESSION AND CORRELATION

Fitting Relationships Between Variables

The data consist of n pairs of measurements, $\{(x_1,y_1), \dots, (x_n,y_n)\}$, and we consider the question of dependence between x and y, and what form the dependence takes. To illustrate the type of situation under consideration suppose we have recorded, for 12 male patients, ages (x years) and weights (y pounds). The data are given in Table 8. A fairly strong degree of statistical dependence would be expected since the distributions of weights within age groups are quite different. Usually the main feature of interest is just the behaviour of the mean value of y as x varies, and not the whole distribution. A *scatter diagram*, or *dot plot*, as in Fig. 8 helps to clarify the discussion. It appears that as x increases the mean of y at first increases quite steeply and then tails off to a constant value around 170, though the variation about the

it and the i-th point (x_i, y_i) is $(y_i - \mu_i)$, μ_i denoting $\mu(x_i)$. We wish to make these distances small and a reasonable method is to minimize the sum of their squares, $Q(\theta) = \Sigma(y_i - \mu_i)^2$, the summation being over all the data points for $i = 1, \ldots, n$; as usual, squaring avoids negative contributions to Q by points

TABLE 8
AGES AND WEIGHTS OF 12 MALE PATIENTS

Age (x)	23·7	8·9	51·6	5·2	12·4	47·3	28·6	18·3	46·3	38·4	32·6	63·5
Weight (y)	156	83	164	49	96	157	180	152	198	175	169	161

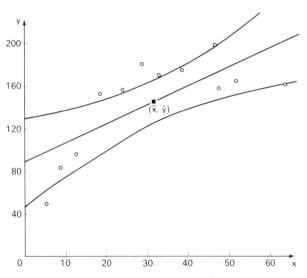

Fig. 8 Scatter plot for the weight/age data.

mean level for any given x is large (strictly speaking, we would need to have several y's recorded at each x to substantiate this last conclusion). Such behaviour is conveniently described in terms of a curve, say $\mu(x)$, whose value for given x is the mean level of y for that x; $\mu(x)$ is called the (mean) *regression curve* (of y on x). Unfortunately, when a set of data is collected one still has the problem of deciding which equation describes $\mu(x)$, and this is often difficult. There is little formal guidance available mainly because the variety of possible mathematical forms is so vast. The usual methods are to choose a *model* derived from the underlying physical or biological theory, or more commonly to use a simple type of curve which will satisfactorily describe the data but which makes no claim to being true in any sense. In the latter category the most popular curves are straight lines, quadratics and sometimes higher order polynomials, and also other curves such as hyperbolae and exponentials.

Let us suppose that a suitable form for $\mu(x)$ has been chosen, say a quadratic $\mu(x) = \theta x^2$. The constant θ will be adjusted so that the curve lies close to the points on the scatter plot. There are many criteria which could be used for closeness, probably the most common being that of *least-squares*. If the curve $\mu(x)$ is plotted with the data the vertical distance between

below the curve. We write $Q(\theta)$ to indicate that it is a function of the *parameter* θ, and the least-squares value of θ is that which minimizes Q. In our quadratic example the minimization is easily accomplished by the usual calculus technique of equating derivatives to zero; we have $Q'(\theta) = -2\Sigma(y_i - \theta x_i^2)x_i^2$, giving the least-squares estimate of θ as $\Sigma y_i x_i^2 / \Sigma x_i^4$.

The idea can be extended to the case where y is related to several other variables $x, z, \ldots$ and the curve μ contains several parameters $\theta_1, \theta_2 \ldots$; we simply minimize $Q(\theta_1, \theta_2, \ldots) = \Sigma(y_i - \mu_i)^2$, where $\mu_i = \mu(x_i, z_i, \ldots)$, with respect to all the θ's. Of course, some curves are more easily fitted than others and unless μ has the so-called linear form (that is, a plot of μ against any one θ, for any given constant values of the others, is a straight line), the minimization process can be difficult. For all but the simplest problems it is necessary to use a computer.

An important point to make about regression curves is that even when a very clearly defined relationship exists between x and y *causation* cannot be inferred purely from the data; only *association* can be established. For instance, any two variables which tend to increase with time, like the standard rate of income tax and the number of patients undergoing psychiatric treatment, will show an association which may or may not be spurious.

Straight-line Regression and Correlation

The most commonly used form for $\mu(x)$ is a straight line: $\mu(x) = \alpha + \beta x$, where the two parameters are α (the *intercept*) and β (the *slope*). Given a sample of n points $\{(x_1, y_1), \ldots, (x_n, y_n)\}$ the least-squares estimates of α and β, which we will denote by a and b, are found by minimizing the sum of squares

$$Q(\alpha, \beta) = \Sigma\{y_i - \mu(x_i)\}^2 = \Sigma\{y_i - \alpha - \beta x_i\}^2$$

with respect to α and β. This problem has an easy solution (equating derivatives to zero),

$$b = T_{xy}/T_{xx}, \quad a = y - b\bar{x},$$

where $\bar{x} = \Sigma x/n$, $\bar{y} = \Sigma y/n$, $T_{xx} = \Sigma(x_i - \bar{x})^2$, $T_{xy} = \Sigma(x_i - \bar{x})(y_i - \bar{y})$. The new quantity T_{xx} is recognizable as the sum of squared deviations of the x's about their mean $\bar{x}$; the corresponding T_{yy} for the y's will be used below. Also T_{xy} is similar in form to T_{xx} and

T_{yy} but has x and y appearing on an equal footing. From the equation $a = \bar{y} - b\bar{x}$, it is seen that the fitted line passes through the mean point $(\bar{x}, \bar{y})$.

For illustration only the computations will be performed for the weight/age data, though clearly a straight line is not appropriate in this case. We set out the working in Table 9; there are quicker methods but in the space available we concentrate on concepts rather than on computations. From the x-total $\bar{x} = 376\cdot8/12 = 31\cdot4$, and from the y-total $\bar{y} = 1740/12 = 145$. An arithmetic check is to sum the columns $(x - \bar{x})$ and $(y - \bar{y})$ (taking account of signs)—their totals should be zero. The last three columns have entries typified by $(-7\cdot7)^2 = 59\cdot29$,

when a curve appears to fit well it should be borne in mind that, without invoking considerations beyond the data, there is no evidence that it will continue to fit well outside the range of the present observations.

We may sometimes wish to 'correct' a y-value for the corresponding x. For instance, if the weights of two groups of boys are to be compared, we can try to neutralize the effect of one group's being, on the whole, slightly older by standardizing all weights to age 10; this is done by moving the points on the scatter plot parallel to the regression line until they are vertically above 10 on the x-scale. The formula is y(corrected) $= \mu(10) + [y - \mu(x)]$, $\mu(10)$ being the point

TABLE 9

COMPUTATIONS FOR FITTING A STRAIGHT-LINE REGRESSION

	x	y	$x - \bar{x}$	$y - \bar{y}$	$(x - \bar{x})^2$	$(y - \bar{y})^2$	$(x - \bar{x})(y - \bar{y})$
	23·7	156	−7·7	11	59·29	121	−84·7
	8·9	83	−22·5	−62	506·25	3844	1395·0
	51·6	164	20·2	19	408·04	361	383·8
	5·2	49	−26·2	−96	686·44	9216	2515·2
	12·4	96	−19·0	−49	361·00	2401	931·0
	47·3	157	15·9	12	252·81	144	190·8
	28·6	180	−2·8	35	7·84	1225	−98·0
	18·3	152	−13·1	7	171·61	49	−91·7
	46·3	198	14·9	53	222·01	2809	789·7
	38·4	175	7·0	30	49·00	900	210·0
	32·6	169	1·2	24	1·44	576	28·8
	63·5	161	32·1	16	1030·41	256	513·6
Totals	376·8	1740	0·0	0	3756·14	21 902	6683·5

$11^2 = 121$, and $(-7\cdot7) \times 11 = -84\cdot7$. Thus $T_{xx} = 3756\cdot14$, $T_{yy} = 21\,902$, $T_{xy} = 6683\cdot5$; finally $b = 6683\cdot5/3756\cdot14 = 1\cdot78$ and $a = 145 - (1\cdot78 \times 31\cdot4) = 89\cdot11$. The fitted line, $y = 89\cdot1 + 1\cdot78x$, is drawn in Fig. 8.

The alternative regression of x on y will not be immediately obtainable from the one we have found; in general it will be a different line because the distances whose sum of squares is minimized in order to calculate the parameters, say a' and b', are measured horizontally in Fig. 8 instead of vertically. Actually one finds that $b' = T_{xy}/T_{yy}$ and $a' = \bar{x} - b'\bar{y}$, the result of merely interchanging x and y in the above account.

Having fitted the line there are various uses to which it may be put: for a purely descriptive purpose, to summarize the trend of the data; for prediction, for instance, if the line fitted better we might predict that the average weight for 40-year-old male patients is 164 pounds and judge them as over- or underweight on this basis; for deriving 'corrected' values; for comparison with other data where the line may be different. In the case of prediction the danger of extrapolation should be stressed; from Fig. 8 it could be inferred by extending the line to the right that at age 90 the mean weight is 249·3 pounds. Even

on the line corresponding to $x = 10$ (i.e., 106·9 lb) and (x, y) the point to be moved.

To assess how well the curve fits the data, probably the best all-round method is just to look at Fig. 8. However, when there is more than one x-variable this is not possible. There are various techniques based on examining the *residuals*—these are the discrepancies $(y_i - \mu_i)$ between the observed y_i's and the fitted values $\mu(x_i)$. They may be plotted against x and y and various other factors which have not been included explicitly in the model but which might possibly be related to y; for instance, as x increases from 0 the residuals in Fig. 8 are at first consistently negative (points below the fitted line), then all positive, and then negative again, such consistency indicating a distinct lack of fit of the straight line. A single measure of the combined size of the residuals is the *residual sum of squares*. This is the minimized value of Q, i.e., $Q(a,b)$ (with a and b inserted for α and β). For straight-line regression this can be shown to be equal to $T_{yy} - bT_{xy}$. We defined the *residual mean square* $s^2 = $ (residual sum of squares)/$(n - 2)$ as an average measure of variation of the data points about the fitted line—the choice of divisor $(n - 2)$ comes about because two parameters, α and β, have been estimated (s^2 is said to have $(n - 2)$ degrees of freedom). For the weight/age data the residual sum of squares is 21 902 − (1·78 × 6683·5) = 10 010·17, so $s^2 = 10010\cdot17/10 = 1001\cdot017$; the residual standard deviation is the square root $s = 31\cdot639$.

When straight-line models are under consideration the sample *correlation coefficient r* is often quoted. This is calculated as $r = T_{xy}/(T_{xx}T_{yy})^{1/2}$; it is symmetric in x and y. It can be shown that r always lies between −1 and +1, a value near zero implying that a (non-horizontal) straight line does not fit the data

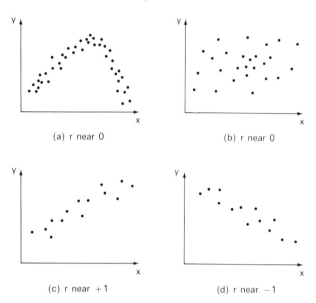

(a) r near 0   (b) r near 0

(c) r near +1   (d) r near −1

Fig. 9 Interpretation of sample correlation coefficient.

well. Figure 9 illustrates the correlation in some assorted situations. The sample correlation r is usually regarded as being useful for differentiating between situations like (b) versus (c) or (d), but it is important to remember that since r is linked to straight-line models, it fares badly as a general measure of the strength of relationship between x and y in cases such as (a) where the dependence is strong but the correlation weak (since the best-fitting line there would be nearly horizontal); a complementary case to (a) is the weight/age data where $r = 6683\cdot5/(3756\cdot14 \times 21902)^{1/2} = 0\cdot74$ is quite large, but the relationship is clearly not of straight-line form. It is best always to plot a scatter diagram from which the usefulness of the quoted r-value can be assessed. In cases such as (b), where it is not clear to the eye whether or not the general spread of the points is enough to obscure any underlying straight line, the null hypothesis that the (population) correlation is zero can be tested by computing $t = \{(n-2)r^2/(1-r^2)\}^{1/2}$ and referring to the t-tables with $\nu = n - 2$ degrees of freedom. For the weight/age data $t = 3\cdot48$ which exceeds the value 3·17 in Table 4 and so $p < 0\cdot01$; however, this procedure assumes an underlying straight line and Normal distributions and merely tests within this framework whether or not that

line is horizontal—the scatter plot in this instance (and knowledge of the biological situation) shows the test to be inappropriate at the outset.

More About Regression Lines

So far the treatment has been fairly informal. To derive more information and to extend the usefulness of a fitted curve we have to be more specific about the underlying assumptions. The details are given for the straight line but analogous techniques hold for any fitted model.

We note briefly that x and y are both regarded as random variables in this section, that is, no values are fixed beforehand. An individual is examined and, whatever the resulting (x,y) pair, it is accepted as the observation for that individual. An alternative common set-up is when the x's are not random: a specific x-value is chosen and then the corresponding random y is observed—for instance, in calibration solutions of given concentration (x) are subjected to analysis, and the instrument provides a reading (y). The methods described here are all regularly applied to such data, although, strictly speaking the interpretations are different—for instance the terms regression and correlation really only apply when both variables x and y are random.

It is assumed that the 'true' form is $y = \alpha + \beta x + \varepsilon$, where α and β are unknown parameters, and ε is a random departure or error term. When a pair (x,y) is observed x and y will not generally satisfy $y = \alpha + \beta x$ precisely, otherwise all points on the scatter diagram would lie exactly on a line. For a single x-value there will be a distribution of y-values centred at $\alpha + \beta x$, i.e., ε has a probability distribution with mean 0. Also, it is usual to assume that the variance σ^2 of the ε-distribution is the same at all x-values— this property is called *homoscedasticity*, the converse being *heteroscedasticity*. These assumptions about the mean and variance of ε are sufficient to provide much of the justification of the least-squares method, but we will need more. We further assume that the ε-distributions, for each fixed x, are Normal. In summary, the underlying model for our data is that $y_i = \alpha + \beta x_i + \varepsilon_i$, where the ε's are independent $N(0,\sigma^2)$ variables.

With the above framework it can be shown mathematically that b is $N(\beta,\sigma^2/T_{xx})$, a is $N(\alpha,\sigma^2\Sigma x_i^2/nT_{xx})$ and $(n-2)s^2/\sigma^2$ is χ^2_{n-2}. Briefly, this means that in repetitions of the data-gathering, each with the same x-values, the various values of b (similarly a and s^2) emanate from the stated distribution; strictly speaking, the statistical inference is made conditional on the observed values of $\bar{x}$ and T_{xx}. This theory justifies the following procedures.

We use s^2 as an estimate of σ^2, the residual variance. Thus standard errors (s.e.) for the estimated regression parameters are

$$\text{s.e.}(b) = s/T_{xx}^{1/2}, \text{ s.e.}(a) = s\{\Sigma x_i^2/nT_{xx}\}^{1/2}$$

Using these we can construct a confidence interval for the slope β as $b \pm t \times$ s.e.(b), where t is the appropriate tabulated t-value with $\nu = n - 2$ degrees of freedom; for the weight/age data, s.e.$(b) = 31\cdot639/(3756\cdot14)^{1/2} = 0\cdot52$, and the 95% t-value for 10 degrees of freedom is $2\cdot23$ from Table 4, so a 95% confidence interval for β is

$$1\cdot78 \pm (2\cdot23 \times 0\cdot52), \text{ i.e., } 1\cdot78 \pm 1\cdot16.$$

Similarly, using the algebraic identity $\Sigma x_i^2 = T_{xx} + (\Sigma x_i)^2/n$, we have

$$\Sigma x_i^2 = 3756\cdot14 + 376\cdot8^2/12 = 15\,587\cdot66,$$

so s.e.$(a) = 31\cdot639 \times \{15\,587\cdot66/(12 \times 3756\cdot14)\}^{1/2} = 18\cdot61,$

and a 95% confidence interval for α is

$$89\cdot13 \pm (2\cdot23 \times 18\cdot61), \text{ i.e., } 89\cdot13 \pm 41\cdot50.$$

Significance tests may also be made, for instance under $H_0: \beta = \beta_0$, $t = (b - \beta_0)/$s.e.(b) has the t-distribution with $n - 2$ degrees of freedom.

A confidence interval for the whole regression line can also be derived as follows. We first require the standard error of $(a + bx)$ for any given value of x; this can be derived as

$$\text{s.e.}(a + bx) = s(n^{-1} + (x - \bar{x})^2/T_{xx})^{1/2}$$

Then, at the given value x, a 95% confidence interval for the 'true' value $(\alpha + \beta x)$ on the line is $(a + bx) \pm t$-$\times$ s.e.$(a + bx)$. Using the weight/age data again, at $x = 50$ years,

$$\text{s.e.}(a + bx) =$$
$$31\cdot639 \times \{0\cdot0833 + (50 - 31\cdot4)^2/3756\cdot14\}^{1/2} = 13\cdot25$$

so the 95% interval for $(\alpha + 50\beta)$ is $\{89\cdot13 + (50 \times 1\cdot78)\} \pm (2\cdot23 \times 13\cdot25)$, i.e., $178\cdot13 \pm 29\cdot55$. Such an interval may be calculated for all values of x within the range of interest, thus constructing two curves, one above and one the same distance below the regression line, as in Fig. 8.

ACKNOWLEDGEMENT

It is a pleasure to thank Peter Wood for his help with the data used as illustrative examples.

REFERENCES

1. Lindley D. V., Miller J. C. P. (1970). *Cambridge Elementary Statistical Tables*. Cambridge University Press.
2. Sokal R. R., Rohlf F. J. (1973). *Introduction to Biostatistics*. San Francisco: W. H. Freeman and Co.
3. Snedecor G. W., Cochran W. G. (1967). *Statistical Methods*, 6th edn. Iowa: State University Press.

FURTHER READING

Armitage P. (1971). *Statistical Methods in Medical Research*. Oxford: Blackwell Scientific Publications.

6. Quality Assurance
P. M. G. Broughton

INTRODUCTION

Quality assurance is essentially concerned with the reliability of information about patients. Although the laboratory is responsible for the reliability of the analytical data it produces, many different factors and a variety of staff are involved between the initial request and the final laboratory report. The *patient* must be correctly identified and, for some investigations, specially prepared. The *specimen* must be properly collected into a suitable container, adequately labelled, transported to the laboratory and stored so that it will not deteriorate. The *analysis* must be reliable and the results correctly calculated and expressed without ambiguity. The *report* must reach the ward or clinician for whom it is intended, together with all the information needed to interpret it. Although some of these factors are outside the direct control of the laboratory, the clinical biochemist must consider them all because often nobody else will do so. His responsibility is not limited to providing correct results on the specimens he receives, but he must be involved in all stages from sampling to reporting and interpretation. The term '*quality assurance*' (which has now replaced 'quality control') emphasizes the need for a comprehensive view of the whole process of investigation.

Quality assurance is concerned with the study of errors and the procedures used to recognize and minimize them. This involves three stages: measurement of aspects of quality, such as accuracy or precision; comparison of the results of these measurements with some standard of desirable performance; and control of this quality at the desired level during each analysis. It is a complex process which uses two main techniques. *Internal quality control* is the set of procedures used by laboratory staff for continuously monitoring the quality of analytical results in order to decide whether these are sufficiently reliable to be reported to the requesting clinician. *External quality assessment* is a system for retrospectively and objectively comparing the results from different laboratories by an external agency. Both require special types of specimen, techniques and statistical methods, and demand understanding of analytical chemistry as well as initiative in applying this to the correction and prevention of errors. Quality assurance also requires knowledge of biological variation in health and disease so that analytical variation can be seen in its correct perspective. Despite the pressures of increasing workloads, demand for faster analyses and the limitations of finance, space, staff and equipment, quality assurance should always be seen as an obligation to the patient.

WHAT IS QUALITY?

The primary aim of the laboratory is to produce correct results, not by chance, but at all times, and it uses quality assurance procedures to achieve and demonstrate this. Most of the methods used for internal quality control and external quality assessment have a statistical basis and monitor only two aspects of quality, namely accuracy and precision. Whether the laboratory achieves quality, and manages to control it, depends on a number of factors, the most important being the selection of the analytical method used. This choice is often difficult to make from a survey of the literature because of inadequate information, doubts about its relevance and lack of understanding of the factors which should be considered. No system of quality assurance is likely to improve a method which is fundamentally unsound and before attempting to control quality it is necessary to decide which performance characteristics are relevant.

An analytical method defines the procedure, materials and equipment necessary to obtain a result. The method is judged by the results obtained with it and all its components and characteristics contribute to the quality of the result. The same performance characteristics apply to simple kit methods and to complex automated systems, and these can be grouped into two types—those concerned with practicability and those which relate to reliability.[1]

Practicability

The criteria by which a method is judged to be practicable are speed, cost, safety, the analytical skill required and the risk of failure of the method. Thus a method may be accurate and precise but unsuitable for routine use because it is too slow, requires expensive equipment, employs hazardous reagents or is satisfactory only when used by highly skilled analysts. These factors are usually judged subjectively and, although there have been few attempts to apply control methods to them, they should not be ignored. Even with an apparently simple method, the accuracy and precision of results may depend on the skill and experience of the operator. A record of machine downtime will measure its dependability. Some laboratories have instituted methods of monitoring the speed at which routine results are reported. Measurements such as these will often indicate where control or improvement is required.

Reliability

This comprises four interrelated factors:

1. *Precision* is defined as the agreement between replicate measurements. It is a measure of variability, dispersion or scatter between results due to random error, that is, error occurring by chance. Variability is inevitable in any measurement, but all random errors should not be regarded as unavoidable: sometimes their cause can be identified and the error reduced or eliminated. It is usually assumed that random errors have a Gaussian distribution (Fig. 1) and variability can then be expressed in terms of the standard deviation (SD) or coefficient of variation (CV). Both these factors increase numerically as precision deteriorates, and consequently terms such as high or low precision should be avoided because the SD and CV are measures of imprecision. Some authors distinguish two types of precision: repeatability, referring to the precision obtained by one operator over a short period of time, and reproducibility for analyses over a longer time interval with different analysts, instruments and reagents. Similarly the optimal conditions variance refers to the imprecision obtained when one analyst measures a series of replicates under optimal conditions (i.e., in sequence), whereas routine conditions

variance refers to the imprecision obtained when the analyses are made routinely and replicates interspersed with other specimens in different batches.[2,3]

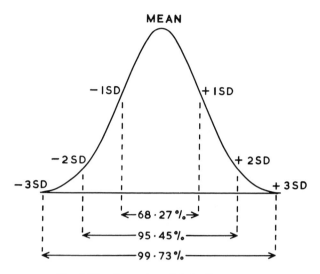

Fig. 1 The Gaussian distribution curve.

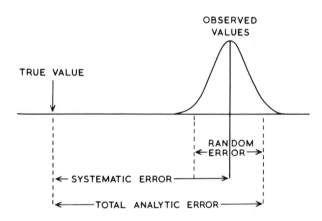

Fig. 2 Relation between random, systematic and total analytic errors.

2. *Accuracy* is defined as the agreement between the best estimate of a quantity and its true value. As with precision, adjectives such as high or low should be avoided, since it is inaccuracy or bias which is usually measured. Inaccuracy is due to systematic error and, to avoid the contribution of random errors, it can only be assessed from a mean value and not by a single measurement. The relationship between random, systematic and total analytical error is shown in Fig. 2 and it can be seen that accuracy becomes more difficult to assess when precision is poor. For some tests, it is impossible to specify the true value, and in these circumstances the laboratory can only monitor changes in accuracy with time or compare the relative accuracy of two alternatives, either or both of which may be inaccurate.

3. *Specificity* is defined as the ability of a method to determine solely the component it purports to measure. It has no numerical value, but is assessed from evidence about the components which contribute to the result and on the extent to which they do so. Specificity has a marked effect on accuracy and if it varies (for example with different specimens) it will also contribute to imprecision.

4. The *detection limit* is the smallest single result which, with 95% probability, can be distinguished from a suitable blank. At this point the analysis becomes just feasible, but it is imprecise and may be inaccurate. High blank values increase the detection limit and variation between blanks affects precision. The term 'sensitivity' is sometimes used for this concept, but it may also be used to denote the slope of the calibration curve and, in a different context, as a measure of the ability of a test correctly to detect disease.[4] Consequently this term should not be used as a reliability characteristic of an analytical method.

In selecting an analytical method, all these practicability and reliability criteria need to be considered. Thus a method may have good precision, but be nonspecific, or it may be accurate, precise and specific but be unable to detect small quantities of the analyte. Speed of analysis may influence precision and analytical skill may affect accuracy. The selection of a method is usually a compromise made after assessment of all these factors and their relative importance to the laboratory.

CONTROL MATERIALS

Control specimens are analysed solely to obtain information about quality. They have three main applications:

1. in internal quality control, to measure and control precision by comparing the analytical results found over a period of time; it is not necessary to know the true value for the specimen;

2. in internal quality control, to measure and control accuracy by comparing the value found with the true value or with some stated value, such as that given by the manufacturer. The same material can also be used as a calibration standard, but it cannot at the same time function both as a control and as a standard. This means that the accuracy of a method cannot be tested with a control specimen which, directly or indirectly, was used for calibration.

3. in external quality assessment the same specimen is analysed in a number of laboratories and the results compared.

Control specimens are essential for the reliable performance of any laboratory test and a wide variety of commercial preparations are available, including both liquid and lyophilized serum and urine. Manufacturers specify the concentrations of various constituents, which may be normal or abnormal, and most types can also be purchased without stated values. The main advantages of commercial products are that they can be obtained with stated values and they are stable, so that a large batch can be used over a long period. However, it is important to understand the inherent limitations of these materials which are imposed by their nature and method of preparation.[5]

Preparation of Control Specimens

Most commercial products are derived from horse, bovine or human serum. To obtain elevated concentrations, chemicals or extracts of animal tissues are added during manufacture. Some preparations are dialysed or deionized to remove glycolytic agents or compounds of low molecular weight; the residue is then analysed and chemicals weighed in to give the desired concentrations. Liquid control materials usually contain a preservative to ensure stability, but most are stabilized by lyophilization: exact amounts of liquid serum are dispensed into vials, and lyophilized before sealing the container under vacuum. Individual specimens are reconstituted by adding a known amount of water.

Preparations of control serum can also be made in the clinical laboratory, but these tend to be less stable. Glucose and urea decompose rapidly if there is any bacterial contamination.

Control materials derived from human sources may contain Australian antigen or other dangerous pathogens. Consequently all specimens, including those specifically used for quality control and assessment should be treated by laboratory staff as if they were capable of transmitting infection.

Urine specimens for use as control materials can usually be preserved with acid or a bacteriocidal agent such as thiomersal; tests should be made to ensure that these additions do not interfere with the analysis.

Most lyophilized control products are stable when dry and stored in the cold; preparations containing bilirubin should be protected from light. Except for enzymes, the stability of reconstituted serum is similar to that of human serum: glucose and bilirubin decompose unless the specimen is frozen or preserved, but other constituents are usually stable for about a week if the specimen is stored in the refrigerator. Best results are obtained with freshly reconstituted serum and specimens should never be frozen and thawed more than once.

Source of Control Specimens

When using control specimens, it is assumed that any errors in the analysis will affect control and patients' specimens equally. Consequently these specimens should resemble each other as closely as possible, but in practice they may show differences which affect their behaviour. Unlike most patients' specimens, control samples are usually not turbid and contain neither fibrinogen nor haemoglobin. Products which have been subjected to intensive pre-treatment may be clear non-viscous solutions with different physical characteristics from those of serum. The preservatives, antibiotics, coagulants and anticoagulants used in manufacture can interfere with some analytical methods, but are rarely named. Components of animal origin may differ significantly from those in human serum; for example, some methods for the measurement of serum iron-binding capacity give incorrect results with lyophilized animal serum. Immunological methods, designed for use with human material, cannot be used with products of animal origin.

The matrix in which the analyte is dissolved in the control specimen can affect some types of analytical method. For example, liquid control serum preserved with ethylene glycol should not be used with direct ion-selective electrodes (ISEs) which use undiluted specimens. Lyophilization may produce changes in the matrix, so that the reconstituted material behaves differently from fresh human serum when used with direct ISEs or with some dry reagent film techniques, the latter possibly due to surface tension changes.

Extracts of animal tissues are often used to obtain elevated levels of enzymes. The isoenzymes in these usually have different kinetic properties from those in human serum and the conditions of assay may not be optimal for them. One product may contain several isoenzymes, as well as variable inhibitors, interfering enzymes, cofactors, chromogens and artefacts, so that different results are obtained by different methods. Commutability is a term which refers to the ability of an enzyme material to show inter-assay activity changes comparable to those of the same enzyme in human serum.[6] The ratio of activities of the enzyme in the control material to that in human serum should be constant for different analytical methods. Since different factors may be involved for each enzyme, each may require a different control material. For accuracy control the product is only applicable to the method stated by the manufacturer, and it is only suitable as a precision control if that method is optimal for the isoenzymes in the product. Changing the control specimen can lead to an apparent alteration in precision because the conditions of assay have not been adjusted to the different isoenzymes. For some isoenzyme analyses it appears that only human serum can be properly used as a control specimen.

Lyophilization can introduce artefacts which affect enzymes. The alkaline phosphatase activity of freshly reconstituted serum increases to a variable extent if the serum is allowed to stand at room temperature for 24 h before assay; reproducible results are, however, obtained if the serum is mixed for 30 min after reconstitution, and then stored for not more than 4 h at 4 °C before assay. Creatine kinase in some control preparations is light-sensitive and may need the addition of activators to regain its full activity. Enzymes in reconstituted serum are usually less stable than in human serum, but this may depend on the source and method of manufacture of the product.

All these factors may not be specified by the manufacturer, and the user should always make preliminary tests on any control material to make sure that it is applicable to his analytical method.

Inter-vial Variability

The variability between samples of a control material will determine the amount of analytical variation which can be detected. Consequently it is essential that different vials of the same product are identical and, if lyophilized, each vial must contain exactly the same amount of dried material. It has been proposed that the CV between vials, due to lack of homogeneity or of reproducible delivery volume, should not exceed 0·25% and present production technology is capable of achieving this.[5] However, since variability between vials is usually much less than the analytical SD, it cannot be measured by analysis of a number of vials. Reconstitution of the serum will also introduce some variability and precautions should be taken to minimize this.

Accuracy of Stated Values

If manufacturers' values are used for accuracy control or calibration, they must be accurate. Most manufacturers use several reference laboratories or consensus values (*see* later) in deriving their stated values, but rarely quote all the data or explain how the value was obtained in a manner which would increase the user's confidence in the product. Since this value may depend on the analytical method used, most manufacturers quote values obtained by different methods. However, since each method value may have been obtained in only a few laboratories, it is doubtful whether it is typical of that method. A range of values for several methods is of limited use to the analyst who uses none of these methods. The user may thus be tempted to believe that it is the manufacturer who is wrong. Repeated analyses of several different products, will soon make apparent any discrepancies between them (Table 1). If the results for different products agree, the user will gain confidence in them and in his own analytical accuracy.

PRECISION

Two experimental designs can be used to measure imprecision.[4,7,8]

TABLE 1
RESULTS FOR DIFFERENT COMMERCIAL PREPARATIONS OF CONTROL SERUM ANALYSED CONCURRENTLY IN ONE LABORATORY

Component	Mean value found (no. of assays in parenthesis)	Manufacturer's stated value	Difference
Calcium (mmol/l)	2·22 (4)	2·27	−0·05 (−2·2%)
	2·59 (5)	2·63	−0·04 (−1·5%)
	2·97 (5)	3·07	−0·10 (−3·2%)
Iron (μmol/l)	24·3 (23)	25·6	−1·3 (−5·1%)
	26·1 (4)	25·6	+0·5 (+1·9%)
	31·5 (5)	31·3	+0·2 (+0·6%)
	42·1 (5)	56·4	−14·3 (−25·4%)
Potassium (mmol/l)	4·04 (5)	4·0	+0·04 (+1·0%)
	4·17 (28)	4·14	+0·03 (+0·7%)
	4·30 (3)	4·35	−0·05 (−1·1%)
	5·34 (5)	5·3	+0·04 (+0·8%)

The data suggest that the laboratory's calcium results were consistently low (by 1–3%) but those for potassium were satisfactory. The iron results for one sample are discrepant.

1. A series of n replicate measurements are made on the same specimen and their individual values (x) recorded and the mean $(\bar{x})$ calculated. Then

$$SD = \sqrt{\frac{(x - \bar{x})^2}{n - 1}} \quad \text{or} \quad \sqrt{\frac{\Sigma x^2 - [(\Sigma \bar{x})^2 / n]}{n - 1}}$$

2. A series of N different specimens are each analysed in duplicate and the differences (d) between duplicate pairs recorded. Then

$$SD = \sqrt{\frac{\Sigma d^2}{2N}}$$

This method can be modified to use, for example, triplicate analyses which are then treated as two pairs of duplicates.

Usually about 20 replicates are used; the number should be stated as it is needed in calculating the confidence limits of the SD and in testing the significance of the difference between SDs. The mean value should be given so that errors can be expressed in percentage terms using the CV:

$$CV = \frac{SD}{\bar{x}} \times 100\%$$

With a Gaussian distribution, positive and negative deviations from the mean are equally probable and small deviations occur more frequently than large ones (Fig. 1). In practice, the frequency distribution of errors often shows several differences from Gaussian curves, with either skewness (that is, non-symmetrical curves) or kurtosis, where the proportion of results in the middle of the curve is either increased or decreased (see Chapter 5). Some of these effects may be due to observer bias or digit preference in rounding off results, and the SD is then not a true representation of imprecision. Logarithmic transformation has been used to overcome this, but it is doubtful whether the extra time and effort is warranted. Nevertheless it is worth checking that the actual frequency distribution of errors does not differ markedly from that predicted from the SD. For example, from statistical considerations it may be expected that about 0·3% of results will lie outside the limits of the mean ±3 SD. In practice the proportion of these outliers is sometimes higher due, for example, to gross errors in transcription or arithmetic, or to transposition of specimens. Large errors of this type occur infrequently, but should always be recorded. It is best to separate them from random analytical errors by deleting all replicate results which lie outside specified limits (e.g. 3 SD), recording their number and proportion, and then recalculating the SD from the remaining results as a measure of analytical imprecision. A separate record should be kept of the number and proportion of outliers (the 'blunder rate'); some reports suggest that this rate may be as high as 0·5–1%.

In any analytical process, the random errors of each stage or step have a cumulative effect on the total error. This effect can be expressed mathematically by using variances:

$$SD_T^2 = SD_1^2 + SD_2^2 + SD_3^2 \ldots$$

where subscripts 1, 2, 3, etc. refer to components of the total random error (SD_T). Thus the SD over a prolonged period of time will usually be larger because of the variance arising from different analysts, instruments, batches of reagents, etc. Each of these can be studied by an appropriate experimental design but, without full details, statements of SD have little meaning. Thus a within-batch SD refers to replicate measurements within one batch and between-day SD to replicates analysed on different days. Both are important but they must not be confused. Precision depends on the conditions under which the results are obtained and the many factors which can affect it must be considered in some detail when choosing methods for its measurement.

Selection and Arrangement of Specimens

The methods used in clinical biochemistry are applied to specimens from patients, and the specimens used to assess precision should resemble these as closely as possible. Measurements with pure aqueous solutions will often give a smaller SD. The identity of control specimens should not be known to the analyst as this may consciously or unconsciously affect his results. This can be done by giving fictitious patients' names to control specimens. This may be particularly important if imprecision is estimated from differences between duplicates, as the analyst will naturally expect these to agree.

Control specimens should be interspersed with patients' specimens in a random order and not in sequence, so that sample carryover is included.[7] This effect arises when one sample affects the result obtained on another one, usually that immediately following it. If a sample with a true value A is followed by two replicates (B_1 and B_2) of another sample of different concentration, the result B_1 will be affected by carryover from A. This carryover can be expressed mathematically as:

$$K = \frac{B_1 - B_2}{A - B_2}$$

Since the value of K is constant for each analytical system, the error introduced ($B_1 - B_2$) depends on the concentration difference ($A - B_2$), and will be zero if replicates are arranged in sequence.

Effect of Concentration

The SD of most analytical methods varies with concentration, sometimes by more than threefold over the range encountered in routine practice (Fig. 3). The percentage error (CV) is not necessarily independent of concentration. This type of curve has been termed the precision profile and is useful in showing the concentration range over which the method is most precise. Particular attention should be paid to concentrations which are important for medical decisions, such as the upper and lower limits of the reference range.

With colorimetric methods, the effect is probably related to photometric error, and with most conventional instruments the most precise measurements are made at an absorbance of 0·434. Similar effects have been noted with both manual and automated methods. The SD and CV values of Na and K measured by flame photometry or ISEs show less variation with concentration. With most tests the SD is larger and the CV smaller at high concentrations. In general, both the SD and CV should be recorded,

but if one of these is approximately constant, only this value need be stated. Some evidence suggests that precision is more difficult to control and shows greater variability at high concentrations. If the method requires a blank, this should be included with each replicate test, as variations in this have a greater effect on precision at low concentrations.

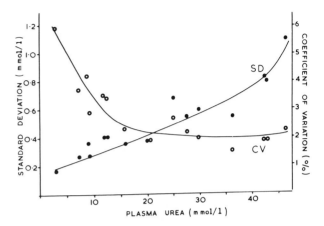

Fig. 3 Effect of concentration on SD (closed circles) and CV (open circles) of plasma urea measurements on the AutoAnalyzer. From data reported by Campbell and Annan. *J. Clin. Pathol.*, **19** (1966) 513.

Precision over Different Analytical Periods

Extending the period of time over which replicate measurements are made tends to increase the SD for two reasons. First, the inclusion of additional sources of variation, such as reagents, standards and analysts, increases the total variance arithmetically and, secondly, it introduces variations due to changes in accuracy.

The second effect is illustrated in Fig. 4, which shows mean and SD values for replicate plasma sodium analyses made during one week. The within-plate SD averaged 0·60 mmol/l but varied inexplicably from 0·3 to 2·1 mmol/l for individual plates. The mean value of the replicates within each plate varied from 134·3 to 137·3 mmol/l in a similar random manner which was unrelated to changes in SD. When discrepant mean values (marked A) or high within-plate SD values (marked B) were found for sodium, there were no parallel changes in the results for urea, potassium, chloride or bicarbonate, which were measured concurrently on the same equipment. When all the results for one day were combined, the within-day SD was usually greater than any of the within-plate SDs for that day. Similarly, the SD calculated from the complete week's results was greater than any of the within-day SDs. For some tests, the week's SD may be three times the average within-plate SD.

The SD does not always increase with the period of time over which replicates are measured, but only when two series of replicates with different mean values are combined. Long-term levels of precision thus depend both on the short-term precision and on changes in accuracy. Within-batch variation is smaller than the variation over a series of batches or days, because accuracy is more constant over a shorter period. However, the within-batch SD is not constant for all batches. Laboratories have good and bad days affecting, often independently, both accuracy and precision. Manual methods are particularly

sequence, the SD reflects the optimal conditions variance. This procedure can only be used when large batches can be processed and the results may not be typical of all batches.

2. Analyse at least 20 specimens in duplicate, placing the duplicate specimens in random order in the same run or batch. The differences between duplicate results are used to calculate the SD and, since this may depend on concentration, separate calculations should be made

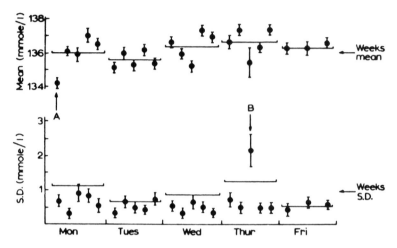

Fig. 4 Mean and SD values for plasma sodium concentration calculated for each AutoAnalyzer plate tested over 5 consecutive days. The vertical lines indicate ±1 standard error of the mean and SD values. Horizontal lines denote the mean and SD of all results obtained within the day. Reproduced from Broughton and Annan *Clin. Chim. Acta*, **32** (1971) 433.

prone to this if the analyst becomes distracted, tired or bored. Within one laboratory, the between-day SD is more stable than the within-batch or within-day SD, as the effect of good and bad batches or days is evened out. Short-term changes in accuracy will be hidden, and show only as a deterioration in precision if SDs are calculated over long periods.

Evaluation of the Precision of Methods

Information about precision is required when selecting a method or instrument for routine use and, since many factors can affect precision, data must be obtained by well-defined and standardized procedures.

Measurement of Within-batch Imprecision. Two experimental designs are possible and either can be used to make a rapid assessment of a method and to compare two methods.

1. Analyse approximately 20 replicate specimens in one batch or run, and calculate the within-batch SD. If necessary the experiment can be repeated with replicate specimens of a different concentration. If replicates are arranged in

for (a) all specimens, (b) those within the lower (defined) part of the range and (c) those within the upper (defined) part. In each case the mean and number of duplicate pairs are recorded. The results reflect the mean within-batch imprecision over the period of the test.

The SD obtained by each of these methods may depend on the nature and concentration of the specimen(s) and the performance of the analysis at the time, and consequently cannot be used as a definitive measure of precision of the method. Nevertheless, they are useful in deciding whether the method is likely to be satisfactory.

Measurement of Between-day SD. The between-day SD, measured over a period of typical performance, is used as a definitive measure of imprecision of the method which can be compared with that of other methods and with required standards of performance.

Select 3–5 specimens which span the analytical range of the method; at least one should have a low value, one a high value and one intermediate. Specimens must be stable over the 20 working days of the test and they will therefore probably be commercial control specimens. If liquid specimens are used, 20 replicate samples from each should be stored deep frozen and one thawed each day for analysis. If lyophilized serum is used, the reconstitution procedure must be standardized and individual vials shown to be identical; alternatively a number of vials can be reconstituted, the contents pooled and aliquots stored as described for liquid specimens. One sample of each serum is analysed in a random position in a run of patients' specimens once per day for 20 consecutive working days. If analyses are not performed every day, the test should be done on 20 consecutive days on which the analysis is made. The results are checked for drift in accuracy by comparing the mean of the first 10 with that for the second 10, and if these differ significantly further analyses must be made. The between-day SD is then calculated from the 20 results.

If the results are to be taken as typical of the method, they must be obtained under normal routine conditions including both good and bad days. Before recommending or condemning a new method, it is worth repeating these tests in another laboratory. Confirmation of the SDs will provide reassurance that the results are typical; any differences should be further investigated.

ACCURACY

Accuracy is probably the most elusive quality to determine in a method, mainly because of the difficulty of defining the true value for a component in a biological specimen. Although some methods are undoubtedly inaccurate, it is often difficult to prove which is correct because results are affected by random and systematic errors arising within each individual laboratory as well as errors inherent in the method. Although circumstances may make it necessary to use methods of unknown or inferior accuracy, the continued use of these should not be tolerated. Before describing techniques for the assessment of the accuracy of analytical methods, some general problems of measurement in clinical biochemistry must be considered.

Calibration Standards

All quantitative measurements require a calibration standard (sometimes called a calibrant), that is, a material or solution containing a known amount of the component to be assayed. For brevity, this component is termed the analyte. The concentration or other quantity of this component in a sample is determined by comparison with the standard. The accuracy of the standard affects the accuracy of the result, so the concentration of the standard must be known with greater certainty than that required for the result.

The standards used in other branches of analytical chemistry can be classified according to their purity, but many of those used in clinical biochemistry are mixtures or impure and cannot be so classified. A simpler approach is to divide standards into two easily recognizable groups. A *primary standard* solution is one in which the concentration is determined solely by dissolving a weighed amount of primary standard material in an appropriate solvent and making up to a stated volume or weight. Its accuracy depends solely on the purity of the standard material and the accuracy with which the solution is prepared. Primary standard materials must have a defined composition, be stable and capable of being dried without decomposition, and their purity should not affect the accuracy of the analysis. A *secondary standard* solution is one in which the concentration or other quantity is determined by an analytical method of known reliability. Its accuracy depends on the accuracy of the analysis which, in turn, will involve a standard which, ultimately, must be a primary standard. With this classification both potassium permanganate and serum can function as secondary standards.

Serum standards (i.e. control specimens which have been reliably assayed) are sometimes referred to as reference specimens or materials, but care should be taken that this term is not confused with the specimens used to derive reference values. Standard Reference Materials are a group of primary and secondary standards with certified values produced by the US National Bureau of Standards. The word 'standard' can also mean uniform (e.g. standard method) or quality (e.g. a standard of performance) and whenever ambiguity could arise the term calibration standard or calibrant should be used.

An internal standard is a substance not normally present in the specimen and clearly distinguishable from the analyte, which is added in known amount to the sample, or to both the standard and the sample, in order to correct results for inaccuracy. For example, a radioactive substance may be added to the sample in order to correct for losses in chromatography. Lithium is added to both standards and samples in the flame photometric determination of sodium and potassium in order to compensate for changes in instrumental response during an analytical run.

Accuracy of Analytical Methods

Analytical methods can be classified into four types according to their accuracy.[4,9]

1. A *definitive method* is one with no known source of inaccuracy which has been exhaustively investigated and shown to give unambiguous results. The isotope dilution–mass spectrometry method for serum calcium is an example. The result given by these methods is the definitive value.
2. A *reference method* is one which after exhaustive testing and comparison with a definitive method has been shown to have negligible inaccuracy in comparison with its imprecision. One

method of this type is the determination of serum calcium by atomic absorption spectroscopy, and the result it gives is termed the reference method value.[10] Both definitive and reference methods require high quality standards, either primary standards or Standard Reference Materials.

3. A *method of known bias* should be tested against a reference method. Often this bias will be shown to be small or close to zero, but if it is significant this must be clearly stated. Methods which have been thoroughly tested and shown to be reliable, with little or no bias, are sometimes referred to in the literature as Selected or Standard methods.

4. *Methods of unknown bias* are not uncommon with assays of complex analytes which are not available in purified form. For these, external quality assessment is often the only practical way of approaching the measurement of bias.

The method used to calibrate a secondary standard is of vital importance, and the practice of standardizing one serum against another will perpetuate any errors in the analysis. In clinical biochemistry, biological solutions are used as secondary standards for a variety of reasons:

1. Since most methods are non-stoichiometric, one or more calibration standards must be analysed with each batch of specimens. Sometimes aqueous standards cannot be treated in exactly the same manner as specimens, for example, in methods involving protein precipitation or enzymic hydrolysis of conjugates.

2. The method may not be specific. In this case the sample generates a reading due to some component which is not present in the standard. Interference by non-creatinine chromogens and some drugs are examples of this. To overcome this, the analyte may be incorporated in a biological matrix in an attempt to make the standard resemble the sample and to introduce an equal amount of interference. However, non-specific components may be quantitatively or qualitatively different in standards and samples and may vary between samples for example, when lipaemia, hyperbilirubinaemia or drugs are present. Consequently the use of non-specific methods will introduce varying inaccuracies with different type of calibration materials: pure standards could be used if methods were specific.

3. A pure solution of a compound may react differently from that present in human serum. Bilirubin in chloroform, for example, reacts more rapidly with diazotized sulphanilic acid than that in serum and the product has a slightly different absorption maximum. Dialysis of some compounds through the membrane of the Auto-Analyzer® is slower when protein is present.

4. Many automatic analysers require serum standards, particularly if enzymes and proteins are measured concurrently with other components.

On some occasions it may be impossible to analyse a pure standard with every batch of specimens because it is unstable, expensive or non-existent. Standardization of enzymes, for example, must be made indirectly. In these cases, the specimen concentration can be calculated by using some other characteristic of the standard, such as its molar absorptivity. When calibration standards do not exist for an assay, the result must be calculated from instrument readings of time, temperature, mass, volume, pressure, etc., any of which may be inaccurate.

Specificity

Although a method may give accurate results with pure aqueous solutions, it may prove to be unusable with biological specimens containing interfering materials. These materials can vary in kind and quantity between specimens, so that the accuracy of the result depends upon the specimen as well as the method. Correction for known inaccuracies in a method can be erroneous because it is usually assumed that inaccuracy is constant.

Assessment of accuracy must therefore be made with both normal and abnormal specimens and by testing for interference. Substances which are likely to interfere can sometimes be predicted from a study of the method. For example, in colorimetric methods other coloured substances such as bilirubin and haemoglobin may interfere and this can be investigated by adding them to see whether they increase the result. Interference by turbidity from lipaemic serum can be tested by adding latex particles to produce an artificial turbidity. In the presence of bilirubin some kinetic methods for creatinine assay give low results; conversely, spuriously elevated bilirubin values may be found by the dichlorophenyldiazonium method in patients with renal failure. It is sometimes useful to distinguish between non-specificity and interference. *Non-specificity* always produces high results because some feature in the method, such as the wavelength, has failed to discriminate between two substances. *Interference* is usually more complex and can lead either to high results (enhancement) or low results (inhibition). For example, emission flame photometry for the determination of potassium is, with adequate wavelength resolution, highly specific, but the addition of large amounts of sodium will enhance the results by producing an ionic interference. Similarly phosphate can cause interference (inhibition) in the highly specific atomic absorption method for calcium. Glucose oxidase methods are specific but may nevertheless be inaccurate due to the presence of inhibitors which may occur in some specimens but not others. Non-specificity and interference can occur together: haemoglobin can produce falsely high results in the determination of bilirubin, due to the failure of the method to distinguish between the colours of haemoglobin and azobilirubin, but it can also interfere by inhibiting the reaction of the diazo reagent with bilirubin.

Understanding the cause of the inaccuracy will often suggest a method for overcoming it by, for example, incorporating a blank measurement, using a different wavelength or adding equal amounts of the interfering substance to the standard.

Drug Interference

This is becoming a major problem in clinical chemistry and Young, Pestaner and Gibberman[11] have listed over 9000 effects of drugs on laboratory tests. Many drugs can affect biochemical results in a manner which can mislead the clinician. These effects may either reflect a change taking place only during the analytical procedure (*in vitro* effects) or they may reflect a true *in vivo* change in the analyte.[12]

In vitro effects arise during the analysis and cause inaccuracy. These effects can be due to the drug or its metabolites. Examples are:

1. The drug may directly simulate the component to be measured, particularly with colorimetric and fluorimetric methods. Coloured drugs such as bromsulphthalein may mimic the substance to be measured. α-Methyl dopa, used in the treatment of hypertension, gives a fluorescence in some methods which is indistinguishable from that produced by catecholamines.
2. The drug may disturb the conditions of the assay by, for example, preferentially reacting with a reagent. Large doses of ascorbic acid can do this with several methods.
3. The drug may act directly or indirectly on the substance to be measured and thus interfere with the analysis. For example, EDTA may be given as a drug and will chelate with calcium, which cannot then be measured by methods which employ a chelating agent. Salicylate will bind to albumin and this may cause interference with some methods of determining albumin which depend on dye-binding.

In vivo effects are more complex. Some are well known and predictable from even a superficial knowledge of the action of the drug. Thus insulin lowers plasma glucose, thiazide diuretics lower plasma potassium and increase uric acid. However, many others are unexpected and the clinician may not be aware of them when interpreting a result. Examples are:

1. The drug may react directly on or compete with the substance to be measured, for example, by binding. Thus oral contraceptives influence the plasma concentration of many hormones, mainly through effects on their binding proteins: total T3, total T4 and TSH concentrations are all increased.

2. The drug may cause direct inhibition or activation of one or more steps in the metabolism of the substance. Thus, phenobarbitone induces liver enzymes which result in a lowering of the plasma bilirubin level, and vitamin B_{12} stimulates erythropoesis in megaloblastic anaemia, leading to a fall in the plasma iron concentration.
3. The drug may have an indirect effect on metabolism by affecting the synthesis of specific enzymes or by interfering with cofactors necessary for the metabolism of the substance. Antibiotics affecting the intestinal flora can alter the urinary pattern of oestrogen and indole metabolites.
4. The drug may interfere with physiological processes which influence the concentration of the substance in body fluids. Thiazide diuretics, for example, affect the renal excretion of oestrogens, and phenytoin reduces calcium absorption.

In vivo and *in vitro* effects can occur together. Thus L-dopa can elevate urine oestrogen values if enzymatic hydrolysis is used in the method, and it can also increase oestrogen production by causing release of gonadotrophins from the hypophysis.

These effects have important implications in quality assurance. In most cases it is not practical to ask for therapy to be discontinued whilst laboratory investigations are completed. The major problem is to recognize when interference is occurring and this is made more difficult when the laboratory does not know what drugs the patient is receiving. It is essential that details of all the patient's drugs are entered on the request form. *In vitro* interference can only be overcome by modification or change of analytical method. *In vivo* interference is often unrecognized and, although it is not usually considered part of quality assurance, the biochemist should be aware of all the factors which can influence his results. At present the only safeguard is constant vigilance for unexpected results which might be related to the presence of a drug.

Accuracy of Enzyme Assay

At present pure enzymes cannot be used as standards, and calibration must be made by measuring enzyme activity under rigorously controlled standard conditions. The result is recorded in units which are a function of the method used, i.e. pH, temperature, buffers, etc., and any deviations from the prescribed conditions can alter the result. By definition, the result is only accurate if it is identical with that obtained by the method used to define the unit. The lack of comparability between laboratories is probably due to the use of minor modifications of the method, whilst retaining the unit defined by it.

Two methods of calibration are possible. Primary methods depend on measurement of changes in con-

patients' home. Often these tests are performed by persons who are inexperienced in laboratory work, using different methods or equipment, but without any form of quality control. In these situations the immediate need is for speed, but sometimes this is only achieved by sacrificing some precision and accuracy. This may not be regarded as important in a clinical emergency; for example, a rapid but approximate blood glucose result is valuable in a case of suspected diabetic coma. However, this result may later be used to assess the effect of treatment and results must therefore be precise if sequential tests are to be correctly interpreted. Laboratory staff should therefore be involved as much as possible in tests done outside the laboratory—in the selection of methods and equipment, in training staff, and in monitoring the quality of their results. The laboratory itself should maintain a high standard at all times which is sufficient to meet the most stringent requirements of any of its users.

Precision Requirements

The laboratory may regard the precision and accuracy of its results as under control if they all fall within defined limits. These limits are usually based on what the laboratory can achieve routinely, rather than what is clinically necessary. Although some manufacturers of control materials quote acceptable limits for their assay values, these are not based on biological or clinical requirements. They are usually the limits found by the laboratories which assayed the material, or those which the manufacturer believes the user should be able to achieve, and therefore depend on the accuracy and precision of both the manufacturer and the user.

The laboratory must have some standard of performance at which to aim. Acceptable levels of accuracy are difficult to define, but in the long term, no inaccuracy can be considered acceptable.

In general, there are four schools of thought on the specification of precision requirements. The first school maintains that the levels of precision achieved by good laboratories should be used as the target (Table 2). The publication of data such as these showing the state of the art tends to encourage competition between laboratories to do better, and this has undoubtedly helped to improve performance. However, these achievable levels are capable of almost limitless improvement, possibly at additional cost or by sacrificing speed, so the laboratory may be striving for a standard of precision which is clinically unnecessary.

A second school of thought relates precision requirements to biological variation. For example, Tonks proposed that the allowable limits of error should be defined as plus or minus one quarter of the reference interval, and expressed as a percentage of the mean reference value. This was probably an oversimplification, in that the choice of one quarter, instead of some other fraction, was arbitrary, and the reference interval often depends on age, sex, etc. A more satisfactory method of assessing requirements is to relate these to the mean physiological day to day variation of the analyte.[15] Thus if the true biological variance is S_B^2, and the analytical variance is S_A^2, the observed variance (S_o^2) will be equal to $S_B^2 + S_A^2$. When $S_A = 0.5 S_B$ the analytical variation will contribute less than 20% to the total observed variability. This increase is considered to be tolerable. Using this approach, several authors have quoted recommended analytical CVs based on half the biological CV (Table 2).

The disadvantage of this method is that biological variation in sick patients may be different from that in healthy subjects. Furthermore, a variety of factors can affect biological variation, for example, food, time of day, posture, etc., and in hospital practice these cannot be entirely standardized.

A third approach uses a consensus of clinicians' views on the levels of precision that they require.[17] Naturally, these vary widely and are probably

TABLE 2

ESTIMATES OF PRECISION REQUIREMENTS, EXPRESSED AS COEFFICIENTS OF VARIATION (CV%)

Serum analyte	Achieved by top 20% of UK labs, 1981 (Stevens and Cresswell quoted by Fraser[15])	Recommended analytical CV (= half the physiological CV)[16]	Medically useful CV (consensus of physicians' opinions)[17]
Albumin	2·4	1·6	—
Calcium	1·6	0·9	4·8*
Cholesterol	2·6	2·6	12·3
Creatinine	2·5	2·2	10·1*
Glucose	1·9	3·0	11·2*
Iron	3·0	13·3	17·2
Phosphate	2·2	3·7	14·3
Potassium	1·1	2·3	4·8
Sodium	0·6	0·4	1·7*
Total protein	1·5	1·4	8·3
Urea	1·7	6·0	12·2*
Urate	2·1	4·1	—

* In these cases the CV depended on concentration, and the *lowest* value is quoted.

influenced by the levels each clinician is accustomed to. Nevertheless, these opinions are useful in high-lighting clinical situations where important decisions are made. However, the data given in Table 2 show large differences in what the average clinician believes he wants, and what the laboratory believes he ought to have (and what can be provided).

A fourth school of thought maintains that precision requirements will inevitably vary, depending on the clinical problem at the time, and that it is impossible to specify a single universal requirement of acceptability.[18] For example, the precision required for blood glucose assays is much more stringent when per-formed during a pituitary function test than in testing a patient in suspected diabetic coma. Requirements may vary so widely that they cannot be expressed as a single figure, whether this be a CV or SD. In general, requirements are more demanding when the clinician has little other relevant data about the patient and the result is pathognomonic. Higher stan-dards of performance are also required when the results are used for research purposes or in epidemio-logical studies of populations.

Taking all these views into account, it seems likely that most laboratories can now achieve satisfactory levels of precision for the commonly measured ana-lytes, where reliable analytical methods are readily available. There is probably little to be gained by further improvement in the precision of potassium assays for example. However, this should not be allowed to lead to complacency. The measurement of calcium, for example, will always require the high-est standard of performance and for many of the more complex assays (such as peptide hormones) consider-able improvement is still required. Quality is never static: improvement in methods not infrequently leads to improvement in medical techniques and patient care. As a general rule, the laboratory should always strive for the best: it is thoroughly bad practice for the laboratory to regard its results as 'good enough for clinical purposes' when it is not in a posi-tion to judge what these purposes are, or the use to which the clinician, either at the time or later, may make of them.

Reference Values

Traditionally laboratories measured reference ranges by analysing specimens from apparently healthy volunteers, usually laboratory staff or blood donors. The distribution of results was assumed to be Gaus-sian and the range expressed as the mean ± 2 SD, which includes 95% of the population. The observed SD (S_o) is related to the true biological variation (S_B) and the analytical variation (S_A) by:

$$S_o^2 = S_B^2 + S_A^2$$

Analytical variation can therefore widen reference intervals and blur the distinction between normals and abnormals. However, S_A is not constant and is larger between-days than within-days, so the appar-ent reference range may be larger if the specimens are analysed over a long period, particularly if the accuracy changes during this time. Similarly, the apparent range will be narrower if specimens are ana-lysed in duplicate or within a short period.

Evidence has shown the limitations of this approach. For some tests the distribution of reference values is non-Gaussian.[19] Values depend on age, sex and race, and possibly other uncontrollable factors. Some tests are influenced by posture, diet and exer-cise and affected by diurnal and circadian variations. Specimens must, therefore, be collected under care-fully controlled conditions. Consequently, for many tests a single set of reference values is no longer appropriate, and most laboratories use published data to derive their reference values. However, this assumes that the analytical methods used to obtain these values were of similar accuracy and precision to those used in the laboratory. This is not easy to verify. For some tests, such as enzyme assays, there is no agreement on accuracy, and different reference ranges must be used for each method. For the clini-cian this is highly confusing, even if the ranges are reliable for the particular variant of the method used.

In general, the use of analytical methods which give method-dependent values and therefore differ-ent reference ranges is to be deprecated. If the labora-tory needs to determine its own reference values it should take into account the factors discussed in this section.

Clinical Uses of Precision Data

The clinician should not normally need to question laboratory accuracy, although it may be necessary to reassure him of this. He may, however, need to know the confidence limits of a result and these can be calculated from precision data. The 95% confi-dence limits of a single observation are ±1·96 SD and for the mean of duplicate observations ±1·38 SD.

The laboratory should publish the SD or CV values of its tests and revise these regularly. This informa-tion can be used as a basis for answering three ques-tions frequently asked by clinicians:

1. **Is this result abnormal?** The reference range includes both analytical variation and the bio-logical variation between individuals and is usually expressed as the mean ±2 SD. Thus there is a 1 in 20 chance that a healthy person will give a result outside this range, and a 1 in 40 chance that he will give either a high or a low result. A result which is 3 SD from the reference mean has only a 0·2% chance of being 'normal'. Because of the complexity of factors determining reference values, this explanation is an over-simplification, and it assumes that both the analytical accuracy and precision at

the time are equal to those used in deriving the reference range.

2. **Does this second result differ significantly from the previous result?** The difference between two results on the same patient is unlikely (1 in 20 chance) to be due to analytical variation if it is greater than 2·7 times the analytical SD. Significant differences could, however, be due to normal biological (e.g. diurnal) variations rather than to a clinically significant change. The problem is to decide which analytical SD to use in making this calculation. If accuracy is constant, the SD for the two batches or days should be used. If accuracy is not constant, this must be taken into account, as well as the random error. This may not be possible, and many laboratories therefore base the assessment on the between-day SD, which will include a component due to accuracy change. This is not entirely satisfactory from a scientific viewpoint, as it does not take into account the actual precision on the two occasions, and it averages out the differences between good and bad days. Whenever small changes are sought, it is best to analyse the specimens in the same batch (e.g. in dynamic function tests) or to examine trends rather than only two values.

3. **Is this result different from a specified value of assumed clinical or therapeutic significance?** Such a critical value or action limit may be plasma bilirubin of 340 μmol/l in a newborn infant or plasma potassium of 3 mmol/l in a patient receiving diuretics. If the difference between the observed and stipulated values is more than 2·0 times the analytical SD, it is unlikely (a 1 in 20 chance) to be caused by analytical variation. This assumes that the analytical SD is constant and that the method used has the same accuracy as that used to establish the specified value.

METHODS OF INTERNAL QUALITY CONTROL

The main purpose of internal quality control methods is to detect errors and thereby ensure the reliability of laboratory results. These methods involve two stages: the accumulation of analytical data, followed by statistical treatment to determine whether the results are under control. To be effective, data must be available and shown to be satisfactory before patients' results are reported. In most of these methods it is assumed that the control data reflect changes in the results of patients' specimens, but in most cases it is impossible to be certain that an error affects all patients' specimens to the same extent. Therefore control data should not be used to correct for inaccuracies. Preventive maintenance should prevent many errors, but once an error is detected its source must be identified and the fault corrected as quickly as possible. The aim should be to detect and identify incipient errors before they affect patients' results. Quality control methods must be regarded as less than efficient if it is necessary to reject and repeat a batch of analyses or, even worse, to correct a result which has already been reported.

Acquisition of Quality Control Data

No single method of quality control is adequate alone, and none is infallible. The methods chosen depend on the test, and in general should include methods for monitoring both inaccuracy and imprecision. All results should be recorded and a note made of any changes in reagents, standards or equipment which may affect performance. This may be useful retrospectively in tracing the probable cause of a change in performance. Each method should be tried with different control chart techniques and reviewed regularly to ensure that it is giving useful information.

Control Specimens. Two types of control specimen are used—one to monitor precision and another, for which the stated value is known to be reliable, to monitor inaccuracy. At least one precision control specimen should be included in every batch and this should preferably have a concentration close to that at which important medical decisions are made (e.g. at the limit of the reference range). The SD should be calculated as soon as sufficient data are available. Although it is useful to measure imprecision at different concentrations, for daily control purposes it is better to have a large amount of data for one concentration, so that the within-batch or within-day SD can be calculated, than to have fewer results at several different concentrations. Ideally, both the accuracy and precision of every batch should be monitored, but as a rough working guide the number of control specimens should be about 5% of the number of patients' specimens. Both normal and abnormal values should be included for accuracy control. To avoid bias, specimens should be disguised, for example, with fictitious patients' names. Control specimens with known values ('bench controls') can be used to check for drift or to demonstrate that an instrument is performing satisfactorily before the rest of the batch is processed. Since the analyst knows the expected values, these are not objective measures of inaccuracy and imprecision.

Duplicate Specimens. It is sometimes possible to make routine analyses in duplicate, and the difference between duplicates (the range) can be used as a measure of within-batch imprecision. Sometimes the patient's specimen is divided into two portions immediately after collection, coded, and then analysed independently. If laboratory staff do not know that this is being done, it is a rigorous test of performance.

Exchange of specimens between laboratories is a

useful method of detecting differences in accuracy. This is particularly important if patients move between two hospitals. The two laboratories exchange specimens, standards and reagents and work together until they resolve any systematic differences.

Daily Mean. For many tests the overall distribution of patients' results obtained each day is remarkably constant and in some circumstances their mean value can be used as a quality control statistic. Alterations in this value from day to day could be due either to changes in accuracy or to alterations in the population studied.

The sensitivity of this quality control method to changes in accuracy is determined by the standard error of the daily mean, which depends on the range of values included and their variation, and the number of results used. Some authors include only those results within the reference range or which have a Gaussian distribution. These have a narrower distribution and therefore require fewer results to achieve a stable daily mean (sometimes only 10), but this procedure only monitors accuracy changes within the reference range. If the distribution of results is highly skewed, or the range is wide, or the proportion of abnormal results is variable, the variation in the daily mean can be reduced by including only those values which lie within truncation limits; these limits can be quite arbitrary.

The daily mean can be a useful method of quality control for tests which are done in large numbers, and where the population sampled each day is relatively constant and not affected by, for example, seasonal variations. Patients who are investigated at week-ends usually have more abnormal results than those tested during the week and for some tests mean values may therefore be different. The method is also useful for tests where other types of control specimen are either not available (e.g. whole blood) or unstable. It is the only quality control method which includes sources of variation arising outside the laboratory, such as the cleanliness of syringes and specimen containers. In one report, changes in the daily mean were traced to the introduction of a batch of blood-collecting tubes containing potassium EDTA instead of heparin. It can also be used to monitor the efficiency of specimen transport, separation and storage. One laboratory noticed that the daily mean for plasma potassium was lower on Saturdays than during the week. This was traced not to a change in the population, but to shorter centrifuging of blood specimens, which, during the week, became overheated from prolonged centrifuging. The method is independent of any operator bias and requires no additional analyses, although extra labour is involved in making the calculations.

Reference Values. Regular measurement of reference values can sometimes be used as a method of quality control. If reference intervals for a test are narrow, reference specimens from laboratory staff can be used to check accuracy (or changes in accuracy). This is sometimes useful for components which are absent (e.g. erythrocytes in urine) or unstable (e.g. CO_2 and pH) in other types of control specimen. A normal urine specimen and a positive control should be included in every batch of qualitative tests. For tests in which the majority of results are normal (e.g. urine catecholamines and their metabolites), it is useful to plot the last 100 or so results on a histogram to see whether the distribution fits the stated reference range.

In one version of this method, the frequency distribution of approximately 500 patients' results is calculated and the cumulative relative frequency plotted against concentration on probability paper. The line joining the plotted points will show a change in slope at values which divide different populations. If patients' values comprise two overlapping Gaussian distributions (normal and abnormal), the line will show a single inflection. Changes in the concentration value at the point of inflection indicate either an alteration in the population or a change in accuracy.

Other Methods. Quality control of blood pH and gas analyses presents special problems because the components are unstable and measurements are made on whole blood. Special control solutions are commercially available for these tests. However, the use of control buffer solutions for checking the performance of electrodes will only detect errors in calibration, but the response of the electrode may be different with a protein-containing solution. Calibration of P_{CO_2} by direct-reading methods can be checked with a gas of known CO_2 content. Methods for determining oxygen tension are usually calibrated with two gases, one with a known oxygen content and the other oxygen-free; air, with a P_{O_2} of approximately 10 kPa, can be used to check this calibration. Probably the best quality control method for blood gas analysis is the use of whole blood which has been freshly equilibrated in a tonometer with a gas of known P_{O_2} and P_{CO_2} tensions. Since these components are unstable, specimens must be analysed within 30 min; air bubbles in the syringe will invalidate results. Some laboratories insist on the use of glass syringes, as there are reports that gases diffuse through plastic ones. These analyses all depend on accurate and precise temperature control and these should always be checked independently, preferably with a certified thermometer.

Special methods are used for the quality control of instruments. Stopwatches and thermometers can be checked by comparison with other, preferably certified, instruments. Spectrophotometers are checked for linearity and absorbance accuracy with solutions of potassium dichromate, and for wavelength accuracy with appropriate solutions or special filters (see Frings et al.[20] for details).

Control Charts

All quality control information should be plotted on control charts so that it can be seen by all staff as well as by clinicians who visit the laboratory. Computers make calculations easier and on-line control possible, but the greatest problem is not in acquiring data but in interpreting it, and this is made easier by the method of display used. The software provided with many automatic analysers gives a very clear display of control data. For a more permanent record, one useful technique is to use a plastic laminated swivel chart with coloured self-adhesive spots and tapes, which is updated each day.

The chart consists of a graph in which a measured quantity, or a statistic derived from it, is plotted against the time or date of analysis.[21,22] Any of the following statistics can be used, and different combinations should be tried to see which is the most useful:

1. the result obtained from a control specimen or, alternatively, the difference or percentage difference between the result and a mean or target value; (Sometimes the results of specimens with different concentrations can be plotted on the same graph as the difference or percentage difference from their expected value.)
2. the mean of duplicate analyses of a control specimen;
3. the difference between duplicate analyses of the same control or patient specimen, or between two different control specimens;
4. the SD or CV calculated for the batch, day, week or month; (A running SD can be calculated from the last 15 replicate analyses.)
5. the daily mean;
6. reference values;
7. readings of standards and blanks.

Initially, the variation of the quantity or statistic with time is measured, preferably with at least 20–30 degrees of freedom, during a period in which the performance of the method is judged to be satisfactory. From the observed distribution of data, control limits are calculated which include most (customarily 95 or 99%) of the values, and these limits are also plotted on the graph. Usually two sets of limits are used: 95% (2 SD) probability limits for warning and 99% (3 SD) as action limits. The method is regarded as under control as long as values outside the control limits occur less frequently than one in 20 or 100 times. The control limits are recalculated at suitable intervals from the performance data accumulated over periods of satisfactory operation.

Occasionally an observed change may be just large enough to be significant in terms of the statistical test used, but for practical purposes is so small that it can be disregarded. The biochemist, not the statistician, must decide what is an important change in the context. In each case, all staff must know the action to be taken when limits are exceeded. How-ever, a consistent trend or change should not be ignored merely because the control limits are not crossed.

Charts can be used to indicate precision and accuracy, as well as changes in each of these. The commonest is a chart of control specimens results (Fig. 6). This should show a sequence of points randomly distributed about the central line, with 1 in 20 outside the 95% limits. An increasing random distribution of points outside these limits indicates deterioration in precision.

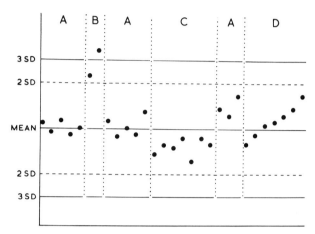

Fig. 6 An example of a control chart with 2 SD warning limits and 3 SD action limits. During the periods marked A the method was in control. At B there was a jump in the control chart with points outside the limits. In the period C there were 7 successive points below the mean, and in period D seven successive points showed an upward trend.

Non-random patterns may be of several different types (see Fig. 6):

1. Extreme variations due to gross errors are obvious. Within any set of control results there will be occasional grossly discrepant results or outliers, due to mistakes of specimen identification, calculation or transcription. Statistically, these are unlikely to have occurred by chance, and some authors therefore omit them from the control chart. This makes the chart look better, but since outliers can also occur among patients' results, the impression is misleading. The frequency of outliers is therefore important, but frequently disregarded, and they should be included on control charts: the magnitude of the error usually makes it obvious that these are gross errors or blunders rather than random analytical variations.
2. Jumps in the control line indicate a sudden alteration in accuracy due, for example, to a change in standard or a reagent, which should be indicated on the chart.
3. A sequence of points may lie on one side of the central line, rather than being randomly distributed about it, but are still within control

limits. This indicates inaccuracy, and seven successive points on one side of the line indicate that the method is out of control. Plotting the running mean of, say, the last 4 results or 10 daily mean values, helps to show trends in accuracy whilst the method is still ostensibly in control.

4. Seven successive results showing a regular upward or downward trend indicate that the method is going out of control. Trends may not be easily apparent on the usual control chart,

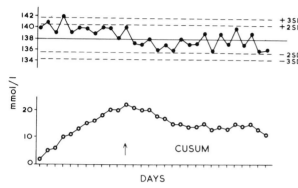

Fig. 7. A cusum chart for the daily mean of plasma sodium measurements. The upper chart shows the original data with 2 SD warning and 3 SD action limits. The lower cusum chart shows the cumulative sum of these values about a baseline value of 138 mmol/l. At the point marked, new calibration standards were prepared, and the cusum graph changed slope.

but are enhanced by plotting accuracy data on a cumulative sum ('cusum') chart. The statistic plotted is the accumulating algebraic sum of the positive and negative deviations of the results from their expected value. If x_1, x_2 and x_3 are sequential values and k the expected value, then the value plotted (S) is

$$S_1 = x_1 - k$$
$$S_2 = S_1 + x_2 - k$$
$$S_n = S_{n-1} + x_n - k$$

Accuracy is constant as long as the points are scattered randomly about a line of constant slope; a change of slope indicates a change in accuracy (*see* Fig. 7). In practice the graph often shows random variations which make it difficult to recognize changes in slope early enough for the method to be useful.

5. Cyclic variations may occur due, for example, to change of analysts on different days or weeks. These can be difficult to detect, and may only be revealed by a close inspection of the data.

Even if it only uses a few of these techniques, a laboratory which takes its quality control seriously will often accumulate so much data that it is difficult to interpret before patients' reports are due to be

dispatched. To assist this, some authors have recommended that relevant control data should be combined into separate accuracy and precision indices, and changes in these can be monitored each day.[3] A laboratory computer is probably essential for this data reduction, and it also enables conventional quality control information to be calculated and displayed clearly and rapidly.

Finally it must be remembered that there are many stages in the investigation of patients which cannot be covered by statistical methods of quality control. Patients' results should always be checked for plausibility and a close watch kept for unexpected results. The object of these methods is not to accumulate large amounts of retrospective data, or to prepare impressive graphs, but to ensure reliability of results. Control charts and statistical techniques merely indicate the probability of error, but do not correct it.

EXTERNAL QUALITY ASSESSMENT

Although the general principles of quality assurance are well known to clinical biochemists, some laboratories believe that participation in external quality assessment (EQA) schemes makes internal quality control unnecessary. This view is particularly common with some of the newer and more complex assays, where there is a lack of commercial control materials for internal quality control, whereas external techniques have been a major feature in the improvement of analytical methods. This confusion has been partly due to the use of the word 'control' for both, suggesting that the two techniques fulfil the same function and are therefore interchangeable. In fact, because of their relatively slow turn-round of results, external techniques cannot usually be used for daily quality control, and their primary function is for assessment of methods, equipment, laboratories, etc. The terms internal quality control and external quality assessment make this difference explicit.[23]

External quality assessment programmes were originally developed to survey the state of the art of analytical work in a group of laboratories in a region or country. Identical specimens were analysed in participating laboratories and the results returned to the organizer, who then sent a report to participants comparing their results. Participation was voluntary and usually the identity of participants was known only to the organizer. Locally organized schemes are sometimes used to investigate special problems, such as the need for common calibration standards, and are particularly useful if participants meet regularly to discuss their results. Anonymity is then abandoned by common consent. In some countries laboratory work is controlled by legislation and participation in EQA programmes is mandatory; proficiency is then tested before a certificate or licence to practice is granted.

In EQA schemes, the same specimen is sent to all participating laboratories, who must have complete confidence that it is stable, homogeneous, and suitable for use with their methods. It may be a clinical specimen, but with large numbers of participants, the need for large volumes and guaranteed stability requires the use of lyophilized or preserved specimens, usually prepared commercially. Sometimes a set of such specimens is distributed and participants are requested to analyse one at specified intervals. In all cases, it is essential that participants analyse EQA specimens by their routine procedures and do not give them special treatment. Participants must provide the organizer with details of the analytical methods used so that the results obtained by each method can be reviewed.

Results are processed by computer, usually after dividing them into method-groups, and the mean and SD of all results calculated. In order to exclude gross errors, outliers are usually removed by rejecting all results more than 3 SD from the mean, and the recalculated mean and SD are computed from the remaining results. These are returned to the participants usually with a histogram showing the laboratory's result in relation to the others and to the mean result or target value. With good organization, reports are returned promptly, at regular intervals, before the next EQA specimen is due to be analysed.[24]

Several procedures have been used to classify the results of individual laboratories. Individual results can be expressed in terms of the SD or CV of all participants, so that the performance of each laboratory can be seen in relation to the others. Results can then be graded as good, acceptable or unacceptable on the basis of deviations from the mean value of all participants, method-mean values or some other target value. If disguised duplicates are included in a set of specimens, the results can be used to assess imprecision. The SD of each laboratory can then be arranged in a league table of performance in the hope that this will stimulate improvement by competition. In another method, each result is given a score (Variance Index Score, VIS) based on the difference between the result (x) and the method mean ($\bar{x}$), expressed as percentage, divided by a chosen CV for that analyte (CCV), and again expressed as a percentage.

$$\text{VIS} = \frac{x - \bar{x}}{\bar{x}} \times \frac{100}{\text{CCV}} \times 100$$

The Mean Running Variance Index Score (MRVIS) is the mean VIS for the last 10 results for the analyte. This can be plotted graphically and displayed in the laboratory with internal quality control data. Unlike some scoring systems the MRVIS is relatively insensitive to a single poor result. Graphs of this type provide an excellent illustration of changes in performance with time, and the data have been used to show an overall improvement of performance in UK laboratories since the inception of EQA. The VIS represents a composite of bias from the target value

(that is, systematic error) and imprecision, but gives no information about the relative contributions of these two types of error.[2,3]

In the earlier years, the mean results reported by participants depended on the methods used, and there was no evidence to show which (if any) was correct (Table 3). Methods with poor interlaboratory agreement were, however, identified and in many cases were replaced. As a result, agreement between methods improved and for many analytes the mean of commonly used methods is close to the overall

TABLE 3

RESULTS OF SERUM CHOLESTEROL ASSAYS BY PARTICIPANTS IN THE UK NATIONAL EXTERNAL QUALITY ASSESSMENT SCHEME

	n	Mean (mmol/l)	CV (%)
March, 1979			
Liebermann–Burchard and			
AutoAnalyzer methods	88	5·78	14·5
Enzymic methods	99	4·83	7·7
Overall	234	5·30	15·0
December, 1979			
Liebermann–Burchard and			
AutoAnalyzer methods	13	8·46	8·2
Enzymic methods	232	7·65	6·0
Overall	248	7·74	6·3

mean. Can this overall mean or consensus value then be taken as the true value? Obviously participants must have confidence in the target value used in scoring their performance. The results of analyses of the same serum in different EQA schemes show that consensus values for many analytes are reproducible. In addition, several authoritative reports have shown close agreement between the consensus value and that obtained by definitive methods.[23] Although such agreement should not be assumed for all analytes or for all specimens in all EQA schemes, it demonstrates the power of EQA in deriving reliable consensus values which can be confidently used as a target. Many commercial companies now quote consensus values for their control materials.

When EQA is applied to new and technically demanding assays, problems inevitably arise in deciding on suitable target values for each specimen. When there are relatively few participants and a diversity of methods, consensus values may not be reproducible and there is no reason to assume that they are correct. Nevertheless, they do serve as a provisional target (when there is no other), and enable a start to be made on the elimination of methods with poor precision. The organizer can then arrange additional experiments (such as recovery or dilution studies or analysis by reference methods) and encourage participants to begin to reduce their bias.

External quality assessment provides an opportunity for each laboratory to assess its own performance and make its own judgement on it. In the UK the professional associations offer help and advice on a confidential basis to laboratories which consistently perform badly. In most cases, the revelation of differences between laboratories acts as an incentive to improvement. External quality assessment is also recognized as a powerful tool for investigating the factors which contribute to the quality of laboratory work: for example, choice of methods and equipment; good internal quality control; and, perhaps above all, the need for sound laboratory management and efficient organization.

SOURCES OF ERROR

Internal quality control procedures are designed to detect and distinguish between systematic and random errors. The analyst must then identify the source of the error before he can hope to eliminate it.

The selection of analytical methods (which include automatic analysers) is the most important factor in determining the frequency and magnitude of errors. Even when correctly performed or used, some of these are still inadequate. Local modifications, made for reasons of speed or convenience, are probably responsible for the differences found between those using ostensibly the same method. For a method to give reliable results in all competent hands, the analyst requires complete and adequate written instructions, specifying the critical factors and tolerances in the method; he must not then make unauthorized modifications. Even with the best automated techniques, differences can still occur between laboratories or days, indicating the presence of some uncontrolled factors. Simple methods are easier to control and reliability is improved by work simplification, particularly with complex methods or when working conditions are made difficult by overcrowding or a heavy work load. Despite automation and mechanization, human fallibility still accounts for the majority of errors, and the importance of adequate technical skill, knowledge and supervision cannot be overstressed. Human errors, arising from the stress of overwork in poor conditions and the boredom of repetitive procedures, also lead to faulty manipulation, observation, calculation, recording and transcription. Many laboratories designate a quality control officer with responsibility for reviewing quality assurance data and identifying and removing errors. All mistakes and errors should be documented, as the most frequent ones arise from a limited number of sources.

In order to decide whether a change in a laboratory result is clinically significant, it is necessary to understand the sources and magnitudes of variation which occur independently of any change in health. These variations may be classified as follows:

1. analytical variation, which comprises both within-batch and between-batch components;
2. pre-analytical variations arising from the technique of venepuncture, centrifugation of the blood, separation and storage of the plasma, as well as potentially controllable variations within the individual due to posture, time of day, diet, exercise, etc.; (*Note.* In order to assess differences between individuals, as well as changes within individuals, these sources of pre-analytical variation should be minimized by, for example, standardizing the technique of collecting blood specimens. When studying short-term (e.g. within-hour) changes in a subject, specimens should be analysed in the same batch, thereby removing the between-batch analytical variation.)
3. post-analytical variations arising after the analysis has been completed; these include calculation, preparation and despatch of the report, etc.

One study found that the prevalence of pre- and post-analytical errors was 0·5%, half being due to transcription errors and the remainder being mainly due to chart reading and calculation errors. Although the laboratory's quality control results may be excellent, patients' results should always be checked for plausibility before the report is despatched to make sure that there are no obvious pre- or post-analytical errors, most of which cannot be detected by conventional quality control techniques. A laboratory computer is invaluable in identifying reports which require special scrutiny—for example, those in which one or more results exceed specified limits or those in which results have changed significantly from previous values (the 'delta check').

The checklist given below is intended as a reminder of some common sources of these types of error, and to stimulate the search for others, but it should not be regarded as exhaustive:

The Patient

1. Incorrectly identified, particularly if unconscious, confused, deaf or named John Smith.
2. Incorrectly prepared; for example by not fasting or not ingesting the 75 g glucose he should have received for a glucose tolerance test.
3. Receiving drugs which interfere with the analysis or cause unexpected changes in the analyte.

The Specimen

1. Collection at the wrong time, for example in a tolerance test. Some components show a marked circadian variation and should be collected under standard conditions.
2. Dilution of the blood specimen by collecting from a vein close to an intravenous infusion.
3. Prolonged occlusion of the upper arm with a tourniquet, resulting in ultrafiltration of blood in the forearm to produce spurious increases

in the concentration of plasma proteins and substances bound to them, notably calcium.

4. Contamination of the syringe or specimen container. This is particularly important with trace elements: zinc is leached from the rubber cap of some plastic disposable syringes and urine will extract lead from some types of glass bottle.

5. Interaction of the specimen with its container. On storage of plasma samples, up to 10% of calcium is lost by adsorption onto the walls of some polystyrene cups when the pH increases due to loss of CO_2. Mercury is lost from urine by adsorption onto the walls of plastic containers but not glass ones.

6. In function tests, failure to empty the bladder completely, or incomplete or inaccurately timed collection of urine or faeces. As a check, the total volume (or mass) of these specimens should always be recorded. The creatinine content of supposedly 24 h urine collections can be used to check their completeness.

7. Incorrect urine preservative or blood anticoagulant. The same type of blood (arterial, venous or capillary) and anticoagulant should be used for sequential tests. Fluoride used as a preservative for glucose inhibits many enzymes. Blood specimens collected in EDTA show high potassium, low calcium and alkaline phosphatase levels.

8. Incorrect labelling of the specimen with the name or time; given a wrong accession number or transferred to mislabelled tubes within the laboratory.

9. Haemolysis of blood specimens, producing spurious increases in plasma potassium, phosphate and LDH.

10. Delays in the blood specimen reaching the laboratory, allowing time for loss of CO_2 and diffusion of substances out of erythrocytes, giving high values for plasma phosphate and potassium (for which specimens should be separated within 2 h of collection). Delays cause rapid autolysis of cells in urine and CSF.[25]

11. Instability of enzymes like acid phosphatase that rapidly lose their activity at room temperature. Specimens should be kept cool and analysed as soon as possible.

12. Destruction of bilirubin by exposure to light.

13. Interchange of specimens or samples during analysis. This is particularly liable to occur when an urgent specimen needs to be fitted into a run on an automatic analyser. During analysis, unlabelled tubes may be transposed during loading or unloading from the centrifuge or when a full rack of tubes is inadvertently reversed.

14. Evaporation of the specimen (and standard) whilst standing in cups awaiting analysis.

Reagents and Standards

1. Impure or unstable. If in doubt always check the stability.

2. Improperly prepared by, for example, using the hydrated salt when the anhydrous one was intended, or diluting with distilled water instead of buffer. New solutions should be checked against old ones, either by analysing specimens with both, or with independent tests such as absorbance or pH.

3. Illegibly or inadequately labelled.

4. Incorrectly stored, for example in light or at room temperature. Since many have a limited shelf life, the date of preparation should always be given on the label.

5. Contaminated. Discard if turbidity or mould appears.

6. Poor quality distilled or deionized water.

Equipment

Written instructions should always be located with the equipment and read and followed by all who use it. The laboratory should have a programme of regular inspections, preventive maintenance and performance checks, and keep written records of these and the actions taken in response to a fault. Good records help to pinpoint sources of error. Instability, drift and excessive carryover are common indications of faults.

Pipettes, dispensers, etc.—contaminated, dirty or incorrectly calibrated. Calibration of automatic dispensers and diluters should be checked regularly, as the manufacturer's settings may not be accurate and can change with use.

Centrifuges—dirty or overheating, producing a safety hazard as well as causing transfer of potassium from erythrocytes to plasma and loss of labile substances.

Spectrophotometers—shift in wavelength accuracy, selection of wrong filters or a mismatched pair of filters. Non-linearity due to the use of the wrong wavelength or a wide bandwidth arising, for example, from a dirty lamp. Inaccurate absorbance scale. Excessive stray light due to dust causing wavelength and linearity errors. Changes in the ambient temperature, for example, from draughts, affect the absorbance of some solutions and may require the insulation of the instrument.[20]

Cuvettes—dirty, scratched or mismatched (particularly in the ultraviolet region). Errors in pathlength can be checked with cuvettes of certified pathlengths (e.g. 10 mm ± 0·02 mm).

Flame photometers—dirty, non-linear or incorrectly calibrated; partial blockage of nebulizer; contaminated air supply; low gas cylinder pressure.

Readings can be affected by direct sunlight. Ageing of the hollow cathode lamp affects readings with atomic absorption spectrometers.

pH meters—standardized with wrong buffer; faulty or dirty electrodes; inadequate temperature control.

Clocks and thermometers—inaccurate or inadequate for the purpose. Incorrect times and temperature will result in inaccuracy, but excessive variability due to failure to control them will produce imprecision. For enzyme assays some authors recommend that temperature should be controlled to within $\pm 0.05\,°C$. A one-hour alarm clock is inadequate for measuring a 15 min reaction time.

Automatic analysers—dirty membrane; clot in line; manifold lines worn or improperly installed; improperly adjusted probe; excessive heating leading to sample evaporation; sample or reagent carryover.

Calculation

1. Failure to correct results for dilution, particularly when one analyst sets up the test and another calculates the result. Ambiguous instructions can lead to a dilution of 1 *to* 2 when 1 *in* 2 was intended.
2. Arithmetical error or a misplaced decimal point. All readings should be recorded on work sheets so that results can be checked before reports are issued.
3. Out-of-date or incorrect calibration.

The Report

1. Transcribing error, so that a serum sodium of 142 mmol/l is reported as 124 mmol/l.
2. Transposition of two specimens or results leading to incorrect reports on *two* patients.
3. Error arising from telephoning of results. These should always be read back for checking and it is useful for wards to be provided with pre-printed notepads for recording telephoned results.
4. Misunderstanding the units used (which should always be specified), so that a result in mmol/l is interpreted as if it were in mg/dl.
5. And, finally, is the report legible and unambiguous and will it reach the person intended, in sufficient time to be useful, and include all the information (such as reference values) needed to interpret it?

REFERENCES

1. Büttner J., Borth R., Boutwell J. H., Bowyer R. C., Broughton P. M. G. (1979). Approved (IFCC) Recommendation (1978) on Quality Control in Clinical Chemistry. Part 1, General principles and terminology. *Clin. Chim. Acta*; **98**: 129F.
2. Whitehead T. P. (1977). *Quality Control in Clinical Chemistry*. New York: Wiley.
3. Whitehead T. P. (1977). Advances in quality control. *Adv. Clin. Chem*; **19**: 175.
4. Büttner J., Borth R., Boutwell J. H., Broughton P. M. G., Bowyer R. C. (1979). Approved (IFCC) Recommendation (1978) on Quality Control in Clinical Chemistry. Part 2, Assessment of analytical methods for routine use. *Clin. Chim. Acta*; **98**: 145F.
5. Büttner J., Borth R., Boutwell J. H., Broughton P. M. G., Bowyer R. C. (1981). Approved (IFCC) Recommendation (1979) on Quality Control in Clinical Chemistry. Part 3, Calibration and control materials. *Clin. Chim. Acta*; **109**: 105F.
6. Fasce C. F., Rej R., Copeland W. H., Vanderlinde R. E. (1973). A discussion of enzyme reference materials: applications and specifications. *Clin. Chem*; **19**: 5.
7. Broughton P. M. G., Gowenlock A. H., McCormack J. J., Neill D. W. (1974). A revised scheme for the evaluation of automatic instruments for use in clinical chemistry. *Ann. Clin. Biochem*; **11**: 207.
8. Percy-Robb I. W., Broughton P. M. G., Jennings R. D. *et al.* (1980). A recommended scheme for the evaluation of kits in the clinical chemistry laboratory. *Ann. Clin. Biochem*; **17**: 217.
9. Tietz N. W. (1979). A model for a comprehensive measurement system in clinical chemistry. *Clin. Chem*; **25**: 833.
10. Pickup J. F., Jackson M. J., Price E. M., Healy M. R. J., Brown S. S. (1975). Use of the reference method for determination of serum calcium in a quality-assurance survey. *Clin. Chem*; **21**: 1416.
11. Young D. S., Pestaner L. C., Gibberman V. (1975). Effects of drugs on clinical laboratory tests. *Clin. Chem*; **21**: 1D.
12. Siest G., Dawkins S. J. (1984). IFCC Expert Panel on Drug Effects in Clinical Chemistry. Part 1. The basic concepts. *J. Clin. Chem. Clin. Biochem*; **22**: 271.
13. Bretaudiere J. P., Dumont G., Rej R., Bailly M. (1981). Suitability of control materials. General principles and methods of investigation. *Clin. Chem*; **27**: 798.
14. Westgard J. O., Carey R. N., Wold S. (1974). Criteria for judging precision and accuracy in method development and evaluation. *Clin. Chem*; **20**: 825.
15. Fraser C. G. (1983). Desirable performance standards for clinical chemistry tests. *Adv. Clin. Chem*; **23**: 299.
16. Statland B. E. (1980). The relationship of biological variation and clinical decision levels to quality assurance. In *Quality Assurance in Health Care: A Critical Appraisal of Clinical Chemistry* (Boutwell J. H., ed.). Washington, DC: American Association of Clinical Chemists.
17. Skendzel L. P., Barnett R. N., Platt R. (1985). Medically useful criteria for analytic performance of laboratory tests. *Am. J. Clin. Pathol*; **83**: 200.
18. Büttner J., Borth R., Boutwell J. H., Broughton P. M. G., Bowyer R. C. (1981). IFCC Approved Recommendation (1979) on Quality Control in Clinical Chemistry. Part 6. Quality requirements from the point of view of health care. *Clin. Chim. Acta*; **109**: 115F.
19. Flynn F. V., Piper K. A. J., Garcia-Webb P., McPherson K., Healy M. J. R. (1976). Biological and analytical variation of commonly determined blood constituents in healthy blood donors. *Clin. Chim. Acta*; **70**: 179.
20. Frings C. S., Broussard L. A., Fendley T. W., Lodmell

J. D., Rand R. N. (1979). Calibration and monitoring of spectrometers and spectrophotometers. *Clin. Chem*; **25**: 1013.

21. Büttner J., Borth R., Broughton P. M. G., Bowyer R. C. (1983). Approved (IFCC) Recommendation (1983) on Quality Control in Clinical Chemistry. Part 4, Internal quality control. *J. Clin. Chem. Clin. Biochem*; **21**: 877.

22. Westgard J. O., Barry P. L., Hunt M. R., Groth T. (1981). A multi-rule Shewhart chart for quality control in clinical chemistry. *Clin. Chem*; **27**: 439.

23. Whitehead T. P., Woodford F. P. (1981). External quality assessment of clinical laboratories in the United Kingdom. *J. Clin. Pathol*; **34**: 947.

24. Büttner J., Borth R., Boutwell J. H., Broughton P. M. G., Bowyer R. C. (1983). Approved (IFCC) Recommendation (1983) on Quality Control in Clinical Chemistry. Part 5, External quality control. *J. Clin. Chem. Clin. Biochem*; **21**: 885.

25. Wilding P., Zilva J. F., Wilde C. E. (1977). Transport of specimens for clinical chemistry analysis. *Ann. Clin. Biochem*; **14**: 301.

FURTHER READING

Rodbard D. (1974). Statistical quality control and routine data processing for radioimmunoassays and immuno-radiometric assays. *Clin. Chem*; **20**: 1255.

7. The Relevance of Biological Rhythms to Clinical Biochemistry

J. R. Daly*
revised and updated by
J. Arendt

INTRODUCTION. THE NATURE OF BIOLOGICAL RHYTHMS

Although biological rhythms such as the succession of seed-time and harvest, the mating cycles of animals and the menstrual periods of women have been known from time immemorial, it is only relatively recently that they have been studied scientifically. It is now recognized that many physiological, biochemical and psychological variables show a distinct rhythmicity with a regular period, and their study is a rapidly growing discipline with the somewhat grandiose title of Chronobiology.

The study of rhythms is evolving its own terminology and statistical theory. These will be of concern only to biologists who wish to make rhythmicity a special research interest, but, as the study of rhythms advances, their investigation is increasingly relevant to the clinical biochemist, who should therefore have some awareness of the nature of these rhythms and the terminology used in their description, as well as the extent to which their investigation has already proved diagnostically valuable.

Biological rhythms are often described as *exogenous* or *endogenous*. The former are direct responses to a rhythmic change in the environment and disappear if the varying environmental factor becomes constant. An endogenous rhythm, however, is an inherent property of the organism and has a periodicity of its own. This periodicity is often modified by a rhythmic environmental variable and may become coupled to it. Thus a rhythm with an endogenous periodicity of about 24 hours may become linked to the alternation of light and darkness. In such a case, the environmental variable is known as a *synchronizer* or *Zeitgeber* and is said to *entrain* the rhythm.

Rhythms can be graphically represented by fitting sine curves to the data.[1] The *mesor* is the name given to the central value around which the individual levels vary, and if the observations of the levels have been made at equal intervals throughout the period it will be represented by the mean of all the levels. The *amplitude* is the maximum excursion of the sine wave above and below the mesor. The *acrophase* is the time at which the sine wave has its peak value. The *period* of the rhythm is the time interval between two corresponding points of consecutive oscillations (Fig. 1).

These variables are sometimes expressed diagrammatically by means of a *cosinor*. For a circadian rhythm this consists of a 24-h clockface in which an arrow points to the acrophase, and the length of the shaft of the arrow is proportional to the amplitude of the oscillation. Halberg has described the construction of such cosinors and given an account of the statistical procedures which may be used to determine whether fluctuations in level are random or truly rhythmic.

* Deceased

In human physiology two main rhythms have been clearly defined and intensively investigated, namely menstrual and circadian. Menstrual rhythms have a period of about 28 days and circadian of about 24 hours. Circadian rhythms are also known as nyctohemeral or diurnal. Diurnal is a term with a certain ambiguity, as it is sometimes used in contrast to nocturnal. It is therefore best avoided. Human annual rhythms have also been noted, but usually only with large sample numbers.

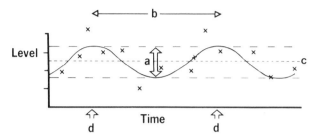

Fig. 1 Sine wave fitted to individual data points *x*. (*a*) represents the amplitude of the oscillation, (*b*) the period, (*c*) the mesor, (*d*) the acrophase.

The endogenous nature of many human circadian rhythms has been amply demonstrated by hundreds of studies in environments free from time cues.[2] Such free-running rhythms usually assume a period length somewhat longer than 24 h: around 25 h is commonly cited. In such environmental isolation, all circadian rhythms may remain coupled together running with the same frequency. Alternatively the sleep–wake cycle may assume a much longer period than, for example, temperature. Such internal desynchronization can be forcibly induced in all subjects, and provides evidence for the 'multi-oscillatory' nature of the circadian system.

An area of the hypothalamus, the supra-chiasmatic nucleus, is considered to be the major central rhythm-generating system, or, in common parlance, the anatomical site of the biological clock. Destruction of this area in animals leads to the loss of a large number of circadian rhythms, together with ovulatory cyclicity.[3] By extrapolation it is therefore considered to be the major site of rhythm generation in man although it remains possible that other sites exist, notably in neighbouring areas of the brain, and in the eye.

The synchronization of free-running endogenous rhythms to the periodicity of the environment (e.g. daily and seasonal rhythms) is effected by means of various time-cues or zeitgebers. In animals the daily variation of light and darkness is by far the most important zeitgeber, followed by temperature variations, social factors, food availability and humidity. In man, until recently, light and darkness were not thought to be of major importance. Social cues and a knowledge of clock-time appeared to override light–dark cues. In fact light is a strong time-cue in man but only if it is sufficiently bright. Using the pineal hormone melatonin as an index of acute human response to light, it has been possible to show that normal domestic lighting (~ 500 lux) will not suppress melatonin production at night, whereas the intensity of light seen, e.g. on a bright spring day (> 2500 lux) will.[4] Further work has shown that it is possible to entrain human circadian rhythms with bright light,[5] and that human seasonal rhythms may also be light-dependent.

Under normal circumstances all our rhythms remain entrained and coupled together. Various situations arise, however, in which desynchronized rhythms occur, or are induced. Desynchronization can either be external, i.e. with respect to the external environment, internal, i.e. rhythms are desynchronized with respect to one another, or both external and internal simultaneously.

Common situations where desynchronization is induced are encountered in jet-lagged travellers and in shift-workers. The circadian system cannot, for example, adapt rapidly to an abrupt change of time zone of several hours. Various rhythms take different times to re-entrain to local time, up to three weeks in some cases (e.g. cortisol), and during this period desynchronization is present.[6] An analogous situation is seen in shift workers where, following each change of shift, circadian rhythms must adapt to the new schedule.

Whether or not disturbed circadian rhythms are detrimental to health is open to debate. There is little evidence that shift work or frequent travel across several time zones leads to ill-health. On the other hand such populations are self-selected: intolerant individuals will opt out leaving, in all probability, those with a particularly robust circadian system. Nevertheless the disturbed sleep, disorientation, inappropriate timing of body needs and of mental and physical performance in susceptible individuals in a state of circadian dysrhythmia can be incapacitating. Recent work suggests that melatonin, the hormone of the pineal gland, is able to alleviate jet-lag and rapidly to resynchronize some circadian rhythms following time-zone change and should thus prove of considerable benefit to large numbers of people.[7]

Disturbed circadian rhythms are also associated with various clinical conditions. The most important to date appear to be depression and 'delayed sleep phase' insomnia; in both conditions there is some evidence that resynchronization is of benefit to the patient. In old age the circadian system also appears to be less robust.

Where a patient is undergoing clinical tests, involving variables with marked daily rhythmicity such as cortisol, it is essential that the clinical biochemist should be aware of a possible state of desynchronization. The timing of samples, and the interpretation of results can then be modified appropriately.

It is remarkable that so many biological variables

should show a circadian rhythm: indeed Aschoff[8] has listed no less than fifty. He points out that such rhythms, being entrained by the 24 h period of the principal rhythmic variable of the environment, may be of value to the organism by helping it to adapt to the changing conditions of a temporally programmed world. Sollberger[9] has suggested that an endogenous circadian rhythm might originate as a response to a rhythmic environmental variable, and that once the oscillation has become self-sustained it could be inherited through evolutionary selection. It would have survival value for the species because the endogenous rhythm would to some extent prepare the organism in advance for the rhythmic environmental changes of the 24 hours, thus helping it to do the right thing at the right time.

Biochemically, the most striking known rhythms are those of hormone levels, and this applies both to menstrual and circadian cycles. As biological rhythms become more clearly understood and more precisely defined, so disturbances in them caused by disease will become more frequently recognized. Thus their investigation may provide a delicate diagnostic indicator. To date, however, they have been little studied clinically.

CLINICAL APPLICATIONS OF THE STUDY OF BIOLOGICAL RHYTHMS

Chief among the reasons why exploration of any alteration in rhythms has been so little used in diagnostic clinical chemistry, has been the impracticability of very frequent sampling. Traditionally diagnostic techniques have been centred on the 'one-off' blood sample, which really gives very little information indeed. There is no way of telling from a single sample whether the blood level of the substance analysed represents a peak or a nadir, or whether it is on a rising or a falling curve. Additional information, it is true, can be obtained from analysing a 24 h urine sample. This may give an approximation to the integrated circulating level of the substance throughout the 24 h, but it can still give no idea of the frequency or temporal direction of fluxes. Furthermore, the relationship between the level of a substance in the plasma and its concentration in the urine may be a complex and indirect one. Inferences from urinary concentrations are therefore subject to a number of imponderables. There is, in addition, the notorious difficulty of obtaining accurately timed urine collections.

Attempts to overcome these difficulties have been for the most part confined to repeated blood sampling at intervals for a relatively short time following the administration of a specific challenge to a metabolic or endocrine system. Obvious examples of this approach are the glucose tolerance and insulin hypoglycaemia tests, in which blood is sampled before, and at say, 30 min intervals after, the administration of glucose or insulin for a period of about 2 h. It

is only in very recent years that a technique has been applied for very frequent sampling, every five minutes or so, which is continued for up to 24 h. In this way a great deal of new information is already being obtained about naturally occurring rhythms. Such techniques have been applied particularly in endocrinology, and have revealed the pulsatile nature of the secretion of many pituitary and other hormones, a discovery that has necessitated reconsideration of many of our ideas of their secretory mechanisms and effects on target organs.

It remains to be seen whether application of these very frequent sampling techniques to other areas of clinical biochemistry will prove diagnostically helpful. Their use depends on a recently developed technology, and this is the reason why their application has until now been so limited.

This technology is based on highly sophisticated sampling and analytical methods. The sampling requires very narrow-gauge, flexible catheters that can be simply and safely inserted into a peripheral vein, and retained in position with a minimum of inconvenience to the patient and with virtually no restriction of his movement. It is even possible to run the catheter through a wall so that sampling is performed from an adjacent room. In this way sampling can be continued throughout the night without it being necessary to approach the patient, who continues to sleep undisturbed. It is then possible to monitor continuously other functions such as the electroencephalogram, pulse rate or respiratory rate in parallel with blood sampling. Thus, the relationship of plasma hormone levels to electroencephalographically defined sleep stages has been studied in some detail.

The development of these sampling methods offers a complex challenge to the laboratory. First, methods are needed which can be carried out on very small volumes of blood for each analysis—they must therefore be extremely sensitive. Secondly, they must have sufficient precision to discriminate between small fluctuations of level, and thirdly, the methods should be capable of handling large batches. New automated and semi-automated procedures and radioimmunoassay methods are meeting this challenge, although still more sensitive methods are required to define the lower limit of some hormone levels. The combination of rapid sampling and advanced analytical methods will no doubt lead to the discovery of new rhythms and of ways in which their study may serve diagnostic needs.

Very frequent sampling procedures would in themselves be far too great a strain on both clinical and laboratory resources to be applied widely to individual diagnostic problems at present, and are suitable only for research. In order to detect a rhythm, sampling must be at least double the frequency of the oscillation, which may otherwise be missed (Fig. 2). However, once a rhythm has been identified, and its amplitude and period defined, it may be possible to use it as the basis of a diagnostic investigation with relatively limited sampling. There is a danger, however, in reducing the frequency of sampling too drastically, that spurious frequencies may appear, or true ones be deleted. This is a particular risk when there is a great deal of 'noise' in the system. Such

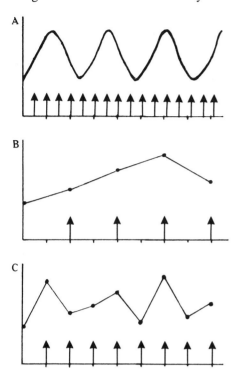

Fig. 2 How the rhythm of a regular oscillation (A) may be completely lost (B) or distorted (C) if sampling, represented by the arrows, is insufficiently frequent.

a problem may arise, for instance, in the diagnosis of Cushing's syndrome and will be discussed in more detail later (*see* Fig. 13).

The two major areas in which the study of rhythms is important in diagnostic clinical biochemistry are the hormonal changes of the menstrual cycle and of the circadian function of the hypothalamic-pituitary-adrenal (HPA) axis.

The Menstrual Cycle

By a study of the inter-related patterns of hormone levels circulating in the blood or excreted in the urine throughout the menstrual cycle, clinical biochemists have been given a means of evaluating clinical problems manifested by amenorrhoea and infertility, and for monitoring the results of therapy.

A number of hormones have been investigated in the study of the endocrinology of the menstrual cycle. Among them are the glycoprotein gonadotrophic hormones of the anterior pituitary, luteinizing hormone (LH) and follicle-stimulating hormone (FSH), together with the ovarian steroids oestradiol and progesterone.

Radioimmunoassay has made possible the determination of LH and FSH on small plasma samples, and these have been measured throughout the cycle. It should be pointed out at this stage, however, that the measured pattern is normally that of *immunoreactive* gonadotrophins, and not of *bioactive*. Bioassays are also available now with sufficient sensitivity to permit measurements of plasma gonadotrophin levels during the menstrual cycle, and the pattern observed is not altogether identical to that obtained by immunoassay. Indeed, to add to the problems, the patterns obtained when different bioassays are employed are not always identical either. It is not possible at present to interpret these anomalous findings, which are being actively investigated in many centres. One serious source of difficulty in gonadotrophin assay, particularly bioassay, arises from the complexities of standardization, because pure synthetic standards with structures identical to those of the circulating forms of the hormones are not available. Despite these problems, and whatever may be the precise significance of immunoactive hormone, a distinct and reproducible pattern has been observed, which is characteristic of the normal menstrual cycle and which correlates with the other events of the cycle in an apparently significant way.

Until fairly recently, studies of ovarian steroids could be undertaken only by measuring their urinary excretion. In the case of progesterone this meant that the direct measurement of the hormone was not undertaken, but rather that of its principal urinary metabolite, pregnanediol. However, radioimmunoassay is now applicable to steroids as well as to peptides; and, furthermore, as the synthetic substances can be obtained pure, steroid radioimmunoassay is free from the standardization problems found in gonadotrophin assay. The ovarian hormones themselves can therefore be measured in plasma. Just as with the gonadotrophins, a distinct and reproducible pattern of oestradiol and progesterone has been observed (Fig. 3).

For approximately one week after the onset of menstrual bleeding, the blood levels of oestrogens, progesterone and LH are very low, with a slight elevation of FSH. During the following week FSH declines to a nadir, progesterone remains low and oestrogens begin to rise. These hormonal events correspond to the phase of follicular development in the ovary, and of repair and proliferation in the endometrium. By mid-cycle the oestrogens have reached a peak and there is then a sudden and abrupt surge of gonadotrophin secretion, the LH level exceeding that of FSH. This mid-cycle LH peak is one of the most characteristic features of the normal menstrual cycle, and the other events of the cycle are often timed relative to it. Clinically, these events are normally timed from the first day of menstrual bleeding, as this is a readily identifiable occurrence. However, from an endocrinological viewpoint it is more apposite to take the day of the LH peak as day 0, and count the days backwards (with a negative sign) and forwards (with a positive sign) from that, as in Fig. 3.

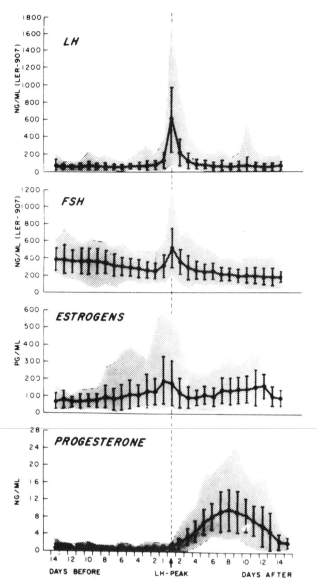

Fig. 3 Changes in key hormone levels in the plasma during a normal menstrual cycle. The data represent the mean, standard deviation and full range of values seen (shaded area) in 40 normal menstrual cycles. From Dyrenforth et al.[10]

The LH surge is believed to be triggered by the preceding oestrogen rise. It is more or less synchronous with ovulation. At the time of the LH peak oestrogens fall, and this decline may persist for a day or two, to be followed by a second rise. Coincident with this second rise of the oestrogen, there is a marked rise in the progesterone level, both these steroids being the product of the growing corpus luteum, their increased secretion corresponding to the secretory phase of the endometrial cycle. The gonadotrophins fall abruptly after the mid-cycle

surge. Towards the end of the fourth week of the cycle both oestrogens and progesterone fall as the corpus luteum regresses, and this fall leads to the onset of menstrual bleeding.

For practical purposes it is not necessary to study every hormone, still less every hormone every day, in order to diagnose most menstrual abnormalities. To determine whether a cycle is ovulatory two or more blood samples may be taken at intervals during the latter half and analysed for progesterone. If the level of any one of them is more than 5 ng/ml the presence of a corpus luteum is indicated and this is presumptive evidence of ovulation. Failure of the progesterone to reach this level suggests failure of ovulation.

The centre controlling the menstrual rhythm is believed to lie in the hypothalamus, and the stimulus to gonadotrophin secretion is passed to the anterior pituitary by hypophysiotrophic hormones which are secreted by nerve endings from cells arising in hypothalamic nuclei. At present there is believed to be only one gonadotrophin releasing hormone, a decapeptide, which regulates the secretion of both gonadotrophins. The property of the female hypothalamus to 'cycle', i.e. to stimulate a rhythmic secretion of gonadotrophins, is a major difference between the central nervous system of the sexes, and results in the overall lifetime pattern of their gonadotrophin secretion being different (Figs. 4 and 5).

There are confused and contradictory reports about whether, in adults, there is a circadian rhythm of gonadotrophins, as well as a menstrual rhythm. It is agreed, however, that the secretion of these hor-

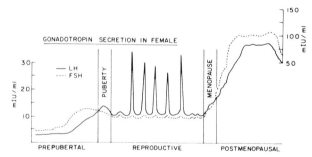

Fig. 4 The life cycle of gonadotrophin secretion in the human female, represented diagrammatically, showing how the secretory pattern falls into three distinct phases. From Yen et al.[11]

mones occurs in episodic bursts, following the pulsatile release of hypothalamic gonadotrophin releasing hormone (GnRH or LHRH), and 20 min sampling reveals marked fluctuations of the level. During puberty, but not adult life or childhood, a regular pattern does appear in the daily secretion of gonadotrophins. Then, a direct association appears between sleep and augmented bursts of secretion: plasma levels are thus appreciably higher during the night than during the day in adolescents of both sexes (Fig. 6). This relationship between sleep and

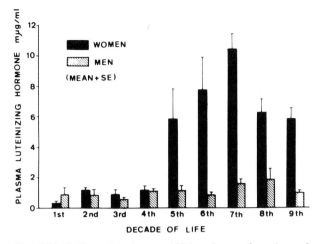

Fig. 5 Variations in plasma LH level as a function of age. Between five and twelve normal subjects were studied in each group. The marked difference in LH secretion during the lifetime of males and females is apparent. From Vermeulen et al.[12]

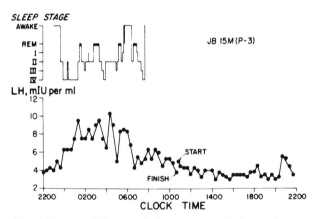

Fig. 6 Plasma LH sampled every 20 min for 24 h in a 15-year-old boy. The episodic secretion of the hormone is apparent, as is the nocturnal rise which is characteristic of puberty. The top part of the illustration is a sleep histogram recording the stages of electroencephalographically defined sleep. The peaks of LH appear to coincide with 'slow-wave', i.e. stage III and IV, sleep. From Weitzman and Hellman.[14]

hormone secretion has been recognized with other pituitary hormones in addition to the gonadotrophins, as will be discussed later.

Circadian Hormonal Rhythms

The best known and most widely studied human circadian rhythm is that of the activity of the adrenal cortex. This was first observed over 30 years ago by Pincus,[13] who found that the urinary excretion of 17 oxo-steroids was uniformly lower at night than during the day. The circadian rhythm of adrenal activity has subsequently been confirmed many times, and is apparent if either plasma or urinary coticosteroids are measured. In people maintaining normal life patterns, i.e. sleeping at night and being active during

the day, the plasma cortisol reaches a peak of about 15–25 μg/100 ml (c. 420–700 nmol/l) between 0600 and 0800 h and falls to less than 7 μg/100 ml (195 nmol/l) at around midnight. The plasma corticosterone and aldosterone levels follow a similar rhythm at much lower concentrations, although the level of aldosterone is influenced by a number of other variables, notably sodium and potassium intake and posture.

Early studies showed the circadian rhythm of plasma cortisol to have remarkable regularity, both from subject to subject and from time to time in the same subject. However, these studies all employed relatively infrequent sampling; perhaps every four hours or so (Fig. 7). In recent years very frequent sampling (several times per hour) has been employed in rhythm studies and has revealed that cortisol is secreted episodically (Fig. 8). The circadian variation

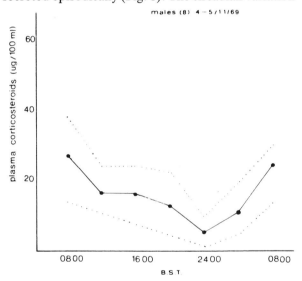

Fig. 7 Plasma corticosteroid levels in 8 healthy males sampled every four hours throughout the 24. Mean and range are shown. From Daly.[15]

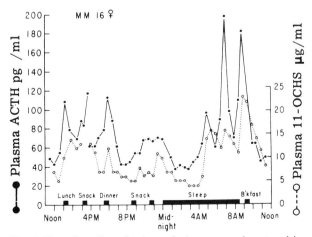

Fig. 8 The circadian rhythm of plasma corticosteroids and ACTH in a young healthy female. The episodic nature of the secretion is apparent. From Krieger et al.[16]

in the mean plasma cortisol level appears to be determined by the number and duration of these secretory episodes and the manner in which they are clustered throughout the 24 h. It has been estimated that there are about twelve of these episodes during each 24 h, and that most of them occur during the latter part of the night. About half of the total cortisol secreted during the 24 h is produced during that period.

There is some evidence that the adrenal cortex varies throughout the 24 h in its sensitivity to corticotrophin (ACTH), and also that there may be variations in the metabolic clearance rate of cortisol. It is clear, however, that the circadian variations in the secretion of cortisol conform to a similar pattern to that of the secretion of ACTH from the anterior pituitary, and that the variation in cortisol secretion is in response to this (Fig. 8). ACTH secretion in

which is the major, although probably not the sole, synchronizer of the HPA circadian rhythm. Secretion of cortisol is virtually zero at about the time of onset of sleep and for 2 to 4 h thereafter. From mid-sleep onwards there are increasingly frequent and prolonged bursts of secretory activity, bringing about the peak level of plasma cortisol at, or shortly after, the time of awakening. Nevertheless, the HPA circadian mechanism is not directly linked to the neurological changes of sleep for the pattern of the rhythm is maintained if the subject stays awake all night (Fig. 10), and readjustment of the rhythm following sleep-reversal (e.g. brought about by rapid east–west air travel across a number of time zones) takes several days. More recent evidence also suggests that bright light is a strong synchronizer of the HPA axis. The pattern may sometimes be altered in the blind,

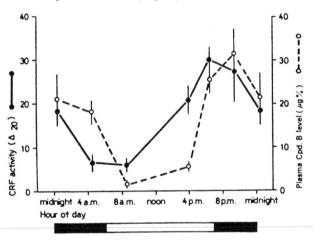

Fig. 9 The circadian rhythm of plasma corticosteroids and hypothalamic CRF activity in the rat. The corticosteroid level follows a similar pattern to that of CRF, with some delay. The rat, being a nocturnal animal, has a circadian rhythm of the HPA axis almost exactly 12 h out of phase with that of man. From Hiroshige and Sakakura.[17]

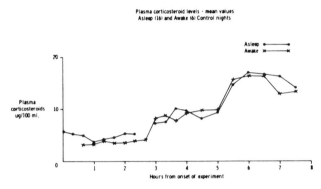

Fig. 10 The rise in plasma corticosteroids throughout the night. The experiments in each case began at about 2300 h. The data represent the mean of 16 nights during which the subjects slept and of 6 nights during which they remained awake. The graphs are almost superimposable, indicating that the circadian rise in cortisol is not directly related to sleep.

its turn is probably dependent upon stimulation by corticotrophin releasing factor (CRF) from the hypothalamus, and it has been shown in experimental animals that there is a circadian rhythm in the CRF content of the hypothalamus (Fig. 9). Thus, the ultimate stimulus for the cortisol circadian rhythm lies in the central nervous system.

A large number of studies has been carried out in order to determine whether the rhythm of the HPA axis is synchronized by a regular environmental variable. These studies have included investigation of the circadian rhythms of blind individuals, night workers, volunteers isolated in caves who have been exposed to continuous light or continuous darkness, or who have had their sleep/wake cycle altered or reversed. The principal conclusion revealed by these studies is the amazing things that people will put up with in the interest of science. However, the results also suggest that it is the alternation of sleep and wakefulness

appearing to 'free run' with a period slightly different from 24 h.

The indirectness of the relationship of the HPA circadian rhythm to sleep contrasts interestingly with the rhythm of growth hormone secretion. In normal people there is a significant rise in the level of circulating growth hormone (GH) during early nocturnal sleep. Frequent sampling throughout EEG-monitored sleep has shown that this GH peak is associated with stages 3 and 4 of slow-wave sleep as defined electroencephalographically; in other words, with 'deep' sleep (Fig. 11). This relationship between GH secretion and slow-wave sleep is a close one, and if the subject is kept awake the GH peak does not occur (Fig. 12). Similarly, if sleep onset is delayed the GH peak will also be delayed, occurring when the subject reaches stage 3 or 4 sleep. Following travel across time zones the GH peak appears normally as soon as the subject enters slow-wave sleep.

The circadian rhythm of the plasma cortisol is ultimately regulated by the CNS and lesions in the suprachiasmatic nucleus of the hypothalamus have been reported to abolish it. Furthermore, patients with an altered state of consciousness or a disturbed sleep pattern may have an altered rhythm, and it is therefore seen in certain psychiatric diseases, notably depression.

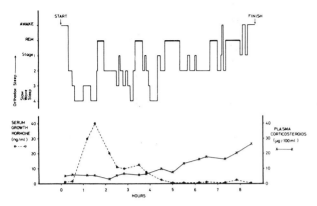

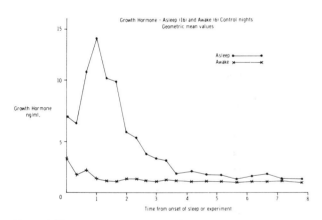

Fig. 11 GH and corticosteroid rise during sleep. The rise in GH occurs early in sleep when, as shown by the sleep histogram, 'slow-wave' sleep predominates; the rise in cortisol occurs late, when REM sleep is prominent.

Fig. 12 The nocturnal rise in GH. The data represent the mean of 16 nights asleep and 6 nights awake. Unlike the cortisol (Fig. 10) the GH peak is entirely abolished if the subject stays awake.

Disturbances of the rhythm may also occur in less specific situations. Any acute illness, particularly if accompanied by pain or fever, and also trauma or major surgery, may cause stress activation of the HPA axis, and this may over-ride the circadian rhythm.

In none of these instances is the alteration of the circadian rhythm of plasma cortisol sufficiently specific a change to be of any diagnostic assistance. However, the possibility that a non-specific factor of this type is present must always be borne in mind when the plasma cortisol is being assessed in the diagnosis of Cushing's syndrome, which is the only pathological state in which loss of the circadian rhythm of cortisol is of specific diagnostic importance. This is the case whether the Cushing's syndrome be due to adrenal

hyperplasia consequent upon hypothalamo-pituitary overdrive or the ectopic ACTH syndrome, or to a tumour of the adrenal leading to autonomous cortisol secretion.

It is frequently the case that the plasma cortisol is estimated only at 0900 h and midnight as a test of the circadian rhythm in the diagnosis of Cushing's syndrome. If the midnight level is high and the points mentioned above about non-specific loss of the rhythm are borne in mind, then this may be of considerable diagnostic help. However, it is important

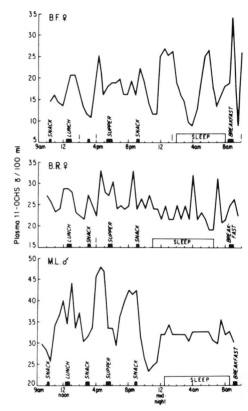

Fig. 13 The oscillations in plasma corticosteroids in three cases of Cushing's syndrome. The circadian rhythm is lost, but there are apparently random fluctuations of wide amplitude. From Krieger et al.[16]

to realise that the episodic secretion of cortisol is maintained in Cushing's syndrome (Fig. 13). The amplitude of each secretory episode is greater than normal, and the troughs may bring the cortisol level into the normal range. As the secretory episodes apparently occur randomly in this disease it does not require a remarkable coincidence for a morning and midnight sample to show a spurious circadian rhythm.

The author recently investigated a proven case of Cushing's syndrome due to a benign adrenal adenoma, in whom on two consecutive days the morning plasma cortisols were 18 and 16 μg/100 ml (500 and 440 nmol/l), and the midnight levels 7·5 and 3·0 μg/100 ml (210 and 80 nmol/l). This was shown not to be a 'true' circadian rhythm, indeed the plasma cortisol level did not respond to exogenous ACTH nor did the morning value suppress after dexamethasone, thus showing the adenoma was independent of pituitary control and hence 'disconnected' from the circadian 'clock'. The diagnosis of Cushing's syndrome should therefore never be excluded on the basis of an apparently normal circadian rhythm revealed by only two samples, and results of a rhythm study should be considered in conjunction with those of other investigations such as dexamethasone suppression.

Circadian Variation in Response to Adrenal Function Tests

Not only does the secretion of cortisol show a circadian rhythm itself, but there is a circadian variation in the response of the HPA axis to a number of clinically useful function tests.

Infusion of the 11β-hydroxylase inhibitor, metyrapone, between 0600 and 1200 h is followed by a prompt rise in urinary 11-desoxycortisol, indicating a brisk response of ACTH secretion to the decline in circulating cortisol caused by the metyrapone. Infusion of a similar dose during the afternoon produces a smaller and slower response, suggesting the feedback stimulus to the hypothalamus and pituitary, effected by a lowered plasma cortisol, is greater in the morning when the level is usually high, than in the afternoon, when it is lower.

Similarly, there is a rhythmic variation in the feedback responsiveness of the hypothalamus-pituitary to increased levels of circulating corticosteroids. Dexamethasone in an oral dose of 0·5 mg at 0800 or 1600 h causes only brief suppression of cortisol secretion, whereas the same dose given at midnight produces marked suppression for 24 h. This variability is made use of in the 'one-dose' dexamethasone suppression test used in the diagnosis of Cushing's syndrome. Dexamethasone, in a dose of 1 mg, is administered orally at or about midnight and this, in a healthy subject, will result in suppression of the normal peak of plasma cortisol the following morning. In Cushing's syndrome the suppression does not occur.

Sleep Related Hormone Secretion

The fact that LH in adolescents and GH are secreted in close association with certain neurological events related to sleep has already been mentioned. The sleep associated secretion of GH has been used in the diagnosis of dwarfism. A blood sample is taken 60–90 min after the patient has been observed to go to sleep, and, if the level is 10 ng/ml or more, GH deficiency is excluded. A lower level is not diagnostic of GH deficiency, however, but indicates the need for further testing.

Prolactin is another pituitary hormone which shows rhythmic secretion (Fig. 14), its highest levels

occurring in association with sleep, but this observation has not so far been put to diagnostic use.

Finally, it has also been shown that the plasma testosterone level is high in the early hours of the morning, and it has been suggested that this is

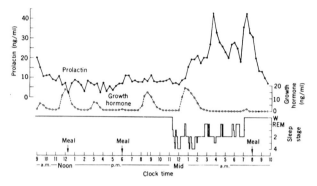

Fig. 14 The 24 h patterns of GH and prolactin secretion and their relationship to sleep in a healthy 23-year-old male. From Sassin et al.[18]

associated with periods of REM sleep, which predominate in the latter half of the night. There has been some disagreement about whether there is a true circadian rhythm of testosterone, but the consensus of opinion is that one does occur, which is similar to that of cortisol (Fig. 15).

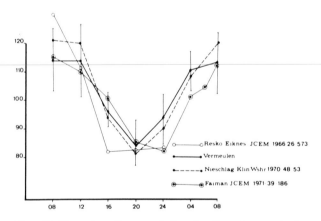

Fig. 15 The circadian variation in the plasma testosterone level in normal males derived from the work of several authors. The data are expressed as percentage deviation from the mean level (100%). From Vermeulen et al.[12]

Thyroxine and TSH

Frequent plasma sampling has revealed that there are acute fluctuations in the levels of both thyroxine and TSH in normal subjects. No clear circadian rhythm has been demonstrated for thyroxine, and there is a conflict of opinion as to whether such a rhythm exists in TSH secretion. The size of fluctuations in thyroxine level vary from subject to subject, but in some individuals may cover the whole of the normal range, the lowest values being around

4 µg/100 ml (about 50 nm/l) and the highest 10 µg/100 ml (about 125 nm/l) in the course of a single day. The values, however, fluctuate around a mean which remains fairly constant throughout the 24 h, although there is a tendency for them to be higher at night.

Melatonin and the Pineal Gland

Probably the most robust and high-amplitude circadian rhythm is that of the pineal hormone melatonin. Although it is not yet of diagnostic importance, except possibly in the case of pineal tumours, it is likely to prove useful in the assessment of rhythm disorders. Furthermore, it has therapeutic potential in the rapid resynchronization of disturbed rhythms.

Virtually all melatonin production occurs at night in a normal environment (Fig. 16). The pineal is the major source of circulating melatonin. The rhythm of production is generated in the suprachiasmatic nucleus (SCN) and entrained by the light–dark cycle. The neural pathway from the SCN to the pineal passes via the superior cervical ganglion, terminating in noradrenergic α- and β-receptors on the pinealocyte. Adrenergic stimulation at night leads to a 30 to 70-fold increase in the activity of the rate-limiting enzyme in melatonin synthesis, serotonin *N*-acetyltransferase, and production of melatonin itself.

In animals melatonin is a photoperiodic messenger molecule, i.e. it transmits information about the length of light and darkness. It enables photoperiod-dependent species to time their seasonal activity (e.g. reproduction) to an appropriate time of year. In some species it is intimately concerned with the organization of the circadian system, and this may well also be true in humans.

The circadian rhythm of melatonin is highly endogenous, robust, and resistant to minor metabolic variations and stress. It is thus ideally suited to be a marker of rhythm disturbance, and of the human response to zeitgebers such as bright light. Radioimmunoassays exist for the measurement of both melatonin and its principal metabolite 6-hydroxy melatonin sulphate: the latter has the advantage of being easily measurable in urine,[19] thus opening the way to extensive clinical investigations.

Early studies suggest that melatonin production is modified in affective disease, insomnia, and a number of other CNS-related pathologies. A possible causal relationship of melatonin production to pubertal development has been postulated. In old age the amplitude of its secretory rhythm is drastically reduced and may be related to the circadian disturbances found in the elderly. At present its secretion is being used to 'phase-type' disturbed rhythms in depressive illness as a guide to possible treatment.

The most interesting aspect of the pineal, however, is the apparent ability of melatonin in small, but pharmacological, doses to entrain rest–activity (wake–sleep) cycles and to alleviate jet-lag.[7] Although it has proved difficult to demonstrate an essential role for the pineal in man, these effects of melatonin on the biological clock do suggest that the pineal plays a central role in circadian organization in humans. Moreover, the resynchronizing ability of this mysterious hormone should also prove of considerable importance in shift-work, affective disease, old-age, insomnia and to the military.

Non-hormonal Circadian Rhythms

It will be clear from previous sections that rhythmicity forms an integral part of the secretory mechanism of many hormones. Plasma levels of the more commonly measured substances other than hormones, however, show little evidence of distinct periodicity.

Plasma Inorganic Phosphorus. This is perhaps the substance with the most distinct circadian rhythm. Here the rhythm is defined most clearly by the minimum level rather than by a peak. The minimum occurs shortly before noon, and thereafter the level tends to rise throughout the day, but with no clear peak. The amplitude of the variation can be quite marked, however, with levels sometimes oscillating

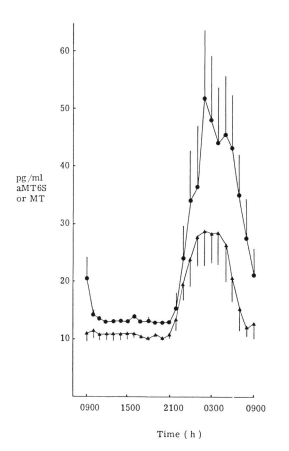

Fig. 16 aMT6S (●——●) and melatonin (▲——▲) plasma levels in 9 subjects (7M, 2F) sampled hourly over 24 hours ($\bar{X}$ + SEM, pg/ml).

throughout the whole of the 'normal range', from about 2·5 to 4·5 ml (0·8–1·5 mmol/l).

Plasma Sodium, Potassium, Calcium, Magnesium and Chloride. These substances show small and irregular oscillations throughout the 24 h. Some workers have reported a regular rhythm of some of these (Fig. 17), but there is not universal agreement on this, and the amplitude of the oscillations is usually so small as to approach the limit of discrimination of

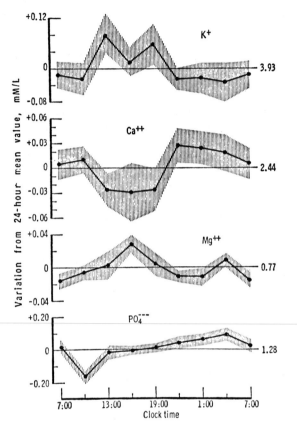

Fig. 17 Variations in plasma calcium, potassium, magnesium and phosphate in 12 healthy subjects (mean ± SD). From Wesson.[21]

standard analytical methods. The potassium level tends to fall following a meal, presumably consequent upon the rise in plasma insulin, and the calcium level falls during recumbency (Fig. 17).

Plasma Protein. Concentrations of plasma protein are lower at night than during the day, but this appears to be a consequence of changes in posture rather than a true circadian rhythm (Figs. 18, 19). As about 50% of circulating calcium is bound to plasma protein the postural changes seen in its level are presumably secondary to those in the protein level. However, the lowest level of plasma calcium does not appear to be during the night (Fig. 17) so other factors must influence it besides postural variations in protein concentration.

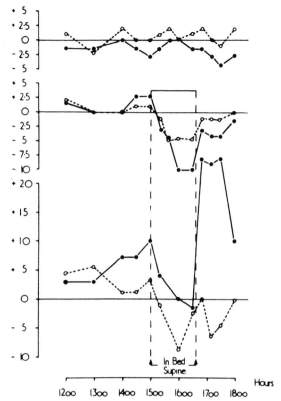

Fig. 18 Changes in plasma calcium (---○---○---) and protein (●——●——●) due to recumbency in two subjects. The top graph represents a control subject who remained sitting or standing. The data are plotted as percentage deviation from the mean value. From Pollard.[20]

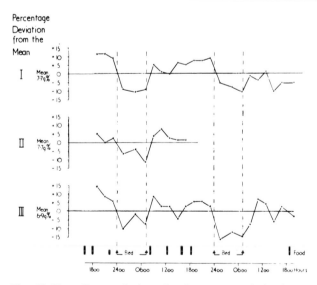

Fig. 19 Circadian variations in plasma protein in three healthy subjects. From Pollard.[20]

Rhythms in Urinary Excretion

It is a matter of universal experience that normal people have a diminished rate of urinary flow at night. Although it might reasonably be supposed that this is due to a diminished fluid intake, experiments carried out nearly a century ago showed that, even when fluid intake is evenly spread throughout the 24 h, urine flow falls during sleep. Paradoxically, recumbency of itself *increases* urine flow.

Excretion of both water and solutes does not normally follow intake closely, but varies cyclically so that at times excretion exceeds intake and at times falls below it. These cyclical variations usually persist even if intake of the substance being investigated is held constant throughout 24 h.

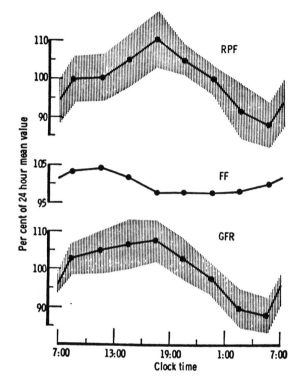

Fig. 20 Circadian rhythm of glomerular filtration rate (GFR), effective renal plasma flow (RPF) and filtration fraction (FF). Mean ± SD of 12 healthy subjects. From Wesson.[21]

The glomerular filtration rate (GFR) and effective renal plasma flow (RPF) show very clear circadian rhythms, the most distinctive feature of which is a nadir in both, occurring between 0400 and 0600 h (Fig. 20), which follows a gradual decline throughout the evening.

Creatinine also shows a low amplitude circadian rhythm in its rate of excretion which, not surprisingly, parallels that of the GFR, with a minimum in the early hours of the morning, and a peak about mid-afternoon. The amplitude in normal subjects does not usually exceed ± 10%. It is important to bear this variation in mind despite its small amplitude when relating the urinary excretion of some substances to that of creatinine. This is a technique commonly used to quantify urinary excretion without the inconvenience and potential errors involved in collecting 24 h urine samples. The urinary 'substance'/creatinine ratio may give a perfectly valid estimate of the total amount of the substance excreted during 24 h, provided its excretion does not vary significantly throughout the 24 h, or varies in parallel with creatinine. If, however, the variations are opposite in phase to those of creatinine the method may give rise to misleading results.

It is perhaps worth pointing out that there are considerable day-to-day variations in the urine creatinine content and that its use as an index of completeness of 24 h urine collections, still widely practised, may be misleading.

Creatine shows a low amplitude rhythm, similar to that of creatinine, with highest excretion during the day.

Sodium and chloride excretion in normal subjects shows a peak at about mid-day, or somewhat earlier, and has a nadir shortly before waking, i.e. corresponding approximately both to the minimum of GFR, and also, perhaps significantly, to the circadian rise in corticosteroids. This rhythm of sodium and chloride excretion appears to be independent both of salt intake and time of feeding, in that it persists during fasting, during precisely regular feeding, and on diets of either high or low sodium content. However, the rhythm may be lost, or apparently reversed, during cardiac, hepatic, or cerebral disease.

The rhythm of **potassium** excretion is similar to that of sodium and chloride. There appears little doubt that the circadian rhythm of adrenocortical activity is essential for the normal rhythm of potassium excretion, although other factors may disturb it even though the adrenal rhythm remains normal. Pathological conditions which alter the adrenal rhythm alter the rhythm of potassium excretion, and following shifts of the sleep–wake schedule, such as may occur in rapid travel across time zones, the rhythm of potassium excretion settles into the new phase at about the same time as the plasma cortisol. The relation of sodium and chloride excretion to the adrenal rhythm is not quite so well defined, but is disturbed in Addison's disease, Cushing's syndrome, primary aldosteronism and high-dosage corticosteroid therapy.

Calcium excretion also appears similar in phase to that of sodium and chloride.

Acid and ammonium excretion is high at night and falls in the morning, and this appears to be the case whether the subject be asleep or awake, recumbent or active. There appears to be a definite inverse correlation between the excretion of hydrogen ion and that of potassium.

Phosphate excretion roughly parallels that of hydrogen ion, being greatest at night and lowest late in the morning.

CONCLUSION

Circadian rhythms occur not only in the plasma and urine levels of biochemical substances but also in various physiological and psychological functions. Many of these have been studied in detail, not merely because of their intrinsic interest, but because unpleasant symptoms and impaired functional efficiency may occur when circumstances result in dissociation of a biological rhythm from its environmental synchronizer. Such dissociation occurs most commonly as a result of rapid east–west travel, giving rise to a condition popularly known as 'jet-lag'. It is therefore clearly of importance to those concerned with the competence of air-crew. Despite much research, however, few clear correlations between circadian rhythms and functional disturbances have emerged. Neither are there any definite symptoms consequent upon alteration in biochemical rhythms, other than the obvious inconvenience occasioned by increased urinary flow at night. Thus, although the suggestion that circadian rhythms 'enable the organism to do the right thing at the right time' by anticipating environmental changes is a highly plausible one, it is not at present clear, at least in the case of biochemical rhythms, what they enable the organism to do, or how they help it to do it.

Nevertheless, even if they cause no well-defined symptomatology, disturbed circadian rhythms, may be a diagnostically helpful sign of disease. This is particularly the case in endocrine disease, as has been described. Outside the field of endocrinology, however, the investigation of circadian rhythms has so far produced little of diagnostic help. The main concern of the clinical biochemist with such rhythms must be to bear them in mind when following results from day to day in an individual patient. Where the amplitude of the oscillation is wide compared to the extent of the normal range, as in plasma inorganic phosphate for instance, he must ensure that samples are taken at the same time each day. In general, it should be the rule that all samples be marked with the time (using the 24 h clock) at which they are taken as well as with the date.

The hormonal rhythms of the menstrual cycle are more clearly related to function, and disturbances of the rhythms may lead to obvious problems such as clinical menstrual disorders or infertility.

REFERENCES

1. Fort A., Mills J. N. (1970). Fitting sine curves to 24 h urinary data. *Nature*; **226**: 657.
2. Wever R. A. (1979). *The Circadian System of Man: Results of Experiments under Temporal Isolation*. New York: Springer Verlag.
3. Rusak B., Zucker I. (1979). Neural regulation of circadian rhythms. *Physiol. Rev*; **59**: 449.
4. Lewy A. J., Wehr T. A., Goodwin F. K., Newsome D. A., Markey S. P. (1980). 'Light suppresses melatonin secretion in humans', *Science*; **210**: 1267.
5. Wever R. A., Polasek J., Wildgruber C. M. (1983). Bright light affects human circadian rhythms. *Pflügers Archiv*; **396**: 85.
6. Arendt J., Marks V. (1982). Physiological changes under-lying jet-lag. *Br. Med. J*; **284**: 144.
7. Arendt J., Aldhous M., Marks V. (1986). Alleviation of 'jet-lag' by melatonin: preliminary results of a controlled double-blind trial. *Br. Med. J*; **292**: 1170.
8. Aschoff J. (1965). *Science, NY*; **148**: 1427.
9. Sollberger A. (1969). Circadian rhythms. *Exp. Med. Sur*; **27**: 80.
10. Dyrenforth I., Jewelewicz M., Warren M., Ferin M., Van de Wiele R. L. (1974). Temporal relationships of hormonal variables in the menstrual cycle'. In *Biorhythms in Human Reproduction* (Ferin M., Halberg F., Richart R. M., Van de Wiele R. C., eds) pp. 171–201. New York: John Wiley.
11. Yen S. S. C., Vandenburg G., Tsai C. C., Siler T. (1974). Causal relationship between the hormonal variables in the menstrual cycle. In *Biorhythms in Human Reproduction* (Ferin M., Halberg F., Richart R. M., Van de Wiele R. C. eds) pp. 427–45. New York: John Wiley.
12. Vermeulen A., Verdonck L., Comhaire F. (1974). Rhythms of the male hypothalamo-pituitary-testicular axis. In *Biorhythms in Human Reproduction* (Ferin M., Halberg F., Richart R. M., Van de Wiele R. C., eds) pp. 427–45. New York: John Wiley.
13. Pincus G. (1943). A diurnal rhythm in the excretion of urinary ketosteroids by young men. *J. Clin. Endocrinol*; **3**: 195.
14. Weitzman E. D., Hellman L. (1974). Temporal organisation of the 24 h pattern of the hypothalamic-pituitary axis. In *Biorhythms in Human Reproduction* (Ferin M., Halberg F., Richart R. M., Van de Wiele R. C., eds) pp. 371–95. New York: John Wiley.
15. Daly J. R. (1970). The effect of time zone displacement on the circadian rhythm of plasma corticosteroids. *Clin. Trials J*; **7**: 56.
16. Krieger D. T., Allen W., Rizzo F., Krieger H. P. (1971). Characterisation of the normal temporal pattern of plasma corticosteroid levels. *J. Clin. Endocrinol. Metab*; **32**: 266.
17. Hiroshige T., Sakakura M. (1971). Circadian rhythm of corticotropin-releasing activity in the hypothalamus of normal and adrenalectomised rats. *Neuroendocrinology*; **7**: 25.
18. Sassin J. F., Frantz A. G., Weitzman E. D., Kapen S. (1972). Human prolactin: 24 h pattern with increased release during sleep. *Science*; **177**: 1205.
19. Arendt J., Bojkowski C., Franey C., Wright J., Marks V. (1985). Immunoassay of 6-hydroxymelatonin sulfate in human plasma and urine: abolition of the urinary 24-hour rhythm with atenolol. *J. Clin. Endocrinol. Metab*; **60**: 116.
20. Pollard A. C. (1964). The quantitative changes which occur throughout the day in some commonly determined plasma constituents. *Technicon International Symposium*, London.
21. Wesson L. G., jr. (1964). Electrolyte excretion in relation to diurnal cycles of renal function. *Medicine*; **43**: 547.

FURTHER READING

The following symposia and reviews are recommended for those wishing to obtain further details.

Aschoff J. (1976). Circadian systems in man and their implications. *Hosp. Pract*; **11**: 51.

Colquhoun W. P. (ed.) (1971). *Biological Rhythms and Human Performance*. New York and London: Academic Press. *Contains much information on non-biochemical rhythms.*

Daly J. R., Evans, J. I. (1974). Daily rhythms of steroid and associated pituitary hormones in man and their relationship to sleep. *Advances in Steroid Biochemistry and Pharmacology* (Briggs M. H., Christie G. A. eds), Vol. 4, London and New York: Academic Press.

Ferin M., Halberg F., Richart R. M., Van de Wiele R. L. (eds) (1974). *Biorhythms and Human Reproduction*. New York: John Wiley.

Krieger D. T. (ed.) (1979). *Endocrine Rhythms*. New York: Raven Press.

Minors D. S., Waterhouse J. M. (1981). *Circadian Rhythms and the Human*. Wright, P. S. G., Bristol, pp. 143–8.

Moore-Ede M. C., Czeisler C. A., Richardson G. S. (1983). Circadian timekeeping in health and disease, Part 1, Basic properties of circadian pacemakers. *New Engl. J. Med*; **309**: 469.

Moore-Ede M. C., Czeizler C. A., Richardson G. S. (1983). Circadian time-keeping in health and disease, Part 2, Clinical implications of circadian rhythmicity. *New Engl. J. Med*; **309**: 530.

8. Reference Values and the Concept of Normality

G. S. Challand

Introduction
   Development of concept of normal range
   Statistics of normality
Laboratory factors influencing results
   Collection, transport and storage of specimens
   Imprecision of analysis
   Laboratory (and clinical) mistakes
Biological factors influencing result distribution
   Intra-individual factors
   Interindividual factors
Reference values
Interpretation of results

INTRODUCTION

Development of Concept of Normal Range

Two independent developments have contributed to the concept of the normal range in medicine: one linguistic; and one statistical. The word 'normal' was used in chemistry in 1857, and physics in 1859, to mean the average of observed quantities. By 1890 the term was used to mean the usual state or condition.[1] By 1896 the term 'normal range' was in common currency in medicine and required no explanation.[2] In 1931 Peters and Van Slyke[3] used 'normal values' to mean the total range of values obtained from healthy adults. In 1946 King[4] defined 'normal value' as 'the amount of a constituent present in ... a healthy human being' but stated that some healthy individuals showed divergent figures. He therefore defined the normal range as the range of values encompassing 80% of the normal values. In

1964 Henry[5] defined the normal range as that which included 95% of values from healthy human beings. He also pointed out the influence of sample size on a measured normal range, and suggested that a correction should be used based on this. By 1976 the definition had been modified to 'the concentrations of the constituent ... in ... clinically normal (apparently healthy) persons'.[6] A minimum sample size of 100 was suggested, but the normal range was still 'the interval into which the central 95% of the apparently healthy persons fall'.

From a statistical viewpoint, the original Gaussian (also called normal, Gaussian normal, error, or Gaussian error) curve is commonly associated with Karl Friedrich Gauss, who derived it in a study of errors of measurement. However, similar curves had been derived a century earlier by de Moivre in connection with probability theory. The Gaussian curve extends to infinity in both directions, but has the property that most values lie close to its centre. Thus, 68·1% of values lie within 1 SD of the mean, 95·4% lie within 2 SD, 99·7% lie within 3 SD, and 99·99% lie within 4 SD.

There is no theoretical reason why the distribution of any analyte should follow a Gaussian curve, and Reed and co-workers,[7] among others, have shown how estimates of the normal range are affected by this assumption.

Statistics of Normality

The measured distribution of any analyte is the result of two main factors. Biological variation itself is unlikely to give rise to a distribution which is exactly Gaussian; but it frequently gives rise to a distribution in which most values lie close to the mean. When an analyte is measured, superimposed upon biological variation is analytical error. This may well follow a Gaussian curve, but if an occasional random error occurs, more values may fall in the tails of the distribution than would be expected by chance. The combination of biological variation and analytical error therefore frequently gives rise to a distribution which is or can be transformed to a distribution not significantly different from a Gaussian curve (*see* Fig. 1).

When a normal range is derived, the common practice is to measure an analyte in a large number of apparently healthy people, and to check that the distribution of values is not significantly different from Gaussian. The mean and SD are calculated, and the

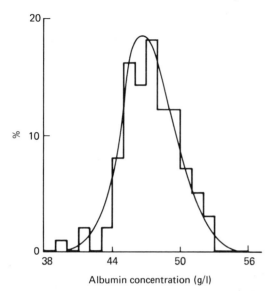

Fig. 1 The distribution of serum albumin values in 100 healthy blood donors.

limits of the normal range are derived as the mean plus or minus 2 SD. It is accepted that this is likely to exclude 4·6% of normal values. The reasons for this exclusion may be summarized as:

1. Biological variation may on occasion give rise to an extreme value;
2. Analytical or other error may give rise to an extreme value;
3. There may be a hidden (or sub-clinical) pathological cause affecting the analyte in a small proportion of apparently healthy people.

There is of course no reason for these factors to affect exactly 4·6% of the population. Although it may be justifiable to exclude some values from a distribution because of a hidden pathological cause, the extremes of biological variation and analytical error inevitably mean that some healthy people will yield results outside the normal range defined in this way. If a normal range is used to distinguish between health and a given disease, two factors affect the decision on where the limits of the normal range should be placed. The first is the degree of overlap between the distributions of results characteristic of health, and of results characteristic of disease. The second is the prevalence of the disease.

For a diagnostic measurement such as the concentration of thyrotropin in serum (TSH, Fig. 2), there is no significant overlap between values obtained

from healthy people, and values characteristic of primary hypothyroidism. Since few other pathological conditions cause TSH to rise, it is commonsense to include all of the values obtained from healthy people in the normal range, and indeed the upper limit of the normal range can be increased to some extent without weakening the diagnostic power of the test.

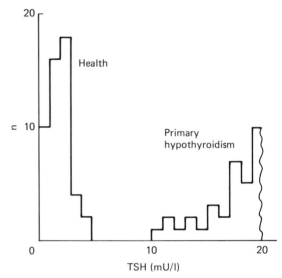

Fig. 2 The distributions of serum thyrotropin (TSH) values in healthy people and in patients with primary hypothyroidism.

For a measurement such as urea in plasma, the situation is different (Fig. 3). There is considerable overlap between the distributions from healthy people and those from people with renal disease. In addition, conditions unrelated to renal disease can increase plasma urea concentration. In this case, an

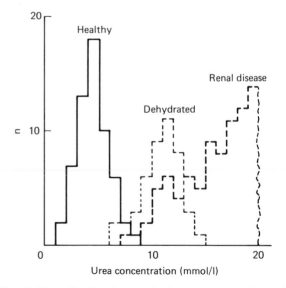

Fig. 3 The distributions of plasma urea values in healthy people, in dehydrated patients, and in patients with renal disease.

appropriate choice of where the upper limit of a normal range should be set can only be made if the relative prevalences of each condition are known, together with the consequences of generating either false positive or false negative results. This is because the relative numbers of false positive and false negative results are affected by the degree of overlap, by the prevalence of the condition, and by the upper

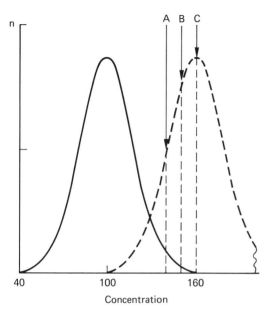

Fig. 4 Overlapping distributions in health and in disease.

limit of the normal range. Galen and Gambino[8] among others have rationalized concepts and definitions in this area.

To take a simple example, Fig. 4 shows overlapping distributions for a diagnostic test from healthy people and from people with a defined disease. The upper limit of the normal range can be set conventionally at A, the mean +2SD of results from the healthy population. Both false positive and false negative results will be produced. If set at C, virtually no false positives will be produced by the test, but half the people with the disease will be given results regarded as normal. B is a compromise between these. Table 1 shows the consequence of choosing A, B, or C as the prevalence of the disease changes. At an upper limit of the mean +2SD (A), the greater the proportion of false positives to true positives as the prevalence decreases. If the upper limit of the normal range is increased to minimize this effect, then the greater the proportion of false negatives to true negatives.

LABORATORY FACTORS INFLUENCING RESULTS

Collection, Transport, and Storage of Specimens

Poor venesection technique, and prolonged or inappropriate storage of samples before transport to a

TABLE 1
THE INTERACTION BETWEEN THE UPPER LIMIT OF THE NORMAL
RANGE AND DISEASE PREVALENCE

Take a hypothetical analyte with in healthy people, a Gaussian distribution with mean 100 and SD 20. In diseased people the distribution is Gaussian with mean 160 and SD 20. If the analyte is measured in 1000 people taken at random, the following results will be expected.

		Prevalence of disease					
		50%	10%	5%	1%	0·5%	0·1%
No. healthy		500	900	950	990	995	999
No. diseased		500	100	50	10	5	1
Upper limit of normal range							
	True +ve	418	84	42	8	4	1
+2 SD	False +ve	12	21	22	23	23	23
(140)	True −ve	488	879	928	967	972	976
	False −ve	82	16	8	2	1	0
	True +ve	327	65	33	7	3	1
+2·5 SD	False +ve	3	5	6	6	6	6
(150)	True −ve	497	895	944	984	989	993
	False −ve	173	35	17	3	2	0
	True +ve	250	50	25	5	2	0
+3 SD	False +ve	2	3	3	3	3	3
(160)	True −ve	498	897	947	987	992	996
	False −ve	250	50	25	5	3	1

laboratory, can markedly affect the concentration or activity of many analytes. It is unfortunate that in the majority of hospitals these factors are outside the control of the laboratory. However, laboratory staff should be involved in the education of nursing and junior medical staff, who often do not realise that for many analytes, transport of the sample to the laboratory takes considerably longer than its analysis.

Imprecision of Analysis

The imprecision of analysis affects directly the measured normal range: the larger the imprecision, the wider the normal range estimate. For some analytes, e.g. plasma potassium, analytical imprecision is much smaller than biological variation, so that changes in imprecision have little effect. For other analytes, e.g. plasma sodium, analytical imprecision is of similar magnitude to biological variation. For these analytes, an increase in imprecision significantly increases the proportion of results falling outside the normal range. In addition, a normal range derived in one laboratory is only transferable to another laboratory if both have identical bias and imprecision. This factor, rather than differences in populations, is likely to be the major factor causing different laboratories to produce slightly different normal ranges, although sample sizes and sampling error also make significant contributions.

Laboratory (and Clinical) Mistakes

Mistakes occur in all laboratory analyses. Some of these are outside the control of the laboratory, e.g. misidentification of patient; incorrect patient preparation; or sample contamination. Others may be due to the analysis, e.g. incorrect reagents; or to laboratory data handling, e.g. incorrect calculation of result. Early estimates of the incidence of mistakes were as high as 3%.[9] Advances in work simplification and in analytical and data handling automation have reduced this incidence, so that now it can be as small as 0·3%.[10] However, a blunder almost by definition is a sizeable error, and gives a misclassification of patient from normal to abnormal, or worse (and more difficult to detect) from abnormal to normal.

BIOLOGICAL FACTORS INFLUENCING RESULT DISTRIBUTION

The factors which can affect intra- and interindividual variation are summarized in Table 2. The relative effects of these can have significant consequences for

TABLE 2
FACTORS INFLUENCING BIOLOGICAL VARIATION

Diet	Age	Hormonal changes
Exercise	Sex	Physical size
Postural factors	Race	Environment
Temporal changes	Stress	Medication
Genetic differences	Pathology	

the estimation of the normal range.[11] However, some, e.g. diet, medication, and age, have significant effects both within and between individuals. Factors which are considered to affect intra-individual variation therefore tend to be short-term effects.

Intra-individual Factors

Diet. Food affects the concentration of many analytes in blood. Some post-prandial effects are well known and well described, e.g. rises in glucose and triglycerides. Diet may also have long-term effects, e.g. dietary iodide and blood thyroid hormone concentrations; vitamin D intake and serum alkaline phosphatase activity.

Postural Factors. A change in posture from a period of recumbency to an upright stance rapidly leads to haemoconcentration. This increases by up to 15% the plasma concentration of many proteins. Many small-molecular-size substances are to a greater or lesser extent bound to plasma proteins, e.g. calcium, iron, cortisol, and the total concentrations of these can also increase. This is probably the most important single reason why normal ranges determined on hospital in-patients are usually lower than normal ranges determined on ambulatory out-patients. It may also explain why some analytes, e.g. iron, can show a

diurnal variation even when there is no obvious hormonal or neuronal explanation for this.

Exercise. Exercise can have direct effects on the concentration of, for example, lactate, and on the activity of relatively muscle-specific enzymes such as creatine kinase. Exercise also increases the plasma concentration of hormones such as growth hormone, which in turn affect the circulating concentration of many intermediate metabolites.

Hormonal Factors. The most obvious hormonal changes which an individual is subject to are those occurring during the menstrual cycle; and those occurring at puberty and the menopause. In general, different normal values through the menstrual cycle have only been demonstrated for hormones themselves, such as progesterone and luteinizing hormone. It is likely that there are changes in many other analytes, caused by factors such as fluid retention.

Puberty is associated with changes in hormone concentrations, and also with changes in many other analytes such as serum alkaline phosphatase activity. At the menopause, the hormonal changes are such that a wide variety of blood analytes are affected: pituitary and steroid hormones; albumin and many other proteins; and many smaller molecules bound to plasma proteins.

Pregnancy. Pregnancy is of course a major cause of intra-individual variation. Most hormones are affected; pregnancy- and fetal-associated proteins appear in the maternal circulation; and the concentrations of most proteins and many smaller analytes are changed. Some of these changes are hormonally mediated, e.g. an increase in the concentration of thyroxine-binding globulin. For others the mechanism is not clear.

Temporal Changes. The temporal changes occurring in analytes have been reviewed by Simpson[12] among others. Many analytes show temporal changes. These vary from the short-term pulsatile release of many pituitary hormones such as adrenocorticotropin (ACTH); through the diurnal variation associated with cortisol; the monthly variation seen in some hormones in men as well as women; annual variation seen with androgens and cholecalciferol; and longer-term changes which may reflect an ageing process. Those occurring in the neonatal period are well documented;[13] others are less well so. The detection of small long-term changes in an individual is critically dependent upon the ability of a laboratory to maintain long-term accuracy despite changes in methodology and equipment.

Interindividual Factors

Sex. Sex-related steroid hormones obviously have different concentrations in males and females. Many other constituents also have marked sex differences: for example uric acid and calcium in young and middle-aged adults, and the concentrations of a range of plasma proteins.

Race, Diet, Environment and Genetic Factors. It is usually very difficult to separate out these different factors when different analyte concentrations are found in different groups. For example, the reason why many people of Asian origin living in the UK have a markedly raised serum amylase concentration is unknown. For some analytes there are quite well described dietary or environmental factors, e.g. iodide intake affecting thyroid hormone concentrations; vitamin D intake and exposure to sunlight affecting calcium homeostasis. Similarly, the difference in cholesterol concentrations found in different racial groups is probably due to diet or race rather than other environmental factors.

Physical Size. The physical size of an individual has little effect on the measured concentration of analytes. However, the total quantity of analytes in the body is related to body volume; and derived indices such as renal clearance are related to surface area. These therefore show a variation with physical size. Similarly, the 24-hour excretion of many analytes should show a variation with body size. This has not been demonstrated, presumably associated with the imprecision of collection of a 24-hour urine sample, and the day-to-day variation in excretion.

Medication. Drugs, and many other dietary factors such as alcohol or ascorbic acid, may affect the measured concentration of analytes in many different ways. They may induce an increased rate of synthesis or of breakdown of an analyte. They may give a similar analytical signal and thus increase the apparent concentration of an analyte. They may accelerate or inhibit the reaction of an analyte. They may influence the binding of an analyte to a circulating binding protein and thus influence its total concentration. For the clinical biochemist, the problem is even more complex, since metabolites or conjugates of the drug produced *in vivo* may be the active moieties. In general, these are not readily available for testing.

The amount of information about drug effects on laboratory tests is now very large: summarized information has been produced;[14] and much information is now available as computer databases.

REFERENCE VALUES

The normal range came into use as a convenient way of converting results on a continuous scale into two groups: one group of 'normal values'; and one or more groups characteristic of disease. As laboratory tests became more accurate, and as the practice of screening the apparently healthy population

increased, it became apparent to clinical biochemists that this simple concept needed some refinement. With better definition, more accurate information could be given to a clinician.

To standardize terminology and to provide a rational basis for interpretation of results, the International Federation of Clinical Chemistry has defined the following terms.

1. A *reference individual* is an individual selected using defined criteria.
2. A *reference population* consists of all possible reference individuals.
3. A *reference sample group* is an adequate number of reference individuals selected to represent the reference population.
4. A *reference value* is the value obtained by observation or measurement of a particular type of quantity on a reference individual.
5. A *reference distribution* is the distribution of reference values.
6. A *reference limit* is derived from the reference distribution and is used for descriptive purposes.
7. A *reference interval* is the interval between, and including, two reference limits.
8. An *observed value* is the value of a particular type of quantity, obtained by observation or measurement, to be compared with reference values, reference distributions, reference limits or reference intervals.

A subsequent series of recommendations of the International Federation of Clinical Chemistry have dealt with the selection and preparation of individuals for the production of reference values;[15] the control of analytical variation; the determination of reference limits;[16] and the presentation of observed values.[17]

These definitions and recommendations are undoubtedly an advance; and serve three main purposes.

1. They avoid all the connotations associated with the word 'normal'.
2. They provide a means of standardization for laboratories attempting to express values characteristic of health or disease.
3. Reference ranges can be derived in a uniform way for individuals characteristic of a defined disease state, as well as for those characteristic of a healthy population.

In practice, since these definitions and recommendations were produced, there has been little positive advance in the majority of hospitals and laboratories. The term 'reference range' is slowly gaining acceptance as an alternative to the term 'normal range'. Unfortunately many laboratories deriving reference ranges have used the same techniques with which they derived normal ranges, and have adhered to the old concepts. In medicine generally, the two terms are regarded as synonymous. There are several reasons for this:

1. It is very difficult to select reference sample groups which are characteristic of a reference population. 'Health' is more of a theoretical concept than a practical reality; diagnosis is in practice an art as well as a science; and it is seldom possible to find a reference individual suffering from a single definable disease at a defined state in its natural history.

2. Although many laboratories now have access to computers which are capable of building up data files on reference individuals, in practice it is difficult to retain enthusiasm in the laboratory long enough to build reasonably sized reference groups. The sampling error associated with the production of reference limits from small groups may be larger than the uncertainties introduced by calculating normal ranges from less well-defined, larger groups. In addition, it is difficult to ensure that the bias and imprecision of an analysis remain constant as the data file is built up. In a laboratory, both methodology and equipment are subject to quite frequent change.

3. Different laboratories are subject to different levels of inaccuracy, and reference ranges cannot therefore be readily translated from one laboratory to another, although possible solutions to this have been suggested.[18]

4. Clinicians are not yet generally aware of the increase in discriminatory power which better-defined reference ranges could give. As a result, it is difficult for a laboratory to obtain information from a clinician to define properly a reference individual.

In laboratories, it is often forgotten that a request form is a request for a consultative opinion. The majority of reports produced by a laboratory are consultative opinions expressed in numerical form. The problem facing laboratories is that of making reports sufficiently intelligible to a clinician so that appropriate action is taken. The definition of reference ranges is a solution to part of this problem. By itself, it does not solve the problem.

INTERPRETATION OF RESULTS

The normal range and its subsequent refinements were produced to translate numerical values on a continuous scale to a simple 'yes–no' answer for a diagnostic test. As such, they are widely used and accepted by clinicians, even though there has been considerable criticism of such use on conceptual, analytical, statistical and clinical grounds. And, of course, the majority of patients are diagnosed and treated appropriately even where inappropriate normal or reference ranges are applied. All clinicians are aware that however accurately a laboratory establishes reference ranges, false positive and false negative results occur, and laboratory (and other) errors are sometimes made. This does not nullify the importance of a laboratory attempting to produce the most accurate reference ranges that it can (bearing in mind the uncertainty introduced by small sample sizes). Computers are now widely used for producing laboratory reports, and providing that the appropriate information can be input, the appropriate reference range for an individual can be printed as part of his report. There are of course three limitations.

The first is that an exact definition of a reference limit is only of importance in a small minority of patients. The majority of patients receive appropriate diagnosis and treatment with no recourse to laboratory data, or present sufficiently strong clinical evidence for a diagnosis to be made irrespective of laboratory data (whether correct or not), or produce results sufficiently abnormal irrespective of an exact reference limit.

The second limitation is that any attempt to impose an upper limit of normality or an upper reference limit is of course an oversimplification. The factors causing biological, analytical, or pathological variation are so complex that a continuous numerical scale cannot be transformed into a simple 'yes–no' answer. To overcome this problem there have been several attempts to transform analytical results into alternative forms to give a better guide to their diagnostic power. The best-known example is probably the 'surprise index' of Healy.[19] This is to transform results in terms of the number of standard deviations each is away from the mean of a reference range. Thus, any result of $+2 \cdot 0$ corresponds to a result on the upper limit of a conventional normal range. The larger the surprise index, the greater the probability that a result is not indicative of health. So far, none of these suggestions have met with general acceptance.

The third limitation is that the majority of useful laboratory results are not used to assist with a diagnostic process: they are used to monitor therapy or progress. Reference limits are almost irrelevant to this: what is important is whether a significant change has occurred from the previous result. To establish this, both analytical and individual biological variation have to be known. Most laboratories are aware of their analytical variation from quality control data (except this can change with time). There is little information on individual biological variation for the majority of analytes; or for the combination of analytical and biological variation in a stable hospitalized individual. There are major differences, even among experienced clinicians at the same hospital using the same laboratory, in the assessment of the significance of a change in results, and it is common to find that what is regarded as a significant change by some clinicians is well within the laboratory's acceptable analytical variation. This limitation in interpretation is probably of greater consequence to the treatment of more patients than conceptual or numerical differences between normal and reference ranges. Its assessment, and its interpretation by the laboratory to the clinician, is probably the greatest statistical problem facing clinical laboratories today.

REFERENCES

1. *Shorter Oxford English Dictionary*, 3rd edn (1972). Oxford: Oxford University Press.
2. Oliver G. (1896). A contribution to the study of the blood and the circulation. *Lancet*; i: 1699.
3. Peters J. P., Van Slyke D. D. (1931). *Quantitative Clinical Chemistry*. Vol. 1. *Interpretations*. London: Bailliere, Tindall and Cox.
4. King E. J. (1946). *Micro-analysis in Medical Biochemistry*. London: J. & A. Churchill.
5. Henry R. J. (1964). *Clinical Chemistry: Principles and Technics*. New York: Harper & Row.
6. Bermes E. W., Forman D. T. (1976). Statistics, normal values, and quality control. In *Fundamentals of Clinical Chemistry* (Tietz N. W., ed.). Philadelphia: Saunders.
7. Reed A. H., Henry R. J., Mason W. B. (1971). Influence of statistical method used on the resulting estimate of normal range. *Clin. Chem*; **17**: 275.
8. Galen R. S., Gambino S. R. (1975). *Beyond Normality*. New York: John Wiley.
9. McSwiney R. R., Woodrow D. A. (1969). Types of error within a clinical laboratory. *J. Med. Lab. Technol*; **26**: 340.
10. Chambers A. M., Elder J., O'Reilly D.St J. (1986). The blunder-rate in a clinical biochemistry service. *Ann. Clin. Biochem*; **23**: 470.
11. Harris E. K. (1974). Effects of intra- and interindividual variation on the appropriate use of normal ranges. *Clin. Chem*; **20**: 1535.
12. Simpson H. W. (1976). A new perspective: chronobiochemistry. In *Essays in Medical Biochemistry* (Marks V., Hales C. N., eds.), Vol. 2, pp. 115–87. London: The Biochemical Society and The Association of Clinical Biochemists.
13. Clayton B. E., Jenkins P., Round J. M. (1980). *Paediatric Chemical Pathology. Clinical Tests and Reference Ranges*. Oxford: Blackwell Scientific Publications.
14. Young D. S., Pestaner L. C., Gibberman V. (1975). Effects of drugs on clinical laboratory tests. *Clin. Chem*; **21**: no. 5.
15. International Federation of Clinical Chemistry (1978). Provisional recommendations on the theory of reference values. *Clin. Chim. Acta*; **87**: 459F.
16. International Federation of Clinical Chemistry (1984). The theory of reference values. Part 5. Statistical treatment of collected reference values. Determination of reference limits. *Clin. Chim. Acta*; **137**: 97F.
17. International Federation of Clinical Chemistry (1982). Presentation of observed values related to reference values. *Clin. Chim. Acta*; **127**: 441F.
18. Strike P. W., Michaeloudis A., Green D. J. (1986). Standardising clinical laboratory data for the development of transferable computer-based diagnostic programs. *Clin. Chem*; **32**: 22.

given most concisely by the equation bearing his name, $E = hv$, where E is the energy of a quantum of radiation having frequency v. h is known as Planck's constant.

High Energy Radiation

It is clear from the preceding section, and from Fig. 1, that the very high frequency cosmic or gamma radiations contain extremely high energy quanta. Indeed the way in which these radiations interact with matter is characterized by this very high energy. One expects and observes considerable damage at the molecular level when such high energy radiation is passed through matter. Interactions of this kind which are irreversible and result in chemical as well as physical changes are not spectroscopic. If an analytical process were to be developed with these radiations, it would lead to very great experimental problems.

X-rays, which constitute the next region of the spectrum down the frequency ladder, interact with matter in several ways. These include radiation damage effects similar to those found in the γ-ray region; in addition genuine quantized spectroscopic interactions also occur at well defined wavelengths or frequencies. The origin of these interactions lies in the excitation of some of the orbiting electrons of the constituent atoms from their lowest 'ground-state' energy to a higher 'excited-state', the difference between the two states being exactly the same as the energy of the absorbed quantum of radiation. The electrons concerned are the innermost ones, those which are closest and therefore most strongly attracted electrostatically to the positively charged nucleus within. With elements of greater atomic number and consequently higher nuclear charge, a greater attractive force on the inner electrons results and we find that the *energy* of excitation of these electrons is characterized by the nuclear charge. The information that one is likely to obtain from spectroscopic data obtained in the x-ray region is therefore going to be related to the elements present and not to the way in which they are bonded, i.e. information of a molecular nature is not to be expected, molecular bond formation having almost no effect on the inner electrons in their 'closed shells'.

The Ultraviolet and Visible Regions

The ultraviolet and visible regions are found next in the frequency scale. The uniqueness of the visible region is of course that the human eye is sensitive to it, but as the origin of the spectroscopic interactions in both the ultraviolet and the visible regions is the same, spectroscopists consider these two areas together for nearly all purposes.

From Planck's equation it can be seen that the energy per quantum is much less in these regions than in the x-ray region and as a result the only inter-actions to be observed are those associated with the least firmly bound electrons, those which are most easily excited. These outermost electrons are also the ones associated with chemical bonding, either directly or indirectly, and so absorptions in the ultra-violet-visible region should be characterized by the molecular nature of the groups present as well as by the constituent elements.

It is instructive to extend the argument further. In organic compounds there are four main 'types' of electron. The first and from our present point of view the least important, are the inner closed-shell electrons, the ones which require high energy x-ray radiation for excitation and which are therefore unaffected by the ultraviolet-visible frequencies. The second are those represented by the chemists' single bond, the σ (sigma) electrons. The shape of the orbital in which σ electrons are to be found is illustrated in Fig. 2, the region of greatest electron density lies

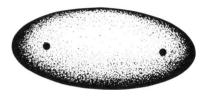

Fig. 2 A σ-orbital.

along the bond axis, between the two positively charged nuclei. These electrons are strongly attracted electrostatically by the nuclei and require the greatest energy of all the bonding electrons for excitation from their ground state to the first excited state. For excitations involving the *greatest* energy and therefore the highest *frequencies*, absorption is at the *shortest* wavelengths.* σ-electron absorptions are all to be found at wavelengths less than 180 nm, this region is known as the vacuum or far ultraviolet, an area in which it is experimentally very difficult to work. For this reason, and because of the fact that all organic compounds possess σ-electrons which are thus rather non-specific, absorptions in this region are not normally used for analytical purposes.

The third main classification of molecular electrons includes the π-electrons, two of which contribute one-half of the chemists' 'double-bond'. A π-orbital may be thought of as constructed from the overlap of two adjacent p-atomic orbitals, the region of highest electron density is somewhat further from the two bound nuclei than was the case before (*see* Fig.

* For many purposes spectroscopists refer to wavelengths rather than frequencies when describing the position of an absorption in the ultraviolet-visible region of the spectrum. The relationship, $c = \lambda v$ where c is the velocity of light (a constant for all frequencies) and λ the wavelength, holds for all electromagnetic radiation. There is therefore an inverse relationship between frequency and wavelength. The nanometre (nm) is 10^{-9} metres and is an accepted SI unit of wavelength. It is numerically equal to the now obsolete unit, the millimicron (mμ) which has sometimes been incorrectly written (mu).

3a) and hence the attraction by the oppositely charged nuclei is less strong than in the case of the σ-electron. The expected excitation energies are therefore somewhat lower for π-electrons than for σ-electrons, and the corresponding absorption wavelengths are greater. This is found in practice, π-electrons have strong absorptions lying mostly in the region 180–400 nm.

Now if all compounds possessing π-electrons absorbed at the same wavelength another non-specific interaction would render this region useless for the analyst. Luckily this does not happen and a reason for the variable absorption wavelength must be sought.

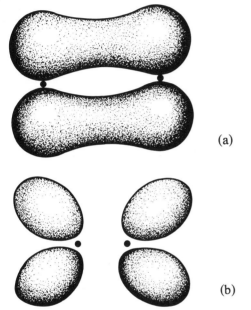

Fig. 3 (a) A bonding π-orbital. (b) An antibonding π^*-orbital.

Consider first the simplest unsaturated hydrocarbon with π-electrons, ethene $CH_2{=}CH_2$. Radiation of wavelength 181 nm promotes the π-electrons into an excited π-orbital, the shape of which is illustrated in Fig. 3b. Though this orbital is antibonding the molecule as a whole does not fly apart as the two carbon atoms remain bonded by the two unexcited σ-electrons. For clarity this orbital is not included in the illustration. In a matter of 10^{-8} seconds the promoted π-electrons return to their ground state π-orbital re-emitting a photon of the radiation previously absorbed.

It may appear that no absorption has taken place in this model as there has been no *net* loss of energy. However, as viewed by an observer facing the source of the initially absorbed radiation a loss of energy *is* observed as the re-emitted photons emerge from the sample in all directions with equal probability and not just in the original direction of the incident beam.

A simple alkyl substituent replacing one of the hydrogen atoms of ethene in the compound propene

$CH_3CH{=}CH_2$, has a small effect on the wavelength of the absorbed ultraviolet light, which is 184 nm in this case. A more dramatic effect is produced however in a compound such as butadiene $CH_2{=}CH{-}CH{=}CH_2$, where two classical π-orbitals are separated from each other by one σ-bond. The absorbed radiation in this compound has a wavelength of 217 nm showing a considerable reduction in the energy difference between ground and excited states compared with ethene. Briefly, the reason for this change is that some overlap of the two π-systems with each other occurs and a delocalization of the π-electrons over all four carbon atoms can take place. This has the effect of lowering the energy of the electrons in both the ground state and even more in the first excited state. The difference between the energy

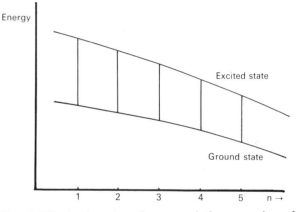

Fig. 4 Effect of conjugation on relative energies of ground and excited states.

states is thus reduced and an increase in the absorption wavelength results.

Butadiene is the first of a series of 'conjugated' compounds which have alternating double and single bonds and where the π-electrons are able to delocalize over more than just two adjacent atoms. If one examines a series of such conjugated compounds one finds that the effect of reducing the energy of the electrons as a result of delocalization continues in a regular way with trienes, tetraenes, etc. Figure 4 shows the way in which ground and excited state energies decrease with increasing delocalization, the abscissa plots the number, n, of the ($-CH{=}CH-$) groups, and Fig. 5 shows the regular way in which the absorption wavelength increases with increasing n. The compound absorbing at 450 nm is trans-β-carotene having 11 conjugated double bond units, its characteristic orange colour demonstrating the considerable absorption of light at the blue end of the visible region. It absorbs continuously over the range 370–540 nm with a maximum at 450 nm.

We see from this that π-electrons are able to absorb throughout the easily available ultraviolet range and indeed into the visible region as well.

The last remaining category of electronic orbitals found in organic compounds, the non-bonding or lone-pairs, have a very large effect on the absorption spectrum of a π-electron compound if a substituent with non-bonding, 'lone-pairs' replaces one of the constituent hydrogen atoms. Thus, ethene absorbs at 181 nm but the compound $CH_2{=}CHNMe_2$ absorbs at 228 nm illustrating the effect on the absorption wavelength of the π-electrons in close proximity to the lone-pair electrons on the N atom. In addition, these electrons have a characteristic absorption irrespective of the presence of unsaturated π-electron groups.

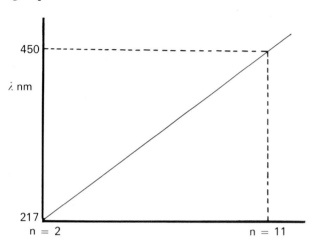

Fig. 5 Absorption wavelengths against conjugation number.

It is seen that absorption of light in the ultraviolet-visible spectrum is largely dependent on the π-electrons, either on their own or in association with atoms or groups of atoms having lone-pair electrons. The *position* or wavelength of these absorptions depends on the chemical nature of the compounds being examined, and determination of the wavelength serves as a *qualitative* indication of the material present. The *intensity* of absorption depends on two factors:

1. the probability that a photon of the light is absorbed by a molecule which lies in its path, and
2. the number of such molecules to be found in the light path.

We will return to this in more detail, later.

Infrared Spectra

The electromagnetic spectrum in Fig. 1 shows the infrared region at lower frequencies than the ultraviolet and visible regions. In accordance with Planck's relation, this region radiates quanta of lower energy than those considered above, and, because we have accounted for all the possible electronic excitations in the higher frequency regions, we might therefore expect to find no further absorption of radiation at these and lower frequencies. This is not found in practice. There is within this region a profusion of sharp and intense absorption lines, but as the energy of infrared radiation is so much lower than that required for electronic excitation we have to seek the origin of these absorption interactions elsewhere.

The explanation for infrared absorption lies not in the constituent electrons but in the vibrational motion of the atoms within the molecule. If two atoms are bound together and vibrating relative to each other along their bond direction and if one atom is slightly more electronegative than the other, then a vibrating electric dipole moment will be set up. It is this electric dipole moment that will couple with electromagnetic radiation present, provided that the frequencies are identical. Molecular vibrational frequencies and hence the corresponding dipolar frequencies lie in the infrared. This region would therefore appear to be a profitable area to examine in greater detail as it is clearly of potential interest for spectrophotometric analysis. It should be noted that bonds with no permanent dipole, usually ones with high symmetry such as the C—C bond in ethane CH_3—CH_3, are in continual vibration but will not absorb infrared radiation. Such vibrations can be studied by Raman Spectroscopy, a branch of the subject which as yet is little used in clinical analysis.

Let us first examine which factors are likely to affect the frequency of molecular vibrations and the corresponding absorptions. In this it is convenient to consider the analogy of a weight suspended by a vertical spring. If the weight is allowed to vibrate, vertically, the spring will alternately compress and extend. The frequency of this vibration will depend on two factors, (i) the mass of the suspended weight and (ii) the elasticity of the spring. If one were to replace the weight with another of twice its mass, the vibrational movement would be much slower and the frequency would be reduced, in fact it would be reduced by a factor of $\sqrt{2}$. Similarly in a molecule consisting of two atoms A and B held together by a bond (the spring) the vibrational frequency will also depend on the masses of the atoms. The vibrational frequency of a C—O bond in an alcohol is therefore expected to be very much lower than the frequency of the C—H vibration as oxygen is 16 times heavier than hydrogen. Though the weight-on-spring analogy is useful the molecular situation is more complex. In the former case only the weight is in motion while in the latter both atoms would be moving, furthermore complicating effects due to other atoms two bonds away also have to be considered.

In the analogy referred to, the elasticity of the spring was expected to have a considerable effect on the vibrational frequency. For any given weight, a stronger spring would cause the vibration to be more rapid than a weaker one. The bond strength in molecules is found to have the same influence, so that the carbonyl bond C=O in ketones and aldehydes vibrates more rapidly than the single bonded C—O found in ethers or alcohols.

To sum up this very rapid survey of the origins of infrared spectroscopy,

1. all atoms within molecules are in constant vibration,
2. all bonds with a permanent dipole will absorb infrared radiation at the vibration frequency, and
3. the vibrational frequency will depend on the atoms associated with the bond as well as the bond strength.

We have referred so far only to the stretching frequency of two atoms bonded together. If we consider a triatomic molecule, a bending vibrational motion is also possible and, if this is associated with a change in a dipole moment as it very frequently is found to do, then an absorption in the infrared region will take place. It is clear from this that a molecule of just 10 to 20 atoms is likely to give rise to a very complex infrared spectrum and this is indeed found to be the case. Furthermore, the spectrum is usually unique for a particular compound, even chemically very similar materials are usually found to have easily distinguishable spectra. For this reason, the spectral region is known as the 'fingerprint region', and is of immense value for qualitative analysis in organic chemistry when applied to pure single compounds.

In clinical biochemistry however the usefulness of infrared spectra is not so clear cut largely because one is usually dealing with a mixture of many components.

All compounds will give rise to their own IR spectra, which are not only unique but also quite complex—consisting of perhaps 6–10 major absorption lines or bands and another 10–20 weaker but easily detected lines. One is therefore likely to have an embarrassment of information as the spectra from many components are present and all hopelessly mixed up together. One is forced, reluctantly, to leave infrared spectroscopy to the organic chemists—except for certain specific situations. These might include, for example, analysis following GLC. Also computer-assisted spectral identifications involving 'reverse searches', which compare hundreds of standard data records with an unknown record, have opened up the subject. We consider whether any other region in the electromagnetic spectrum is going to be of help in the analysis of compounds of clinical biochemical interest.

The Lower Frequency Spectra

Microwave Absorption. In the microwave region of the spectrum, the frequencies are far lower than those encountered in the normal vibrations of molecules. They correspond to the *rotational* frequency of molecules and absorptions in this region may be observed. Rotational spectra in the microwave region are not used for routine analysis for two reasons. The first is that the spectrometers applicable in the microwave region are far more complex—and therefore expensive—than in the infrared region; the second, determining factor, is that in order to obtain satisfactory, sharp, absorption lines in rotational spectra one must have the absorbing material in the form of a low pressure gas. This latter restriction, together with the lack of any great analytical advantages in this region over any other has meant that most microwave work has been and still is primarily of theoretical interest.

Electron Spin Resonance. Electron Spin Resonance (ESR) is the name given to another branch of spectroscopy using microwave frequency radiation. A large magnetic field has to be applied to the sample under study while it is simultaneously being radiated with the appropriate frequency. The magnetic field has the effect of aligning the magnetic moments of the electrons within the sample along two directions, each having a slightly different energy. Transitions between these two energies give rise to spectroscopic interactions of interest.

The only materials which exhibit ESR contain 'unpaired electrons', but in most molecules electrons are paired and no absorption can then be observed. Unpaired electrons occur in paramagnetic materials, the more important being organic free radicals, complex molecules containing transition metals such as iron, manganese, etc., and radiation damaged substances.

An area of increasing interest in Clinical Biochemistry is that of 'Spin Labels'. A spin label is an organic free radical which is capable of being chemically attached to biochemically important molecules such as antigens, antibodies, enzymes, etc. These may all be studied by ESR, which because of its selective nature, is able to ignore all the other non-paramagnetic material that may be present.

Nuclear Magnetic Resonance. Nuclear magnetic resonance (NMR) is superficially similar to ESR, but uses transitions arising from the aligned magnetic moments of the nuclei present rather than the electrons. The electromagnetic radiation frequencies used are in the short-wave radio region, somewhat lower than ESR but the magnetic field strengths are considerably higher.

Only those nuclei that are magnetic will be aligned by an applied field but among those that are, the proton—the nucleus of the hydrogen atom—is by far the most important. Instrumental advances have allowed the routine investigation of other isotopes such as ^{13}C, ^{15}N and ^{39}P. The common isotopes of carbon and oxygen are both non-magnetic.

By the nature of the technique, all substances containing the nucleus under consideration (hydrogen, say) are potentially able to give rise to an NMR spectrum even if it is rather weak. The situation is therefore similar to that of infrared spectroscopy. If a mixture of several chemically different compounds is being investigated an extremely complicated overlapped set of spectra will result. This is unfortunate for, as with infrared, a wealth of analytically important information would be available to the clinical biochemist if each component were to be examined in a pure isolated form. In addition NMR spectra give useful quantitative, as well as qualitative, information. This, therefore, is another area mainly of potential, rather than actual, analytical interest for the clinical biochemist.

BEER'S LAW

In this section we show the quantitative relationship between the concentration of a substance in solution and the amount of light absorbed.

The relationship, known as the Bouguer-Beer-Lambert Law (more popularly, Beer's Law) is concise and well known. Despite its wide application there are a number of popular misconceptions concerning Beer's Law as well as a number of cases of its misuse, even abuse. To appreciate more fully the conditions under which the Law holds so that concentration determinations may be made not only with confidence but also with precision we must start with a derivation of the basic Beer's Law equation.

Derivation

Let us consider a transparent cell containing a solution of light-absorbing solute dissolved in a totally transparent solvent (Fig. 6). The incident radiation

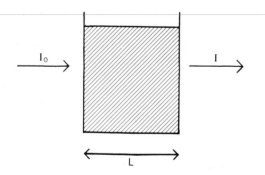

Fig. 6 Idealized absorption cell.

has intensity I_0 and the transmitted radiation has a weaker intensity I. The thickness of the light-absorbing material is L. The fraction of light transmitted by a particular material, I/I_0, varies according to the colour (wavelength) of the light being used. If a solution appears red, then red light will pass through almost completely unattenuated, but blue or green radiation will be strongly absorbed. It follows that to obtain meaningful values of I/I_0, a very narrow range of wavelengths must be used in order that all the light to be absorbed at any particular moment has the same fraction transmitted. This narrow range of wavelengths is known as *monochromatic* or single coloured light. In practice there will always be pres-

ent a small wavelength range but this will not generally affect the results.

If we have chosen the monochromatic wavelength correctly so that absorption by the solute is not insignificant, it is clear that the light intensity will drop continuously over the whole length of the light path within the absorbing medium. We must determine how this intensity varies along the light path.

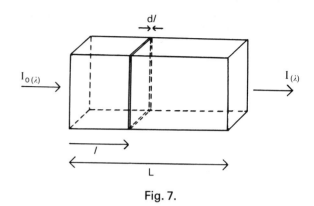

Fig. 7.

Imagine a very thin slice of the absorbing solution of dl thick, with unit cross-section area at distance l from the leading edge; let the concentration of the light-absorbing solute be C. (So far the units of thickness, area and concentration have been avoided, we will return to this point later, but for our present purpose the units used are not important.)

The total number of solute molecules within the thin slice will depend on the concentration and on the volume of the slice, i.e.,

$$\text{the number of molecules} = kCN \cdot volume$$
$$= kCN \cdot (1)\mathrm{d}l$$

where N is Avogadro's number and k is a constant which depends upon the units of concentration used.

Let the effective area that one absorbing molecule presents to the light beam be a and let the probability of absorption by a photon which falls within this effective area, be w.*

The *fraction of light* that will be absorbed by this thin slice will depend on the total effective area of all the absorbing molecules present and on the prob-

---

* The part of a molecule which absorbs radiation of a particular wavelength is called a 'chromophore' and its effective area is not necessarily the average cross-sectional area of the complete molecule for if the absorbing particles in a molecule are, say, the π-electrons associated with a carbonyl bond (as in urea) then the effective area, assuming no conjugation, will be very small. On the other hand the extended conjugated π-orbital in a molecule such as trans-β-carotene with eleven conjugated double-bonds presents a much larger effective area. Furthermore, the probability of a photon's being absorbed by the electrons in such a bond will depend on the relative orientations of the π-orbital in the molecule and the polarization of the light. This probability of absorption, expressed as a fraction, will take some value between 0 and 1, which correspond respectively to zero and complete absorption.

ability of absorption of a photon falling within this total area. This is given by

F = Total number of molecules . a . w

$= kCN . \mathrm{d}l . aw.$

If the intensity of monochromatic light of wavelength λ falling on the thin slice is i (which must lie in the range $I_0 > i > I$), the intensity leaving the slice will be slightly smaller and given by $i - \mathrm{d}i$. The fraction of light absorbed by the slice is then $-\mathrm{d}i/i$, the negative sign indicating a decrease in intensity.

We can now equate these fractions and obtain

$$-\frac{\mathrm{d}i}{i} = kCN . \mathrm{d}l . aw$$

or

$$-\frac{\mathrm{d}i}{i} = \varepsilon' C \, \mathrm{d}l,$$

where $\varepsilon' = kNaw$. This has a constant value at a fixed wavelength for any particular material and includes all the factors so far considered.

This simple differential equation may now be integrated, the intensity i running between the limits I_0 and I and the thickness l running from O to L. The definite integral then becomes

$$\log_e I_0 - \log_e I = \varepsilon' C L$$

or rearranging,

$$\log_e \frac{I_0}{I} = \varepsilon' C L$$

In order to work with logarithms to base 10 the equation can be rewritten,

$$\log_{10} \frac{I_0}{I} = \varepsilon C L$$

where the decadic extinction coefficient $\varepsilon = 0 \cdot 4343 \varepsilon'$.

If the concentration is measured in moles/litre and length in cm, ε is known as the molar extinction coefficient, or molar absorptivity.

The equation in this form shows us the function of the intensities which is directly proportional to the concentration C. This function is given the name 'absorbance' A, and is defined as

$$A = \log_{10} \frac{I_0}{I}$$

so that our equation, the Beer-Lambert equation, reduces to

$$A = \varepsilon C L,$$

which is the most concise form the law can take.

(Other terms for *absorbance* that will be met commonly in the literature are 'Optical Density', 'Absorption' and 'Extinction'. The word 'absor-

bance' should not be confused with *absorptivity* which is an alternative for the extinction coefficient.)

Let us consider now the implications of using this relationship in analysis.

Optical Path Length Variation

It is clear from the equation that doubling *either* the concentration of the solute, C, *or* the length of the absorbing light-path, L, will have the same effect, namely doubling the absorbance. For reproducible and accurate determinations of concentrations therefore, one must either know precisely the dimensions of the absorption cell or use an accurately known standard solution; the former is usual. The standard cell or cuvette, consists of two parallel transparent pieces of glass (or fused silica for use in the UV region), held precisely one centimetre apart by two further pieces of frosted glass or silica. The sides and the square base are all firmly sealed together with an appropriate cement, the transparent windows being optically parallel for any 'wedging' would badly deflect the light beam to different areas of the light-sensitive surface of the detector. Reproducibility of results would be very poor under these conditions.

Though the 1 cm cell is by far the most usual and useful, cells can be obtained with solution path-lengths for 1 mm up to 10 cm.

Wavelength Variation

As the ratio I_0/I varies with wavelength, so also will the absorbance. We deduce from the Beer's Law equation that as A varies with wavelength so also must the extinction coefficient ε, as the values of C and L are clearly independent of such changes.

Let us assume that the variation of A with wavelength λ in our hypothetical solution follows a plot similar to that given in Fig. 8. The wavelength in nanometres corresponding to the maximum absorbance is usually given the symbol λ_{max}. If we now consider the plots obtained from a series of increasingly more dilute solutions of the same material, a

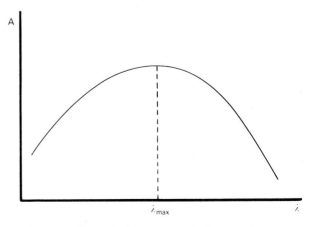

Fig. 8 Plotting absorbance against wavelength.

family of curves of similar shape but decreasing absorbance results (Fig. 9). The absorbance values measured at any particular wavelength (λ_{max}, say) plotted against the corresponding concentrations will in many instances give a linear or straight line relation (Fig. 10). Indeed plots of absorbance at any other wavelength against concentration will also result in straight lines, but the slopes of the graphs will all be different. It is clear that once such a graph has

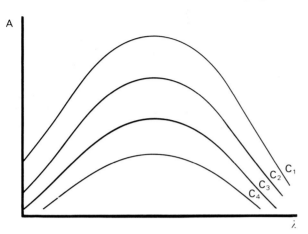

Fig. 9 Absorbance/wavelength curves.

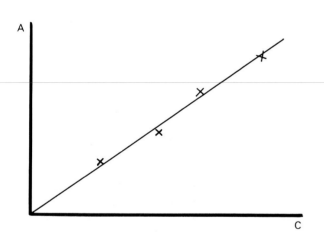

Fig. 10 Plotting absorbance against concentration—Beer's law obeyed.

been constructed an unknown solution of the same substance could be examined at the *same wavelength* and from its measured absorbance value the concentration may be determined.

The fact that in many cases a plot of A against C gives rise to a straight line is not surprising when one considers the form of the Beer's Law relation, $A = \varepsilon C$, which is mathematically a linear equation. (L is taken to be numerically equal to 1 (cm) and is henceforth ignored.) The slope of the plotted graph above gives us the value of ε, the extinction coefficient, and we note that this slope, and hence the ε value, varies according to the wavelength chosen.

A very important point and one that is occasionally misunderstood, is that for a particular substance there is *no one* value of the extinction coefficient. Any value quoted *must* be associated with the appropriate wavelength as well as the units used, i.e. SI, cgs, etc. The base of the logarithms are assumed to be 10 but if otherwise, this should also be stated. Without a reference to the wavelength used, one might perhaps assume that λ_{max} is implied; however this is at best ambiguous and is in any case a dangerous practice.

As was seen above, the concentration of an unknown solution may be obtained by reference to a constructed A versus C graph, but this is unnecessary if a reliable extinction coefficient (together with the units and appropriate wavelength) is available from the literature, as the Beer's Law equation may be applied directly once the absorbance value for the unknown has been found.

Situations in which Beer's Law is not Obeyed

The above argument provides the theoretical basis of the analytical technique, but in practice we find that for many materials a plot of A versus C gives a non-linear relationship, as for example illustrated

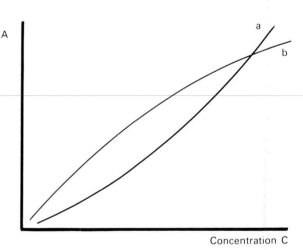

Fig. 11 Plotting absorbance against concentration—Beer's law not obeyed.

in Fig. 11. The curved plots clearly do not correspond to the linear equation $A = \varepsilon C$ and under such circumstances it is said that Beer's Law is not obeyed. There are several possible reasons for non-linear plots, some chemical and some instrumental. We will consider a few of the more important reasons and whether it is necessary or possible to reduce the effect.

A major cause of non-linearity is to be found in the chemical *association* of solvent or other compounds with solute molecules. Another is the *dissociation* of some compounds, perhaps into ions, which becomes more and more marked with decreasing concentrations. Let us consider the latter case in more detail.

Suppose an acid, *HA*, partially dissociates in solution to form ions according to the formula,

$$HA \rightleftharpoons H^+ + A^-.$$

An equilibrium is set up between the concentrations of the three components, *HA*, H^+ and A^-. At high concentrations *HA* predominates but with increasing dilution the relative amounts of the ionic forms become more important. This is normally expressed in terms of the *degree of dissociation* of the acid α given by the equation

$$\alpha = \frac{[H^+][A^-]}{[HA]}$$

where the symbols [····] imply 'the concentration of'.

In a solution of the acid only a fraction is in the undissociated form *HA*, the fraction depending on α which in turn depends on the stoichiometric concentration.

Let us assume that we wish to construct the graph of absorbance against concentration previously described. An appropriate wavelength has to be chosen and a convenient one would be λ_{max} for undissociated *HA*. In general the ionic form A^- will have a different absorption spectrum and a different λ_{max} from *HA*. It is clear from this that the absorbance by *HA* is always going to be less than it would have been in the absence of dissociation and that this effect will become more and more important with increasing dilution. The result is therefore a curved plot similar to Fig. 11a. The various types of chemical association and dissociation effects cannot be avoided and the resulting curved plots are inevitable.

This situation, which is fairly common, does not invalidate the analytical technique for it will be readily appreciated that if one can construct an absorbance/concentration plot then, linear or non-linear, it may be used as a 'working curve' or 'standard curve' from which an experimentally obtained absorbance value (at the appropriate wavelength from an unknown solution of the same substance) will immediately lead to the determination of the corresponding concentration. Of course under these conditions as Beer's Law is not obeyed, the equation $A = \varepsilon C$ cannot be used because there can be no single value for the extinction coefficient. It is not acceptable to refer to 'an extinction coefficient at a particular concentration', indeed the concept of ε when Beer's Law is not obeyed cannot be used.

In some instances the absorbance/concentration curve is essentially linear over a wide range of dilutions but deviates at higher concentrations. It is legitimate to quote (or use) extinction coefficient values for the linear portion provided the applicable concentration range is clearly stated. If there is any doubt a working curve must be constructed.

In conclusion we have found that for analyses in which there is only one light-absorbing component,

published extinction coefficient values (if Beer's Law is obeyed) together with an experimentally obtained absorbance may be used to determine the concentration, or a working curve can be constructed from the absorbance values and the corresponding concentrations of a series of standardized solutions. One is obliged to use the latter method when Beer's Law is *not* obeyed.

Two Component Mixture Determinations

Let us consider the case where two different light absorbing solutes are present in a transparent solvent. The absorption spectra of the two solute materials are different but may overlap with each other to such an extent that at no wavelength can one measure an absorbance of one compound without the interference from the other. A typical situation is illustrated in Fig. 12.

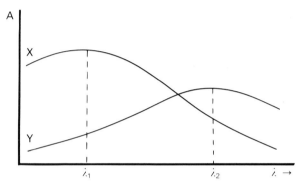

Fig. 12 Absorbance plots in two-component mixture.

λ_1 corresponds to the maximum absorbance of compound *X* and λ_2 to compound *Y*. The problem, then, is to determine both concentrations by a spectrophotometric method.

It will be recalled that, in the derivation of Beer's Law, the absorbance of a solution is directly proportional to the *number* of absorbing particles in the light beam. Thus doubling either the concentration or the path length doubles the number of absorbing solute molecules and this results in doubling the absorbance. Absorbance then is an additive property depending on the total number of absorbing particles in the light beam. In the present problem we have two different absorbing species *X* and *Y* which, considered separately, have quite different absorbance values at any general wavelength. The total absorbance of the two in the presence of each other will therefore be the sum of the individual absorbances. At any particular wavelength, such as λ_1, the total absorbance of the mixture will be equal to the sum of the absorbance due to the amount of *X* and due to that of *Y*. If the concentrations of the two components are C_X and C_Y respectively, we may now write

$$A_{\text{Total}(\lambda_1)} = A_{X(\lambda_1)} + A_{Y(\lambda_1)}$$
$$= \varepsilon_{X_1} C_X + \varepsilon_{Y_1} C_Y.$$

Experimentally we can measure A_{Total} at λ_1 for the mixed solution while the extinction coefficients of pure X and pure Y at λ_1 have yet to be determined but we already know in principle how to find their values. One requires samples of the pure materials X and Y which have to be made up into a series of solutions of standard concentrations and from which plots of absorbance (at λ_1) versus concentrations can be constructed. We have already seen that the slopes of these plots measure directly the values of extinction coefficients of the materials at that particular wavelength. Hence ε_{X_1} and ε_{Y_1} can in principle be obtained. It may often occur that the extinction coefficient of a substance at its own λ_{max} has previously been published. Thus the value of ε_{X_1} may be available and its determination by the above method becomes unnecessary.

The only unknown quantities left are C_X and C_Y. In order to solve for two unknowns we require a second equation and this can be obtained by considering and in practice measuring the absorbance of the mixture at any different wavelength, say λ_2.

Thus we have,

$$A_{Total(\lambda_2)} = \varepsilon_{X_2} C_X + \varepsilon_{Y_2} C_Y$$

As before, ε_{X_2} and ε_{Y_2} can be found from solutions of the pure materials or perhaps one or other of the values may be known from previous work. In any case, these values together with the second experimentally obtained absorbance, A_{Total} at λ_2, give us our second equation. These simultaneous equations can now be solved for the unknowns C_X and C_Y. These become

and

$$C_X = \frac{A_1 \varepsilon_{Y_2} - A_2 \varepsilon_{Y_1}}{\varepsilon_{X_1} \varepsilon_{Y_2} - \varepsilon_{X_2} \varepsilon_{Y_1}}$$

$$C_Y = \frac{A_2 \varepsilon_{X_1} - A_1 \varepsilon_{X_2}}{\varepsilon_{X_1} \varepsilon_{Y_2} - \varepsilon_{X_2} \varepsilon_{Y_1}}$$

These equations appear somewhat complex but all the factors on the right-hand side are known, and so C_X and C_Y can be calculated easily.

The principle is thus established that one may determine the concentrations of a binary mixture using the method described.

Clearly this method is somewhat tedious if only one such mixture is to be analysed. Two absorbance values of the mixture have to be measured and four different extinction coefficients have to be obtained. On the routine basis though, the technique is much more viable. Once the four extinction coefficients have been obtained for any given pair of absorbing substances (at the two appropriate wavelengths) they may be used for *all* subsequent determinations. This problem is eminently suitable for computerization. The four ε values may therefore be included in a suitable program as four items of data and then a set of pairs of experimentally obtained absorbance values are introduced. There will be one pair of absorbance values for each solution mixture, and a set of pairs of concentration values are thus obtained so that the results of many hundreds of analyses may be immediately computed. The results from a continuous-flow analyser, for example, may be stored and then processed very rapidly. If one wishes to change to a different pair of absorbing substances only four variables in the program (the four extinction coefficients) need to be replaced.

It is important to consider the limitations of the method. The assumptions made above in dealing with the simultaneous equations are that A_1, A_2 and all the ε values are known or are at least experimentally obtainable but this is not the case if either of the components fails to obey Beer's Law. A small deviation from the straight line absorbance/concentration plot means that there is no one good value for ε at that particular wavelength and probably not at any other wavelength either. This introduces another unknown factor into the simultaneous equations and so renders them insoluble. It is important therefore that both substances strictly obey Beer's Law over the concentration ranges that are likely to be encountered. Furthermore one must ascertain that this situation still holds when the substances are in the presence of each other. If there is a small and perhaps reversible chemical reaction between the components then Beer's Law will not be obeyed by either when in the presence of the other, though it may be obeyed by each when they exist as single substance solutions.

The easiest way to check that there is no interaction between the components is to run an absorbance against wavelength plot on solutions of each pure component separately and to compare these with a plot, run under the same instrumental conditions, of a 50/50 mixture of the two. The sum of the absorbances of the two materials taken at, say, five or six different wavelengths should be exactly the same as twice the absorbance values of the 50/50 mixture, if Beer's Law is obeyed. If it is not, considerable differences will be observed. The reason for the factor of two difference is that when making up a 50/50 mixture of two solutions, each component becomes diluted by one half.

Clearly this is a very sensitive way of testing not only that Beer's Law is obeyed in straight dilution but that there is no subtle chemical reaction between the solute molecules.

Multi-component Mixtures

Finally we must consider the application of this procedure as a general analytical technique for a solution containing any number of light-absorbing solute components. For *two* absorbing substances in a mixture one requires two absorbance measurements at two different wavelengths; two simultaneous equations are thereby set up. To solve for the concentrations of *three* substances one requires three equations which clearly require three absorbance measurements to be made. In general, n absorbing materials require n absorbance measurements at n different wavelengths to set up n simultaneous equations.

In principle there is no limit to the number of light-absorbing materials which may be simultaneously analysed, but it is found that three substances to be analysed by this method is about the practical limit. The reason for this is that the *accuracy* of the concentration values derived by the simultaneous equations becomes poorer as the number of components (and therefore equations) increases. Indeed even with only three components it is often found most convenient to compensate for one of the components in the mixture by placing a pure solution of that particular material (with a judiciously chosen concentration) into the reference beam of the spectrophotometer in place of the more usual pure solvent. This has the effect of reducing the problem once more to a two-component one. The choice of reference concentration is difficult but important. Over-compensation with an excessive concentration in the reference beam will produce a negative absorbance at those wavelengths corresponding to maximum absorbance, under compensation on the other hand leaves a residual absorbance due to the third component in the mixture which will affect the determinations of the other two values.

This is one example of a broader subject known as 'difference spectroscopy' which provides a sensitive way of detecting small changes in one of several components. Two solutions are compared, one is taken as the sample, the other as the reference. All the common features of the two solutions cancel out but small changes in absorbance due to temperature or solvent or pH effects immediately show up and may be recorded.

INSTRUMENTATION

In the first sections of this chapter we considered the theoretical background to spectrophotometry and have seen that limitations are necessarily imposed on the technique by the nature of the subject. In this section the physical equipment used for measuring absorbance, the spectrophotometer, is discussed and once more we will find that several limitations are imposed.

Single-beam and Double-beam Spectrophotometers

Spectrophotometers may be divided into two basic types, the single beam and the double beam instruments.

The former were inconvenient and time-consuming in use and are now almost completely replaced by double-beam machines. In appreciating the working of the more complex instruments it is useful first to consider the operation of the single-beam spectrophotometer. In these, radiation from an appropriate source is passed into a monochromator where the desired wavelength is selected. The monochromatic radiation then passes through a sample chamber and onto a phototube where it is detected and its intensity determined. For an absorbance measurement to be made both I_0 and I are required (we use the convention already referred to that the intensity of radiation incident on the cell is I_0 and that of the transmitted radiation is I). The intensity of I_0 is not constant with wavelength, for various reasons which we will consider later, so a compensation has to be made for each determination at each wavelength. This may be done by altering the gain of the total amplifier, including the gain of the photomultiplier if appropriate, or by changing the slit width to vary the total radiation emerging from the monochromator. In addition to changes of I_0 with wavelength there are also changes in the sensitivity of the phototube/photomultiplier detector and, furthermore, some wavelength-dependent absorption by the solvent and/or cell material may also be present. In order to overcome all these variables the operation of a single-beam instrument involves for each wavelength, a determination of an *effective* I_0 by passing the appropriate monochromatic radiation through the solvent cell as a reference and recording the output from the phototube. Secondly, the cell containing the solution to be examined (the sample cell) is moved into the light beam. Assuming a finite absorption of radiation by the sample at that wavelength, a reduction in the intensity reaching the phototube will give rise to a reduced output from the detector. This gives a value for I. In practice neither of these intensities is determined independently. Their ratio I/I_0 or the *fraction transmitted* and, more importantly, the logarithm of the reciprocal of that fraction (the absorbance), *are* obtained.

In a *double-beam instrument* the light from the monochromator passes through a 'beam splitting' device which causes pulses of light to fall alternately on the reference cell and the sample cell by means of a system of light-choppers and mirrors. After transmission through the cells the two beams are recombined before falling on the phototube detector. When there is no absorption in the solution the two beams retain the same relative intensities and a continuous, uniform, but not necessarily constant intensity is incident on the phototube. The electrical output from the phototube is therefore also continuous. At wavelengths where an absorption does take place the intensity of the beam transmitted through the sample cell will clearly be less than that through the reference and the recombined beam will no longer be of uniform intensity but will flicker and will produce an AC voltage from the detector. This signal, after amplification through an amplifier tuned to the modulation (beam splitting) frequency, can be used directly for transmission measurements (proportional to I) and displayed on some recorder or

pass through and onto the sample. If the slit width is very narrow the range of wavelengths emerging will be small but finite. The wavelength range will run from λ to $\lambda + \delta\lambda$, the 'purest' monochromatic light having the least range $\delta\lambda$. This range, measured in nm, is the spectral slit width and correlates strongly with the slit width itself.

The *dispersion* of a prism or diffraction grating is a measure of the linear separation of the different wavelengths emerging from the exit slit. In a prism, the dispersion becomes much greater at shorter wavelengths and so the spectrum is much more crowded at the red end. For this reason one finds that in prism instruments it is usually necessary to have a variable slit width. With a constant slit width one would find a very much greater total intensity emerging from the monochromator at the red end of the spectrum than the blue but also the spectral slit width in a region of poor dispersion will be much greater than where the dispersion is better—even though the slit width is constant throughout.

The consequence of large spectral slit widths are reduced resolution and reduced absorbance accuracy when narrow absorption bands are encountered or when one is forced to work at a wavelength where the absorbance is rapidly changing. Under these circumstances the spectral slit width range, $\delta\lambda$, would correspond to a range of different absorbance values which, if too great, would lead to highly misleading results.

In contrast to the variable dispersion of a prism, the diffraction grating gives a constant dispersion over the complete wavelength range. There are complications in the use of gratings such as with the overlapping orders of spectra but these are easily sorted out by the use of appropriate light filters and for many purposes the uniform dispersion obtained gives a great advantage over the use of prisms. At the long wavelength end of the spectra where the prisms give the poorest dispersion a grating instrument is likely to give less trouble from the spectral slit width, however at the short wavelength or blue end of the spectrum the dispersion from a prism instrument may well be greater than that from a corresponding grating. Dispersion is not a major problem for the clinical biochemist as the absorptions tend to be rather broad. For these reasons grating instruments are now almost universally used.

Photodetectors

Radiation detectors with sufficient sensitivity and speed of response for incorporation into spectrophotometers do not give a constant voltage output when activated by light of different wavelengths even if the intensity is the same. This is due to a non-uniform 'quantum efficiency' in the photo-active effect taking place within the detector at different wavelengths and if uncorrected would lead to distorted base lines.

The construction of a phototube incorporates a photo-active surface which consists of a metal plate coated with an easily ionized material, usually containing the heavy alkali metal caesium, held behind a wire screen through which the radiation passes. These 'electrodes' are held apart within a quartz envelope containing a low pressure inert gas. Figure 14 gives a schematic diagram of the phototube and its associated electrical circuit.

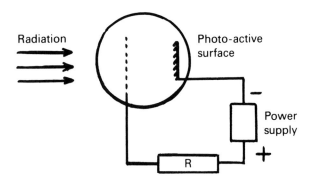

Fig. 14 Photocell circuit.

When the radiation falls on the photo-active plate, some of the outer electrons of the caesium atoms will receive enough energy to escape from the surface. In the absence of a power supply this would leave the metal surface positively charged and fairly rapidly the electrons would be attracted back towards the plate so that an equilibrium situation would establish itself. However, if a power supply is attached to the phototube as indicated, the electrons expelled from the surface will become attracted towards the positively charged, wire grid. The circuit is completed through a resistance, R, which allows a continuous (DC) current to flow for as long as the radiation and power supply remain.

The quantum efficiency of such devices is not good, 20% is considered exceptional, which means only one electron completes the jump across to the grid for every 5 photons arriving at the photo-active surface. It is this primary excitation which is wavelength dependent.

The output of a phototube is the small voltage created across the resistor by the minute primary current. A suitable amplification of the voltage is necessary before enough power is available to drive recorders or servo motors, etc., as appropriate, but it is clear that this voltage, which is directly proportional to the current through R, is also directly proportional to the number of photons (that is, the intensity) of the radiation incident on the detector.

As the output is directly proportional to the intensity of the received radiation it gives direct readings of *transmittance* or percentage transmittance. To obtain readings of absorbance the output must be passed through suitable logarithmic converters which in modern instruments are invariably solid state integrated circuit devices, though in the past various mechanical techniques were used. The photodetector device discussed so far, the 'phototube', has been used extensively in the cheaper spectrophotometers and amplification of the voltage generated by the primary current is necessary in order to obtain enough power to drive the various recorders.

A more satisfactory photodetector, the *photomultiplier*, is now found in nearly all automatic spectrophotometers, and has a fast enough response to follow the modulation frequencies. The output voltage is many orders of magnitude higher than the simple phototube. The photomultiplier consists of a photo-detecting surface rather similar to that previously described but in place of the anode which in the phototube collects the primary electrons, another positively charged electrode called a dynode is included. The dynode is coated with an active surface which releases 3 to 5 electrons for every 1 that arrives from the primary cathode. These in turn are attracted towards a yet more positively charged dynode, again releasing 3 to 5 electrons for every 1 which arrives. This process is continued inside the photomultiplier with some 9 dynodes, the final anode collecting perhaps 10^5 electrons for every 1 primary electron released from the cathode.

It is clear that as each dynode has to be held at a more positive electrical potential than its previous one (about 100 volts in each case), about 1000 volts separates the cathode from the anode. A practical point that follows from this is that if one is tempted to service a spectrophotometer, great care should be taken of the lethal voltages to be found within the instrument. In fact, servicing one's own instrument is not to be recommended and should only ever be undertaken in unusual circumstances, that is where perhaps the problem is too urgent to allow a delay until the firm's service engineer is able to help.

In addition to drawing attention to the personal danger to which the unwary can be exposed when handling live electronic circuitry within spectrophotometers, this is an appropriate point to underline the importance of never allowing daylight or, even worse, direct sunlight into the phototube or photomultiplier compartment when the high voltage is connected. The extremely high current that would be so generated would irreversibly damage the photoactive surface so that a new photodetector would have to be purchased. Without the high voltage connected no current can pass and there would be no damage to the photosurface if daylight is present. In all instruments with photomultipliers, a safety device is incorporated which automatically closes a shutter to the detector when the operator opens the lid to the sample cell compartment. In some of the older single-beam instruments no such safety device was included and care has to be taken that the cell compartment is not opened until the photodetector has been isolated.

Dark Current Compensation

When the shutter of the photocell compartment is closed and no radiation is incident it might be supposed that no electrons would be expelled from the photoactive surface and that the primary current would be zero. This is not the case. A small residual current is always to be found if the appropriate power supply is connected, and this is known as the *dark current*. The origin of the dark current lies mainly in the random thermal excitation processes within the photoactive material. An electron in an individual atom will, from time to time, acquire enough thermal energy to become ionized. Once such an electron has escaped from the surface the accelerating voltage will cause it to move to the anode and contribute to the dark current. This is a small and random process and as such gives rise to a 'noisy' non-uniform, fluctuating, current. In addition, dark current can be caused by imperfect insulation due to dust particles, etc., at the base of the phototube.

It is important to compensate for this dark current because otherwise inaccurate absorbance measurements would result. A 'true' absorbance depends ultimately on a measure of the ratio I_0/I but the dark current still exists in the presence of genuinely photo-generated currents. The intensity ratio actually measured would thus be

$$\frac{I_0 + I_{DC}}{I + I_{DC}}$$

which is clearly not the same as the ratio required. Furthermore, as with most other problems in spectrophotometry, this error becomes worse under high ($A > 2$) absorbance conditions. Under these circumstances the transmitted intensity (I) is considerably reduced (for A greater than 2, I has been reduced to less than 1% of I_0) and I_{DC} is then a very much greater fraction of I and has a correspondingly larger effect.

Some instruments allow for a manually operated electrical bias or offset to compensate for or to reduce the effects of dark current. In other instruments the input amplifier is automatically adjusted during a small part of the modulation cycle which corrects for the dark current effect.

Because of the random nature of dark current, it is not possible to compensate for it completely. For this reason cooling the detector compartment (thus reducing the thermal excitation process) has been advocated. However, in general the advantages expected have not been fulfilled and only in exceptional circumstances is the additional cost worthwhile. In this context it is worth stating that it is bad policy to locate a spectrophotometer near a radiator, a window, or any other potential source of heat. Apart from the increase in noise (and consequent reduction in sensitivity) which may result from a temperature rise of the photomultiplier, the 'bellows effect' caused by temperature cycling would allow dust particles more readily to pass into the spectrophotometer. As we will see later this may increase stray light problems but in addition dust can increase dark current by collecting around, or near to, the base of the photomultiplier. Ideally spectrophotometers should be kept in dust-free, air-conditioned environments.

Accessories

A very wide range of accessories is available from the various instrument makers and space will only allow a discussion of a few of these. New accessories and up-dated versions of old ones come onto the market every year so one is in danger in such a discussion of rapidly becoming out of date. However, some important basic points do emerge.

Micro Sampling. The clinical biochemist may be required to analyse extremely small samples but in a typical spectrophotometer the cross-section area of the light beam leaving the monochromator and passing through the sample holder measures perhaps 5×10 mm. Clearly for the standard 10 mm (1 cm) pathlength cell this represents a required minimum volume of about 500 mm^3 (0.5 ml).

The micro sampling accessory masks the light beam or focuses it down so that a much smaller cross-section area is presented to the sample and, with an appropriately shaped sample holder, the standard 10 mm pathlength can be maintained. This is important for, though a shorter pathlength would reduce the sample volume, the reduced absorbance that would result would give rise to sensitivity problems. Using 10 mm pathlength and a masked beam, volumes of a few tens of microlitres can be examined.

The disadvantage of a focused beam is associated with sample heating problems and subsequent decomposition of reactive materials. The masking method however leads to some loss of energy and the instrument becomes insensitive or sluggish. A slower scan rate then becomes necessary.

Variable Temperature Accessory. Various designs of thermostatting equipment are available on the market. An important point to note is that if the sample is to be held at a temperature in excess of ambient then care must be taken to ensure that adequate thermal isolation from the rest of the spectrophotometer is satisfactory. The problems arising from overheated detectors have already been emphasized but errors caused by stray light can also be influenced adversely by thermal cycling in the monochromator.

PRACTICAL CONSIDERATIONS

In this section we deal with those aspects of spectrophotometry which are essential for those wishing to obtain the highest degrees of accuracy and reproducibility in their analyses. We deal not only with what might be called 'good laboratory practice' but also with some of the considerations given to instrument design by the manufacturers and their implications for the user.

Stray Light

Stray light presents us with perhaps the largest potential source of error in the technique of analysis using spectrophotometers. The definition of stray light is that radiation which reaches the detector at any wavelength other than that set by the monochromator. We will see that it arises from two main sources. It is difficult to be precise at this stage about what is an acceptable stray light fraction as it varies somewhat from circumstance to circumstance. As a rule of thumb, however, it may be assumed that anything greater than about 0.01% stray light is liable to cause unacceptably high errors in absorption measurement. We will see just how this occurs in the section on the effects of stray light but before that it seems appropriate to include a few paragraphs on its origins.

The Causes of Stray Light. A major source of stray light is from within the monochromator. We saw in the Instrumentation section that in order to produce monochromatic light, 'white' light passes through a slit into the monochromator where it is refracted by a grating. The resulting continuous spectrum is played onto the exit slit wall and in principle only the desired wavelength actually emerges through the exit slit. In practice there is some reflection of the spectrum back into the monochromator, although such reflections are kept to a minimum by painting all the inside walls of the monochromator with a matt black paint. A small fraction of light is reflected and ultimately emerges through the slit and will constitute the stray light as it will be made up of all wavelengths present in the original white light. Any chips or other damage to the inner paint surface will enormously increase the amount of spurious reflections and for this reason only manufacturers' service engineers should handle or adjust the internal parts of the monochromators. Other sources of stray light within the monochromator are dust particles which find their way inside and deposit both on the paint surfaces (thus increasing the random reflectance) and on the optical surfaces of the mirrors, or gratings. Dust particles on these optical surfaces will very rapidly increase the random reflectances and the resulting stray light becomes unacceptably high.

The importance of reducing to a minimum the amount of dust which enters the monochromator is obvious and instruments are gasket-sealed in order to achieve this. (Gaskets also serve to eliminate light leaks into the monochromator which would otherwise give hopelessly high stray light figures.) Despite all precautions, some movement of air—together with dust—into and out of the monochromator always seems to occur. The 'bellows effect' referred to before, with alternate expansion and contraction of air within the monochromator due to thermal cycling, on perhaps a daily rhythm, clearly increases the rate of deposition of dust particles. The need for a stable temperature environment is re-emphasized.

If the user suspects that the stray light in his instrument is unacceptably high (for its measurement, see the following section on the effects of stray light) there is little in practice that can be done other than having the instrument serviced or purchasing a new spectrophotometer. The precautions already referred to will help to maintain an instrument in good condition and should be borne in mind when siting a new instrument or planning a new laboratory.

One device used by the manufacturers to reduce stray light in some of the more expensive instruments is to incorporate a double monochromator. In this, two similar monochromators are placed physically next to each other but optically in series so that the exit slit of the first monochromator is the entrance slit of the second. If we assume that the stray light figure in each monochromator separately is 0.5% (enough to give a very high error in some concentration determinations), then the stray light in the double system would be only 0.0025%. This system is superior to the single monochromator instrument, but is more expensive.

Another quite different source of stray light can arise from a spectroscopic process within the sample solution itself. This is a phenomenon known as *fluorescence* and can cause considerable problems to the spectrophotometric analyst. Compounds which are fluorescent are capable of absorbing radiation at one wavelength and then almost instantaneously re-emitting quanta of lower energy at longer wavelengths. This is a property of the electronic orbitals within these particular molecules and involves an excitation from the ground state energy to an excited state (E_2 in Fig. 15). The electrons rearrange and in so doing

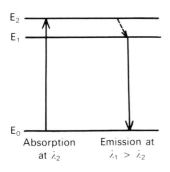

E_2
E_1

E_0

Absorption   Emission at
at λ_2 $\lambda_1 > \lambda_2$

Fig. 15 Origin of fluorescent emission.

drop to a lower excited state (E_1) releasing a small amount of energy in the form of heat. Subsequently the electrons return to the ground state and the lower energy quantum is emitted. The absorbed radiation at λ_2 is the monochromator wavelength, and so λ_1 which is capable of being collected by the detector

(together with any unabsorbed λ_2) is the stray light radiation. The intensity of this stray light can be quite high and can totally invalidate a concentration measurement whether one is trying to determine the fluorescent material itself or some other component in its presence.

Chapter 11 deals with an analytical technique which exploits the phenomenon of fluorescence, where the intensity of the re-emitted (λ_1) radiation gives a measure of the quantity of fluorescent material present. In absorption spectrophotometry, however, fluorescence is a major interference and *must* be avoided at all costs and to underline this, let it be remembered that fluorimetry is several orders of magnitude more sensitive, as an analytical technique, than is spectrophotometry.

The Effect of Stray Light in Spectrophotometers. Let us first consider an example. Assume that we wish to measure the concentration of a material which has a single strong absorption maximum at 200 nm. This is close to the short wavelength limit of many instruments and slightly beyond it for others so let us assume that we can just reach this wavelength with our spectrophotometer. Now to obtain a value of concentration we must first measure the absorbance and, following normal practice, we set the monochromator to λ_{max}. The radiation emerging from the monochromator at λ_{max} (200 nm) is not as intense as one would wish for the emission characteristics of deuterium lamps fall off considerably at these short wavelengths. To compensate for this the slit width of the monochromator of many instruments is opened further to allow more radiation (greater integrated intensity) to emerge. There are two drawbacks to this. First the spectral slit width, discussed in some detail in the section on monochromators, becomes greater and this reduces the instrument's resolution. Second and even more damaging to concentration measurements, the stray light which also emerges from the monochromators is further increased. To make matters much worse, the stray light which contains all wavelengths other than λ_{max} will pass through the sample almost unattenuated as there are no other absorption bands, while the intensity at the absorption wavelength itself will be reduced considerably. The effect of stray light is therefore expected to be most marked at high absorbance values where I_0 is very much larger than I. It is also most important near to the instrument's wavelength limits where sensitivity is falling.

Put algebraically, the ideal absorbance $\log_{10} I_0/I$ becomes, with stray light, $\log_{10} (I_0 + I_{SL})/(I + I_{SL})$. If we are dealing with a 'true' absorbance of 2.00, I_0 becomes $100I$ and if we also assume that the stray light figure for our instrument is 0.1% (it could be even higher than this for it will be recalled that the slit width is unusually wide due to the extreme wavelength range we are using) then the actual absorbance, including stray light, becomes

$$A = \log_{10} \frac{I_0 + 0.001I_0}{0.01I_0 + 0.001I_0}$$

$$= \log_{10} \frac{1.001}{0.011}$$

$$= 1.96.$$

Thus 0.1% stray light, under these conditions, gives a 2% error in absorbance. Further, if the absorbance had been a little higher at 2.50, then 0.1% stray light would give an error of 4.8% while at an absorbance of 3.00, the error rises to 10%. With a stray light figure of 0.2%, the errors at $A = 2.00$, 2.50 and 3.00 rise to 4%, 8.5% and 15.9% respectively.

We see from this illustration that a small amount of stray light can produce an unacceptably high error in concentration determinations, the measured values always being lower than the actual values.

The example assumed that the stray light originated in the monochromator. This as we have seen is not the only possible source of stray light and we should consider now the case of a fluorescent sample. Here the stray light originates within the sample chamber and will differ from the previous case in having a rather narrow band of stray light wavelengths. However, the intensity of the emitted radiation can easily be a sizeable fraction of the exciting intensity. Spectrophotometers are invariably made with the monochromator preceding the sample chamber so the only possibility of reducing stray light originating in the sample chamber is by use of a well-chosen light filter inserted between the sample and the photodetector. This helps, but it will be clear that even with a filter a large fraction of the detected radiation could be stray light if the sample is fluorescent.

To illustrate how far a fluorescent sample can affect the measurement, if we take an absorbance of 3.00 and assume the *equivalent stray light* is 1%, then the error reaches 35%. The phrase 'equivalent stray light' takes into account the fact that the photodetector may be more sensitive to the stray light wavelength than the wavelength the instrument is nominally set at, a situation that often obtains in practice.

However good the spectrophotometer may be and however small the fraction of stray light originating from the monochromator, if the sample is fluorescent, the results will be quite hopeless.

How can one tell if a sample is fluorescent, and if it is, what can be done about it?

Well-known examples of fluorescent materials are those which absorb ultraviolet radiation and re-emit in the visible region. These appear visibly to glow rather brightly compared with their non-fluorescent surroundings and such materials are easily recognized for what they are. It is more difficult to identify clinical samples where both the excitation (absorbed) wavelength and the re-emitted wavelength occur in

the ultraviolet and cannot therefore be seen by eye. Also difficult are samples which fluoresce too feebly to be detected by the human eye. If fluorescence is suspected the quickest test is to measure two absorbances at an appropriate wavelength, one with the sample tube close to the monochromator exit slit, the other with the tube as close to the photodetector as possible. As the light beam from the monochromator is parallel (or nearly so) there should be no change observed in absorbance wherever the sample tube is placed along that beam in the sample chamber. If fluorescent materials are present however, the detector will receive a different stray light signal depending on the angle subtended by the sample on the detector aperture (Fig. 16). This is due

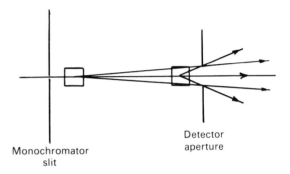

Monochromator slit

Detector aperture

Fig. 16 Effect of sample cell position on the stray light at the detector due to fluorescence.

to the emitted fluorescent radiation no longer following the original parallel beam but being re-emitted from the sample tube in all directions with equal intensity. As the stray light figure depends on the position of the sample tube, so also will the apparent absorbance.

If the material is found to be fluorescent extreme caution should be taken in using spectrophotometry for concentration determinations. It is probably better to say that this technique should never be used if one is dealing with fluorescent samples.

If one is forced to work with a fluorescing absorption band then to minimize the stray light effect, first use a light filter to absorb the fluorescent wavelength but not the incident radiation, and secondly place the sample tube as close to the monochromator and hence as far from the detector aperture as possible.

Turbidity

Turbidity is frequently coupled with fluorescence in being a major interference of spectrophotometry and for this reason it is included under 'Practical Considerations' though as no wavelength change is involved it is not stray light.

Turbidity occurs whenever a solution contains particles which have dimensions of the same order of magnitude as, or larger than, the wavelength of the radiation being used. As we are dealing with wavelengths between 200 and 800 nm we are going to observe turbidity only when giant polymeric molecules, with molecular weights of 10 000 or more, are present. Thus nucleotides and many proteins will give turbid solutions, so also will aqueous colloidal suspensions of lipids or solids where the droplet or particle size is sufficiently large.

Under these circumstances photons entering the sample become scattered in all directions and so reduce the intensity of the collimated beam reaching the photodetector. This reduction in intensity would be interpreted by the instrument as an absorbance even though no actual absorption of radiation may occur.

Two different analytical problems may be considered, first where the scattering material is the substance to be analysed, the second where the scattering substance is an interference in the presence of a genuine solute which is to be determined. In the first case the scattering, and hence the *apparent absorbance*, is proportional to the concentration of the suspended particles. As the apparent absorbance is roughly proportional to the concentration this would appear not to have a disastrous effect on concentration measurements. However, scattering usually produces a very high apparent absorbance and so greatly reduces the sensitivity of the instrument. A 'scattered transmission accessory' is available with some instruments. This works by moving a specially designed detector close to the sample tube so that the maximum amount of scattered radiation can be collected.

The second situation, where one is trying to determine the concentration of a light-absorbing solute in the presence of a scattering material, is clearly untenable as extremely high errors are almost certain to be encountered.

The accessory mentioned above will not help in this situation as the concentration of the scattering material will have as much effect on the detected intensity, as will the concentration of the absorbing solute.

All in all, turbid samples are better avoided unless one has otherwise ideal conditions.

BIBLIOGRAPHY

The following list includes a few reference books which will be of use to those who wish to follow up this subject in more detail. The list makes no pretence at being complete and in some cases the publications are becoming rather 'middle-aged'—they are still nonetheless very useful sources of information.

Bashford C. L., Harris D. A., eds. (1987). *Spectrophotometry and Spectrofluorimetry*—A Practical Approach. Oxford: IRL Press. Useful for the new researcher faced with an unfamiliar instrument or assay—also for an experienced scientist hoping to develop new approaches to existing problems.

Bauman R. P. (1967). *Absorption Spectrophotometry*. New York: John Wiley and Sons. This book covers not only spectrophotometric matters but also some of the underlying spectroscopic theory. Somewhat advanced in places but well worth examining.

Burgess C., Knowles A., eds. (1981). *Standards in Absorption Spectrophotometry*. Compiled by members of the UV spectrometry Group. London: Chapman and Hall. An authoritative and practical guide for biochemists who use these techniques routinely.

Christian G. D., O'Reilly J. E., eds. (1986). *Instrumental Analysis* 2nd edn. Chapter 7. Hemel Hempstead: Allyn and Bacon. A more up-to-date basic coverage with some interesting newer techniques described.

Edisbury J. R. (1968). *Practical Hints on Absorption Spectrometry 200–800 μm*. Bristol: Hilger and Watts. Written in a somewhat unorthodox but very acceptable style, this book includes a wealth of useful practical suggestions for the spectrophotometrist. A 'must' for anyone with instrumental difficulties.

Lothian G. F. (1969). *Absorption Spectrophotometry*. Bristol: Adam Hilger. Another classic publication covering the whole field, well worth reading.

Stearns E. I. (1969). *The Practice of Absorption Spectrophotometry*. New York: Wiley-Interscience. A good, general and readable coverage of the subject.

10. Analytical Atomic Spectroscopy

J. B. Dawson

INTRODUCTION

Most metals can be determined by the methods of classical inorganic analysis. These techniques are, however, frequently inapplicable to biological and particularly clinical samples, mainly because the amounts of material available for analysis are limited and the results are required within a few hours. Alternatively, modern methods of analysis such as colorimetry, fluorimetry, electrochemistry (ion selective electrodes, polarography and anodic stripping voltametry), neutron activation and mass spectrometry are feasible, but none can be readily applied in the clinical laboratory to as many elements as analytical atomic spectroscopy. For the purposes of this chapter the term 'spectrochemical analysis' will be regarded as synonymous with 'analytical atomic spectroscopy' and either may be used when referring to analysis based on the emission or absorption of radiation in the 170–900 nm waveband by a free atom.

The principles of spectrochemical analysis have been recognized for well over 100 years. Emission spectroscopy has been known as a method of identifying elements by the characteristic spectrum of the free atom since the work of Herchel and Talbot in the 1820s; the dark Fraunhofer lines in the spectrum of the sun first noted by Wollaston in 1802 and explained later by Bunsen and Kirchoff in 1860, provided the first example of absorption spectroscopy. However, it was not until the 1930s that the use of emission spectroscopy as an analytical tool became widespread and only in 1955 that Walsh[1] suggested the application of the absorption principle as the basis for a quantitative method of elemental analysis in the laboratory.

The use of spectrochemical methods for the analysis of biological materials began on a significant scale in the early 1930s. At that time arc and spark techniques using photographic recording of the spectrum were predominant and required a specialist spectrographic laboratory. In these techniques the sample is placed either on a metal or graphite electrode or in a recess in the electrode. An electrical discharge is initiated between the sample containing electrode and a counter electrode. The sample is vaporized into the electrical plasma where its emission spectrum is excited. (An electrical plasma is a region of highly ionizd gas generated either by a discharge between electrodes or by a high frequency alternating electromagnetic field.)

More appropriate to the chemical laboratory and for use by the clinical chemist were flame excitation methods using simple photoelectric instruments. These instruments in which the sample is continuously fed to a flame as an aerosol were initiated by Lundegardh[2] in 1928; they eliminate the errors and complexity of electrical excitation and photographic recording and speed the analysis by producing an analytical signal which can be instantly read from a meter. Laboratory versions of such instruments were operating in the late 1930s, but the first widely available commercial instruments did not appear until the late 1940s. These instruments were generally limited to the measurements of sodium and potassium and possibly calcium. However, before the use of more advanced forms of emission flame photometers was established, flame atomic absorption instruments became available and revolutionized the determination of many elements. In contrast, atomic fluorescence analysis, proposed by Winefordner[3] in 1964, has not been widely applied to biological materials because the potential of atomic emission and absorption spectrometry has not yet been fully exploited and commercial atomic fluorescence spectrometers have been slow to appear on the market. The inductively coupled plasma (ICP) method was first used in quantitative analysis for the excitation of the emission spectra of elements in a nebulized solution by Greenfield[4] in 1964. Again exploitation of the technique has been delayed. A range of commercial instruments is now available, however, and when simultaneous multi-element analysis (<5 elements) is required the ICP technique may be the method of choice.

The commonest elements determined by emission flame photometry were sodium and potassium but currently many laboratories use ion-selective electrodes. Calcium is determined by a variety of methods including colorimetry, ion-selective electrodes and atomic absorption spectroscopy. The choice of method depends upon the biochemical information required and the facilities available. For elements present at lower concentrations, e.g. aluminium, cadmium, copper, iron, lithium, lead, magnesium, selenium and zinc, the sensitivity and selectivity of atomic absorption spectrometry offers undoubted advantages. In view of the known essential role or toxicological properties of some 25 elements, an increasing demand for the measurement of elements in biological materials is inevitable.

Principles of Spectrochemical Analysis

Spectrochemical analysis is based on the excitation of electrons in the outer shell of a free atom to higher energy levels by collisions with other atoms or direct absorption of radiation. The energy changes involved in these transitions are determined by the atomic structure of the element. The energy, ΔE, of the photon emitted or absorbed is characteristic of the element and may be calculated from equation (1).

$$\Delta E = E_1 - E_2 = h\nu \qquad (1)$$

E_1 and E_2 are the energies of the electron in the upper and lower states respectively, h is Planck's constant and ν is the frequency of the radiation. The selectivity of spectrochemical methods derives from the narrowness of the distribution of photon energies about their mean value. The wavelength, λ, of the radiation is related to the energy change in the atom by equation (2), where c is the velocity of light.

$$\lambda = \frac{hc}{\Delta E} \qquad (2)$$

A *spectral line* is the monochromatic image of the entrance slit of a spectrometer produced by the objective lens after dispersion of the radiation into its components by a prism or grating; radiation of different wavelengths forms images at different positions in the focal plane of the instrument. The *natural* width of a spectral line due to atomic processes corresponds to variations in the wavelengths of emitted photons of ~0.002 nm. The limiting band pass of instruments used in clinical chemistry is much greater than this (≥ 0.1 nm).

The presence of a given element in a sample may be deduced from the wavelengths of the photons emitted or absorbed by an atomized sample. When the atomization conditions are carefully standardized and the intensities of the spectral lines are measured, quantitative analysis of that element can then be carried out. *Emission methods of analysis* are based on the thermal excitation of the atom and the measurement of the radiation emitted as the atom returns to a lower energy state. In *atomic absorption analysis* the atom absorbs radiation at the wavelength of a resonance transition, i.e. a transition from the ground state, and the analytical signal which is measured arises from the decreased transmission of the atomic vapour. The absorbance of the vapour, A, which obeys the Beer–Lambert law (3), is proportional to the amount of the element in the sample.

$$A = \log_{10}\frac{I_o}{I} = kCL \qquad (3)$$

where I_o = intensity of the incident radiation, I = intensity of the transmitted radiation, k = absorption coefficient, C = concentration of atomic vapour, L = absorption path length.

Atomic fluorescence analysis depends upon the measurement of radiation emitted after excitation of the atomic vapour by radiation of either the same (resonance fluorescence) or differing wavelength.

Advantages of Spectrochemical Methods

The principal advantages of analytical atomic spectroscopy are: specificity, sensitivity, accuracy, speed, flexibility, availability and low cost. The specificity of the technique leads to simpler sample preparation by reducing the need for preliminary separation of the element from the sample matrix. Interactions between element and matrix which lead to enhanced or reduced analytical signal are generally known as 'interferences'. Elements may be detected in solutions containing as little as 100 ng/l or 10^{-12} g absolute of the metal. This great sensitivity enables trace elements to be measured, analyses carried out on small amounts of material and solutions to be diluted to minimize interference effects. Measurements can be made with a reproducibility (coefficient of variation, CV) of 0.5 to 1.0% with an accuracy of 2%. In a routine laboratory, up to 100 analyses per hour can be carried out on a single instrument. Instruments are relatively inexpensive, widely available and easily installed in a clinical laboratory. The technique is applicable to a wide range of elements and sample materials. As expensive reagents and highly trained staff are not necessary, the cost per analysis is low when a large number of analyses are carried out.

The greatest problem in the application of atomic spectroscopy to clinical material arises from the fact that it is not an absolute method of analysis and therefore requires careful calibration to obtain accurate results. It is not possible to produce a synthetic standard which is identical in composition with that of a biological material, hence when developing a new analytical procedure it is always necessary to investigate the possibility of errors arising from differences between the standard and sample materials. It is usually possible to modify the composition of the standard or sample, or both, to eliminate the effect of these differences. When this is not possible, the 'standard addition' method may be used. In this technique the sample is measured alone and again with known increments of the element; the concentration in the original material is deduced by extrapolating the response curve backward until it intercepts the concentration axis. Implicit in this approach is the assumption that the increment of the element behaves in the same manner as the indigenous element.

Detection Limits and Precision of Measurement

The analytical signal is measured against a background signal which may be generated either in the atomic vapour or within the instrument. Both signals are to some extent unstable for even with perfect instrumentation there is the random nature of the emission of light quanta. The detection limit of an analytical method is determined by the magnitude of the background, its stability and the sensitivity of the analytical signal, it is the quantitative answer to the question—'What is the least concentration or amount of a substance whose presence can be reported with a chosen degree of certainty by a complete analytical procedure?' The sensitivity of an analytical procedure is the rate of change of output signal with change in concentration or amount of the element to be determined, i.e. the slope of the calibration curve. Commonly the detection limit is expressed as that concentration or amount of the element which will generate a signal equal to the average blank plus three times the standard deviation, SD, of the blank. As the average blank is subtracted from all measurements, detection limits are often expressed in terms of the SD of the blank. Three times the SD of the blank is, for practical purposes, equal to twice the SD of an analysis at zero concentration. This derives from the fact that in the analysis of a sample, the blank is measured twice, once alone and once when the sample is measured hence the contribution of the blank to the total error in the measurement of the sample will be $\sqrt{2}$ times that of the blank alone.

$$\text{Detection limit} = 2\sqrt{2}\,\sigma_B/S \qquad (4)$$

where σ_B = standard deviation of background, S = sensitivity = signal/unit mass or concentration.

In the analysis of a sample containing none of the element to be measured, the probability of a value equal to the detection limit appearing by chance is nearer 1 in 10, not the 1 in 20 predicted from the normal error curve. This is because the distribution of errors at low concentration is not Gaussian.

Detection limits may be used as figures of merit of analytical systems, either to compare one method with another, or to monitor the performance of a selected method. By adopting standard procedures, detection limits can be used to determine or even predict the effect of changes in analytical conditions and to compare one instrument or laboratory with another. Published data on detection limits may be used as the basis for selecting a possible analytical method and for this purpose it is frequently adequate to know the order of magnitude of the limit. If the desired analysis appears to be feasible, other factors such as specificity, instrument availability, ease of analysis, and the risk of contamination or loss of element during sample processing, should then be considered before a final choice is made.

From the point of view of the clinical biochemist it is often the *determination limit*, i.e. the lowest concentration or amount of an analyte that can be measured with the required precision which is important. In practice, this limit is commonly approximately ten times the detection limit.

If the sensitivity of an analytical procedure changes with time, particularly in emission analysis, an internal standard may be used to improve the reproducibility of the measurements. An internal standard is an element which is added in a known amount to the sample to monitor changes in the analytical performance of the system. It should not be naturally present in the sample and should be chemically similar to the element to be determined. The wavelengths of the spectral lines of the two elements should be close and the excitation schemes similar. The calibration curve is a plot of the *ratio* of the intensities, or absorbances, of the spectral line of the analytical element to that of the internal standard against the *concentrations* of the element in samples of known composition.

The relative sensitivities of emission and absorption methods for the determination of an element using the same atomic vapour have been predicted by Alkemade[5] to be in the same ratio as the spectral radiances of black bodies at the temperatures of the atomic vapour and the effective excitation temperature of the absorption light source. A curve of the wavelength dependence of the detection limit ratio derived from this theory on the assumption of an atomic vapour temperature of 2500 K and a light source temperature of 6000 K is shown in Fig. 1. The experimentally measured values lie close to the theoretical curve. It is apparent that when elements with

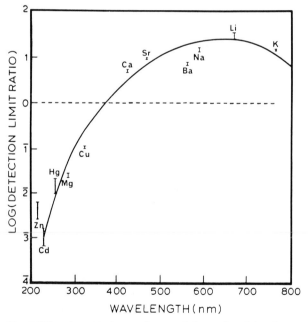

Fig. 1 Wavelength dependence of the ratio of the detection limits in absorption to those in emission, (A/E). Absorption light source temperature 6000 K; atomic vapour temperature 2500 K. Theoretical curve, error limits (SD) on experimental points.

resonance lines at 400 nm or greater are to be measured the sensitivities of emission methods are equal to or greater than absorption; however the selectivity of the latter minimizes spectral interferences and therefore it may still be the preferred method. If the temperature of the atomic vapour is raised to 4000 K then the cross-over point will be in the region of 200 nm. Such temperatures are obtained in electrical plasmas and lead to the excitation of complex spectra.

also excite atomic emission, and for selecting and measuring the intensity of the analytical spectral line; instruments for absorption and fluorescence analysis also incorporate a light source to irradiate the atomic vapour. The inter-relationships between the basic functions of an instrument are illustrated schematically in Fig. 2. The construction and operation of the individual components will be presented in groups depending on their function.

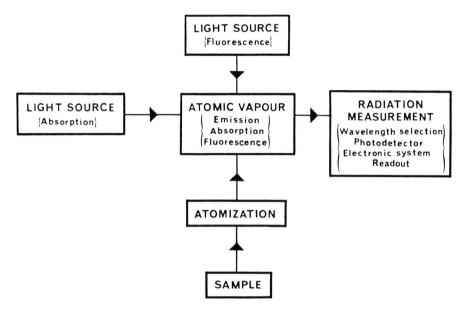

Fig. 2 Block diagram of instrumental configurations in analytical atomic spectroscopy.

Atomic fluorescence analysis is a very sensitive technique and has proven detection limits as low as 10 ng/l. It is most suitable for the measurement of dilute solutions where fluorescence-quenching processes, background scatter, and emission from other components of the sample are minimal. High-intensity light sources such as lasers may be used to achieve greater sensitivity but the concomitant increase in the intensity of the scattered radiation tends to offset the gain in analytical sensitivity. While it may be feasible to dilute biological samples to reduce the amount of scattered light, the problem of contamination then arises. Atomic fluorescence techniques have been applied to the determination of arsenic, cadmium, copper, lead, magnesium, mercury, selenium and zinc in biological material. The procedure and results obtained by this method for copper, magnesium and zinc were no improvement on those obtained by atomic absorption and in view of the limited availability of suitable instrumentation the discussion in this chapter will be directed principally towards the established techniques of atomic emission and absorption.

FUNDAMENTALS OF INSTRUMENTATION

All instruments for spectrochemical analysis consist of a means for vaporizing the sample, which may

Atomizers

These devices convert the sample as presented to the instrument into an atomic vapour. The energy for this process may be provided by a flame or electric current. The efficiency with which the atomic vapour is generated is an important factor in determining the sensitivity of the analysis. Interaction between the element to be determined and its matrix during atomization is one of the principal causes of interferences.

The ideal atomizer is one in which the sample is completely converted into an atomic vapour in a reproducible manner, the vapour produced is of a high atomic density and there are no interactions within the vapour which could lead to impairment of the emission, absorption or fluorescence of radiation. The sample may be presented to the atomizer either in a continuous process, which is used when the sample size is relatively large (1 ml or more) or in discrete aliquots with samples of less than 100 μl. Continuous-flow systems are simple to use and more precise (CV 0.5–2.0%), but they are less sensitive. They employ either a nebulizer in association with a flame or gas plasma, or a rotating electrode or drip feed with the arc or spark. Discrete systems require accurate measurement of small sample volumes or small amounts of tissue. After *in situ* drying and ashing, the sample is thermally atomized by one of the following: a flame, the passage of an electrical current through the support, striking an arc to the support or irradiation with a pulse of energy, e.g. a laser. The coefficient of variation of these methods is 1–10%. Automatic sample dispensing is necessary to obtain the greatest precision.

The shape of the atomic cloud generated from the sample is determined by thermal expansion of the vapour and the surrounding gas flow. As the vapour expands and mixes with flame or shielding gases the atomic density is reduced. This vapour forms a dynamic 'cell' in which the analytical signal is generated. Atoms pass through the 'cell' at high speed (~200 cm/s) and thus at any one instant the number of atoms emitting or absorbing radiation within the optical aperture of the system is relatively small. In atomic absorption, this number may be increased by passing the atomic vapour through a tube sited on the absorption axis of the instrument and thereby increasing the residence time of an atom in the absorption cell. The tube may be heated by a flame, an electrical heater or by the passage of an electric current through the tube wall.

Flames.

Sample introduction. The flame is the most commonly used energy source for atomization in clinical chemistry. Liquid samples are fed to it as aerosols generated by pneumatic nebulizers. In these devices the sample is drawn into a near supersonic air flow where the liquid stream is broken down to a heterogeneous cloud of droplets ranging in diameter from 1 μm to 50 μm. Though 85% of the droplets are <10 μm in diameter, only 20% of the sample is contained in them. In one form of automatic sample handling, flow injection analysis (FIA) the sample is pumped to the nebulizer and may be diluted or concentrated en-route.

In the pre-mix burner system (Fig. 3) nebulization takes place in a chamber designed to remove the larger droplets. The resulting aerosol has a mean diameter of 2 μm and contains only 5–10% of the original sample. Various devices such as impact beads, counter-jet gas flows and pumped sample flow have been used to increase the proportion of the sample carried to the flame but this is rarely greater than 15%. This improvement frequently arises from the inclusion of larger droplets in the aerosol fed to the flame which can lead to increased interference due to incomplete vaporization of the larger particles before entering the observation zone of the flame.

Other nebulizer systems such as ultrasonic and electrostatic devices have been used in attempts to improve nebulizer efficiency. Though fine homogeneous aerosols and efficiencies of well over 50% have been achieved, the additional complexity of the instrument and the significant cooling of the flame which results from the transport of larger volumes

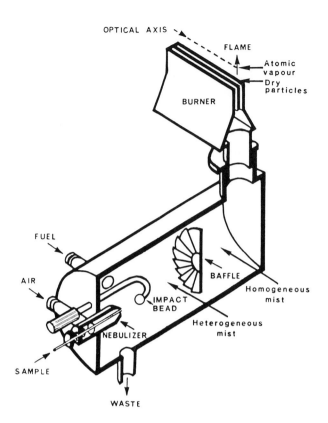

Fig. 3 Pre-mix or laminar flow burner system.

of solvent have militated against widespread use of these alternatives.

The use of heated spray chambers overcomes some of the cooling problems and has led to 8-fold improvements in sensitivity. This process is known as 'desolvation' of the aerosol. The addition of organic solvents such as ethanol and propanol to aqueous solutions improves the efficiency of sample transfer to the flame by a factor of up to three by reduction of surface tension, which leads to the production of a greater proportion of fine droplets. The increased dilution of the sample will, in part, off-set the gain in sensitivity.

As an alternative to introducing the sample into the flame as an aerosol, it may be dried on a suitable support and then inserted into the flame. Using this technique the efficiency of sample utilization is increased to 100% and solvent cooling of the flame eliminated. In the most successful of these techniques for the determination of lead in blood, the Delves' cup (Fig. 4a), the sample, 10 μl whole blood, is dried and oxidized with hydrogen peroxide in a small nickel, noble metal or silica crucible of capacity ~0.2 ml which is then inserted into a flame below an orifice in the centre of a heated absorption tube (10 cm long, 1 cm internal diameter). By this means the residence time of the atomic vapour in the absorption path is increased 5–10-fold compared with that in a conventional flame. Overall a gain in sensitivity of up to 100-fold is obtained with a precision of 5–10% which can be improved by repeated measurements. An intermediate system in which the sample may be continuously aspirated into the flame employs a slotted quartz tube into which the atomic vapour is directed (Fig. 4b); the improvement in sensitivity is of the order of 3-fold. These methods are only suitable for volatile metals, e.g. cadmium, lead and zinc. Most commercial flame atomic absorption instruments can be fitted with attachments for these forms of analysis.

supply. Cylinders of flammable gases should be stored and used according to local safety regulations.

The pre-mixed or laminar flow burner is the type in universal use at the present time. In this system (see Fig. 3) the fuel gas, oxidant and the sample as an aerosol, are mixed prior to passage to the burner. Atomic absorption analysis is usually carried out using a premixed flame burning from either a slot 10 cm long or an array of holes. In a laminar flame the secondary reaction zone may be 'separated' from the primary zone by means of a clear silica tube or

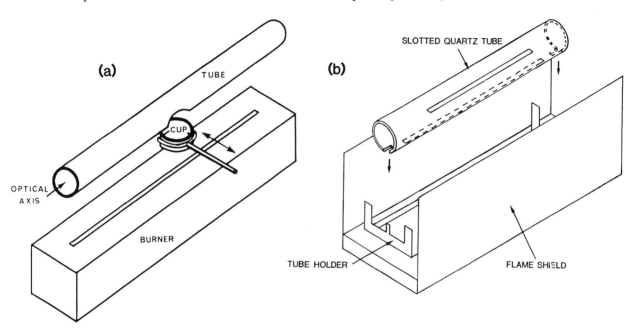

Fig. 4 Attachments to increase sensitivity in flame atomic absorption spectrometry: (a) Delves' cup atomizing system; (b) slotted quartz tube atomizer.

TABLE 1
CHARACTERISTICS OF GAS MIXTURES USED FOR FLAME ATOMIZATION

Gas mixture	Temperature (approximate) K	Flame speed (approximate) cm/s
Air–propane	2100	80
Air–acetylene	2500	160
Air–hydrogen	2300	350
Oxygen–acetylene	3250	1100
Oxygen–hydrogen	2950	900
Nitrous oxide–acetylene	3100	285

Gas mixtures and burners. Table 1 summarizes the characteristics of gas mixtures which have been used in flame photometry. The flame speed, i.e. the rate of propagation of the combustion zone through the gas mixture, has a crucial effect on the burner design as the velocity of the gas mixture emerging from the burner head must be equal to, or greater than, the flame speed if 'flash-back' is to be avoided. Where possible, instruments using flames should be fitted with safety devices which cut off the fuel gas supply in the event of failure of the flame or oxidant gas

an inert gas shield. This procedure reduces the flame background signal by preventing the entrainment of room air which forms the blue secondary reaction zone in the outer mantle of the flame. This is particularly advantageous in atomic emission or atomic fluorescence spectrometry.

Although the processes whereby an element in the aqueous sample becomes a free excited atom in the flame are complex (Fig. 3) and the factors influencing their efficiencies are incompletely understood, remarkably reproducible results can be obtained provided that the pressure and flow rates of the gas supplies are precisely controlled. For emission analysis, the flame temperature must be high enough to excite sufficient atoms to give the required sensitivity but not so high that appreciable ionization occurs. In addition, the emission spectrum of the flame itself should not overlap the wavelengths of the spectral lines to be measured. In atomic absorption analysis the function of the flame is to convert the sample into an atomic vapour. As a general rule the flame temperature should be as low as possible compatible with complete atomization of the analytical element in order to obtain maximum residence time of the atoms in the optical path of the instrument. The air–acetylene flame is adequate for most elements but for those producing thermally stable compounds, or where the matrix contains such materials, the higher temperature of the nitrous oxide–acetylene flame is desirable. This flame produces long-lived CN and NH species which apparently inhibits the formation of oxides. The nitrous oxide–acetylene flame is very transparent at short wavelengths (approximately 180 nm), but only a few elements of clinical interest, e.g. arsenic and selenium, have resonance lines at such short wavelengths. The nitrous oxide–acetylene flame is slightly more difficult to use and requires efficient ventilation, but when used as a separated flame this gas mixture can serve as a very sensitive source for emission flame photometry. The low-temperature, reducing, hydrogen–argon-entrained air flame which is also very transparent at short wavelengths gives the greatest sensitivity for a few elements, e.g. tin, but is subject to numerous interferences.

The rate at which the solvated sample vaporizes either in an aerosol or from a solid support depends on its chemical composition and the flame temperature. High temperature flames give rapid and complete vaporization but result in greater expansion of the flame gases and hence a reduction in the atomic vapour density. Once a sample is atomized the element can react with flame gases and this can lead to a loss of sensitivity if stable compounds are formed. A fuel-rich flame minimizes oxide formation. Since the density of the excited atoms in the flame varies with the height above the burner it is important to select, for each element, the correct zone of the flame in which analytical measurements are made in order that interferences are minimized and sensitivity maximized.

Electrically Energized Atomization. Electrically heated furnaces may produce a neutral atomic vapour only or may, additionally, excite the emission spectrum of the element being analysed. Systems generating the former have a low background emission and are therefore particularly suitable for use in atomic absorption and atomic fluorescence analysis. When a gas is heated electrically it may be used as an emission source and by appropriate choice of excitation

systems such as atmospheric or low pressure gas plasmas, arcs or sparks, effective temperatures ranging from 3000 to 10 000 K can be obtained. These high temperatures reduce matrix interferences and increase excitation of the atomic vapour. Two forms of plasma-generating systems based on a flow of inert gas are in current use. The most widespread is the inductively coupled plasma (ICP) which operates at radio frequencies (5–50 MHz, 1–5 kW) and is used for the analysis of solutions (Fig. 5a), and the microwave plasma (MIP) operated at 2450 MHz and ~200 W and used for gas analysis (Fig. 5b). As the analytical sensitivities of these systems tend to be comparable with or worse than those for atomic absorption methods, the principal justification for the use of plasmas lies either in a special advantage for a particular analysis, e.g. the analysis of the effluent from a gas chromatograph by an MIP, or in their multi-element capability. Because of the high cost and complexity of the excitation system and its associated optical equipment these techniques are not widely used for the analysis of clinical material.

The inductively coupled plasma has also been coupled to mass spectrometers (ICP-MS) to produce a powerful technique for the determination of elements by virtue of its sensitivity, multi-element capability and applicability to stable isotope analysis. It is relatively free from interferences but molecular compounds may be formed in the plasma whose masses are coincident with those of the analyte elements. This effect may complicate the determination of trace elements in untreated clinical materials such as serum owing to the presence of a large excess of proteinous material. The problem may be overcome by preliminary ashing of the sample. Instrumentation for ICP-MS is very expensive and the technique is unlikely to have a major impact on clinical analysis for some time.

In electrothermal atomizers, atomization is effected by resistive heating of the sample support. This support is commonly made of graphite and in the widely used Massmann furnace (Fig. 6a) takes the form of a tube approximately 5 cm long, 0.5 cm i.d., with a small hole in the centre through which the sample is dispensed. In order that atomization may take place in an inert atmosphere the tube is mounted in a chamber on the absorption path of an atomic absorption instrument. An alternative system (Fig. 6b) operates in the open with an inert gas shield and consists of a graphite rod, a few mm in diameter and ~4 cm in length, the centre of which is machined to provide an indent into which the sample is dispensed. This system is claimed to be particularly suitable for atomic fluorescence measurements. The addition of a small amount of methane to the inert gas shield reduces oxidation and increases the lifetime of graphite rods by producing a coating of pyrolytic carbon on the surface of the rod. To contain the atomic vapour for absorption measurements a small graphite tube (Fig. 6c) or cup (0.5 cm deep and

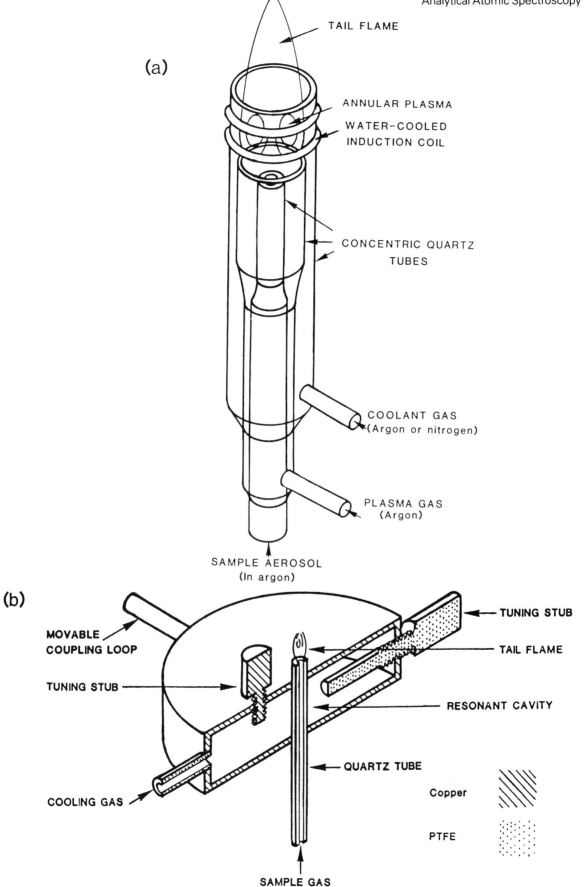

Fig. 5 Electrical plasma generating systems: (a) inductively coupled plasma torch; (b) microwave cavity plasma generator.

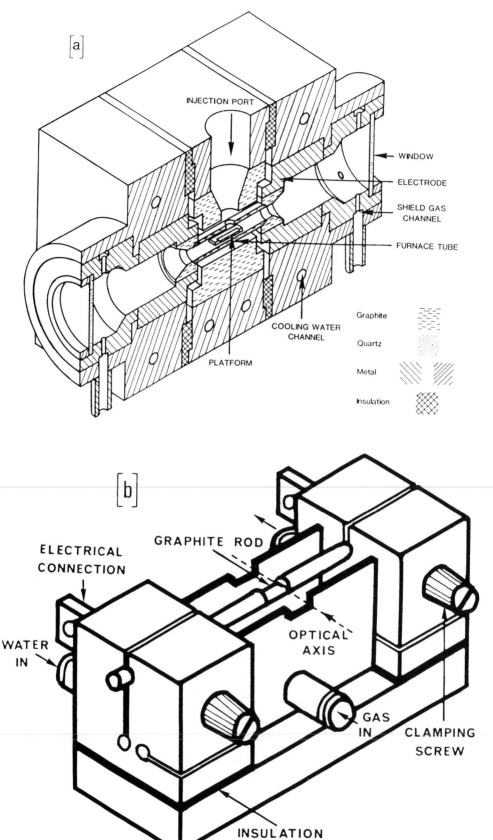

Fig. 6 Electrically heated graphite atomizers: (a) Massmann furnace; (b) carbon rod atomizers.

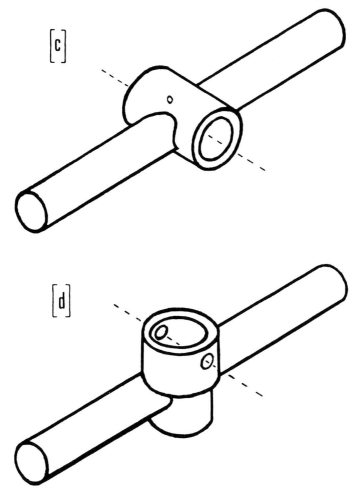

Fig. 6 (*contd.*) Electrically heated graphite atomizers: (c) mini-Massmann furnace; (d) graphite cup. Systems (c) and (d) are mounted in place of the rod shown in (b).

a few mm in diameter) (Fig. 6d) is mounted between spring-loaded graphite rods which also provide electrical connections. The sample is dispensed into the cup or tube and absorption measurements are made either through the tube or a small hole near the upper lip of the crucible. The mass sensitivities of these devices are greater than those of the Massmann furnaces but only small samples can be handled. When using a tubular furnace, matrix interference effects are reduced if the sample is placed on a graphite platform (the L'vov platform[6]) within the furnace (Fig. 6a). This improvement is attributed to atomization taking place into an atmosphere that is hotter than the surface of the platform. The sampling cycle time is slightly increased.

Electrothermal atomizers can accommodate sample volumes ranging from 1.0 to 100 μl. The solution is dried *in situ* by the passage of a small current, the temperature of the support is then raised to ash the sample and finally the residue is atomized by passing a current of 100–300 A. The process cycle time is 1–3 min while the duration of the atomic vapour pulse is less than 1 s. The reproducibility of the atomic

absorbance signal ranges from 1 to 10% depending largely upon the reproducibility of sample dispensing and distribution within the furnace. As the volatility of elements varies considerably it is necessary to optimize the instrumental operating conditions for each analysis. The combustion of organic materials generates smoke and molecular species which may scatter and absorb the analytical line. In some cases this spurious absorption signal is generated before the element vaporizes (Fig. 7, Peak A) and thus does not interfere with the analysis. Commonly, however, some background absorption occurs simultaneously with the analytical signal (Fig. 7, Trace ii, Peak B). To correct for this effect, the background absorbance is measured and subtracted from that of the resonance line (Fig. 7, Trace iii).

Background absorbance can be measured using either the continuum spectrum from a deuterium discharge lamp with the wavelength setting of the instrument unchanged or a nearby non-resonance spectral line emitted by the absorption light source. In the former case it is the average absorbance over the pass band of the monochromator (~1 nm) which is measured while in the latter, though the effective band width is much less (0.002 nm), the measurement is made at a wavelength remote from the resonance line. Measurements of background absorbance very close to the wavelength of the analytical line may be made by the Smith–Hieftje system,[7] In this approach self-reversal of the resonance line emitted by the hollow cathode lamp is produced by passing

Zeeman effects occurring in the background signals and temporal changes in atomic or background absorbances within the cycle time of the magnetic field. The influence of these effects is not likely to be serious. For most analyses, however, deuterium arc background correction combined with matrix modification and platform atomization will produce satisfactory analytical results.

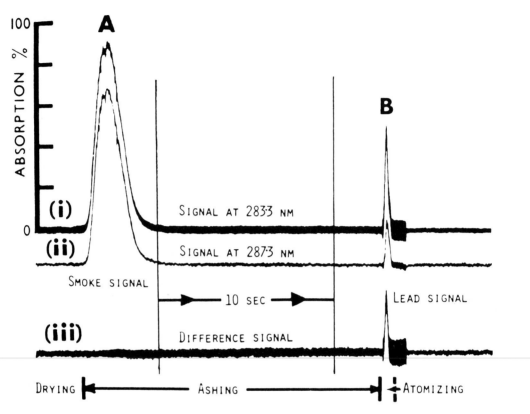

Fig. 7 Absorption traces resulting from the atomization of 2 µl of whole blood containing 580 µg/l of lead in a graphite cup atomizer: (i) absorption at lead resonance radiation wavelength; (ii) absorption at background correction wavelength; (iii) net absorption due to lead, corrected for background. Peak A, absorption due to combustion of organic material. Peak B, absorption due to lead and sodium chloride vapour.

heavy current pulses (100 µs, 300 mA) through the lamp. This removes most of the radiation that can be absorbed by the analyte element in the atomized sample. The absorbance signal produced during the current pulse is thus determined principally by background absorption and during normal low current operation by atomic plus background absorbances. Not all elements readily produce self-reversal of the resonance line. The most complete method of background correction available at the present time is based on generating the inverse Zeeman effect in the atomic vapour by placing the atomizer in an alternating magnetic field.[8] By utilizing the optical polarization effects associated with the Zeeman effect, background correction up to absorbance 2 can be made at precisely the same wavelength as the atomic absorption measurement. The limitations in this method of background correction may arise from

Copper, iridium, silver, tantalum and tungsten metals have been used as current-carrying sample supports. Tantalum has been used in strip form in a sealed chamber, the sample being held in an indent. During an analysis the chamber is filled with an inert gas, or for the measurement of refractory oxides a hydrogen purge is used. The other metals have been used as wires in a variety of atmospheres but the lower melting points of some of these limit the range of elements which can be determined. The most important characteristics of a material to be used in the fabrication of furnace tubes, cups or filaments are: high melting point, very low level of impurities, chemical inertness, high strength, machinability, low thermal expansion, good electrical conduction, and maintenance of a stable shape. For general use carbon in one or other of its forms appears to be the most suitable material. Attempts have been made to improve the performance of graphite furnaces by coating the inner surface with metals such as lanthanum or zirconium. The procedure has not been found to be generally beneficial.

Detection limits in the region 10^{-12} g of element and CVs of 1–10% are obtained using electrothermal atomizers for atomic analysis. When expressed in terms of solution concentration these limits ($\sim 10^{-7}$ g/l) are some 1 to 2 orders of magnitude lower than can be obtained by direct aspiration of the sample. This improvement originates from efficient utilization of the sample and the generation of the atomic vapour in a small volume. As yet, furnace systems are somewhat slow in operation, but mechanized sample dispensing facilitates unattended operation and improved precision.

Atom Vapour Generation by Chemical Means. In these systems chemical reagents are used to release the analyte element from aqueous samples into gaseous form as either the element or a volatile compound. The advantages of this approach are reduced interferences by virtue of separating the analyte from the sample matrix, and lower concentration detection limits because larger volumes of sample can be used.

Cool vapour atomization. Mercury vapour may be generated from an aqueous sample by reduction of its compounds using stannous chloride or, less commonly, sodium borohydride to liberate the metal. The free mercury is removed by passing gas through the solution and is carried in the gas flow to an absorption cell where its absorption or fluorescence signal is measured. The method has a detection limit of ~ 1 ng and a CV of about 5%. Sensitivity can be increased by collecting the liberated mercury on silver or gold wire followed by its rapid release by heating.

Metal hydride generation. Several elements including antimony, arsenic, bismuth, germanium, lead, selenium, tellurium and tin, form volatile hydrides which readily decompose on heating to generate the free atom. A variety of reducing agents including zinc metal, magnesium-titanium (III) chloride, and sodium borohydride may be used. Sodium borohydride has proved to be the most useful and may be applied to all the above elements. The acidified sample is added to dilute sodium borohydride solution in a cell and an inert gas passed over the surface of the liquid. The rapid evolution of hydrogen mixes the hydride with the purge gas. The gas mixture is passed either to an argon–hydrogen–entrained air flame or to a silica atomizing tube heated electrically or by an air–acetylene burner where the hydrides are decomposed. The silica tube either serves as an atom reservoir for absorption measurements or its effluent is excited for fluorescence measurements. It is important that any air in the generator cells should be flushed out of the system prior to injection of the sample. The method has a CV of 5% to 10% and detection limits of 1 µg/l. Elements that are easily reduced by sodium borohydride, e.g. silver, copper, nickel, if present in relatively high concentration can interfere with the generation of the gaseous metal hydrides.

Light Sources

Continuum sources can be used for atomic absorption analysis but, as the absorption bandwidth of an atomic line is very narrow (~ 0.002 nm) the energy absorbed from such a source is relatively small and hence, unless very high quality optical and electronic systems are used, the analytical signal is weak. The theoretical advantage of a continuum source is that it is suitable for the analysis of a wide range of elements. In fact, the only significant application of these sources is in background-correction devices. Most of our discussion will therefore relate to atomic-line sources where considerable energy is available within the narrow absorption band.

The first requirement of an atomic-line light source is that it should emit resonance radiation of the element with a line width less than that of the absorption line. Absorption measurements are simplified when the emission line is intense, stable, non-reversed and free from significant continuum background or interfering lines, which could pass through the monochromator and lead to reduced sensitivity and non-linear calibration graphs. High-intensity radiation is essential for fluorescence measurements but the stability requirement is less stringent. The unwanted effect of light generated in the atom cell entering the detection system may be minimized by the use of either a very intense light source or by modulating that light source prior to its passage through the cell.

Discharge Lamps
Metal vapour discharge lamp. This type of lamp is filled with an inert gas at a pressure of 0.1–0.41 Pa. It contains a small amount of the metal to be excited and a pair of electrodes to supply electrical power either as DC or low frequency AC. The filler gas initially carries the discharge then the metal vaporizes and ionizes, takes over the discharge process and its emission spectrum is excited. This change in the discharge mechanism is demonstrated by the familiar transition from the red neon emission to the yellow sodium emission of some street lighting.

Electrodeless discharge lamp. Internal electrodes are not necessary when lamps are excited at radio or microwave frequencies. The lamps consist of a sealed quartz tube filled with an inert gas and contain the metal to be excited or one of its volatile compounds. Atomic emission is excited following the absorption of energy by ions in the lamp oscillating under the influence of a radio frequency field generated by a coil round the tube or by a microwave field produced in a resonant cavity. The lamps generate intense radiation of volatile elements such as arsenic, cadmium, mercury, selenium and zinc. They are more difficult to operate than hollow cathode lamps and are used mostly in atomic fluorescence where their greater brightness is an advantage.

Hollow cathode lamp. The hollow cathode lamp is the commonest light source used in atomic absorption spectroscopy and is suitable for most metals. The construction of the lamp is shown in Fig. 8. The cylindrical cathode contains the metal to be determined in

power supply should be highly stabilized as the light output of the lamp is very sensitive to changes in current. This output can be increased by up to 100-fold either by incorporating additional electrodes to generate a second discharge or by pulsing the current supply to the lamp (300 mA, $\sim$20 μs, 300 Hz). Demountable and water-cooled lamps have been used in special circumstances but for most applications the normal lamp is adequate.

Multi-element discharge lamps have been developed and offer two advantages: first, a single lamp is adequate for several analyses, therefore it is not

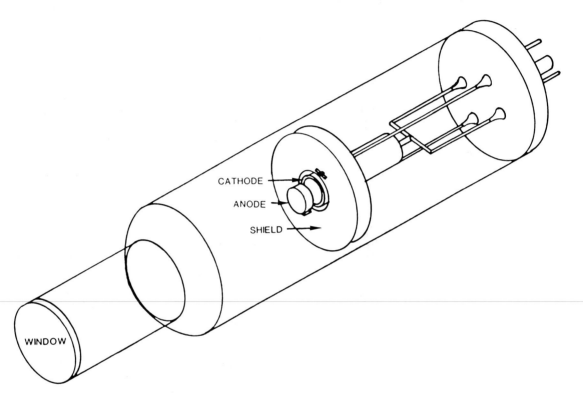

CATHODE

ANODE

SHIELD

WINDOW

Fig. 8 Hollow cathode discharge lamp.

the form of either pure metal, an alloy or in some cases, a coating on a suitable base metal. The anode is of tungsten and the window is borosilicate glass, or silica if the analytical line is in the ultraviolet region. An electrical potential of 350–500 V is applied to the lamp and this accelerates ions of the filler gas to strike the cathode with sufficient energy to eject metal atoms ('sputtering'). Collisions between these sputtered atoms and the filler gas ions lead to excitation of the emission spectrum of the former. As the cathode temperature is low and the interior of the cathode is free from electric fields, thermal ('Doppler') and electrical ('Stark') broadenings of the spectral line are minimized. Self absorption by the atomic vapour in the lamp, which can lead to loss of analytical sensitivity and curved calibration graphs, is minimized by running the lamp at the lowest possible current compatible with an adequate light output, this is frequently between 5 and 10 mA. The

necessary to stock as many lamps and secondly, there is no 'warming-up' when changing from one element to another. Four-element hollow cathode lamps have been operated but owing to preferential sputtering effects, the emission is not as great as that of a single element lamp. The limitations of multi-element lamps are: (1) only certain combinations of elements are possible, (2) the lamp life is no greater than that of a single element lamp, (3) the pressure of the filler gas is a compromise between the optima of the individual elements and (4) the cost of the multi-element lamp is greater than that of the single element lamp.

Radiation Measurement

Most of the sensitivity and selectivity of the analytical system is provided by the atomic process itself. The correct choice of wavelength-selection system, photodetector and electronic system can, however, facilitate the analysis by maximizing sensitivity, linearity and stability while minimizing the risk of errors arising from spurious signals generated by other components of the sample.

Wavelength Selection. The function of the wavelength-selecting device is to accept as much light from the source as possible and isolate the required spectral line. The aim is to obtain the maximum signal-to-noise ratio. The term 'noise' is used to describe the instability, or lack of reproducibility of the analytical signal. Most commonly it arises in the radiation source from the complex interactions in the excitation process which affect the intensity of the spectral line and its background, particularly in the event of weak signals where the randomicity of photon emission is dominant.

Wavelength selection can be achieved by using either a filter or a dispersive device. The light-gathering power or aperture of the filter is generally much greater than that of a dispersion system, but it is less selective. Further, the filter is simpler in construction but less flexible in application. If the signal-to-background ratio is high (≥ 2), though the absolute signal level is low, the signal-to-noise ratio can be improved by increasing the light-collecting power of the system, i.e. enlarging the filter size, widening the entrance slit, and integrating the signal. If the signal-to-background ratio is low (≤ 1) the signal-to-noise ratio can only be improved by increasing the resolution and light-collection efficiency of the system.

Optical filters. These devices may be divided into two groups: (1) absorptive filters such as coloured glass, gelatin and solutions, and (2) interference filters. The latter (Fig. 9a) can be made to transmit at any desired wavelength (λ) by adjusting the thickness (t) of transparent dielectric layers (refractive index, μ_λ) to satisfy the condition $n\lambda = 2\mu_\lambda t$ where n is an integer. Such a filter should be used with parallel light at near normal incidence when its bandwidth may be as little as 5 nm; the pass band of absorptive filters is much greater. When the emission from the element to be determined is very much stronger than that from any other element having a spectral line within the pass band of the filter, a simple filter is adequate, e.g. sodium in serum.

Dispersive systems. When parallel light falls on a prism or diffraction grating, it is dispersed to form a spectrum (Fig. 9b,c); if a single spectral region is observed, the instrument is a monochromator, if a wide region, it is a spectrograph or multichannel spectrometer.

Three parameters are used to measure the performance of a dispersion system: (1) reciprocal linear dispersion, which is usually expressed in nm/mm in the focal plane of the instrument; (2) resolution, the wavelength of measurement divided by the minimum wavelength interval between two spectral lines that

can be distinguished as separate; (3) the light-transmitting efficiency, determined by the aperture (defined as the focal length of the spectrum-forming lens divided by the diameter of the light-limiting orifice), the reflectivity of mirrors, transmission of lenses, and light losses in the dispersing element. The light-transmitting capacity of a prism instrument is greater than that of one using a grating because of the distribution of energy by the grating into several dispersion orders. The dispersion of a grating, is, however, generally greater than the prism and is practically independent of wavelength while that of a prism increases markedly from the visible to the ultraviolet. Unless a good quality grating is used, light scattered by the grating may generate a background signal.

The requirements of a monochromator for atomic absorption analysis are slightly less demanding than those for emission in that light-collection efficiency is less important because of the relatively high brightness of the absorption light sources and the simpler spectrum. Furthermore, up to 2% of non-resonance radiation may pass through the monochromator without detectable loss of either sensitivity or linearity of calibration. Dispersions of 0.1 to 1.0 nm/mm are therefore used in emission analysis while 1 to 6 nm/mm are adequate for absorption. The resolution of a filter flame photometer for the determination of sodium and potassium may be as low as 30, while that of an atomic absorption instrument may be 2000 and of an emission spectrometer 30 000. In emission analysis, rapid repetitive short-range wavelength scanning may be used to modulate the intensity of a spectral line so that electronic means may be used to isolate it from a background continuum.

When large numbers of samples are to be analysed the wavelength stability of the instrument is important. With filter instruments this problem does not arise and can be minimized in a dispersive monochromator by setting the exit slit to be slightly wider than the entrance. In the case of sophisticated spectrometers, computer control is used to stabilize the instrument settings.

Photodetectors. The radiation emitted by an excited atom may be detected and measured by either photographic or photoelectric devices. In the former case, the radiation is dispersed in a spectrograph and the resulting spectrum photographed. In the latter, a single spectral line is selected by means of either a filter or monochromator and is used to activate a photoelectric detector which provides an electrical signal proportional to the intensity of the radiation incident upon it. Photographic recording is rarely used in clinical chemistry owing to the inconveniences of film processing and densitometric measurements, and the poor analytical precision (CV = 10%).

There are four types of *photoelectric detectors*: (1) photovoltaic, the generation of an electromotive

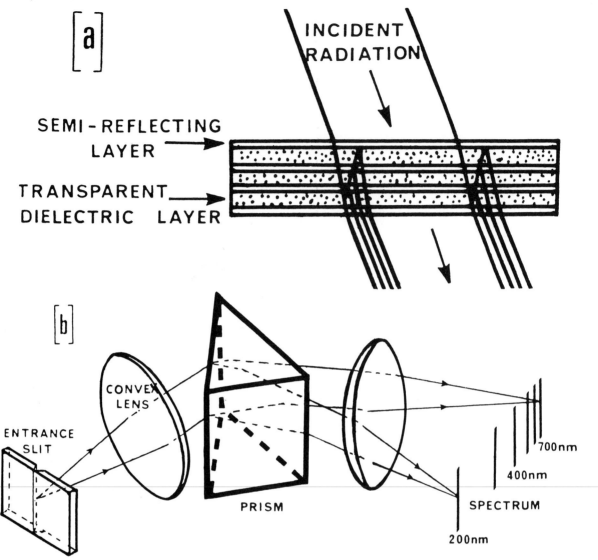

Fig. 9 Wavelength selecting systems: (a) interference filter; (b) prism spectrograph.

force across a junction of two metals; (2) photoemissive, the emission of electrons from a photosensitive surface; (3) photoconductive, reduction in the resistance of an irradiated surface; (4) phototransistor, modulation of current flow through a transistor when radiation falls on its junction. Photoemissive detectors are the ones most widely used in spectrochemical analysis. The vacuum photoemissive cells have greater sensitivity, spectral range and stability than solid state detectors. The latter can, however, be fabricated into a linear array of photodiodes for the simultaneous measurement of radiation at several wavelengths in a dispersed spectrum.

The photomultiplier is a combination of a photoemissive cell with an electron multiplier; it is the most sensitive and widely used detector in spectrochemical analysis. In the photomultiplier, electrons released when light strikes the photocathode are accelerated by an electrical potential towards a sensitive surface, the dynode, which releases an average of five elec-

trons for every electron striking it. By the suitable arrangement of a series of dynodes and accelerating potentials a total electron multiplication of the order of 10^6 may be achieved. Light intensities can be measured with a CV of 0.1% or better.

One of the most important properties of a photodetector is its spectral response. The maximum efficiency of a photocathode (electrons/photon) is of the order of 10–15%. Most photocathodes have a peak in their response at about 400 nm and fall to low values at 200 and 650 nm. Special cathode materials may be used to extend the response to 800 nm on the one hand and to 150 nm on the other. Generally a photomultiplier which is sensitized to respond to red and infrared radiation will suffer from a greater 'dark' current, i.e. a current when the cathode is not irradiated. When measurements are to be confined to the spectral region below 310 nm it is advantageous to use a 'solar blind' photomultiplier (i.e. one which does not respond to visible light) as this reduces the

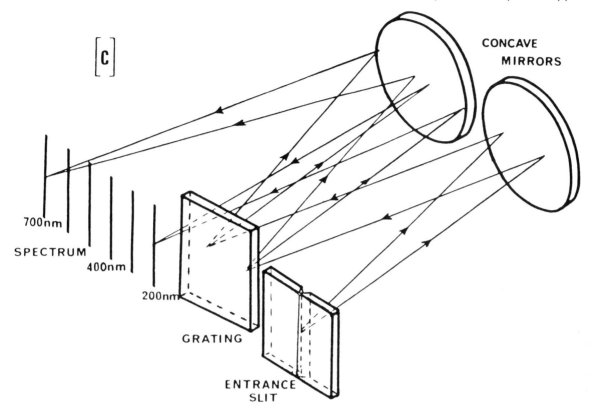

[c]

700nm

SPECTRUM

400nm

200nm

GRATING

ENTRANCE
SLIT

CONCAVE
MIRRORS

Fig. 9 (*contd.*) Wavelength selecting systems: (c) grating spectrometer.

background signals in the system due to stray light and dark current.

The output signal of a photomultiplier is a stream of electron pulses. At low light intensity it is possible to resolve the individual pulses. The frequency of these pulses is a measure of the rate at which photons strike the photocathode. The counting of individual photo-electron pulses can be used to obtain lower detection limits in emission or fluorescence analysis by facilitating the measurement of low light levels. The performance of photomultipliers is further improved by cooling the photocathode to reduce the tube dark current; this does not have any significant effect on its sensitivity to light.

Electronic System and Readout. The ideal measuring system produces an output signal which is proportional to the concentration of the measured element over a concentration range of several orders of magnitude. The analytical signal generated by the emission or absorption of radiation by the element and the response of the detector often do not fulfil this condition. In these cases either the instrument operator draws a calibration curve or the instrument maker incorporates a linearizing circuit in the instrument in order to derive the concentration of the element. For example, in atomic absorption analysis a logarithmic amplifier may be used to convert a signal which is proportional to transmittance to one pro-

portional to absorbance and hence to the concentration of the atomic vapour. For a given set of analytical conditions the range of sample concentration which can be satisfactorily measured is up to three orders of magnitude for emission and fluorescence spectrometry but little more than a single order for atomic absorption. By adjustment of the analytical procedure, a working range appropriate to the samples to be analysed can usually be obtained.

The measuring circuit of the early flame photometers consisted of a photovoltaic cell connected directly to a galvanometer. Modern instruments, using photomultipliers, require amplification of the photocurrent before it is adequate to drive a measuring circuit. The radiation from the light source used in atomic absorption and atomic fluorescence is usually modulated to improve discrimination against background signals. Modulation is effected either by modulating the current passing through the lamp or by using an optical 'chopper' which interrupts the light beam. Demodulation is carried out by tuned or linear gating circuits and lock-in or phase-sensitive amplifiers. These circuits select only that part of the output signal which occurs at the same time as radiation from the light source is passing through the system; they also automatically subtract any continuous background signal. It is important that the response of the electronic system is sufficiently fast to reproduce accurately transient signals. Once the desired signal has been extracted it may require further processing to obtain a more readable output signal. Most commonly this would involve increasing the response time of the circuit to minimize the effects of short-term fluctuations in the signal. The precision of the reading may also be improved by integrating the output signal for a predetermined time. When the anticipated variation in the amount or concentration of the element to be measured is small, scale expansion may be used to facilitate the measurement. Scale expansion consists of increasing the amplification of the output signal and introducing a controllable signal of opposite polarity to 'neutralize' or 'back-off' most of the analytical signal, consequently small changes in the analytical signal are a greater proportion of the net output signal. The incorporation of microcomputers into spectrometers not only has increased the sophistication of the processing of the analytical results, e.g. linearization of calibration curves and correction for matrix interference effects, but also has made possible the automatic adjustment of instrument parameters to accommodate the desired analysis.

The output signal may be presented in analogue form on a meter or chart recorder and digitally on a display or printer. While the most elaborate read-out system may be of the greatest convenience to the analyst, it is also liable to be the greatest trouble in its setting up and servicing and is only justifiable when large numbers of identical analyses are to be carried out. Commonly the most satisfactory system consists of a recorder read-out, for the instrument may then be left unattended with automatic sample feed yet the operator has the opportunity to monitor visually the performance of the equipment. The output signal may also be fed to a separate computer system for more sophisticated data processing.

INSTRUMENTS FOR SPECTROCHEMICAL ANALYSIS

A great variety of instruments is available for spectrochemical analysis ranging from simple single-channel flame photometers for sodium or potassium to complex vacuum direct-reading spectrometers for the simultaneous measurement of many elements. Though general use of the multi-element ICP spectrometer is increasing, its application to clinical analysis is very limited; therefore, for the purpose of this review we will restrict discussion to the single- or dual-channel instruments which have found widespread use in clinical chemistry. These instruments use the flame as the atomizing system with provision for attachments for electrothermal atomization. They are designed for either emission or absorption spectroscopy but some may be adapted by the user for atomic fluorescence work. As a general policy when a large number of identical analyses have to be carried out, best results are to be obtained by

dedicating an instrument to that work and this can often be met by relatively simple instrumentation. Where a greater variety of analyses is required, more expensive instrumentation may be inevitable.

When the purchase of an instrument is contemplated it is highly desirable that the user should carry out trials of at least two instruments over a period of several days in his own laboratory. Factors to be evaluated include: the convenience of operation of the instrument, the precision and accuracy of results, safety, operating costs in terms of capital depreciation, materials and labour, maintenance service by either the manufacturer or an 'in-house' technician and, if the instrument is to be used for a variety of analyses, the ease of conversion from one application to another. If the prospective customer cannot carry out these trials he should at least consult colleagues with experience of the instruments.

Emission Flame Photometers

Simple flame photometers using a filter for selecting the required spectral line are suitable for the determination of sodium and potassium in most clinical samples. In these instruments the sample is nebulized into the relatively cool air–propane flame. Several filter/photodetector units may be mounted round a single flame for simultaneous measurement of several elements. The desirable features of a flame photometer are rapid operation, the use of minimal quantities of sample, high sensitivity, no carry-over, complete linearity and high precision. The use of an internal standard generally reduces the effect of instrumental drift but may increase the random error of measurement. The greater the sensitivity and stability of the instrument, the more dilute the analytical solution can be. This is generally advantageous, except for the risks of contamination or loss of elements by adsorbtion onto the walls of the storage vessel, because interference effects are less and calibration curves more linear.

To obtain the accuracy necessary to meet clinical requirements, standards spanning the range found in practice should be run with each set of determinations and at least one of these should be repeated at regular intervals with the samples. With instruments calibrated to read directly in concentration units, particular care is necessary to ensure that the instrument performance corresponds to the conditions under which the original calibration curve for the instrument was derived. Interferences are generally not a serious problem though in the determination of potassium, to minimize spectral interference by sodium, some instruments incorporate a sodium-rejection filter in the potassium channel.

Calcium and lithium may also be determined using simple filter flame photometers but atomic absorption methods are preferable for the measurement of the low concentrations of lithium in serum and to overcome the interference problems which arise with calcium. The range of elements determined by emission flame photometry can be widened if the high temperature nitrous oxide flame is used, but to take advantage of this system a much more selective monochromator is required to avoid the problems of spectral interference. Further, the analytical signal is dependent on flame temperature and slight changes in flame gas composition can lead to significant changes in sensitivity. The principal advantage of such a system, in comparison with atomic absorption, is the elimination of the absorption light source.

Atomic Absorption Spectrometers

The stability of a single-beam instrument (Fig. 10a) using either an air–acetylene or nitrous oxide–acetylene flame is frequently adequate for clinical analysis provided that a warm-up period prior to measurements is allowed. The instrument can be applied to a wide range of elements. Baseline drift due to changes in output of the light source can be reduced by incorporating a double-beam optical system (Fig. 10b) into the instrument. In such a system radiation

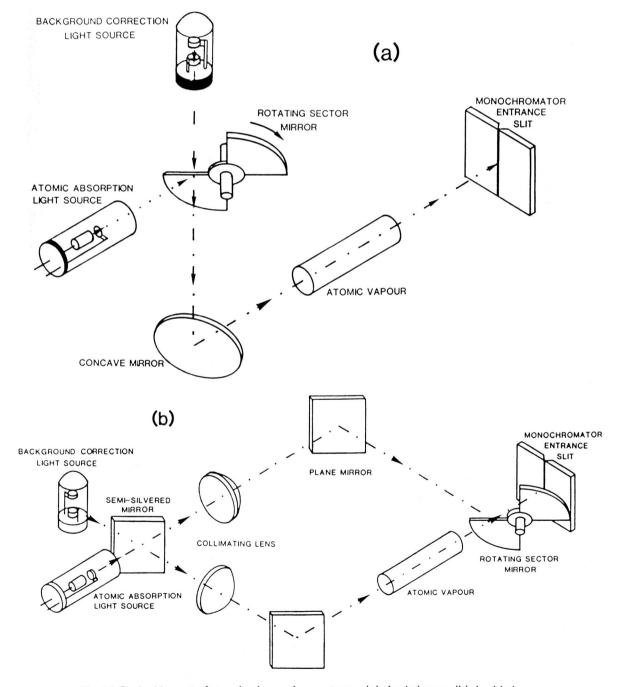

Fig. 10 Optical layout of atomic absorption systems: (a) single beam; (b) double beam.

from the source follows two paths, one passing through the atomic vapour and the other around it. The intensity of the radiation following each path is measured and the resulting signals are combined electronically to give an output which is a function of their ratio, i.e. absorption or absorbance. Though the long-term stability of the baseline is greatly improved, the short-term random fluctuation may even be worse owing to the increased complexity of the instrument. With many instruments satisfactory correction for baseline drift is achieved by means of an automatic zero reset of the instrument at regular intervals during the analysis of a batch of samples. There is little difference between the sensitivities of single- and double-beam instruments when using similar atomizing systems. All instruments may be connected to chart recorders or printers in addition to the analogue or digital display built into the instrument for presenting the output signal.

When transient response and non-flame atomization is used, some form of correction for the background absorption arising from smoke and molecular vapours is usually necessary. Improved background correction is obtained if the absorbances of the spectral line and the background are measured simultaneously by instrumental means. The simplest system is one in which the reference channel of a double-beam instrument is used to accommodate a spectral continuum light source, usually a deuterium discharge lamp. In this system, the compensation for light source instability may be lost but, provided great care is taken over the optical and electronic alignment of the two channels and the instrument is allowed to reach thermal stability, effective and instantaneous background correction is obtained. In dual-wavelength instruments incorporating double-beam operation the electronic circuit of the second wavelength-channel can be used to give background correction. This system corrects for drift in the light output of both the resonance and the spectral continuum lamps. Where background correction is provided by either the Smith–Hieftje or Zeeman systems, the optical system is simple as only a single light source is used. The Zeeman system is the most universally applicable but requires the more elaborate instrumentation. Both systems can produce calibration curves in which the absorbance value rises to a maximum with increasing analyte concentration and then decreases. The origin of this 'roll-over' in the calibration curve is the existence of a significant level of atomic absorption within the background correction signal and stray light within the atomic absorption signal. In this situation it is possible, at high analyte concentrations, for the measured background-correction absorbance to increase with analyte concentration faster than the measured atomic absorption signal. The corrected signal, i.e. the difference between the two measured absorbances, can thus decrease with increasing concentration.

Instruments are provided with facilities for scale expansion of typically up to 50-fold and also for adjusting the time constant of the response of the instrument to match the increased sensitivity. Variable integration times and peak reading facilities may also be available. The operation of some atomic absorption instruments is simplified by

1. the incorporation of automatic flame ignition with safety devices,
2. auto-zero facilities whereby the press of a button sets the instrument to zero absorbance, and
3. read-out displays indicating directly in concentration units.

To reduce the changeover time when measuring several different elements some instruments are provided with stand-by facilities for warming-up hollow cathode lamps. To make full use of the facilities available on an instrument, careful attention should be given to the manufacturer's handbook.

As the absorption of radiation by the atomic vapour obeys the Beer–Lambert law, absorbance should be plotted against concentration to obtain linear calibration curves. In practice, however, the solutions analysed are usually dilute and generate an absorption signal of the order of 10% of the incident radiation. When this is the case, almost linear calibration curves can be obtained by plotting absorption against concentration. To obtain accurate measurements of these low densities, scale expansion with display of the output signal on a chart recorder is necessary. Three- to five-fold expansion is commonly used and may be extended up to fifty- or a hundred-fold. In the latter case, however, unless large time constants are used, the instability of the signal will be such that the results will be no better than those obtained using a scale expansion of 10- to 30-fold.

The range of elements which are measurable by an instrument can be considerably increased with the aid of attachments. These usually take the form of special atomizers such as electrothermal devices and hydride generators which can give up to 1000-fold improvement in sensitivity for some elements. One of the most useful attachments is automatic sample handling as this facilitates unattended operation of the instrument. The simplest system is an independently controlled turntable presenting samples sequentially to a flame photometer, the most elaborate is a turntable with a sampling arm injecting samples into a graphite furnace which also controls the operation of the furnace and the data processing of the atomic absorption spectrometer. While each instrument manufacturer has a range of attachments for his own instrument it is often feasible to assemble a hybrid system.

Most atomic absorption instruments may also be used for emission analysis. If a nitrous oxide–acetylene flame can be used and the instrument contains a relatively high resolution monochromator, then the detection limits for elements with analytical lines at wavelengths $\geqslant 300$ nm are likely to be as low as those using atomic absorption. This facility appears to be overlooked by many users. Similarly, experience suggests that fluorescence attachments, in combination with cool vapour or hydride generators, may be most suitable for a limited range of elements such as arsenic, mercury, lead and selenium.

Instrument Operation

The instrument should be located in a clean, draught-free environment, provided with a fume extraction hood and sufficient space for handling samples. Attention should be given to the safe storage of gas cylinders. Where compressed air is used, the supply must be clean and adequate to meet the demands of the instrument without a significant reduction in the pressure. Cylinders of acetylene should be replaced before becoming completely empty to avoid contamination of the fuel gas with acetone. Electrical interlocks should be incorporated into the gas and water supply lines to ensure safe operation of the instrument and as safeguards against possible leaks.

Most instruments will give better results if allowed to settle down for at least 15 min after switching on. Before commencing an analysis the performance of the instrument should be checked using standard materials to ensure that it is operating under its established optimum conditions. Though an analytical instruction book is supplied with the instrument, it is advisable to examine the effect of changes in instrumental setting whenever a new analysis or new instrument is being established in the laboratory. In the case of a flame-based instrument this procedure involves determining the flow rates of the fuel and oxidant gases and the zone of the flame suitable for the analysis. To obtain maximum sensitivity and stability of an atomic absorption spectrometer the current through the light source may require periodic adjustment particularly when the lamp is approaching the end of its life. Other instrumental controls requiring setting include the wavelength scale, the slit width of the monochromator, the amplifier gain and scale expansion. When using a nebulizing system the sample flow rate may also need adjustment and periodic checking to ensure that blockage has not occurred. Flameless atomizers also require optimization of gas flows and the current and times required for drying, ashing and atomizing the sample. Where continuum source background correction is employed, the intensity of the light from that source will require adjustment to obtain a balance with the absorption light source.

Where a large number of similar analyses are to be carried out by a variety of operators, best results will be obtained if an instrument is dedicated to that analysis alone and its operation standardized as far as possible. If, to accommodate a variety of analyses, it is necessary to alter the operating conditions of the instrument, it is desirable that this should be carried out by one or two operators who specialize in the analyses.

The techniques of analytical atomic spectroscopy are not easily incorporated into automatic clinical chemistry systems because of difficulties in obtaining compatible sample throughput rates, instrumental stability, and the need to maintain a close watch on the performance of the instrument to avoid malfunctions such as nebulizer blockage. The principal merits of automation are reduced operator fatigue and improved precision. These advantages are not likely to be realized on batch sizes of less than 20 to 30 samples or with a throughput of less than 100 samples per week. The most time-consuming operations in spectrochemical analysis are sample preparation and data processing. These processes may be automated but the complexity and expense of doing so in the routine clinical laboratory are generally barely justified by the analytical work load though other factors such as improved precision may be an important consideration.

Instruments in regular use require servicing which, in addition to incorporating performance checks, may include cleaning and replacement of parts. The need for such maintenance, much of which could be carried out by laboratory staff, is likely to be infrequent but should not be overlooked if consistent performance is to be obtained from the instrument.

ANALYTICAL PROCEDURES

To avoid repetitive descriptions of procedures for individual elements, this section will deal with general methods of sample preparation and instrumental technique from which may be selected methods suitable for most metals of interest in clinical chemistry. Flame methods are generally used and a guide to the choice of the combustion gas mixture which will give the greatest sensitivity for a given element is presented in Table 2.

The concentration of some elements in biological tissue and the detection limits for those elements by several spectrochemical techniques are given in Table 3. The purpose of this table is to provide data on the basis of which an analytical method may be selected for the measurement of a given element in particular tissue. It cannot be regarded as a reference source of biochemical information owing to the wide variation in the published values from which it was compiled. Similar variability was found in the reported detection limits whose published values usually relate to pure solutions of the metal, not biological samples. Detection limits in biological samples may be only one-fifth as sensitive as those in pure solutions. To overcome the effects of sample viscosity and surface tension when the sample is aspirated into a flame, serum should be diluted at least 10- or 20-fold. This additional dilution of the sample increases the demand on the sensitivity of the analytical system. The suitability of a method for a particular

TABLE 2

RECOMMENDED GASES FOR USE IN FLAME ATOMIC ABSORPTION SPECTROSCOPY. 1. PREFERRED MIXTURE. 2. ALTERNATIVE MIXTURE

Propane air 1	Propane air 2	Air 1	Air 2	Acetylene oxygen 1	Acetylene oxygen 2	Nitrous oxide 1	Nitrous oxide 2	Hydrogen air 1	Hydrogen air 2
Ag		Au	Ag			Al		As	
Bi			Ba, Bi			Ba, Bi			
						B			
Cd, Cs	Cu	Co, Cu	Ca, Cd			Ca, Ce			
			Cr, Cs			Cr			
		Fe		Eu		Er	Eu		
		Ga		Gd			Gd		
			Hg			Hf, Ho			
		In, Ir							
K			K						
Li			Li		La	La, Lu			
		Mg, Mn	Mo			Mo			
	Na	Na, Ni				Nb, Nd			
		Pb, Pd				Os			
		Pt			Pr	Pr			
Rb		Rh	Rb			Re			
		Se, Sr	Sn			Si, Sc	Sn	Sn	Se
	Sb	Sb				Sm	Sr		
		Te, Tl				Ti, Tm			
						Ta, Tb			
						Th			
						U, V			
						W			
						Yb, Y			
Zn			Zn			Zr			

TABLE 3

CONCENTRATIONS IN HUMAN TISSUE AND DETECTION LIMITS IN AQUEOUS SOLUTION FOR METALS OF PHYSIOLOGICAL INTEREST. OWING TO THE VARIABILITY OF PUBLISHED DATA, NUMERICAL VALUES ARE ROUNDED OFF TO 1, 2 OR 5

Element/Atomic weight	Matrix	Concentration in solution or wet tissue g/l	g/g*	g/day	Method	Wavelength (nm)	Representative detection limit (pure solution) g/l	g†
Ag	Blood, whole.	10^{-6}			Emission, flame	328.1	10^{-5}	
	serum		5×10^{-8}		plasma		2×10^{-6}	
	Tissues				Absorption, flame	328.1	10^{-6}	
					electrothermal		2×10^{-8}	2×10^{-13}
107.87	Intake, food				Fluorescence, flame	328.1	10^{-7}	
					electrothermal		10^{-7}	10^{-12}
	Excretion, urine							
	Total body							
Al	Blood, whole.	5×10^{-6}			Emission, flame	396.2	5×10^{-6}	
	serum	5×10^{-6}			plasma	396.2	10^{-6}	10^{-11}
	Tissues		5×10^{-5} to 2×10^{-7}		Absorption, flame	309.3	2×10^{-5}	
					electrothermal		10^{-6}	10^{-11}
26.98	Intake, food			5×10^{-2}	Fluorescence, flame		10^{-4}	
					electrothermal			
	Excretion, urine	10^{-5}						
	Total body	10^{-1} g						
As	Blood, whole.	2×10^{-4}			Emission, flame	235.0	10^{-2}	
	serum	2×10^{-6}			plasma	278.0	10^{-5}	
	Tissues		10^{-6} to 10^{-7}		Absorption, flame	193.7	10^{-4}	
74.92					electrothermal		10^{-6}	10^{-11}
					cool vapour			
					(hydride)	193.7	10^{-6}	10^{-9}
	Intake, food			10^{-4}	Fluorescence, flame	193.7	10^{-4}	
					electrothermal			
					cool vapour			
					(hydride)	193.7	10^{-7}	
	Excretion, urine	2×10^{-5}						
	Total body	2×10^{-2} g						
Au	Blood, whole.				Emission, flame	267.6	5×10^{-4}	
	serum				plasma			
196.97	Tissues		2×10^{-6} to 10^{-7}		Absorption, flame		2×10^{-5}	
					electrothermal	242.8	10^{-6}	10^{-11}

TABLE 3—Contd.

Element/Atomic weight	Matrix	Concentration in solution or wet tissue			Method	Wavelength	Representative detection limit (pure solution)	
		g/l	$g/g*$	g/day		(nm)	g/l	$g†$
	Intake, food				Fluorescence, flame	242.8	5×10^{-6}	
					electrothermal		5×10^{-7}	5×10^{-12}
	Excretion, urine Total body							
Ba	Blood, whole.				Emission, flame	553.6	10^{-6}	
	serum	2×10^{-5}			plasma	455.4	5×10^{-7}	
137.34	Tissues		10^{-7} to 2×10^{-8}		Absorption, flame	553.6	2×10^{-5}	
					electrothermal		10^{-5}	10^{-10}
	Intake, food			2×10^{-3}	Fluorescence, flame			
					electrothermal			
	Excretion, urine Total body	2×10^{-2} g						
Be	Blood, whole.				Emission, flame	234.9	10^{-3}	
	serum				plasma	234.9	10^{-6}	
9.01	Tissues		10^{-8} to 5×10^{-10}		Absorption, flame	234.9	2×10^{-6}	
					electrothermal		2×10^{-7}	2×10^{-12}
	Intake, food				Fluorescence, flame		10^{-5}	
					electrothermal		2×10^{-8}	2×10^{-12}
	Excretion, urine Total body							
Bi	Blood, whole.	5×10^{-6}			Emission, flame	223.1	2×10^{-3}	
	serum				plasma		5×10^{-5}	
208.98	Tissues		$\leqslant 10^{-8}$		Absorption, flame	223.1	10^{-5}	
					electrothermal		10^{-6}	10^{-11}
					cool vapour			
					(hydride)	223.1	2×10^{-6}	2×10^{-10}
	Intake, food				Fluorescence, flame	223.1	2×10^{-5}	
					electrothermal		10^{-6}	10^{-11}
	Excretion, urine Total body	10^{-5}						
Ca	Blood, whole.				Emission, flame	422.7	2×10^{-7}	
	serum	10^{-1}			plasma	393.4	2×10^{-7}	
40.08	Tissues		2×10^{-1} to 5×10^{-5}		Absorption, flame	422.7	10^{-6}	
					electrothermal		2×10^{-8}	2×10^{-13}
	Intake, food			10^{0}	Fluorescence, flame		2×10^{-5}	
					electrothermal			
	Excretion, urine Total body	2×10^{-1} 10^{3} g						
Cd	Blood, whole.	10^{-6}			Emission, flame	326.1	10^{-3}	
	serum	10^{-7}			plasma	326.1	5×10^{-6}	5×10^{-10}
112.40	Tissues		2×10^{-4} to 10^{-6}		Absorption, flame	228.8	5×10^{-7}	
					electrothermal		10^{-7}	2×10^{-12}
					flame, cup		2×10^{-7}	10^{-11}
	Intake, food			5×10^{-5}	Fluorescence, flame	228.8	2×10^{-7}	
					electrothermal		10^{-9}	10^{-14}
	Excretion, urine Total body	10^{-6} 2×10^{-2} g						
Co	Blood, whole	5×10^{-7}			Emission, flame	345.4	2×10^{-5}	
	serum	5×10^{-7}			plasma		5×10^{-6}	
58.93	Tissues		2×10^{-7} to 10^{-8}		Absorption, flame	240.7	10^{-5}	
					electrothermal		5×10^{-7}	5×10^{-12}
	Intake, food			10^{-4}	Fluorescence, flame	240.7	2×10^{-6}	
					electrothermal		2×10^{-6}	2×10^{-11}
	Excretion, urine Total body	5×10^{-6} 2×10^{-3} g						
Cr	Blood, whole.				Emission, flame	425.4	5×10^{-6}	
	serum	10^{-6}			plasma	357.9	5×10^{-6}	
52.00	Tissues		10^{-6} to 5×10^{-7}		Absorption, flame	357.9	5×10^{-6}	
					electrothermal		5×10^{-7}	2×10^{-11}
	Intake, food			10^{-4}	Fluorescence, flame	357.9	5×10^{-5}	
					electrothermal		5×10^{-7}	5×10^{-12}
	Excretion, urine Total body	2×10^{-6} 5×10^{-3} g						
Cu	Blood, whole.	10^{-3}			Emission, flame	327.4	10^{-5}	
	serum	10^{-3}			plasma	327.4	5×10^{-6}	5×10^{-10}
63.54	Tissues		2×10^{-4} to 10^{-6}		Absorption, flame	324.7	2×10^{-6}	
					electrothermal		5×10^{-7}	10^{-11}
	Intake, food			2×10^{-3}	Fluorescence, flame	324.7	10^{-6}	
					electrothermal		10^{-7}	10^{-12}
	Excretion, urine Total body	2×10^{-4} 10^{-1} g						
Fe	Blood, whole.	5×10^{-1}			Emission, flame	372.0	2×10^{-5}	
	serum				plasma	372.0	5×10^{-6}	5×10^{-10}
55.85	Tissues		2×10^{-4} to 5×10^{-6}		Absorption, flame	248.3	10^{-5}	5×10^{-9}
					electrothermal		10^{-6}	2×10^{-12}
	Intake, food			10^{-2}	Fluorescence, flame	248.3	5×10^{-6}	
					electrothermal		2×10^{-6}	2×10^{-11}
	Excretion, urine Total body	5×10^{-4} 5 g						

TABLE 3—*Contd.*

Element/Atomic weight	Matrix	Concentration in solution or wet tissue — g/l	g/g*	g/day	Method	Wavelength (nm)	Representative detection limit (pure solution) — g/l	g†
Hg	Blood, whole.	10^{-6}			Emission, flame	253.7	10^{-2}	
	serum	2×10^{-6}			plasma	253.7	2×10^{-5}	
200.59	Tissues		10^{-6} to 10^{-7}		Absorption, flame	253.7	5×10^{-4}	
					electrothermal		10^{-5}	10^{-10}
					cool vapour		10^{-7}	10^{-9}
	Intake, food			2×10^{-5}	Fluorescence, flame	253.7	10^{-4}	
					electrothermal		2×10^{-6}	2×10^{-11}
					cool vapour		10^{-7}	5×10^{-10}
	Excretion, urine	5×10^{-6}						
	Total body							
K	Blood, whole.	2×10^{0}			Emission, flame	766.5	2×10^{-7}	
	serum	2×10^{-1}			plasma		10^{-4}	
39.10	Tissues		2×10^{-3} to 2×10^{-4}		Absorption, flame	766.5	5×10^{-6}	
					electrothermal		10^{-7}	10^{-12}
	Intake, food			2	Fluorescence, flame			
					electrothermal			
	Excretion, urine	2						
	Total body	10^{2} g						
Li	Blood, whole.				Emission, flame	670.8	5×10^{-9}	
	serum	2×10^{-5}			plasma	670.8	10^{-6}	
6.94	Tissues				Absorption, flame	670.8	10^{-6}	
					electrothermal		5×10^{-7}	5×10^{-12}
	Intake, food				Fluorescence, flame			
					electrothermal			
	Excretion, urine	5×10^{-6}						
	Total body							
Mg	Blood, whole.	5×10^{-2}			Emission, flame	285.2	5×10^{-6}	
	serum	2×10^{-2}			plasma	279.6 or 285.2	2×10^{-6}	
24.31	Tissues		10^{-3} to 5×10^{-5}		Absorption, flame	285.2	10^{-7}	
					electrothermal		5×10^{-9}	5×10^{-14}
	Intake, food			5×10^{-1}	Fluorescence, flame	285.2	2×10^{-7}	
					electrothermal		10^{-7}	10^{-12}
	Excretion, urine	5×10^{-2}						
	Total body	2×10^{1} g						
Mn	Blood, whole.	2×10^{-5}			Emission, flame	403.1	5×10^{-6}	
	serum	10^{-6}			plasma	403.1	10^{-6}	
54.94	Tissues		5×10^{-6} to 2×10^{-7}		Absorption, flame	279.5	2×10^{-6}	
					electrothermal		2×10^{-7}	2×10^{-12}
	Intake, food			5×10^{-3}	Fluorescence, flame	279.5	10^{-6}	
					electrothermal		5×10^{-7}	5×10^{-12}
	Excretion, urine	10^{-6}						
	Total body	2×10^{-2} g						
Mo	Blood, whole.	10^{-5}			Emission, flame	390.3	10^{-4}	
	serum	2×10^{-6}			plasma	379.8	5×10^{-6}	
	Tissues		2×10^{-7} to 2×10^{-8}		Absorption, flame	313.3	2×10^{-5}	
					electrothermal		5×10^{-6}	5×10^{-11}
95.94	Intake, food			10^{-4}	Fluorescence, flame	313.3	5×10^{-4}	
					electrothermal			
	Excretion, urine			5×10^{-5}				
	Total body	10^{-2} g						
Na	Blood, whole.	2			Emission, flame	589.0	10^{-7}	
	serum	3.2			plasma	589.0	2×10^{-5}	
22.99	Tissues		5×10^{-3} to 10^{-3}		Absorption, flame	582.0	10^{-6}	
	Intake, food			4	electrothermal Fluorescence, flame		5×10^{-8}	5×10^{-13}
					electrothermal			
	Excretion, urine	2						
	Total body	10^{2} g						
Ni	Blood, whole.	2×10^{-6}			Emission, flame	341.5	2×10^{-5}	
	serum	10^{-6}			plasma	352.5	5×10^{-6}	
58.71	Tissues		2×10^{-6} to 10^{-7}		Absorption, flame	232.0	10^{-5}	
					electrothermal		10^{-6}	2×10^{-11}
	Intake, food			5×10^{-4}	Fluorescence, flame	232.0	2×10^{-6}	
					electrothermal		5×10^{-7}	5×10^{-12}
	Excretion, urine	5×10^{-6}						
	Total body	10^{-2} g						
Pb	Blood, whole.	2×10^{-4}			Emission, flame	405.8	2×10^{-4}	
	serum	5×10^{-5}			plasma	405.8	10^{-5}	10^{-10}
207.19	Tissues		10^{-5} to 5×10^{-7}		Absorption, flame	283.3	2×10^{-5}	
					electrothermal		10^{-6}	10^{-11}
					flame cup		10^{-7}	5×10^{-12}
	Intake, food			2×10^{-4}	Fluorescence, flame	405.8	10^{-6}	
					electrothermal		10^{-6}	10^{-11}
	Excretion, urine	10^{-5}						
	Total body	10^{-1} g						
Sb	Blood, whole.	5×10^{-7}			Emission, flame	259.8	5×10^{-4}	
	serum	5×10^{-7}			plasma		2×10^{-4}	
121.75	Tissues		5×10^{-9}		Absorption, flame	217.6	5×10^{-5}	
					electrothermal		2×10^{-6}	2×10^{-11}
					cool vapour (hydride)		5×10^{-4}	5×10^{-7}

TABLE 3—*Contd.*

Element/Atomic weight	Matrix	Concentration in solution or wet tissue g/l	g/g*	g/day	Method	Wavelength (nm)	Representative detection limit (pure solution) g/l	g†
	Intake, food				Fluorescence, flame	217.6	5×10^{-5}	
					electrothermal		10^{-4}	10^{-9}
	Excretion, urine							
	Total body							
Se	Blood, whole.	5×10^{-5}			Emission, flame	196.0	10^{-1}	
	serum				plasma/hydride		10^{-5}	
78.96	Tissues		10^{-6} to 2×10^{-7}		Absorption, flame	196.0	10^{-4}	
					electrothermal		2×10^{-6}	2×10^{-10}
					cool vapour			
					(hydride)		10^{-6}	10^{-9}
	Intake, food			5×10^{-5}	Fluorescence, flame		5×10^{-5}	
					electrothermal			
					colour vapour			
					(hydride)	196.0	10^{-7}	
	Excretion, urine							
	Total body	2×10^{-3} g						
Si	Blood, whole	2×10^{-3}			Emission, flame	251.6	2×10^{-3}	
	serum	10^{-4}			plasma		10^{-4}	
28.09	Tissues		2×10^{-6} to 5×10^{-6}		Absorption, flame	251.6	10^{-4}	
					electrothermal		10^{-5}	10^{-10}
	Intake, food				Fluorescence, flame	251.6	5×10^{-4}	
					electrothermal			
	Excretion, urine							
	Total body	2×10^{1} g						
Sn	Blood, whole.	10^{-4}			Emission, flame	284.0	10^{-4}	
	serum	2×10^{-5}			plasma	303.4	2×10^{-5}	
118.69	Tissues		10^{-7} to 10^{-8}		Absorption, flame	224.6	10^{-4}	
					electrothermal		10^{-6}	5×10^{-11}
					cool vapour			
					(hydride)	224.6		
	Intake, food			2×10^{-3}	Fluorescence, flame	224.6	5×10^{-6}	5×10^{-10}
					electrothermal	303.4	5×10^{-5}	
	Excretion, urine	2×10^{-5}					10^{-5}	10^{-10}
	Total body	5×10^{-3} g						
Sr	Blood, whole.				Emission, flame	460.7	5×10^{-7}	
	serum	5×10^{-5}			plasma		2×10^{-7}	
87.62	Tissues		5×10^{-5} to 5×10^{-8}		Absorption, flame	460.7	5×10^{-6}	
					electrothermal			
	Intake, food			2×10^{-3}	Fluorescence, flame		10^{-5}	
					electrothermal			
	Excretion, urine	2×10^{-4}						
	Total body	10^{-1} g						
Tl	Blood, whole.	10^{-6}			Emission, flame	377.6	2×10^{-5}	
	serum				plasma		2×10^{-4}	
204.37	Tissues		10^{-7}		Absorption, flame	276.8	2×10^{-5}	
					electrothermal		2×10^{-6}	2×10^{-11}
					flame, cup	276.8	2×10^{-6}	2×10^{-10}
	Intake, food			10^{-6}	Fluorescence, flame	377.6	10^{-6}	
					electrothermal		10^{-6}	2×10^{-11}
	Excretion, urine							
	Total body							
V	Blood, whole.				Emission, flame	437.9	10^{-5}	
	serum	5×10^{-6}			plasma	437.9	10^{-5}	
50.94	Tissues		5×10^{-7} to 10^{-8}		Absorption, flame	318.4	10^{-4}	
					electrothermal		5×10^{-6}	10^{-10}
	Intake, food			5×10^{-4}	Fluorescence, flame	318.4	5×10^{-5}	
					electrothermal			
	Excretion, urine	5×10^{-6}						
	Total body	2×10^{-2} g						
Zn	Blood, whole.	10^{-2}			Emission, flame	213.9	10^{-2}	
	serum	10^{-3}			plasma	334.5	5×10^{-6}	2×10^{-12}
65.37	Tissues		10^{-4} to 2×10^{-5}		Absorption, flame	213.9	2×10^{-6}	
					electrothermal		5×10^{-8}	5×10^{-13}
					flame, cup		2×10^{-7}	10^{-11}
	Intake, food			10^{-2}	Fluorescence, flame	213.9	2×10^{-7}	
					electrothermal		2×10^{-9}	2×10^{-14}
	Excretion, urine	5×10^{-4}						
	Total body	2 g						

* Range of values. † The sample size was typically 10 μl.

assay may be assessed if it is assumed that the lowest concentration or amount which can be measured with a CV of ~3% is equal to 10 times the detection limit and the detection limit in a biological material is, on average, twice that in pure solution.

For the measurement of sodium and potassium, serum or urine samples are diluted approximately 200-fold with either distilled water or a diluent containing ~15 μmol/l of lithium if the latter is to be used as an internal standard element. As lithium is present in the sample to a limited extent (~3 μmol/l in serum) sufficient is added to ensure that the indigenous element does not make a significant contribution to the emission signal. For the measurement of calcium, copper, magnesium or zinc by flame atomic absorption the sample requires little pretreatment, e.g. serum requires only dilution with either acid or a solution of lanthanum chloride as a releasing agent. To obtain accurate results it may, however, be necessary to prepare standard solutions whose inorganic composition, at least, is similar to that of the sample.

Sample Preparation

The conditions under which a sample is collected may have a significant effect upon the concentration of the element of interest (*see* Chapter 4). This aspect of clinical chemistry will not be treated here other than to suggest that conditions of sampling should be standardized from one day to the next and should be borne in mind in the clinical interpretations of the results. Some tissues may be analysed directly but this approach presents the problem of standardization; therefore, for most analyses it is advisable to convert the sample to a solution as this is the most convenient form for spectrochemical analysis. A comprehensive review of ashing procedures suitable for use in the determination of trace elements in biological materials has been prepared by Sansoni and Panday.[9]

When handling small samples, care must be taken to ensure that the sample used is representative of the material as a whole. Small samples can also be difficult to manipulate and dispense accurately. Contamination can lead to serious errors as the amount of the element present in the sample may be comparable with that which may be present in a speck of dust or carried by inadequately cleaned laboratory ware.

Blood. For the analysis of blood, serum is preferred as it does not precipitate proteins as readily as does plasma and as the problem of possible contamination from the anticoagulant is avoided. However, plasma is obtained in better yield than serum and can be separated more quickly. If deproteinization of the serum or plasma is necessary it can be carried out with one of the standard reagents such as perchloric, trichloracetic or tungstic acids. It should be ascertained that the elements of interest are not co-precipitated with the proteins and that the protein-bound component of the element is quantitatively released. Whole blood, serum or plasma can be stored at 4 °C for several days or for longer periods if frozen. For the analysis of blood cells, a longer period of centrifugation is required to ensure reproducible packing and elimination of most of the plasma trapped between the cells. The cells may be haemolysed by suspension in distilled water followed by acidification to precipitate cell membranes. Alternatively the cells may be ashed as for other cellular tissue. The cellular concen-

tration of an element may be derived indirectly from the haematocrit of the blood sample, the plasma concentration and the concentration of the element in whole blood. The procedure is simpler but likely to be less accurate than determinations conducted directly on the cells. During the sampling procedure the possibility of contamination by the hypodermic needle, syringe or sample tube should be borne in mind, and the materials used tested by means of 'blank' analyses.

Urine. Urine normally requires less preliminary treatment but specimens of urine should be stored in a refrigerator and preserved by the addition of a bacteriostatic agent if they cannot be analysed within 24 h. Before sampling a specimen for analysis, any sediment should be re-dissolved by acidification to below pH5 with hydrochloric acid. Determination on old and alkaline specimens may give erratic results of doubtful value. Urine specimens can be frozen for prolonged storage.

Tissue and Solid Samples. The analysis of soft and hard tissue, food and faeces necessitates the destruction of organic matter by some form of ashing. This may be accomplished by heating to a relatively high temperature or by wet chemical means. First, the required tissue or bone must be separated from surrounding materials and then can be treated like food or faeces by grinding or homogenizing with distilled water to obtain a uniform mixture from which an aliquot can be taken for analysis. If extended preliminary treatment of the sample is necessary, particular care should be taken to avoid contamination from metal tools and vessels used in the process. If a specimen can be frozen and/or dried, grinding by hand in an agate pestle and mortar is one of the safest procedures. Whatever method of sample preparation is employed, the sampling for analysis, which should aim at being truly representative of the tissue, should be conducted by weight rather than volume.

Ashing Procedures. Following preliminary drying of an aliquot in the crucible on a sand tray, dry ashing is most conveniently conducted in a thermostatically controlled muffle furnace. The temperature of ashing is important if complete destruction of organic matter is to be obtained without loss of volatile metal. In practice, ashing at 500 °C for 16 h (overnight) is convenient for most purposes. The residue from dry ashing is usually leached with a few millilitres of concentrated hydrochloric acid to dissolve the metal oxides. As an ashing aid, magnesium nitrate appears to be advantageous for some elements. Dry ashing procedures can be carried out in platinum, silica or nickel vessels; platinum is generally most suitable but expensive. Silica crucibles are satisfactory for most purposes but should be discarded when the glaze is lost and the walls become rough as some loss of mineral may result. Some losses may also result from chemical combination with the crucible material. Losses due to vaporization of the sample are most severe when the sample size is small. If the temperature necessary to remove organic material leads to the volatilization of metals such as selenium, either closed systems using the oxygen atmospheres of the Schoniger flask and the Parr bomb or the low-temperature, excited-oxygen, ashing device can be used.

Wet ashing procedures are faster than dry ashing and can be completed within one or two hours, but they require more attention; in addition there is a greater problem of contamination due to the quantities of reagents necessary. The most generally useful common acid mixture for wet digestion is a combination of nitric, sulphuric and perchloric acids. There is little danger of explosion from the perchloric acid as long as sulphuric acid is present to prevent the sample from drying and as long as sufficient nitric acid is added initially to dissolve and destroy the bulk of the organic matter. Before using this digestion mixture the reader is advised to acquaint himself of the literature on the use of perchloric acid. An efficient and safe procedure for the wet digestion of organic materials employs a 'Teflon' lined, stainless-steel pressure decomposition vessel. Using this vessel, 1 g of organic material can be dissolved in 5 ml of nitric acid in 30 min at a temperature of 150 °C. A limitation of the technique is the large number of expensive digestion vessels required when many samples are to be analysed in a relatively short time. Several other mixtures have been used for the dissolution of organic material such as nitric acid with potassium permanganate and 50% hydrogen peroxide. An alternative solvent is 'Soluene' (quaternary ammonium hydroxide). This reagent will dissolve 100–300 mg of tissue in 1 ml of 'Soluene' and can be analysed by atomic absorption after 3-fold dilution with toluene. The procedure works well with fatty samples such as brain but not as well with materials with a high protein content such as fish meal. Whatever digestion scheme is used, blanks and samples of known composition should be analysed to determine the extent of contamination and losses taking place during the ashing processes.

Speciation. The biological effect of essential or toxic trace elements is determined by their function in biomolecules such as iron in haemoglobin or copper in ceruloplasmin. Their transport around the body in blood is usually in a loose binding with an organic molecule, e.g. albumin. It is therefore desirable that information such as the ionic concentration, oxidation state, concentration of a metalloprotein, or the nature of organo-metallic complexes be obtained. This necessitates pretreatment of the sample to separate the metallo-compounds prior to the determination of their metal content by atomic spectroscopy. A suitable method should provide rapid and reproducible separation of large and small molecules, with minimum dilution, disturbance of metallo-complex equilibria, or loss of trace element, and be suitable

for automated analysis. A variety of chromatographic methods have all been used for separating the components of the sample. Owing to the sample dilution produced by the eluting fluid the determination of the trace element content of the effluent may be near the detection limit of the analytical method.

Interferences

Interferences occur when the concentration of the element to be determined is apparently altered by the presence of other substances in the sample. The principal sources of interference are:

1. Spectral—arising from incomplete discrimination between the analytical spectral line and other radiation, e.g. in the determination of potassium in serum by emission flame photometry errors will arise unless precautions are taken to prevent intense emission from sodium reaching the detector.
2. Physical—primarily due to the presence of organic materials in the specimen which modifies the viscosity and surface tension of a solution, the flow rate through a pneumatic nebulizer of serum diluted 1:1 with water is 10–20% less than that of water.
3. Chemical—resulting from the presence in the sample of substances which change the atomization or excitation conditions of the element to be determined, e.g. the acidification of an aqueous solution containing 0.5 ppm magnesium, as acetate, to 0.1 M with hydrochloric acid will increase the atomic absorption signal by 6%.

Chemical interference is the major source of error in most analytical problems. In flame methods, the magnitude of the interference may depend upon the zone of the flame used for the analysis and on the anions and cations present in the matrix. A graphical presentation of typical interference effects in the determination of magnesium and calcium is given in Fig. 11.

The occurrence of a particular type of interference will be dependent on the procedure used, perhaps even on the particular instrument. It is therefore important to test for interference under the proposed operating conditions. Spectral or chemical interference can usually be detected by adding to standard solutions of the element, appropriate concentrations of the major inorganic constituents found in the specimens. The cumulative effects of these other ions should be tested as this may be different from the sum of their individual effects. The addition of known amounts of an element to typical specimens and the measurements of its recovery provides a useful indication of a technique's accuracy but, although a satisfactory recovery is essential, this alone does not establish the accuracy of the procedure.

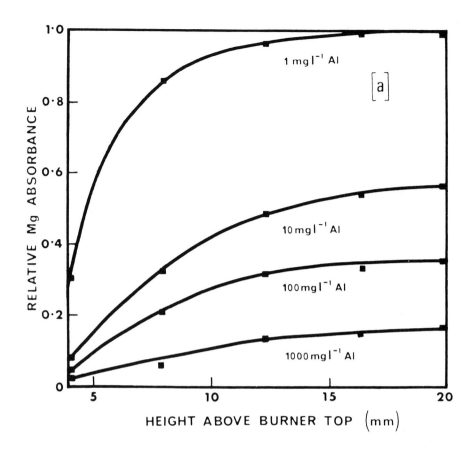

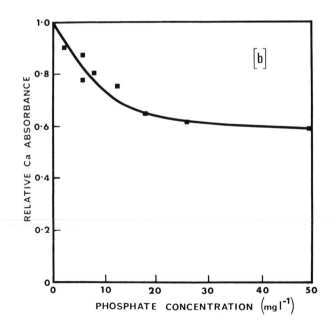

Fig. 11 Interference effects in flame atomic absorption: (a) relative absorbance due to magnesium (0.5 ppm) in aluminium sulphate solutions; (b) relative absorbance due to calcium (2.0 ppm) in phosphate-containing solutions.

The occurrence of physical effects due to organic constituents of the sample can be tested by comparison of the results obtained on aliquots of the same specimen with and without preliminary ashing. Finally, comparison with an established method which employs a different principle is desirable as an independent assessment of accuracy.

If interfering effects are detected the following techniques are available to minimize them: (1) further dilution of the sample; (2) addition of either radiation buffers, chelating agents or releasing agents which reduce the effect of differences between the standard and sample solutions; (3) an excess of the interfering ion may be added to both sample and standard; (4) the standard addition method may be used but it should be borne in mind that the added element may not be treated by the analytical system in precisely the same manner as that already present; (5) either the element to be determined or the interfering elements may be initially separated from the sample. In flame systems if the interference is found to arise in the atomization process it may be best to change the system. For example, the use of nitrous oxide as the oxidant in place of air in emission or flame absorption photometry will overcome many atomization interferences. In analysis using electrothermal atomization, matrix modification is frequently used to improve performance. The function of a matrix-modifying reagent is either to volatilize the matrix before atomization of the analyte element or to stabilize the analyte element to facilitate the use of higher ashing temperatures. Dilute nitric acid serves as a general matrix modifier while nickel is particularly useful for stabilizing arsenic and selenium. Interferences in the generation of gaseous metallo-hydrides is reduced by the use of 'masking agents' such as potassium iodide, EDTA or tartaric acid. Careful adjustment of the sample preparation procedure and reaction conditions can also overcome interference problems. Whichever approach is followed it is likely to be necessary to match the composition of the standard solution to that of the unknown samples if the greatest possible accuracy is to be achieved.

Owing to the prohibitive expense of using specially purified reagents it is often necessary, when carrying out trace element analysis, to measure the amount of that element in the reagents. This is particularly true if composite standards are used in which one or more component is present in a large excess over the measured element, e.g. a standard for the determination of copper in serum may require the addition of a 3000-fold excess of sodium if the standard is to have similar ionic composition to that of the sample.

The stability of dilute standards on storage is somewhat unpredictable and depends upon the composition of the standard and the material of the vessel. The use of aged vessels, i.e. vessels which have previously stored solutions of the required composition for some time, reduces the problem and solutions containing as little as $100 \, \mu mol/l$ may be stable if stored in this way for up to a week. Stronger solutions, e.g. $1 \, mol/l$ are stable indefinitely, but solutions of $1 \, \mu mol/l$ or less are best prepared daily and stored in aged vessels otherwise very rapid changes in concentration can occur.

The resources necessary to establish the accuracy of an analytical procedure are so great that the individual worker developing an analytical method can only carry out a limited evaluation of the self consistency of his method. The use of certified reference materials (CRMs) can reduce this problem but it is unlikely that there will ever be a complete range of CRMs for the determination of elements in clinical samples. In practice, quality control materials whereby the consistency of results within and between laboratories can be maintained may be as important as determining the accuracy of a particular method.

Methods for Improving Sensitivity and Precision

The sensitivity of a procedure can be increased either by more efficient utilization of the sample or by presenting more of the sample to the instrument in the same analytical interval. In systems using nebulization, the addition of a water-miscible organic solvent to the aqueous sample can improve sensitivity up to 3-fold. However, concentration procedures offer the promise of obtaining much greater increases. In some cases the metal may be precipitated by the methods of classical chemistry, or it may be extracted into an organic solvent if a system of favourable partition coefficient is available. If chelation with a suitable reagent, such as ammonium 1-pyrrolidinecarbodithioate (APDC) which complexes with copper and many other heavy metals, is combined with extraction of the chelate into an organic solvent (e.g. methyl isobutyl ketone, MIBK) a considerable concentration and purification of the element can be achieved simultaneously. By means of sequential solvent extraction as many as eleven elements have been determined in 2 ml of whole blood. Metals may also be concentrated by adsorption on a column of cation-exchange resin. When eluted with hydrochloric acid or strong sodium chloride, an effective concentration of 3- to 5-fold may be obtained.

Some variations of instrumental techniques may be used to increase precision and facilitate the measurement of low concentrations. The limit is usually set by the instability of the instrument. When the sample is nebulized into the instrument the effect of baseline drift may be reduced by modulating the sample flow and computing the mean of as many absorption or emission peaks as necessary to give the desired precision. This procedure can also be applied to transient response systems if time and sample size permit multiple measurements. Repeated standardization is also necessary to correct for changes in sensitivity. The effect of rapid fluctuation in the signal is reduced by integration of the area under the emission or absorption curves.

CONCLUSIONS

The methods of analytical atomic spectroscopy are universally applicable to the determination of the elements of interest to clinical chemists. The sensitivity of the technique is such that one of the major problems when measuring the less common elements is contamination from the laboratory environment. The most commonly analysed material is blood and the most frequently determined elements are sodium, potassium, calcium and magnesium. Facilities for determining the first two elements are available in practically all clinical chemistry laboratories and staff are familiar with their operation. Increasingly, however, ion-selective electrodes are being used for these analyses. Atomic absorption instruments for the determination of calcium and magnesium are found in most laboratories. Trace elements such as copper, iron and zinc and the toxic metals lead and mercury can be measured with relatively simple instrumentation provided a member of staff specializes in the applications of analytical atomic spectroscopy, for, in addition to the analysis, advice on sample collection and interpretation of results will be necessary.

As more becomes known of the role of elements in human metabolism it seems inevitable that there will be an increasing demand for analysis. Unless the determination of elements supersedes other analyses, it is unlikely that the average laboratory will have sufficient resources to carry out reliable, wide-ranging trace metal measurements; therefore it may be most economical to set up specialist groups within larger hospital laboratories to carry out metal analysis. The establishment of such a group would justify the installation of more powerful analytical equipment including automatic sample handling and data processing. In addition to carrying out analyses, such central laboratories would be instrumental in developing new methods and establishing the accuracy of selected analytical methods. These centres could also provide reference materials and operate a quality control system in support of analyses carried out elsewhere. The central laboratory could operate an advisory service both in terms of analytical procedures and the metabolic or toxic role of trace elements. A laboratory with a large throughput of urgent samples on complex instrumentation will need either a resident engineer or, at least, a member of the staff who is qualified to take emergency action to repair equipment.

Future developments in the application of spectrochemical analysis to the determination of elements are likely to include:

1. an increase in the number of elements for which well established analytical procedures are available,
2. improved instrumentation, mechanized sample handling and data processing,
3. the combination of atomic spectroscopy with protein separation techniques,
4. the simultaneous measurement of several elements to provide more detailed information on the trace element status of the patient.

Multichannel analytical atomic spectroscopy as practised in, for example, the metallurgical field, has not yet been developed for clinical chemistry owing to the greatly increased complexity of the instrumentation. It is difficult to optimize instrumental conditions for the simultaneous measurement of several elements, therefore at the present time, multi-element analysis is best carried out by sequential measurements of the same sample. This approach may not be feasible when the sample size is limited as in the case of specimens from infants or biopsies. Some of these problems may be overcome by inductively coupled plasma spectrometers. These systems can effectively atomize and excite a wide range of elements without readjustment of the instrument.

Most of the technical problems in the determination of elements in clinical material have been or can be overcome. However, much further study of the relationship between metals and disease is necessary before their true place in chemical pathology can be assessed.

REFERENCES

1. Walsh A. (1955). The application of atomic absorption spectra to chemical analysis. *Spectrochim. Acta*; **7**: 108.
2. Lundegardh H. (1928). Investigation of quantitative spectral analysis. 11. Determination of potassium, magnesium and copper in flame spectrum. *Ark. Kemi. Min. Geol*; **10A**: No. 1.
3. Winefordner J. D., Vickers T. J. (1964). Atomic fluorescence spectrometry as a means of chemical analysis. *Anal. Chem*; **36**: 161.
4. Greenfield S., Jones I. L., Berry C. T. (1964). High-pressure plasmas as spectroscopic emission sources. *Analyst*; **89**: 713.
5. Alkemade C. Th. J. (1968). Science vs. fiction in atomic absorption. *Appl. Opt*; **7**: 1261.
6. L'vov B. B. (1978). Electrothermal atomization—the way towards absolute methods of atomic absorption analysis. *Spectrochim. Acta*; **33B**: 153.
7. Smith S. B., Hieftje G. M. (1983). New background-correction method for atomic absorption spectrometry. *Appl. Spectrosc*; **37**: 419.
8. de Loos-Vollebregt M. T. C., de Galan L. (1978). Theory of Zeeman atomic absorption spectrometry. *Spectrochim. Acta*; **33B**: 495.
9. Sansoni B., Panday V. K. (1983). Ashing in trace element analysis of biological material. In *Analytical Techniques for Heavy Metals in Biological Fluids* (Facchetti S., ed.) pp. 91–131. Amsterdam: Elsevier.

FURTHER READING

General texts
Annual reports on analytical atomic spectroscopy. Vols 1–14, 1971–1984. London: Royal Society of Chemistry.

Barnes R. M. (ed.) (1982). *Development in Atomic Plasma Spectrochemical Analysis*. New York: Wiley-Heydon.

Braetter P., Schramel P. (eds.) (1980, 1982, 1984). *Trace Element Analytical Chemistry in Medicine and Biology*. Vols 1, 2, 3. Berlin: Walter de Gruyter.

Cantle J. E. (ed.) (1982). *Atomic Absorption Spectrometry*. Amsterdam, Oxford, New York: Elsevier.

Christian G. D., Feldman F. J. (1970). *Atomic Absorption Spectroscopy—Applications in Agriculture, Biology and Medicine*. New York: Wiley Interscience.

Ebdon L (1982). *An Introduction to Atomic Absorption Spectrometry—A Self Teaching Approach*. London: Heydon.

Kirkbright G. F., Sargent M. (1974). *Atomic Absorption and Fluorescence Spectroscopy*. London: Academic Press.

Price W. J. (1979). *Spectrochemical Analysis by Atomic Absorption*. London: Heydon.

Current awareness publications
Atomic Spectroscopy. Norwalk: Perkin-Elmer.
Journal of Analytical Atomic Spectroscopy. London: Royal Society of Chemistry.
Progress in Analytical Atomic Spectroscopy. Oxford: Pergamon.

11. Fluorescence and Phosphorescence
J. W. Bridges

Introduction
Theory of the luminescence processes
  Luminescence intensity
  Analytically potentially useful excited state energy changes
  Structural requirements for fluorescence and phosphorescence
  Environmental factors affecting observed luminescence intensity
Instrumentation
  Lamp sources
  The cell compartment and sample presentation
  Detection systems
  Fluorescent standards
  Sensitivity limits of an assay
Practical applications of luminescence measurements
  Analytical applications of luminescence measurements
  Enzyme assays
  Other applications of luminescence

INTRODUCTION

The ability of natural substances to emit luminescence must have been a source of fascination from the time of earliest man.

The first clear description of *fluorescence* properties is generally attributed to the chemist Robert Boyle who observed in the 17th century that when water was left to stand in cups made from lignum nephriticum (Eysenhardtia polystacha), a blue colour developed in reflected daylight. This blue fluorescence was immediately lost when the cup was transferred to transmitted light where the water adopted a clear or yellow-tinged appearance. Boyle further reported that the blue emission was abolished by acid salts of vinegar and was recovered when alkali (oil of tartar per deliquium) was added subsequently. Thus Boyle in a few simple experiments demonstrated that fluorescence is a prompt light emission, which occurs at a higher wavelength than that of light absorption, it is observable in very dilute solutions and it may be pH sensitive.

At about the same time *phosphorescence* was characterized as a slow light emission following light absorption using the mineral Bolognian stone. It was shown to be quenched by traces of iron and other metals. Jacopo Beccari (1682–1766) was probably the first man to report extensively the phosphorescence of biological materials. He concluded that phosphorescence was a property of all plant and animal parts that are well dried (possibly requiring a rigid sample—see p. 151). He also made the important discovery that the intensity of phosphorescence increased when the exciting light was made brighter, thus establishing one of the most fundamental principles of the light emission processes.

Since the time of Boyle and Beccari numerous studies have been made of the light emission characteristics of biological materials. Sadly the majority of these data are of little practical value to the analyst because they were carried out on impure materials. Although fluorimetric assays for several of the B vitamins were developed and fluorimetry was extensively used to identify polycyclic aromatic hydrocarbons and their metabolites in the 1930s and 1940s, it was not until the advent of the first commercial spectrofluorimeters in the late 1950s that attempts were made by scientists in the biological and clinical fields to capitalize on luminescence properties to develop a wide range of assays. The initial stimulus to the awakening of more widespread interest in fluorescence was the need to measure low levels of biogenic amines and antimalarial drugs in blood and urine. In the last decade, largely because of its very high potential sensitivity, fluorescence has gained acceptance as an important tool in the analyst's armoury and has also become extensively employed as a subtle means of investigating macromolecular conformation and small molecule–macromolecule interactions.

In contrast, the development of phosphorimetry for assaying biologically interesting materials has been extremely slow because of the cumbersome requirements of the commercially available equipment for sample handling, namely the necessity of presenting the sample in an organic solvent inside a tube which is then immersed in liquid nitrogen. In recent years several major improvements in sample handling devices have occurred which should enable the more widespread exploitation of this valuable analytical method (*see* p. 159) which should be regarded as complementary to fluorimetry.

kinetic energy to other molecules (termed internal conversion). From this first excited singlet state (lifetime τ of 10^{-6}–10^{-9} s) the electron may return to the ground state, the released energy being given up in further internal conversions, prompt light emission (fluorescence) or as heat through collision with other molecules (quenching). Alternatively the excited molecule may achieve an intermediary, metastable condition through an uncoupling of the normal paired state of the electrons (termed intersystem crossing) to produce a condition of higher multiplicity. The most common conversion is to the lowest triplet state (Fig. 1) which frequently has a lifetime more than 10^6 times longer than that of the excited singlet state.

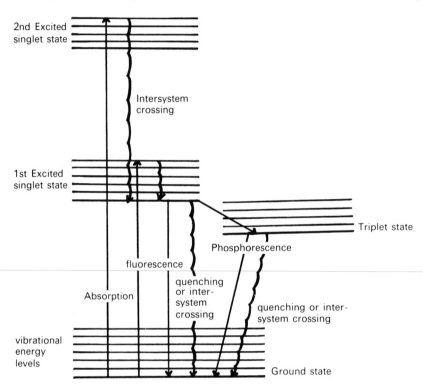

Fig. 1 Schematic diagram of the luminescence processes.

THEORY OF THE LUMINESCENCE PROCESSES[1]

The initial requisite for both fluorescence and phosphorescence is the absorption of ultraviolet or visible light. Provided the wavelengths of light falling on a molecule are suitable (i.e. correspond to those of its ultraviolet/visible absorption spectrum) the energy of some of the electrons in the molecule will be raised from the ground state in which electronic and vibrational energy is minimal to an upper excited singlet state (*see* Fig. 1). Energy is very rapidly lost (within 10^{-12}–10^{-15} s) from all excited states except that of the lowest vibrational level of the first excited singlet state due to thermal or chemical change or radiationless transfer of rotational, vibrational or

(N.B. Direct excitation from the ground singlet state to its triplet state is normally an improbable process, i.e. a forbidden transition.) From the triplet state the molecule may return to the ground singlet state by giving up its energy by internal conversions, through collision with other molecules (quenching) or through a sustained light emission (phosphorescence). Because the phosphorescence lifetime is much longer than that of fluorescence its duration may often be fairly simply measured. This can provide an important characterizing parameter of a compound. From a realization of the mechanisms of light emission certain practically important features of these processes follow: (i) regardless of the level at which the electrons are excited, fluorescence and phosphorescence emissions will normally only occur from the first excited singlet and lowest triplet states respectively thus the wavelengths of maximum fluorescence (λ_{fl}) and phosphorescence (λ_p) are independent of the intensity and wavelengths of the exciting light; (ii) because some of the exciting energy is invariably lost during internal conversion processes the fluorescence wavelength will always be higher than the light absorption wavelength (N.B. energy $\propto$ 1/wavelength). In the process of phosphorescence further radiationless loss of energy will occur during intersystem crossing and hence the phosphorescence wavelength will be higher still.

Luminescence Intensity

The efficiency of the light emission process is defined as the quantum efficiency ϕ where

$$\phi = \frac{\text{the amount of light emitted}}{\text{the amount of light absorbed}}$$

for a molecule under ideal conditions

$$\phi_F + \phi_p + \phi_{int} = 1$$

where ϕ_F = quantum efficiency of fluorescence,
             ϕ_p = quantum efficiency of phosphorescence,
             ϕ_{int} = energy lost by other processes.

Under experimental conditions additional quenching of both phosphorescence and fluorescence is likely to occur. The lifetimes (τ) of the first excited singlet and triplet states are obviously important determinants of the extent of quenching since quenching is itself a time-dependent phenomenon. Because the lifetime of the triplet state is frequently in the ms to s range molecules passing into this state are extremely likely to lose their energy by collision rather than by emitting fluorescence unless they are set in a rigid matrix. For this reason phosphorescence is normally only observed in very viscous liquids or when the sample is set in a solid matrix (e.g. frozen solutions).

(N.B. Although the term quantum efficiency has an important physical meaning, from an analytical viewpoint it is the intensity of the emitted light rather than the efficiency of the conversion of absorbed light into luminescence which indicates whether or not the fluorescence properties are adequate for an assay to be devised. For this reason fluorescence sensitivity $\phi_F \times \varepsilon_{max}$ is the preferred term—see p. 162.)

Analytically Potentially Useful Excited State Energy Changes

Energy Transitions. On occasion the absorption and fluorescence spectra are mirror images of one another (e.g. some aromatic hydrocarbons) but generally these spectra are not super-imposable because of the vibrational frequency differences between the ground

and the excited states. Excited molecules often display quite major differences in chemical and physical properties from those in the ground state due to modifications in their molecular geometry and electron distribution. For example, acetylene in the excited state adopts a trans geometry more akin to that of ethylene. The influence of solvent may be much greater in the excited state than in the ground state. This is because on excitation the electron cloud of a molecule often becomes redistributed giving an increased degree of polarization thereby increasing the interaction with polar solvents. As a consequence a change of solvent may produce a dramatic change in the luminescence properties but little change in the light absorption profile.

From the mechanistic viewpoint excited state molecules can be considered as interacting with their environment in one of the following ways:

(a) excited state ionization

$$DH \xrightarrow[\text{absorption}]{hv_1} \overset{*}{DH} \longrightarrow \overset{*}{D^-} + H^+$$
$$\downarrow hv_2 \quad \text{fluorescence or quenching}$$
$$D^-$$

(b) charge transfer

$$D \xrightarrow[\text{absorption}]{hv_1} \overset{*}{D} \longrightarrow \overset{*}{AD} \xrightarrow[\text{fluorescence or quenching}]{hv_2} A + D$$

(c) energy transfer

$$D \xrightarrow[\text{absorption}]{hv_1} D^* \longrightarrow D^*A \longrightarrow \overset{*}{A} + D$$
$$\downarrow hv_2 \quad \text{fluorescence or quenching}$$
$$A$$

(d) delayed fluorescence

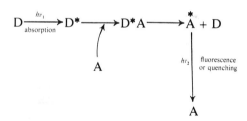

$$D_1 \xrightarrow{hv_1} \overset{*}{D_1} \longrightarrow \overset{*}{D_T} \longrightarrow \overset{*}{D_1} + D$$
$$\downarrow hv_2 \quad \text{fluorescence or quenching}$$
$$\overset{*}{D_T} \qquad D_1$$

(D_1 = singlet state; D_T = triplet state; * depicts an excited state; DH = the molecular form of a molecule and D^- = its anion; A = the ground state and A^* the excited state of a second molecular species.)

Each of these processes is relatively compound specific and therefore can be used for assay purposes and as an extra discriminator for compound identification. Some applications will be discussed later.

A clue to the occurrence of excited state ionization may often be gleaned from the degree of separation of the wavelength of maximal excitation (λ_{ex}) and the wavelength of maximal emission (λ_F). This difference which is referred to as the Stokes shift and defined as

$$10^7 \left(\frac{1}{\lambda_{ex}} - \frac{1}{\lambda_f} \right)$$

is normally below $5000 \, cm^{-1}$. In excited state ionization the Stokes shift may be as large as $10\,000 \, cm^{-1}$. (For further details on these energy transitions see Parker[2].)

Polarized Fluorescence. In addition to these association and dissociation processes molecules may also rotate on their axes between absorbing and emitting light. The extent of rotation can be measured by employing light polarizers. With a light polarizer such as Nicol prism or polarcoat film between the light source and the sample only light of a single plane will fall on the sample molecules. Those molecules with their long axes in the same plane as this polarized light will be preferentially excited. If these molecules are held rigidly or are so large that they can only slowly rotate then their emitted fluorescence will be largely polarized, when monitored by a second polarizer between the sample and the photodetector. In contrast, small molecules in a non-viscous liquid will freely rotate in a random fashion between excitation and emission and hence the fluorescence signal from these molecules will not be polarized. This phenomenon is of particular value for elucidating interactions between small fluorescent molecules and proteins, since a polarized fluorescence signal will only be

lized (π) electron system (involving bonds such as —CH=CH—, >NH, or >O) or from the excitation of a lone pair of electrons (n) associated with bonds such as —N=, C=O, or —N=N—. Generally if the highest absorption wavelength is due to lone pair excitation (termed $n \rightarrow \pi^*$ transition) rather than delocalized electron excitation (termed $\pi \rightarrow \pi^*$ transition) the molecule will tend to be non-fluorescent although it may be highly phosphorescent. (N.B. $n \rightarrow \pi^*$ can often be simply distinguished from $\pi \rightarrow \pi^*$ in a spectrophotometer because they tend to show a weaker ε_{max} and the absorption maximum undergoes a hypsochromic shift, i.e. to lower wavelength, if a more polar solvent is employed.) Conversely if $\pi \rightarrow \pi^*$ transitions constitute the higher absorption wavelength, fluorescence is most likely to be dominant unless the energy transition between the first excited singlet state and the triplet state is small. The presence in the medium of atoms of high atomic number often encourages intersystem crossing and hence phosphorescence at the expense of fluorescence.

An extensive conjugated system of double bonds is generally necessary for a compound to show a high fluorescence intensity (*see* examples below). Molecules containing few π electrons tend to have a low extinction coefficient and a short absorption wavelength (i.e. high energy absorption). On excitation such molecules are particularly vulnerable to photodecomposition.

Molecular rigidity and a planar structure also tend to enhance the efficiency of light emission by reducing thermal loss. Illustrations of rigidity and planarity improving fluorescence efficiency are given below.

Urobilin weak fluorescence
(600 640 nm)

Urobilinogen (non-fluorescent)

Vitamin A
λ_{ex} 345 nm: λ_{fl} 490 nm

Naphthalene
λ_{ex} 286 nm: λ_{fl} 321 nm
ϕ 0.29

Anthracene
λ_{ex} 365 nm: λ_{fl} 400 nm
ϕ 0.46

registered at the photodetector when the small molecules are combined with the macromolecules. It has recently found analytical application in drug immunoassay (*see* p. 170).

Structural Requirements for Fluorescence and Phosphorescence

The excited single state electrons (termed π^*) may arise either from excitation of a molecule's deloca-

Increasing the solvent viscosity or setting the sample in rigid matrix may be used to enhance rigidity and hence fluorescence efficiency. This may account for the frequent observation of fluorescence of a compound on a TLC plate or paper chromatogram which is not seen when the spot is taken up into solution. (N.B. reduction of quenching processes in a more rigid matrix may also contribute to an intensity enhancement.)

Substituents may have a profound influence on the

intensity of light emission. However, because it would be necessary to predict the properties of both the ground state and the highly reactive excited state, the correlation between substituents position and luminescence characteristics is understandably less well defined than that for light absorption. Certain general trends are however apparent. With the exception of paramagnetic atoms and those with a high atomic number, substituents will generally only

fluorescence whereas —NO_2, —Cl, —Br, —I, >C=O, and —N= tend to diminish fluorescence and —SO_3H, —COOH and alkyl substituents usually have little influence. Such guidelines must be treated with caution where several substituents are attached because it is the overall effect of the substituents on the delocalization of the π electron-cloud which governs the fluorescence properties. Molecules of biological interest with a strong native fluorescence

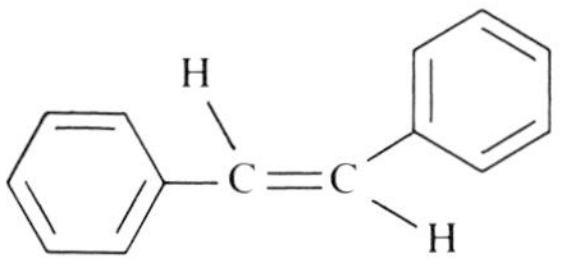

trans stilbene planar
- intensely fluorescent

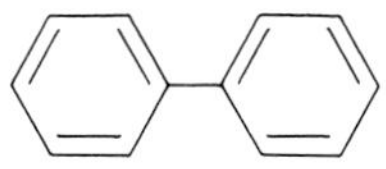

biphenyl non-rigid
ϕ 0.23

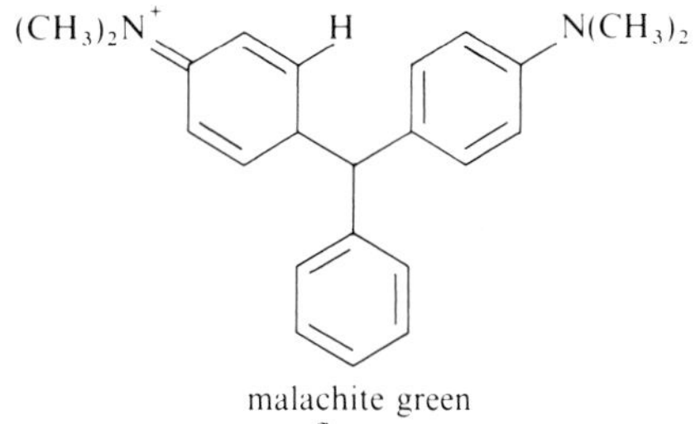

malachite green
non-fluorescent

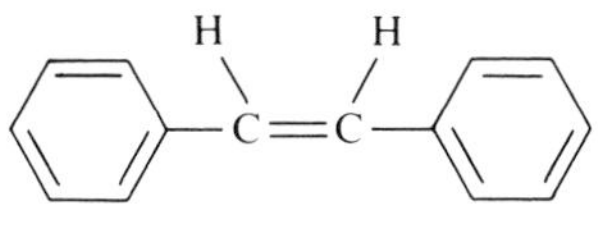

cis stilbene non-planar
very weakly fluorescent

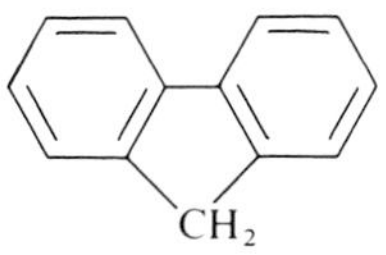

fluorene rigid
ϕ 0.99

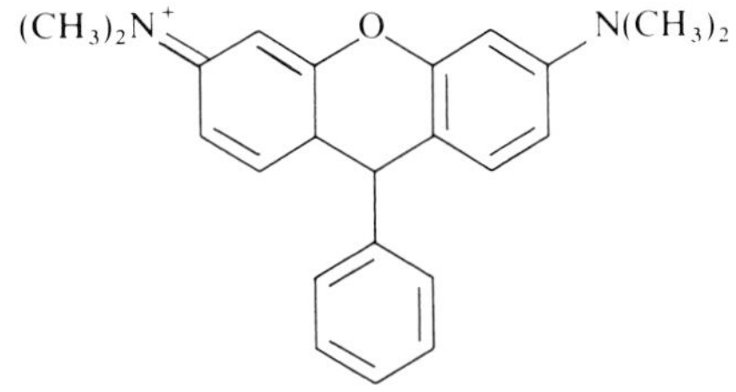

rosamine (fluorescent)

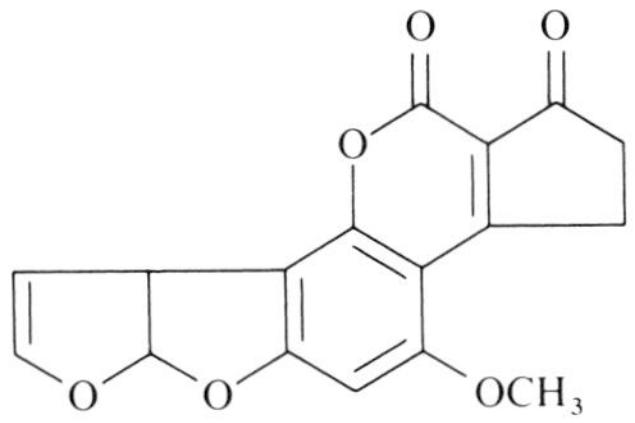

significantly influence luminescence properties if they are directly associated with the conjugated system of double bonds or with the lone pair system responsible for the emitted light.

Normally, —NR_2, —O^-, —OR and —CN enhance

include aflatoxin and many other environmental carcinogens, indoles such as LSD and tryptophan, aromatic amino acids, hydroxyquinolines, acridines such as quinine and $NADH_2$, porphyrins and flavins (Table 1).

Aflatoxin λ_{ex} 365 nm
             λ_{fl} 425 nm

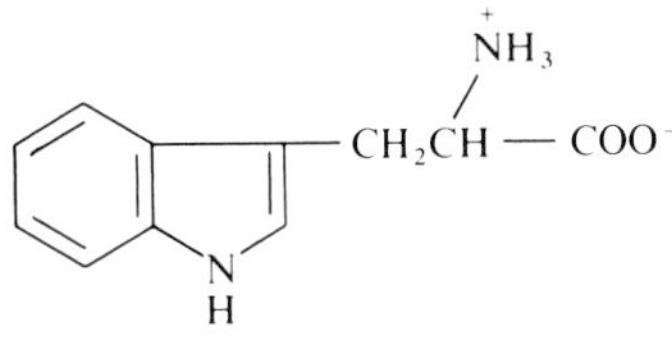

Tryptophan λ_{ex} 290 nm
             λ_{fl} 341 nm

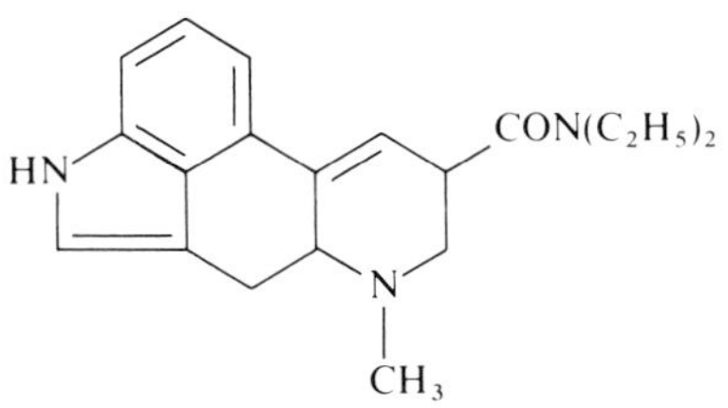

LSD λ_{ex} 335 nm
       λ_{fl} 435 nm

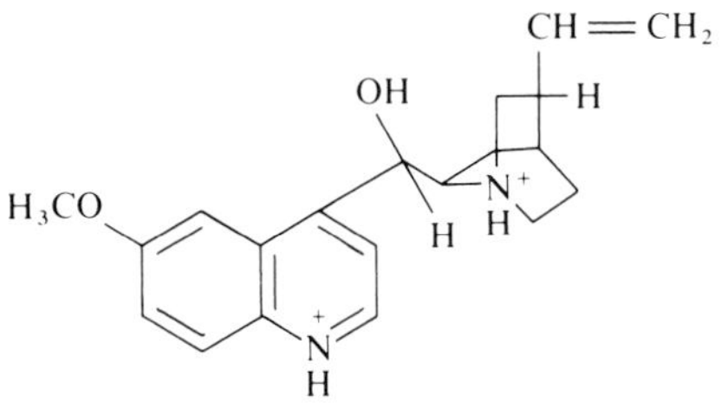

Quinine λ_{ex} 350 nm
           λ_{fl} 450 nm

TABLE 1

NATIVE FLUORESCENCE AND PHOSPHORESCENCE OF SOME BIOLOGICALLY IMPORTANT COMPOUNDS

(N.B. All wavelengths are uncorrected wavelengths and will vary
from instrument to instrument.)

Compound	λ_{ex}	λ_{fl}	Conditions†	Sensitivity*	λ_p	Conditions†	Sensitivity*
Acetyl salicylate	240	nf	—		380	EPA	0·1
Adenine	265	380	5NH$_2$SO$_4$	poor	388	E	good
Adrenaline	295	325	Aq	fair	435	E	fair
Albumin	295	320	Aq	good	440	Aq frozen	good
Amphetamine	270	295	Aq	v. poor	385	EW	poor
ATP	272	390	5NH$_2$SO$_4$	poor	410	Alk. frozen	good
Atropine	260	nf	—	—	410	E	0·1
Benzimidazole	274	290	Aq	fair	na		—
Benzoate	250	375	70% H$_2$SO$_4$	good	400	E	0·005
Benzocaine	310	na	—	—	430	E	0·007
Caffeine	275	317	E	fair	415	EPA	0·01
Chlordiazepoxide	310, 320	435	Aq	fair	450, 470	EW	good
Cocaine	240	na	—	—	400	E	0·01
Codeine	285	350	pH 0	fair	505	E	0·01
Coproporphyrin	402	590	pH 0	good	na		—
Diazepam	290, 325	nf	—	—	440, 470, 510	EW	
Dicoumarol	305			fair	475	E	0·001
DNA							
(*Bacillus subtilis*)		nf	Aq	—	415	E	good
Dopamine	270	325	Aq	poor	420	E	1·0
Ephedrine	225	320	Aq	poor	390	E	0·2
FMN	450	520	Aq	good	na		—
Folic acid	365	455	pH 9	fair	na		—
Imipramine	295	415	pH 14	fair	455	E	fair
Indomethacin	310	410	pH 13	good	485	E	good
Iprindole	310	345	Aq	fair	425, 450, 485	EW	fair
Iproniazid	300, 370	na	—	—	440	EW	fair
Lidocaine	265	na	—	—	400	E	1·2
LSD	325	445	pH 1	good	np	—	—
Morphine	285	350	pH 7	fair	500	E	0·01
NADH	340	460	Aq	0·001	na		—
Phenacetin	310	335	pH 7	poor	499	EPA	0·002
Phenobarbitone	240	420	Alk	fair	380	E	0·10
Procaine	310	345	Alk	good	430	E	0·01
Protoporphyrin	410	595	pH 0	good	na		—
Pyridoxal phosphate	315	370	pH 13	good	410	E	good
Quinine	340	450	0·1MH$_2$SO$_4$	0·0001	500	E	0·04
Salicylate	310	400	Chloroform Acetic acid	good	405	E	poor
Serotonin	295	355	Aq	good	410	E	poor
Sulphacetamide	280	350	W	0·02	410	E	0·0001
Tocopherol	295	340	hexane	good	na		—
Trimethoprim	370	460	on TLC plates	good	410	E	poor
Tryptophan	290	355	Aq	good	440	E	0·002
Tyrosine	295	320	Aq	fair	405	E	0·01
Ubiquinone (reduced)	290	325	Aq	fair	na		—
Warfarin	290, 305	385	methanol	fair	460	E	0·01

† E at 77 K = ethanol. EPA = Ethanol/isopentane/ether (5 : 5 : 2) at 77 K. Aq = water.

* good = detects less than 0·1 g/ml; fair = limit between 0·1 g/ml and 1 g/ml; poor = limit higher than 1 g/ml; nd = not determined; nf = non-fluorescent under conditions specified; np = not phosphorescent under conditions specified; na = results not available.

As might be expected the substituents which diminish fluorescence often enhance phosphorescence. Substituting a molecule with —NO$_2$, —Cl, —Br or —I generally increases its phosphorescence. The greater the atomic number the shorter the phosphorescence lifetime. For example the half-lives of 1-fluoro-, 1-chloro-, 1-bromo- and 1-iodo-naphthalenes are 1·5, 0·3, 0·18 and 0·0025 s respectively. Molecules of biological interest with a strong native luminescence at 77 K include: natural and synthetic purines, tryptophan, acetyl salicylic acid, antibacterial sulphonamides, coumarin anticoagulants and phenothiazines. None of these compounds are phosphorescent in solution at room temperature.

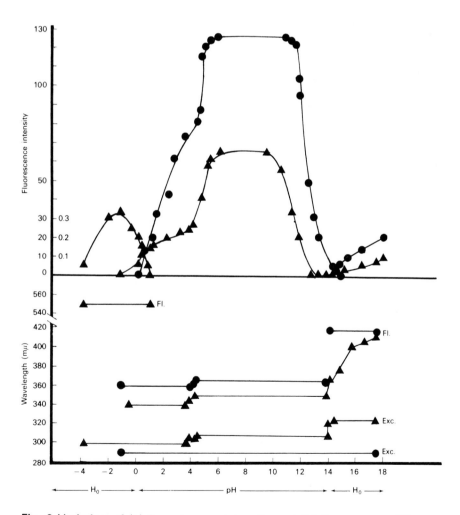

Caffeine ϕ_F 0.22 ϕ_p 0.14

Thiocaffeine ϕ_F 10^{-5} ϕ_p 0.43

Environmental Factors Affecting Observed Luminescence Intensity

Because the emission of luminescence requires the prior generation of an excited and therefore reactive molecular species which can readily react with its surrounds, luminescence is considerably influenced by environmental factors.

pH and Solvent. Alteration of the pH of the solution may lead to a change in the ionization of a compound's substituent groups thereby modifying its fluorescence characteristics. Protonation of —NHR, —N=, or —O⁻ frequently produces profound changes in luminescence properties. Indeed, these changes may often be used to determine the pK of a compound in very dilute solution (Fig. 2). For example, 5-hydroxyindole acetic acid displays a change in both fluorescence intensity and in fluorescence wavelength around pH 11·0 where its phenolic group becomes ionized. Ionization may also give rise to a change in the nature of the luminescence emitted. This is commonly observed on protonation of a pyridine nitrogen. For example, quinoline is phosphorescent at neutral or alkali pH, whereas in strong acid its ring nitrogen is protonated and the resulting cation is fluorescent.

pH-Fluorescence changes are the basis of the so-called fluorescence indicators. These indicators are

Fig. 2 Variation of (a) fluorescence intensity and (b) fluorescence (Fl) and excitation (Exc) wavelength with pH and H_0 of indol-3-ylacetic acid (●) and 5-hydroxy-indol-3-ylacetic acid (▲). Intensity values are arbitrary (from Bridges and Williams (1968) *Biochem. J.*, **107**, 230).

usually phenols which on ionization display a visible fluorescence. They are particularly valuable as indicators in the titration of coloured or cloudy solutions where normal colour indicators such as methyl orange are of little use.[3]

Many molecules display pronounced changes in fluorescence properties which cannot be predicted from simple consideration of the ground state. For example, all 5-hydroxy- and 5-alkoxy-indoles emit a fluorescence at 540 nm in $1.5 \text{ M H}_2\text{SO}_4$ which is not observed with any other indoles. This property may be exploited to estimate serotonin in the presence of other indoles. Benzoic acid, benzoyl glucuronide and hippuric acid fluoresce only in strong acid ($>60\%$ H_2SO_4), conditions under which most other simple benzene derivatives do not fluoresce. Unexpected fluorescence characteristics are also often seen in strong alkaline solution. Excited state ionization or formation of charge transfer complexes are frequently invoked to explain these unusual fluorescences. Although the results are unpredictable, fluorescence studies at extreme pH values are potentially valuable in analysis (*see* pp. 163). It is advisable to try more than one acid or alkali as occasionally quenching results from the counter ion. For example quinine sulphate is very highly fluorescent in 0.005 M H_2SO_4 but is barely fluorescent in 0.1 M HCl due to the quenching effect of the chloride ions.

It is clear from the above discussion that careful selection of pH may enhance both the specificity and/or the sensitivity of a fluorescence assay. Changes of solvent may also give rise to dramatic alterations in fluorescence characteristics; again the effects are not entirely predictable. Commonly the fluorescence wavelength shortens with decreasing polarity of the solvent. For example indole has a λ_{fl} max. of 350 nm in water, 330 nm in ethanol, and 340 nm in dioxan. Occasionally very dramatic changes in emission wavelength (*Stokes shift*) occurs on changing the solvent. For example, 1-anilino naphthalene-8-sulphonic acid (ANS) has a λ_{fl} max. of 513 nm in water, 468 nm in ethanol and 447 nm in hexane. Frequently the fluorescence intensity is also enhanced by selecting a less polar solvent, e.g. in the case of ANS this intensification is some 300-fold. Occasionally, e.g. chlorophyll, the reverse trend is observed. This property of changing fluorescence characteristics in different environments will of course also occur when compounds bind to biologically important macromolecules such as proteins and nucleic acids. Study of these interactions (a technique referred to as fluorescence probing) can give information about small molecule interactions with macromolecules and can be used to assess competition for binding sites by different compounds (*see* p. 170).

The major causes of a hypsochromic shift in λ_{fl} on reducing solvent polarity are usually diminution of hydrogen bonding, suppression of ionization and minimization of dipole–dipole interactions. Non-aqueous solvents are seldom used to assay molecules

of clinical biochemistry interest but this is probably partly a reflection of a conservative approach to setting up fluorimetric assays. The main virtues of using an aqueous medium are that maximal separation of λ_{ex} and λ_{fl} is obtained which minimizes scatter interference in an assay and that assay of ionized forms of molecules can be made. Under conditions where these are not the cardinal considerations, organic solvents should at least be tried because of the possible intensification of fluorescence which may result. Use of an organic solvent should also be considered if there is an overlap between the fluorescence spectrum of the compound under investigation and fluorescent contaminants because a solvent polarity change may enable discrimination between these fluorescences. The main obvious requirement is that the solvent should dissolve the compound under study. Alcohols which, like water, are also proton donating would appear to be especially relevant alternative solvents.

Apart from solvent purity (which will be dealt with in the section on spurious fluorescence, p. 157) the main additional consideration in the selection of solvent is that it should not absorb or fluoresce in the same spectral region as the compound of interest. For example, acetone, benzene and toluene are clearly inappropriate solvents if UV fluorescence is to be measured. For non-rigid molecules, particularly those with potentially interacting π electron systems, e.g. 5-phenyl barbiturates, increasing the viscosity may be helpful in enhancing the fluorescence intensity.

In phosphorimetry the choice of solvent is normally far more restricted than in fluorescence, being limited to those solvents which will form clear, rigid glasses at 77 K. Typically, ethanol, 50% ethan-diol in water or ethanol–isopentane–diethylether mixtures have been employed. A significant development in phosphorimetry was the use of micro sample tubes with which it is possible to use a wide range of solvents, including water. Alternatively the sample may be sited outside the liquid nitrogen cooler thus enabling any solvent to be selected (*see* p. 160).

Temperature. Fluorescence intensity tends to decrease with increase in temperature due in part to the greater propensity for collisions between excited molecules as the temperature is elevated.

Except when measuring enzyme reactions, where small temperature changes can produce a large alteration in enzyme activity, sample temperature variations of 1 or 2 degrees are normally unimportant. For most compounds at 1°C temperature change will cause the fluorescence intensity to fluctuate by only about 1%. However, for some compounds, reductions of up to 5% per degree increase in temperature may occur. Indole-acetic acid, tryptophan, rhodamine B, p-toluene, and 5-phenyl substituted barbiturates are particularly susceptible to temperature changes. In these instances some form of temperature stabilization of the cell compartment may be desirable. A liquid-cooled cell compartment may be essential in fluorimeters where the cell compartment is in very close proximity to the lamp source.

For phosphorescence measurements the effect of temperature on sample rigidity is the overriding determinant, however; lowering the temperature will normally enhance phosphorescence.

Photodecomposition. Many compounds are vulnerable to photodecomposition in very dilute solution but quite stable at higher concentrations. Even established fluorescence standards such as quinine bisulphate will markedly photodecompose at concentrations of $<10^{-8}$ g/ml. The intensity and wavelength of irradiation are the determinants of the extent of decomposition observed. Typically, photodecomposition leads to a lowering of fluorescence intensity; on occasion, however, an increased fluorescence is found, e.g. 4-aminoquinolines, coumarin, various flavins.

In instances where photodecomposition is a problem it is advisable to control the time of sample exposure to the light source by means of a shutter in the exciting light path. Photodecomposition may appear to be much more significant when microcuvettes are used. This is because in the conventional 1 cm^2 cell only a part of the sample is exposed to the exciting light source, thus photodecomposed material will diffuse out of the exciting beam to be replaced by intact molecules. In the microcuvette the whole sample is exposed to the light source thus there is no 'diluent effect' and photodecomposition is more obvious.

Quenching. When one compound reduces the fluorescence of another it is said to quench its fluorescence. Quenching may occur in two principal ways, (a) by inner filter effects, and (b) by true quenching (Fig. 3).

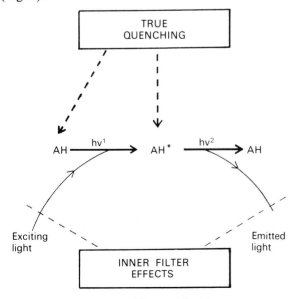

Fig. 3 Quenching mechanisms.

Inner filter effects occur because substances present in the environment of the fluorescent compound either filter out some of the exciting light thus effectively reducing the intensity of light falling on the compound, or filter out some of the emitted fluorescence, thereby diminishing the amount reaching the photodetector. Thus to be effective as an inner filter quencher a substance must display considerable absorption at either the exciting or emitting wavelength of the fluorescing species. A particular example of an inner effect is the phenomenon known as *concentration quenching*. Only in very dilute solution is the intensity of fluorescence proportional to concentration, i.e. only in very low concentrations does the relationship $F = K\phi I_0 \Sigma c$ hold (where Σ = molar absorptivity, K = a constant, I_0 = exciting light intensity, c = molar concentration). This linearity of concentration may extend over a wide concentration range, greater than one thousand-fold in many instances. However, at higher concentrations the intensity : concentration relationship approaches a plateau and at higher concentrations still an inverse relationship between intensity and concentration occurs. The main reason for this loss of linearity is that some of the emitted fluorescence is reabsorbed by other molecules of the compound under examination. Since the quantum efficiency is invariably less than unity, the effective result is that some loss of fluorescence intensity occurs. Also unequal distribution of the exciting light among the molecules occurs, those at the surface being favoured while those in the bulk of the solution may receive very little light. As the concentration of a compound increases, the frequency of these reabsorption events will become greater. The exact concentration at which deviation from a linear intensity/concentration relationship will vary with the optical arrangement of the instrument (right angle or front surface, slit width, etc., *see* Fig. 5) and the fluorescence characteristics of the compound involved. However, a useful rule-of-thumb is that this form of quenching should be carefully looked for if more than 5% of the exciting light is absorbed, e.g. using a conventional fluorimeter phenol concentration quenching may occur above 5 μg/l. Concentration quenching can easily be detected by determining the fluorescence intensity of a sample at two dilutions.

True quenching may occur by the interaction of a quenching agent with either the ground state or the excited states of a fluorescent compound. Because the excited states are more reactive, these excited state interactions are most common. The degradation of excited state energy may occur in several ways, i.e. by conversion of the excited singlet state to the triplet state or by energy, electron or proton transfer. Singlet–triplet conversion may be caused by heavy metal ions, oxygen or halogenated compounds. The extent of quenching observed by these substances is highly dependent on the nature of the fluorescing compound. Quenching by halogens and heavy metal ions appears to be associated with their large magnetic fields. Oxygen quenching, which is frequently accomplished with aromatic hydrocarbons, is due to the fact that the ground state of oxygen is a triplet. In contact with the excited state of the hydrocarbon, oxygen exchanges its triplet state for a singlet state with the consequent intersystem crossing of the hydrocarbon to its triplet state. (N.B. A similar interaction of oxygen with excited bilirubin is the basis for the ultraviolet light therapy used to treat neonatal jaundice. In this case the resultant excited singlet oxygen then goes on to oxidize the bilirubin to excretable degradation products.) Oxygen quenching can of course easily be eliminated by bubbling the sample with nitrogen prior to use. It has proven useful as a means of distinguishing between the dihydrodiol and phenol metabolites of certain aromatic hydrocarbons and has even been employed to measure concentrations of oxygen in solution using benzoin as the fluorescent reagent. Knowledge of the energy levels of the excited states of the fluorescent species and of any contaminants present in its environment is insufficient for more than a very limited prediction of the likelihood of quenching occurring by intersystem crossing. There is considerable selectivity in quenching by intersystem crossing so that the extent of singlet–triplet conversion (measured by changes in the fluorescence : phosphorescence ratio) manifested by various 'quenchers' can serve as a valuable identification criterion. For example, silver ion enhancement of tryptophan phosphorescence has been used to characterize tryptophan in the presence of other substances showing a similar fluorescence while nitromethane has been used to distinguish fluoranthenic hydrocarbons, which are not quenched, from benzo(a)pyrene, anthracene and perylene, which are highly quenched in this solvent. Either electron donation or electron acceptance from the excited singlet state may also occur. Anions which can serve as electron donors include IO_3^-, NO_3^-, $S_4O_6^{--}$, SO_4^{--} and PO_4^{---} while those that may act as electron acceptors include I^-, Br^-, SCN^- and $S_2O_3^{--}$. The direction and extent of electron transfer is of course related to the redox potential of the excited fluorescent compound. Unfortunately this will be different from the redox potential of the ground state molecules and in the light of our present knowledge must be considered to be unpredictable. Despite its unpredictable nature, electron transfer phenomena may be used as identification criteria because particular electron transfer agents tend to be rather selective in their action. For example, the quenching effects of thiosulphate and nitrate can be used to identify tryptophan in tissue fluids.

Quenching by proton transfer is also known as excited state ionization (p. 148). If the fluorescing molecular form of a compound loses a proton in the excited state it will adopt the properties of the anion. This may lead to either enhanced fluorescence (*see* section on pH and solvent) or diminished fluorescence. Very little is known about the factors which will cause an environmental agent to increase the extent of excited state ionization bar the fact that the agent should be an effective proton acceptor.

Quenching by energy transfer may occur without collision between the fluorescing species and the quenching agent. For energy transfer to be effective some overlap is necessary between the emission spectrum of the fluorescing species and the absorption spectrum of the quenching agent. The efficiency of this type of energy transfer varies as the reciprocal of the sixth power of the distance between the two molecules, the distance between them should be less than 50 Å for effective transfer to occur. Energy transfer is commonly observed between monomers within macromolecules or as a consequence of small molecules binding to macromolecules. Intramolecular energy transfer may also occur within small molecules. This will cause some deviations from the structure fluorescence rules cited earlier. NADH-fluorescence is a good example of a light emission arising due to energy transfer (*see* p. 163).

Quenching may occur by simple collision between the quenching agent and the fluorescing species either in the ground state (static quenching) or in the excited state with the subsequent loss of the excited state energy in the form of heat (dynamic quenching). This type of quenching is very dependent on the solvent viscosity. The extent of quenching (Q) can be anticipated from the Stern–Volmer equation:

$$\frac{F_0 - F}{F} = K(Q)$$

where K = constant
F_0 = fluorescence intensity without the quenching agent
F = fluorescence intensity with the quenching agent

If quenching is observed an internal standard (generally a small known amount of the fluorescent species) can often be successfully incorporated in some of the assay tubes to enable the quenching correction factor to be determined. Collisional quenching may be reduced by lowering the sample temperature or increasing solvent viscosity. When the sample is frozen in a solid matrix, which is the situation in phosphorimetry, this type of quenching is minimized.

Scatter. Light scattering may take a number of forms. Tyndall and Rayleigh scattering are characterized by having the same excitation and emission wavelengths—*see* Fig. 4 (peak a). Scattering of this type may be identified by changing the excitation wavelength. The emission wavelength will alter to the same extent if scatter is the source of emission, whereas if it is due to fluorescence (peak c), no change in the optimal emission wavelength will be observed (although the intensity will change). Scatter may interfere with the fluorescence signal by causing the exciting light to be reflected, in which case an enhanced signal may be observed at the detector.

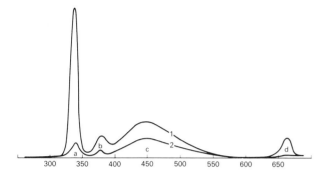

Fig. 4 Emission spectrum of 0·01 μg/ml solution of quinine sulphate in 0·1 N H_2SO_4, λ_{ex} 335 nm (1) in the absence of a polarizing film (2) with a single piece of a polarizing film in the exciting light path in the horizontal position.

If the λ_{ex} and λ_{fl} are close together this reflected light may overlap with the fluorescence emissions thereby causing an apparent increase in the fluorescence reaching the detector. The effects of this type of scatter may be minimized by narrowing the band pass of the excited and/or emitted light paths. Alternatively the exciting wavelength may be lowered to below the λ_{ex} and/or the fluorescence wavelength raised to above its λ_{fl}. Although some resultant loss of sensitivity will accrue this is usually more than compensated for by the great reduction in the scatter interference. The employment of a piece of polaroid film in the exciting light path alone or ideally in both light paths may also be used to reduce the scatter signal (Fig. 4). This approach is based on the principle that the scatter signal has a polarized element which can be eliminated. Some loss of fluorescence signal is also observed though this is small compared with the loss of the scatter signal. The employment of polarizers in this way may frequently improve the potential assay sensitivity. For example in the case of warfarin and quinine sulphate a 10-fold sensitivity improvement may be observed. The orientation of the polaroid film in the light path is important, in the exciting light path it should only pass radiation whose electrical vector is horizontal and in the emission path only light with a vertical vector.

In phosphorimetry scattering problems are considerably less than in fluorimetry. This is because a brief time lapse (mediated by a shutter system) is normally employed in phosphorimetry between exciting the sample and measuring its emitted light. Under these circumstances no reflected exciting light will be able to reach the photodetector.

Raman scattering is fundamentally different from Rayleigh and Tyndall scattering, being characterized by a fixed frequency difference between the exciting and emission wavelengths. Thus if the excitation wavelength is altered the emission wavelength will change, but not by the same number of wavelength units (i.e. the magnitude of change will vary as $1/\lambda_{ex}$). The observed Raman spectrum (peak b) is usually that of the solvent used. The Raman spectrum is normally only a problem when very dilute solutions are being measured and the instrument is near the upper reaches of its sensitivity limits. Sometimes the Raman spectrum will overlap with that of the fluorescence being determined. As in the case of Rayleigh and Tyndall scattering, interference of this type can often be overcome by altering the excitation and/or emission wavelengths. Alternatively the solvent can be changed. Some Raman spectra of commonly used solvents are given in Table 2. The appearance of the Raman spectrum is not always a disadvantage, indeed it can be used as a very rapid, simple and reliable check on both instrumental sensitivity and emission wavelength fidelity.

TABLE 2
RAMAN SPECTRA OF SOME COMMON SOLVENTS

Excitation wavelength (nm)	Raman emission wavelength (nm)		
	Water	Ethanol	Cyclohexane
313	340	344	344
365	416	409	408
405	469	459	458
436	511	500	499

Spurious Fluorescence and Phosphorescence in Luminescence Assays. Additional luminescence signals are often seen which are contributed by contaminants in the sample. These contaminants may arise from the original biological material or they may become accidentally added during the sample work-up procedure. If the biological material is the principal source of interfering agents then some modification in the sample preparation approach is clearly called for. However, all too frequently it is impurities in the reagents and dirty equipment employed in the assay procedure which causes these spurious luminescence problems. Common sources of interference include traces of fluorescent washing powders, materials leached from ion-exchange resins (particularly those incorporating aromatic amines), stopcock grease and inherent fluorescence in the cuvettes and light filters. Impure solvents and reagents are often the culprits. For high sensitivity assay work analar grade chemicals may not be sufficiently pure. It is not especially comforting to be assured that a chemical contains less than 1 ppm of a luminescent contaminant when one is trying to measure nanogram amounts of compound. For similar reasons spectroscopic grade solvents are not always adequate, indeed in the author's experience laboratory grade ethanol frequently contains less luminescent contaminants than spectroscopic grade ethanol. Some fluorimetric grade solvents are commercially available, but the range is at present narrow and the cost high. Solvents that are immiscible with water can often be considerably decontaminated by the simple expedient of washing them with 2 M HCl, then 2 M KOH then glass distilled water. Distilled water may become contaminated if it is stored in polythene containers. Triple-(glass)-distilled water, stored in glass containers, is recommended for high sensitivity work. In studies requiring the assay of materials in strong acid, care must be taken to ensure that pieces of paper tissue do not fall in, for they may react, thereby forming fluorescent products.

INSTRUMENTATION

Although a wide range of fluorimeters is currently available they mostly employ the same fundamental design (Fig. 5). The type of wavelength selection device employed in the exciting light beam strongly influences the form of light source used. If the wavelength selection device has a narrow band pass (e.g. a grating monochromator system) then a continuum lamp, i.e. one that emits light at all wavelengths can be selected, whereas if only crude wavelength selection is accomplished (e.g. a filter) then a line source lamp is normally chosen which only requires of the wavelength selector that it discriminate between well-separated wavelength lines. The specifications for the emission wavelength selector is primarily that it can distinguish between the excitation wavelength (i.e. light scatter signal) and the emission wavelength. Additionally the narrower the band pass the better the prospects of separating fluorescence from the Raman spectrum or from other potentially interfering fluorescence signals. Conventionally in the sim-

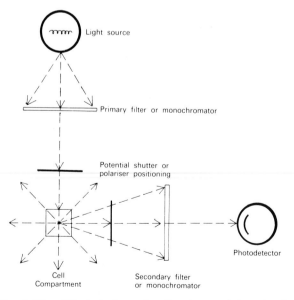

Fig. 5 Simplified design of a fluorimeter/phosphorimeter.

plest instruments a line source lamp is used and cut-off filters are used for excitation and emission wavelength selection.

Interference wedges represent a compromise between this simple light filter approach and the much more sophisticated and expensive grating or prism monochromator. The recent availability of a wide range of interference filters with narrow band passes opens up the prospect of low price fluorimeters employing cheap continuum light sources, e.g. tungsten for operating in the visible region of the spectrum.

Lamp Sources

Line Source Lamps. Mercury lamps are most commonly used as the light source in filter fluorimeters. The principal mercury lines are at 254, 297, 313, 334, 365, 405, 436 and 546 nm, the most useful lines for 'analytical fluorimetry' being at 365 and 436 nm. If the λ_{ex} of a compound falls on, or close to, one of these lines then a mercury lamp source may be as good or better than a continuum source because of its very narrow band width. However, for compounds which do not absorb well at these wavelengths a mercury light source is obviously incompatible with an assay demanding high sensitivity.

Insertion of a phosphor plate in the light path emanating from the lamp can be used to produce a broader wavelength envelope (e.g. the 254 nm mercury line can be shifted by selection of appropriate phosphors to a band around 280 nm thus permitting the excitation of tryptophan and tyrosine); however, some loss of intensity always ensues. As more phosphors are developed the versatility of this approach will improve. A limited range of phosphor-coated lamps which provide a narrow exciting wavelength band is available. Other line lamp sources incorporating elements other than mercury may be purchased. The zinc/cadmium lamp has achieved particularly widespread usage for cortisol assays. The prospect of tailor-made light sources for a number of widely used assays is probably not far distant. The laser is beginning to make an impact in fluorimetry although it has yet to achieve its full potential value.

Continuum Lamps. Xenon lamps are most extensively used in spectrofluorimeters. Although xenon lamps give out a good light intensity between 280 and 500 nm, they suffer from two major deficiencies. The arc is inclined to shift from one striking of the lamp to another, thus the intensity and the focus tends to vary from day to day. Occasionally a shift will occur while the instrument is in use. In a number of spectrofluorimeters, to overcome this problem, a small portion of the exciting light is deflected to a reference photomultiplier which is linked to the fluorescence detector in such a manner that changes in the intensity of light falling on the reference photomultiplier cause reciprocal changes in the response of the detector. Unfortunately, in some instruments this compensating device leads to an appreciable drop in the instrumental sensitivity. This can easily be checked by simply switching the reference system off. An alternative (or additional) approach has been to maintain the lamp in a strong magnetic field so that the tendency of the arc to wander is minimized. This appears to be a fairly effective way round the problem of arc wander.

In spectrofluorimeters in which the light source is finely focused on the cell compartment, it is worth realigning the lamp each time the instrument is used. This can be accomplished by moving the lamp position by means of the adjusting screws until an optimal reading is attained on a reliable light scatter sample (such as a suspension of glycogen).

The second deficiency of xenon lamps is that the light intensity falling on the cell compartment varies at different wavelengths. The intensity normally increases with wavelengths up to 400 nm then plateaus, falling away above 440 nm. As spectrofluorimeters are normally single-beam instruments, there is no automatic compensation for this energy variability. As a consequence the excitation spectra of compounds which absorb in the ultraviolet appear to have their maxima at higher wavelengths than those of the corresponding spectrophotometer-derived absorption spectra. The converse situation pertains for compounds which absorb at wavelengths above 440 nm. Since each xenon lamp will have slightly different characteristics, the excitation spectra derived for a particular compound will tend to vary between instruments. Thus reported λ_{ex} and λ_{fl} values will not necessarily be reproduced on other instruments. If true absorption spectra are required the lamp must be calibrated. A chemical actinometer method has frequently been employed for this purpose (for details see Parker[2] and White and Argauer[4]). Automatic compensating devices are available but these are expensive and their purchase by a clinical biochemistry laboratory cannot normally be justified. Because of the high voltages required to start these xenon lamps and the frequent arcing at the lamp terminals, ozone and nitrogen oxides are produced. These gases are toxic and require effective removal from the working environment.

In some instruments a mirror is placed behind the light source to gather the light which would not otherwise reach the cell compartment. This design modification does tend to increase the intensity of light falling on the sample but the useful lifetime of the mirror is severely limited due to the oxidizing effects of the ozone and nitrogen oxides on the mirror surface which reduce its reflective powers. Regular cleaning with ethanol will marginally prolong the period of usefulness. The xenon lamp loses intensity with age particularly in the ultraviolet region. The useful lifetime of a xenon lamp obviously depends on the sensitivity demands placed on the instrument and varies from lamp to lamp. Between 500 and 1000 h is a reasonable expectation for routine assay purposes.

Cooling the lamp by the blower motor after switching it off will tend to reduce lamp failure rate. Although instrumental sensitivity can theoretically be improved by employing more intense light sources, this approach is limited in practice by the increased photodecomposition of the sample which results.

The Cell Compartment and Sample Presentation

Fluorescence Measurement. Conventionally a 1 cm^2 silica cuvette capable of holding approximately 3–4 ml of solution is used to contain the sample and the fluorescence is measured at right angles to the exciting light source. The logic of selecting a 1 cm^2 cell is less obvious than in spectrophotometry, its main virtue is that the square surface is likely to emanate less scatter than a round surface. If microcells are to be used careful selection to eliminate those with high scattering or fluorescent surfaces is necessary to obtain maximum sensitivity. Meticulous cleaning of these cells with non-fluorescent detergent or with concentrated nitric acid is advisable. Micro-flow cells are increasing in popularity particularly in conjunction with high pressure liquid chromatography.

For highly turbid samples it is advisable to measure the fluorescence originating at the surface of the solution close to the point of excitation (front surface reflectance—*see* Fig. 5). The front surface optical arrangement is also used in many instruments to measure fluorescence on TLC plates and other solid surfaces. The plate is normally either held vertically, close to or in the normal front surface position of the instrument, or it is held horizontally in which case 'light pipes' (wave guides) are used to convey the excited light to, and the emitted light from, the plate. Instruments in which the exciting light is shone through the plate are usually restricted in application to compounds which excite in the visible region of the spectrum because conventional glass plates do not allow the transmission of ultraviolet light. Many of the TLC devices available as attachments for commercial spectrofluorimeters are rather lacking in sensitivity due to poor optical design. Measurement of fluorescence on commercial densitometers is often equally or more satisfactory than employing these TLC plate accessories. Measurement of fluorescence on TLC plates is one of the faster growing methods of fluorescence analysis (*see below*), hopefully this will provide the stimulus for better accessory design.

Phosphorescence Measurement. Phosphorimetric measurement requires two facilities which are not demanded in fluorimetry, namely a means of keeping the sample in a rigid form and a system of enabling alternative excitation of the sample and measurement of its luminescence signal.

Sample rigidity is normally accomplished by freezing the sample at liquid nitrogen temperature. This is achieved in most existing instruments by placing the sample in a narrow silica sample tube and immersing this tube in liquid nitrogen contained in a special Dewar flask which has optically transparent sides (Fig. 6). Because the emissions from the silica samples tubes and the frozen samples contained therein tend to vary according to the orientation of the tube within the Dewar flask, it is advisable to rotate the tube mechanically during the assay. This type of phosphorimetry accessory, although very useful for more fundamental studies, is by no means ideal for routine analytical use because the solvent choice is restricted, the sample tubes tend to crack and bubbling in the liquid nitrogen causes fluctuations in the luminescence signal. Recently the development of several devices in which the sample is located outside

the cooling system has greatly improved the prospects of phosphorimetry becoming acceptable as a routine analytical technique. In one such approach phosphorimetric measurement is made on metal-backed TLC plates which are wrapped around a copper drum containing liquid nitrogen.[5]

However, there is little sign of commercial development of phosphorimeters for analytical purposes. Room-temperature fluorescence employing new forms of solid matrices shows considerable potential.[6]

Because phosphorescence is a relatively slow release of light following excitation of the sample, it is possible to separate the phosphorescence signal from the scatter or fluorescence signals by cutting off the exciting light (so that all prompt emission processes are immediately curtailed) and following the emission signal. This may be achieved by placing a shutter on both the excitation and emission sides of

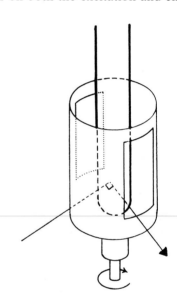

Fig. 7 Rotating shutter for use in phosphorimetry.

the optical path with slots cut in it so that light can only reach the photodetector when the exciting light beam is interrupted (Fig. 7). By varying the speed of rotation of the shutter it is sometimes possible to distinguish slow and fast phosphorescence emissions, thereby improving selectivity. It is also possible by appropriate manipulation of the shutter, to determine the half-life of phosphorescence decay of many compounds. This $t_\frac{1}{2}$, in conjunction with the λ_{ex} and λ_p values, can provide an important identification criterion for a compound.

Detection Systems

Instrumental sensitivity is dictated by the intensity of the exciting light reaching the sample, the amount of fluorescence reaching the detector and the ability of the detector to respond to the signal. The light reaching the detector is obviously determined both

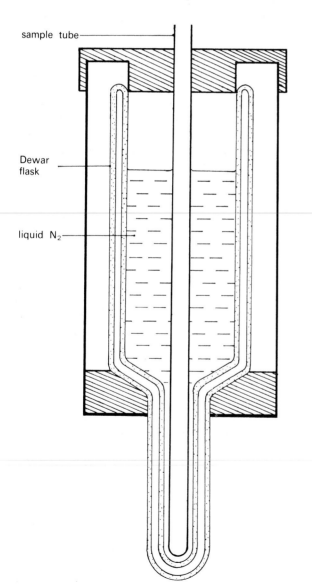

Fig. 6 Dewar flask with optically transparent sides for use in phosphorimetry.

by the emission characteristics of the sample and by the optical geometry of the instrument. The narrower the excitation and emission band passes demanded in the name of specificity the greater are the demands placed on the sensitivity of the detector device. Photomultipliers are normally used as detectors. The sensitivity of their response to the light falling on them will vary with the wavelength of the light. Most phototubes have a peak response between 450 and 500 nm. Phototubes which have an enhanced ultraviolet and infrared sensitivity are available. Ultraviolet tubes are often employed but the infrared sensitive phototube has only limited value in clinical biochemistry, since with the exception of some porphyrins relatively few compounds display fluorescence in the infrared region. Infrared detectors may prove more useful in phosphorimetry. As a consequence of the photodetectors variable response with wavelength the emission spectra produced by most spectrofluorimeters are distorted versions of the true spectra. This means that λ_{fl} or λ_p values determined on one instrument are not necessarily transferable to a second fluorimeter. True spectra can be derived if the emission side of the instrument is calibrated against a light source of known energy distribution or by monitoring detector response using a series of fluorescent standards. Automatic self-correction devices are available but at present the cost of these precludes their widespread use.[4] It is likely that more sensitive phototubes will be used in commercially available spectrofluorimeters in the foreseeable future. Array detector systems (both imaging photon detectors and charge coupled devices) are likely to find an important niche for measuring luminescence changes in tissues, gels, microtitre plates, etc. However, the most useful development is likely to be the incorporation of photon counting devices which will allow the accumulation of the luminescence signal with time (i.e. similar to that used in a liquid scintillation counter). Using biological samples the 'blank' seldom gives a zero signal. Normally the photomultiplier's task is therefore to distinguish between two different light intensities. Thus it is not the overall sensitivity that is important but rather the signal discriminating ability of the instrument. Manufacturers' claims of very high sensitivities for their instruments should be treated with some scepticism by those wishing to use samples of biological origin because the compounds the manufacturers report on are very pure and the requirement for discriminating ability of the instrument is reduced to a minimum.

To optimize the benefits to be derived from photon counting devices they should be linked to simple computer facilities whose task is to discriminate between the desirable and spurious luminescence signals. In principle this could be simply achieved by rapidly measuring the signal at several different excitation and emission wavelengths. In addition, knowledge of the $t_{\frac{1}{2}}$ of individual phosphorescent and fluorescent compounds could be used to improve selectivity, if

fast response electronic shuttering devices were incorporated in the exciting and emitting light paths.

Fluorescent Standards

Because the energy of the lamp output and the phototube response varies with wavelength and the lamp output can vary with usage, fluorescent standards are required both as a check on the performance of the instrument and as a means of comparing results obtained on different instruments. The favoured standards are quinine bisulphate ($1.0\,\mu g/ml$ in $0.05\,\mathrm{M}$ H_2SO_4), fluorescein ($1.0\,\mu g/ml$ in $0.1\,\mathrm{M}$ NaOH), anthracene ($1.0\,\mu g/ml$ in ethanol freshly bubbled with oxygen-free nitrogen) and tyrosine ($1.0\,\mu g/ml$ in water). The use of liquid standards is inconvenient and subject to deterioration on storage. A suitable alternative is to use fluorescent compounds incorporated into plastic blocks. A number of these are commercially available. The Raman spectrum of the solvent (*see* p. 157) may also be used as a monitor of instrumental response.

The luminescence intensities of a sample, derived on a particular instrument can be expressed most readily in absolute terms by relating the fluorescence spectrum of the sample to that, obtained under identical instrumental conditions, for a fluorescent standard. If the λ_{ex}, λ_{fl} or λ_p characteristics of the sample and standard are similar:

$$\phi_{\text{sample}} = \phi_{\text{standard}} \cdot \frac{L_{\text{sample}}}{L_{\text{standard}}} \cdot \frac{\text{OD}_{\text{standard}}}{\text{OD}_{\text{sample}}}$$

where ϕ = quantum efficiency of luminescence, L = luminescence of the sample and standard obtained by determining the area under the emission curve (which can be found simply by cutting out the luminescence spectra plotted on graph paper and weighing them), and OD = the optical densities which for this purpose should be below 0.01 to avoid any possibility of concentration quenching.

If the peak excitation wavelengths of the sample and the standard are rather different, correction must also be made for the different energy output of the lamp at the two excitation wavelengths; this necessitates calibration of the lamp. (For details of calibration methods the reader is referred to references 2 and 4.)

Although quantum efficiency values allow absolute data to be expressed they are not necessarily very helpful in deciding whether or not to exploit a compound's fluorescence properties for analytical purposes. This is because in analysis one is interested in the magnitude of the fluorescence signal, which is determined both by the efficiency of the energy conversion (i.e. quantum efficiency) and by the amount of light adsorbed ($\propto \Sigma_{\text{max}}$). To evaluate its analytical potential fluorescence sensitivity units are preferred, where fluorescence sensitivity of the sample =

$$\frac{\text{quantum efficiency} \times \text{extinction coefficient}}{\text{half band width of fluorescence spectrum}}.$$

Sensitivity Limits of an Assay

As explained above, the limits of sensitivity for the determination of a compound in a biological sample is governed by the ability of the particular instrument to discriminate between the luminescence emitted by the compound and that produced by the biological blank. Some standardization of reported sensitivity limits is necessary. Obviously the instrument used must be clearly specified. One useful way of comparing data between instruments is to report the concentration of the compound which gives a reading of twice the blank value and that which gives a full-scale deflection (usually 100 units). If these figures are determined at the same time as the concentration of a standard required to produce a 50 unit reading is ascertained, then instrumental comparisons and sensitivities of particular assays can be easily made.

PRACTICAL APPLICATIONS OF LUMINESCENCE MEASUREMENTS[7]

The principal uses of luminescence measurements are:

—the analysis identification of endogenous and exogenous compounds in biological tissues and fluids.
—investigations of interactions of small molecules with macromolecules.
—study of enzyme kinetics.
—determination of the subcellular location of chemicals.

Analytical Applications of Luminescence Measurements

Analysis of endogenous and exogenous compounds constitutes by far the greatest application of luminescence measurements in clinical biochemistry. The two volume series *Fluorescence Assay in Biology and Medicine* by Udenfriend[8] and the bi-annual review in *Analytical Chemistry* on 'Fluorimetric Analysis' clearly reflect both the versatility of luminescence techniques and their growing popularity. It is convenient to consider luminescence assays in four categories:

1. assay of native luminescence,
2. chemically induced luminescence assays,
3. quenchofluorimetric analysis
4. analyses involving enzymes.

Native (Intrinsic) Luminescence Compounds which have a strong intrinsic fluorescence or phosphorescence may be assayed directly (*see* Table 2). The likelihood of a compound having suitable characteristics to be assayed by means of its native luminescence can to some extent be predicted from its structure (*see above*). Changes in pH, solvent polarity and viscosity and reduction in temperature should all be considered as means of improving on an assay. Even compounds without obviously apparent native fluorescence may develop luminescence in strong acid or alkali (*see* p. 163).

Tyrosine and tryptophan. Tyrosine and tryptophan have an appreciable ultraviolet native fluorescence which can be used both to assay these amino acids themselves and proteins into which they are incorporated. The intensity of the protein fluorescence depends on both the number of these amino acids and their environment in the proteins. Many proteins which contain both tyrosine and tryptophan exhibit the fluorescence of tryptophan only because the excitation energy of tyrosine is passed on to unexcited tryptophan by a process of non-radiative energy transfer. Other factors will also modify the observed fluorescence, for example cysteine groups in close proximity to tryptophan and tyrosine, will tend to encourage inter-system crossing so that phosphorescence rather than fluorescence occurs. Protein prosthetic groups, particularly those containing metals and porphyrins, can also profoundly influence the fluorescence output.

Metal-containing proteins are usually non-fluorescent although they are often phosphorescent. Determination of the fluorescence : phosphorescence intensity ratio may provide a useful adjunct for the identification of a number of proteins. The additional criterion of phosphorescence lifetime is also valuable in characterizing proteins.[9] Proteins, by virtue of their size, will also emit polarized fluorescence when excited with plane polarized light and this can be used as a further characterization criterion.

Purines and pyrimidines. Pyrimidine and purine are only very weakly fluorescent. Hypoxanthine, xanthine and uric acid are non-fluorescent but adenine is fluorescent at pH 3·0 as its monocation.

(Adenine cation pH 1.0 λ_{fl} 380 nm) (Guanine anion pH 11.0 λ_{fl} 350 nm)

ADP and ATP are weakly fluorescent at pH 1·0 but are more strongly fluorescent than adenine in 2·5 M H_2SO_4. Guanine is fluorescent both at pH 1·0 and at pH 11·0. DNA and RNA also show appreciable phosphorescence which cannot be interpreted simply in terms of their base composition (λ_p 415–430 nm) although at pH 7·0 thymine appears to make the major contribution.

Porphyrins. The porphyrin molecule contains the requisite extensive conjugated system of double bonds for an appreciably fluorescent structure. In acids and in organic solvents porphyrins emit a very strong fluorescence towards the red end of the visible spectrum. For this reason fluorimetry has become one of the principal ways by which porphyrins are assayed. The iron and copper metalloporphyrins are phosphorescent but not fluorescent until the metal ion is removed, whereas the magnesium porphyrin derivatives, e.g. chlorophyll, are highly fluorescent as befits their biological function. Iron can be removed by irradiating the porphyrin with intense ultraviolet light which serves to convert Fe^{3+} into Fe^{2+}. The ferrous iron can then be displaced in the presence of an Fe^{2+} binding agent. Ring opening produces molecules with less intense but nonetheless analytically useful fluorescence. Interruption of the conjugated system of double bonds causes a dramatic reduction in fluorescence intensity. For example, urobilin shows appreciable fluorescence whereas urobilinogen does not (*see* p. 150). Bilirubin and biliverdin develop fluorescence on standing in strong acid.

Pyridines. Pyridine is neither fluorescent nor phosphorescent but some pyridine-based molecules, notably Vitamin B_6 and related compounds, and NADH and NADPH emit considerable fluorescence. The strongest fluorescence of pyridoxine is due to the 3-hydroxypyridine ion although all the forms of this compound are fluorescent to some extent. The reduced but not the oxidized nicotinamide adenine dinucleotides are also strongly fluorescent. The emission characteristics of these reduced compounds are particularly interesting because it is claimed that they are due to radiationless energy transfer from the adenine ring to the reduced nicotinamide ring which then emits the fluorescence. By measuring NADH light emission rather than light absorption a potential increase in assay sensitivity of more than one-thousand-fold can be attained.

3-hydroxypyridine
anion pH 11
(λ_{fl} 365 nm)

NADH   pH 7   (λ_{fl} 457 nm)

Flavins. The flavins display an intense luminescence in aqueous solutions. This luminescence is highly solvent dependent, for example the λ_{fl} shifts to shorter wavelength as the polarity of the solvent is decreased.

As in the case of nicotinamide adenine dinucleotides, in the flavin adenine dinucleotides the adenine moiety greatly influences the flavin fluorescence. In flavins, however, quenching of fluorescence above pH 4·0 is observed due to the formation of donor–acceptor complexes between the adenine and flavin rings. Some of the flavins photodecompose to give more fluorescent materials. Formation of these photodecomposition products can serve as the basis for the fluorimetric assay of these flavins.

Drugs. Many drugs which contain one or more aromatic or heterocyclic rings show appreciable fluorescence or phosphorescence. Some drugs which have a notable native luminescence are listed in Table 1. Because most drugs are metabolized to form products which preserve at least some of the luminescence characteristics of the parent molecules it is often necessary to carry out a metabolite separation procedure prior to making a quantitative measurement. For this reason assay directly on TLC plates following chromatographic separation is becoming increasingly popular. To obtain reliable results careful chromatography and the use of appropriate internal standards is necessary. Pre-washing of the plates and the incorporation of a small amount of non-luminescent antioxidant into the support material is advisable. Improved sensitivity (often 10- to 100-fold) can usually be achieved by spraying the plate with ethanol, triethanolamine, ethylene glycol or water just prior to taking luminescence readings.[4] Other solid surfaces are also amenable for measuring fluorescence, including KBr discs, electrophoretic strips and silicon rubber pads (*see also* p. 169).

HPLC linked to a fluorescence detector may also be used to estimate a fluorescent drug and its metabolites. Overspraying TLC plates with ethanol markedly enhances the sensitivity of TLC phosphorimetric assays.

For further information on native fluorescence characteristics of molecules, the reader is referred to the paper of De Ment[10] who lists the luminescence characteristics of many hundreds of compounds; Bridges[11] provides a largely complementary list of the fluorescence characteristics of many drugs and toxic chemicals.

Chemically Induced Luminescence. Chemical modifications of a compound may be used to enhance its luminescence intensity or change its luminescence characteristics. These modifications may be achieved by extending the conjugated system of double bonds, increasing molecular rigidity and planarity or inserting appropriate substituent groups. In many instances the actual fluorescent products have not been identified. A number of approaches can be used (i) simple chemical manipulation, e.g. oxidation, reduction, hydrolysis[12] or condensation with other molecules; or (ii) tagging the compound with a luminescent label either covalently or through formation of an ion-pair complex. Some examples of these reactions are listed in Table 3. Details of these analytical procedures can be found in Udenfriend,[8] White and Argauer[4] and in the data sheets distributed by the leading manufacturers such as Turners and Aminco.

complex seems likely. Oestrogen fluorescence may be realized by heating with concentrated sulphuric acid or with a less concentrated acid containing hydroquinone. However, because many other organic compounds yield coloured products under these

TABLE 3

SOME EXAMPLES OF CHEMICALLY INDUCED FLUORESCENCE

Compound	Method of inducing luminescence	ex	fl	Sensitivity
Acetylcholine	Reduction to ethanol which is estimated using ADH and NAD	340	460	good
Acetyl salicylic acid	Hydrolysis to salicylate measured at pH 10	313	342	good
Adrenaline	Formation of trihydroxy indole	436	540	good
Amino acids	Couple with fluorescamine			good
Amphetamine	Couple with 9-isothiocyanate acridine			good
Chlorpromazine	Oxidation with H_2O_2 measured at pH 7	360	440	fair
Chloroquine	Photochemical change measured at pH 9·5	360	410	good
Cortisol	Treatment with conc. sulphuric acid	470	525	good
Digitonin	Heat with strong acid	350	490	fair
Fluoride	Quenching of magnesium oxinate fluorescence	420	530	fair
Glucose	Formation of benzonaphthenedione	470	550	good
Glutathione	Coupling with o-phthaldehyde	343	425	good
Histamine	Condensation with o-phthaldehyde			good
Isoniazid	Couple with salicylaldehyde then reduce measure in isobutanol	392	478	good
Librium	Formation of lactam			good
Malate	Condense with resorcinol, mesure at pH 8·5	490	530	fair
6-Mercaptopurine	Oxidation with $KMnO_4$			fair
Methotrexate	Oxidation with $KMnO_4$	280	450	fair
Morphine	Condense with conc. H_2SO_4	365	420	good
Penicillin	Couple with 2-methoxy-6-chloro-9-aminoethyl acridine	420	500	fair
Pyridoxine	Condense with KCN	358	435	good
Pyruvate	Formation of quinoxaline derivative	360	490	good
Reserpine	Treatment with HNO_2			good
Selenium	Couple with 2,3-diamino naphthalene			poor
Serotonin	Condensation with ninhydrin			
Streptomycin	Couple with p-naphthoquinone-4-sulphonate	365	445	good
Sulphonamides	Couple with 4,5-methylene dioxyphthaldehyde	320	375	good
Tetracycline	Couple with Ca^{2+} and barbituric acid	405	530	good
Thiamine	Oxidation to thiochrome	365	435	good
Thiohydantoin	Couple with 2,6-dichloroquinonechloromide			good
Tolamolol	Couple with 4-dichloro-5-triazinyl-1-ethoxynaphthalein			good
Vitamin C	Condense with o-phenylene	350	430	fair
Vitamin D	Complex with acetic anhydride: H_2SO_4	390	470	good

Steroids. Only oestrogens, by virtue of their phenolic groups, possess native fluorescence (λ_{ex} 282 nm; λ_{fl} 330 nm). However, fluorescence can be induced in many steroids by treatment with strong acid or alkali. Specificity is imposed by the work-up procedure.

To assay plasma corticosteroids, for example, the plasma is normally shaken with petroleum ether to remove contaminating lipids, then extracted into methylene chloride and shaken with alkali to remove oestrogens. The methylene chloride is added to a concentrated sulphuric acid/ethanol mixture (3 : 1 v/v) shaken and centrifuged. After 6 min the developed fluorescence is measured. The nature of the fluorescent product(s) is uncertain but a charge transfer

conditions, a subsequent solvent extraction with acetylenetetrabromide containing ethanol and p-nitrophenol is necessary to reduce the blank (Ittrich procedure). Methandrostenolone, progesterone, pregnenolone, testosterone and aldosterone are other steroids which also produce a strong fluorescence in concentrated acid.

Catecholamines. The native fluorescence of most catecholamines is characteristic of catechol (λ_{ex} 285 nm; λ_{fl} 325 nm). Conversion to a highly fluorescent trihydroxy indole normally provides the basis to their fluorimetric assay. This chemically induced fluorescence has several virtues: it enhances the fluorescence sensitivity (by increasing the conjugated system of double bonds, imposing rigidity and inserting appropriate substituent groups), it shifts the λ_{ex} to the visible region and the λ_{fl} to a spectral region in which photomultiplier response is particularly sensitive and it imposes specificity since, by controlling the reaction conditions, formation of trihydroxyindoles is restricted to a very limited number of catechols. Furthermore, trihydroxyindoles derived from individual catecholamines often produce different fluorescent spectra. The trihydroxyindoles are usually formed by oxidation with ferrocyanide followed by alkali treatment. A very large number of modifications to the basic procedure have been published.

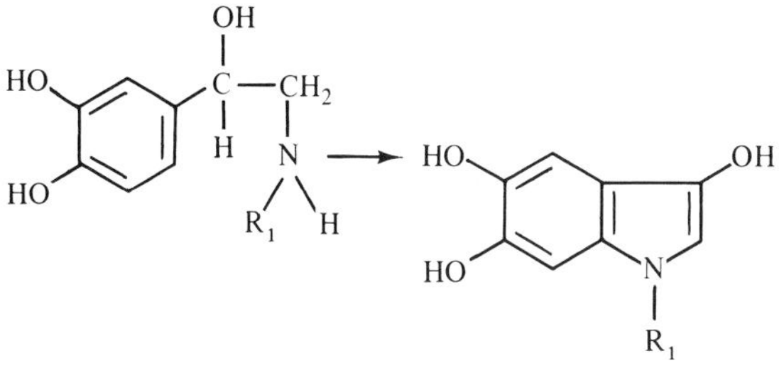

(formation of a trihydroxyindole λ_{fl} 520 nm)

Vitamins. Fluorimetric assays for several of the B vitamins have been available for many years. In one of the earliest procedures still in common use, ferricyanide oxidation is used to convert thiamine into highly fluorescent thiochrome (whose exact structure has not been elucidated). Riboflavin can be estimated as its irradiation product, lumiflavin, while vitamin B_6 may be assayed in its native form, or following either its reaction with cyanide to form the cyanohydrin derivative or its oxidation to pyridoxic acid lactone.

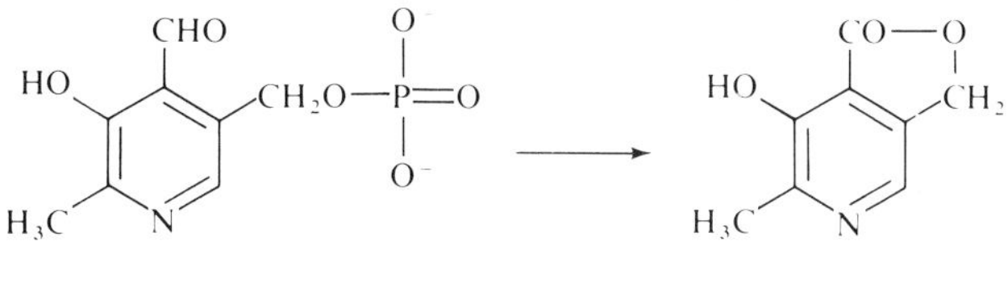

(formation of pyridoxic acid lactone λ_{fl} 450 nm)

Carbohydrates. Carbohydrates possess no native fluorescence. However, on hydration with concentrated acids, reactive materials are produced which will condense with various conjugated double-bond systems to produce fluorescence products. Reagents

which have been used for this purpose include *o*-phenylenediamine, dimedone, 3,5'-diaminobenzoate, resorcinol and 3-hydroxy-l-tetralone. A typical example is the assay method for glucose which depends on its reaction with 5-hydroxy-l-tetralone in concentrated sulphuric acid to form the strongly fluorescent benzonaphthanedione.

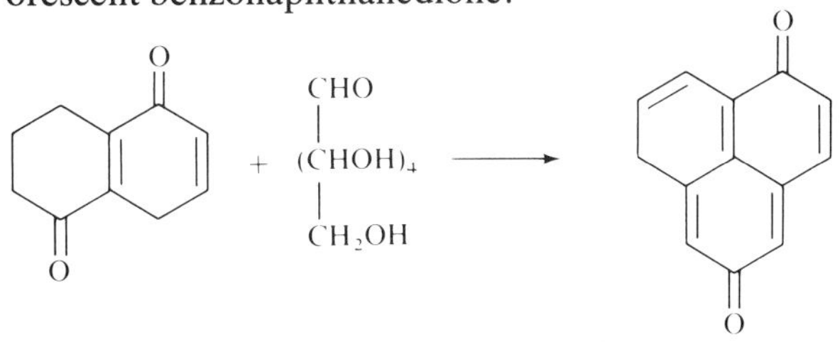

(formation of benzonaphthanedione λ_{fl} 550 nm)

Amino acids and proteins. Only tryptophan and tyrosine have appreciable native fluorescence. To assay other amino acids or proteins containing few, if any, aromatic residues, the favoured approach is to label the amino groups with a fluorogenic reagent. Ninhydrin, 1-dimethylamino naphthalene-5-sulphonyl chloride, *o*-phenaldehyde, fluoresceinisothiocyanate and fluorescamine (fluoram) have all achieved widespread use. Fluorescamine has gained particular popularity because it reacts at room temperature in aqueous solution at near neutral pH. Unreacted material is rapidly destroyed generating non-fluorescent products. Because of the low concentrations at which the fluorescamine-labelled products can be detected, the very mild reaction conditions involved and the versatility of the reaction, assays based on this type of reagent may well replace the routine ninhydrin-based colorimetric analysis of amino acids in the foreseeable future.

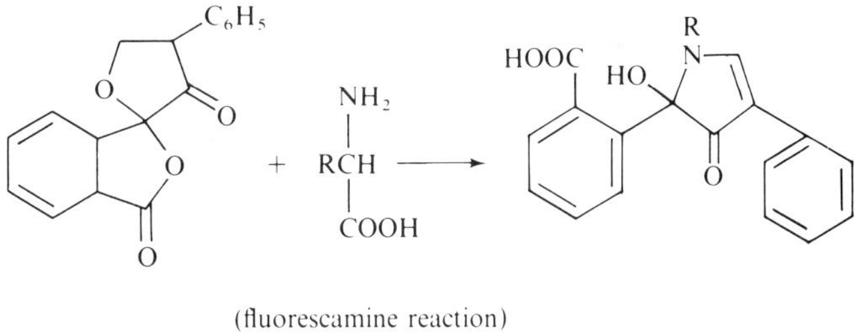

(fluorescamine reaction)

The generation of fluorescence products with ninhydrin is rather less versatile than the colorimetric procedure although for aromatic amino acids, e.g. phenylalanine and serotonin, this method is capable of a very high sensitivity.

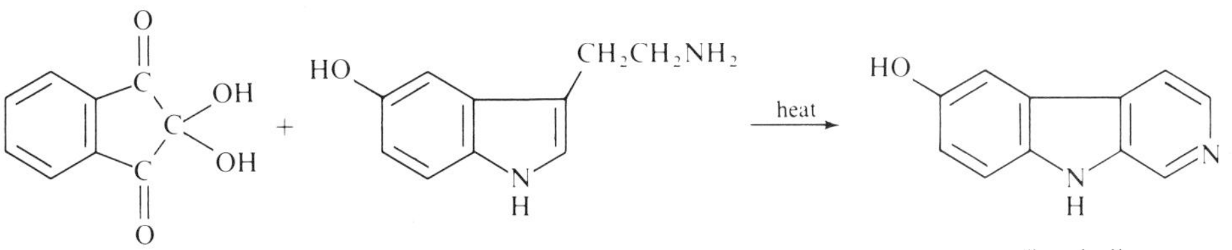

β-carboline

(ninhydrin reaction)

Dansyl chloride (DNS) is also commonly used for labelling the amino group of proteins because it forms highly fluorescent products and it is versatile, reacting with both primary and secondary amines. It suffers from the disadvantage compared with fluorescamine that unreacted dansyl chloride and some of the breakdown products retain their fluorescence in aqueous solution and it is therefore often necessary to subject the labelled protein to a clean-up procedure.

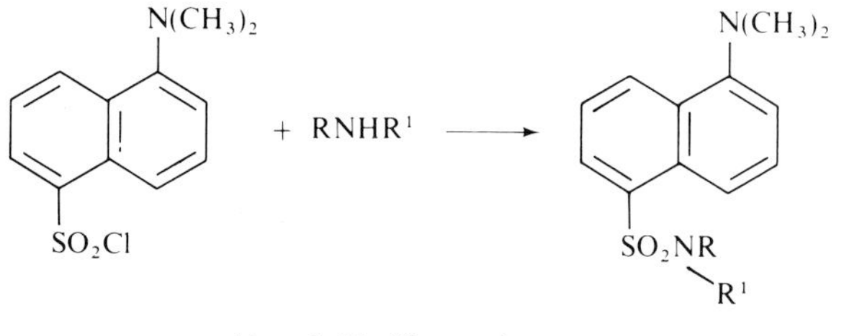

(dansyl chloride reaction)

(N.B. In non-aqueous solution the chloride is less fluorescent and separation may not be needed.)

Fluoresceinisothiocyanate (FIC) has particularly found favour for tagging antibodies. As with DNS, the label itself and some of the breakdown products are fluorescent and often need to be removed once the protein has been reacted. An additional difficulty with both DNS and FIC is that many commercially available samples of these substances are impure and appear to vary in reactivity. A preliminary TLC clean-up of these reagents is often worthwhile.

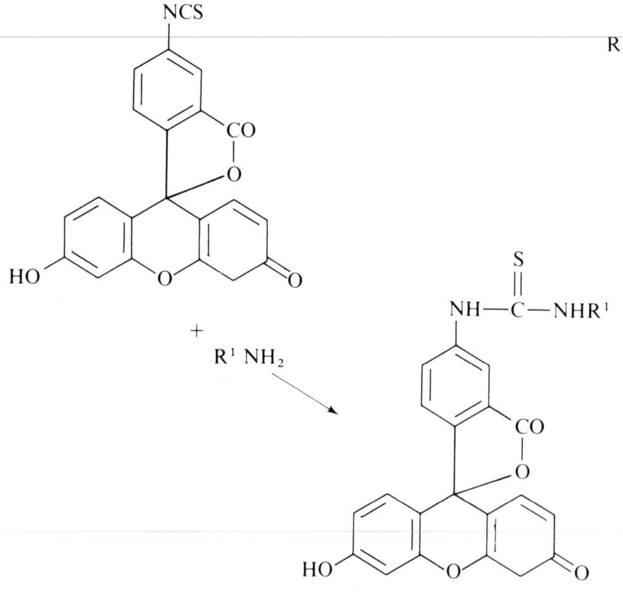

(fluoresceinisothiocyanate reaction)

In addition to the covalent linking of fluorescent labels onto proteins, dyes which change their fluorescence characteristics on binding to proteins (fluorescent probes—*see* p. 170) can also be used for assaying proteins. l-Aniline-8-naphthalene sulphonate (ANS) is particularly suitable for this purpose

because it shows a marked intensification of fluorescence (*see* p. 154). ANS has been used to assay histones, Bence–Jones protein, serum albumin and ribonuclease. In general this method is very sensitive and reliable. Problems may be encountered in estimating samples from jaundiced patients because albumin-bound bilirubin will quench the ANS fluorescence to some extent, presumably by an energy transfer mechanism.

Drugs and other xenobiotics. A very wide variety of methods have been used to induce fluorescence in organic molecules, in many cases they are extensions of methods originally applied in colorimetry. It is only possible in this chapter to outline some of the approaches which are used in order to illustrate their scope. To facilitate this discussion, compounds will be considered according to the functional group involved in the derivatization reaction.

Amino groups. Because primary aliphatic groups can be easily conjugated there are more methods available for assaying compounds containing these groups than for any others. Apart from the reactions listed under amino acids and proteins, many of which are equally applicable to assaying any compound containing a primary aliphatic amino group, methods that are of particular interest are:

1. Hansch reaction

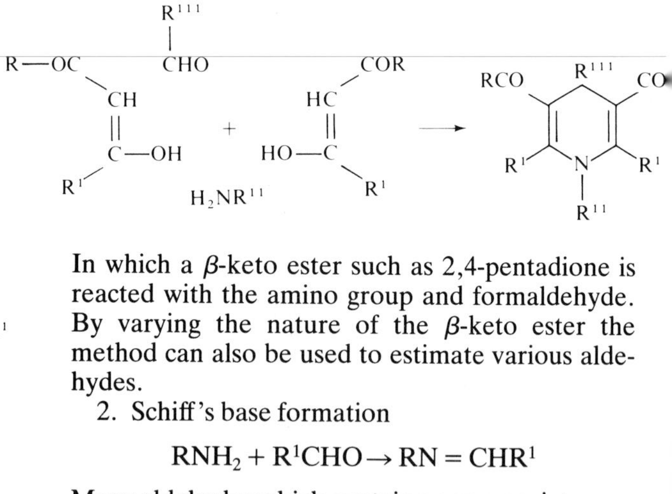

In which a β-keto ester such as 2,4-pentadione is reacted with the amino group and formaldehyde. By varying the nature of the β-keto ester the method can also be used to estimate various aldehydes.

2. Schiff's base formation

$$RNH_2 + R^1CHO \rightarrow RN = CHR^1$$

Many aldehydes which contain an appropriate conjugated system of double bonds may be used; pyrene aldehyde appears to be particularly suitable for primary aliphatic amines. Using this method of tagging with DNS or FIC normally requires a post reaction clean-up procedure. Thin-layer chromatography followed by direct fluorimetric assay on the TLC plate is now finding increasing favour (*see* p. 160). HPLC linked to a fluorescence detector is being increasingly employed to measure this type of derivative. Using fluorescent amines, aldehydes may also be assayed using the above approach.

3. Ion pair formation. The use of ion pair formation to enable charged compounds to be extracted into organic solvents is a widely used technique. By using as the counter ion to the compound a fluorescent species it is possible to determine the concentration of a non-fluorescent compound by measuring the amount of the fluorescent species extracted.

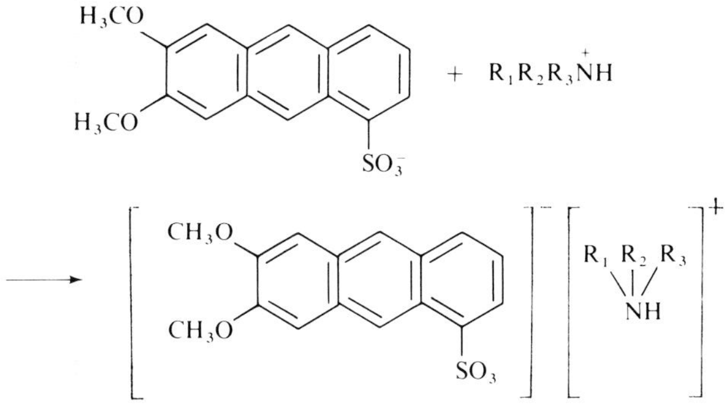

The fluorescent species will not extract into an organic solvent unless the amino counter ion is available. By careful choice of extraction solvent considerable selectivity can be achieved. The selectivity can be improved considerably by combining the formation of fluorescent ion pair derivatives with HPLC separation.

Nitro groups. Nitro groups can be reduced to primary amines using a mild reducing agent such as $LiAlH_4$ which may then be estimated by one of the above methods.

Aldehyde groups. The aldehyde group may quench aromatic and heterocyclic fluorescence. Many aldehydes can be made to fluoresce by adding acidic methanol to form the methyl acetal. For other aldehydes, because of their high chemical reactivity, condensations with a fluorescent amine or hydrazine to form a Schiff's base or with ammonia and a β-keto ester (Hansch reaction—*see above*) may be appropriate. Reaction with 3,5-diamino benzoic acid has also been used rather widely.

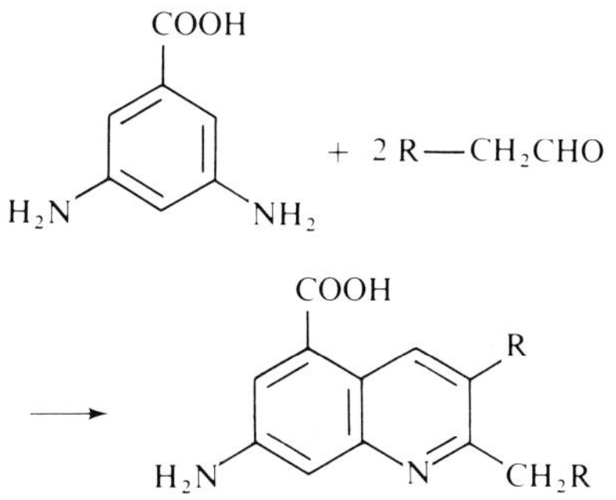

Hydroxy groups. Many phenols show native fluorescence. Primary aliphatic hydroxyl groups may be oxidized to the aldehyde and then estimated by one of the above methods. Alternatively alcohols may be tagged with a fluorescent molecule such as dansyl chloride (DNS) or 4(dichloro-s-triazinyl)-1-ethoxynaphthalene.

Carboxyl groups. Formation of an ester or amide by condensation with a fluorescent phenol or amine and subsequent removal of the unreacted fluorescent reagent is a common approach.

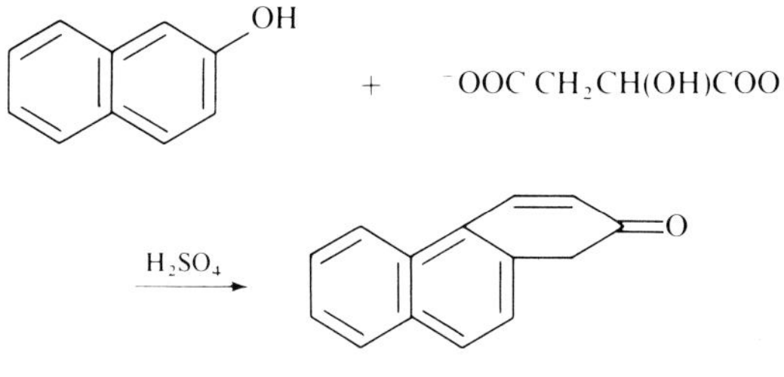

Alternatively by mild reduction the carboxylic acid may be reduced to an aldehyde or to an alcohol and one of the above reactions carried out.

Ion-pair formation using a fluorescent amine counter ion such as dimethylprotriptyline followed by solvent extraction or HPLC chromatography is also suitable. Compounds containing a β-keto acid group can be assayed following their condensation with o-phenylenediamine.

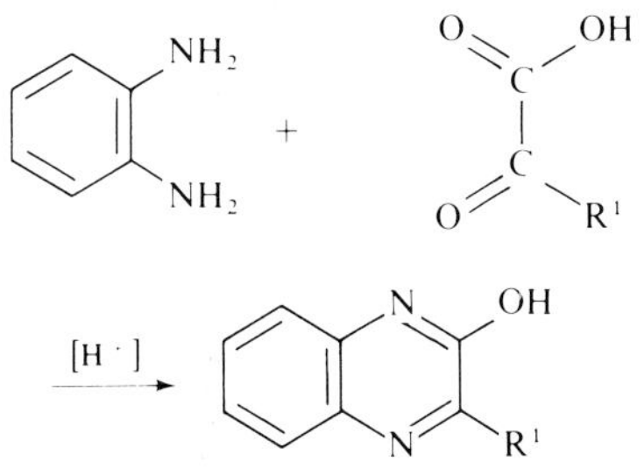

The same reagent can be used to estimate a number of carbohydrates.

The classical book 'Feigl's Spot Tests' describes many qualitative tests for functional groups which involve detection of fluorescent spots on paper chromatograms. Many of these reactions might provide a suitable basis for quantitative analysis. For further details the reader is referred to Bartos and Pesez.[12]

Inorganic substances. On chelation of various metals with 8-hydroxyquinoline fluorescent species are formed. Specificity is produced by controlling the pH of the reaction. This is the basis for the fluorimetric assay of magnesium.

More specific chelating agents are available, e.g. for Ca^{2+} (calcein) and zinc (dibenzothiazoylmethane).

Cyanide may be estimated by its ability to condense with p-benzoquinone derivatives. For further details the reader is referred to Udenfriend[8] and White and Argauer.[4]

Quenchofluorimetric Assay. Non-fluorescent or very weakly fluorescent compounds may often be estimated by their ability to quench the fluorescence of highly fluorescent compounds. Applications of this technique in clinical biochemistry are rather limited and several of the available assays lack specificity. This approach has been successful for assaying various inorganic materials. For example, fluoride has been measured by its quenching effect on magnesium-8-hydroxyquinoline. Macromolecules may also be determined by their ability to quench the fluorescence of a dye. For example, the fluorescent dye tetrabromofluorescein (eosin) is quenched on binding to a number of proteins. This allows many proteins to be assayed in nanogram amounts.

Enzyme Assays

Three types of enzyme reaction have achieved widespread measurement by fluorimetry:

1. enzymes involving NADH, NADPH or FADH as cofactors,
2. hydrolytic enzymes involving synthetic substrates which, on hydrolysis, yield fluorescent products, and
3. oxidation or reduction of synthetic substrates to fluorescent products or to reactive materials which can be made to yield fluorescent derivatives.

Assays Dependent on the Formation of Fluorescent Reduced Cofactors. The fact that the reduced nicotinamide adenine dinucleotides are strongly fluorescent whereas the oxidized cofactors are not has been utilized as the basis for the assay of many dehydrogenases. Very high sensitivities can be achieved, particularly if recycling methods are employed (detection limit of 10^{-9} M). Lowry has introduced microtechniques which permit the detection limit to be reduced to 10^{-14}–10^{-15} mole of these cofactors. The basic principles of assaying the reduced cofactors fluorimetrically are similar to those involved in the spectrophotometric measurement. Enzymes which have been successfully estimated directly by determining the fluorescence of the reduced cofactors include lactate dehydrogenase, glucose 6-phosphate dehydrogenase, glutamate dehydrogenase and 6-phosphogluconate dehydrogenase. In addition using coupled systems many transaminases have been assayed, e.g.

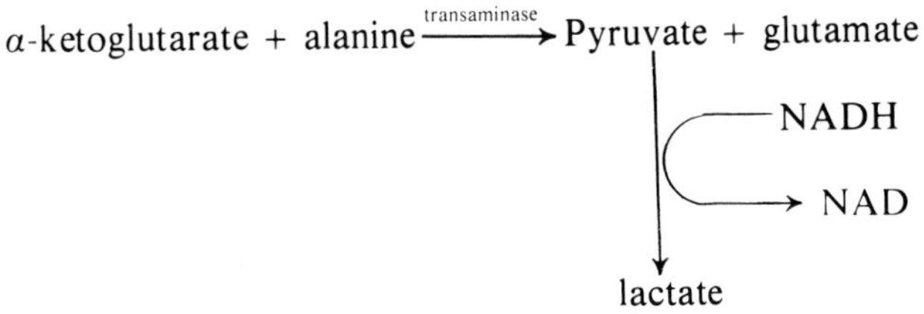

$$\alpha\text{-ketoglutarate} + \text{alanine} \xrightarrow{\text{transaminase}} \text{Pyruvate} + \text{glutamate}$$

NADH

NAD

lactate

(For further references *see* Guilbault.[3])

Hydrolytic Enzymes

Enzymes cleaving esters and ethers. Many phenols are most strongly fluorescent in the ionized form. If the phenolic group is conjugated then ionization is suppressed until the conjugating group is removed, i.e.

$$\text{ROX} \xrightarrow{\text{hydrolysis}} \text{RO}^- + \text{X}^+$$

Most hydrolytic enzymes are highly discriminating in the conjugated group (X) that they will cleave but are able to accept a wide variety of hydroxyl compounds (RO⁻) for the other part of the molecule. Thus it is possible to synthesize artificial substrates which on hydrolysis by these enzymes produce very highly fluorescent products. Umbelliferone, fluorescein, resorufin, 3-hydroxyindole and α- or β-naphthol have been used to provide hydrolytic enzyme substrates. Apart from a high fluorescence sensitivity for the ionized molecule the major dictates for an ideal phenol are:

1. it should ionize at physiological pH to enable assays to be carried out *in situ*;

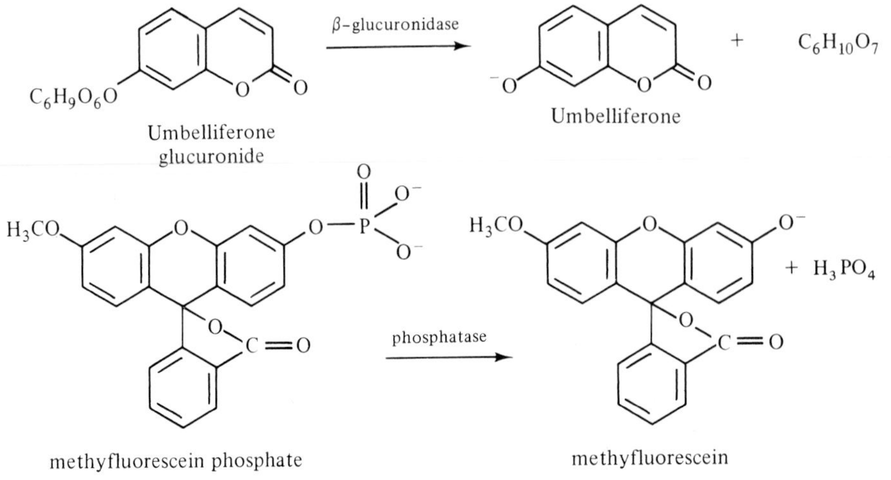

Umbelliferone glucuronide

$C_6H_9O_6O$

β-glucuronidase

Umbelliferone

$+ \quad C_6H_{10}O_7$

methylfluorescein phosphate

phosphatase

methylfluorescein

$+ \ H_3PO_4$

2. its absorption and fluorescence wavelengths should be well separated and should not overlap with those of endogenous compounds likely to be present in biological fluids;

3. it should not be vulnerable to breakdown (chemical or enzymic) or precipitation (i.e. it should be fairly water soluble) in biological fluids, nor should it damage the enzyme system;

4. it should be readily linked to the appropriate conjugate group. Examples of substrates for β-glucuronidase and phosphatase are shown below:

Other enzymes which have been assayed using this approach include β-galactosidase, N-acetylglucosaminidase, β-glucosidase, hyaluronidase, sulphatase, lipase, cholinesterase. The technique is potentially amenable to the assay of any hydrolytic enzyme.

Enzymes cleaving amides. Aromatic amines are often strongly fluorescent whereas the corresponding amides are normally poorly or non-fluorescent.

Using β-naphthylamine condensed with phenylalanine, benzoylarginine, peptidases and proteases have been assayed. It should be pointed out that β-naphthylamine is not ideal for this purpose either in its fluorescence characteristics or in its handling properties (i.e. it is a bladder carcinogen). Other amines, e.g. aminoquinolines or aminoacridines, may be more suitable. For further examples of hydrolytic enzyme assays the reader is referred to the excellent monograph by Leabach.[13]

Other Enzyme Assays. An alternative way of assessing dehydrogenases is to add to the reaction mixture a hydrogen acceptor which becomes fluorescent upon reduction.

resazurin
(non-fluorescent)

resorufin
(λ_{ex} 560 nm; λ_{fl} 580 nm)

Resazurin is particularly useful for this purpose because the fluorescence of its product resorufin is well removed from that of most other biological compounds.

If the enzyme product has a different reactivity from its substrate, the products can often be reacted to form a fluorescent derivative. For example, a very

sensitive assay for amidases could be devised as follows:

$$RNHCOR_I \xrightarrow{\text{amidase}} RNH_2 + R_1COOH$$
$$\downarrow$$

derivatize using fluorescamine
(*see* p. 165)

A particularly interesting assay because it makes use of the differential quenching effects of phosphate buffer on the substrate and the product is that for xanthine oxidase. The substrate 2-amino-4-hydroxypteridine, although fluorescent, is quenched by phosphate whereas the fluorescence of the product isoxanthopterin is not. This type of approach could make an important contribution to other enzyme assays based on fluorimetry (*see* also p. 168).

Guilbault[3] (and subsequent papers) has devised a number of assays for enzyme substrates and enzymes in which the reaction and fluorimetric measurement is carried out on a microscale at the surface of a silicon rubber pad. This approach is well suited to routine application because the pads can be impregnated with the appropriate reagents on a large scale and stored until required, thus the number of manipulations required during an actual assay is minimized. The assay is often rapid because the reagents, although small in amount, are concentrated at the surface of the pad. Many more assays of this type could be developed fairly readily.

Other Applications of Luminescence

To study small molecule/macromolecule interactions. On binding of proteins and other macromolecules a fluorescent small molecule may change its fluorescence characteristics in three ways:

1. it may show enhanced emission of polarized fluorescence (*see* p. 148);

2. it may display an increase or decrease in fluorescence intensity and/or an alteration in its fluorescence wavelength (i.e. act as a fluorescent probe (*see* p. 170);

3. it may pass on its energy to a constituent of the protein which may then emit fluorescence. (Alternatively it may receive energy from the protein.)

Immunoassay. Fluorescence polarization and fluorescence probing are attracting interest as the basis for developing homogenous immunoassays. The antigen is normally labelled with a fluorescent compound (by analogy with radioisotope labelling) such as fluorescamine, dansyl chloride or a fluorescein isothiocyanate (*see* p. 167). This approach is only really suitable for assaying relatively low-molecular-weight compounds (<5000) at concentrations above nanogram levels. However, despite these restrictions the technique is valuable because it is homogenous and readily automated. To obtain optimum results in polarization studies the fluorescent label should be linked to the antigen in such a manner that when the antigen binds to the antibody the fluorescent label is unable to rotate.

The use of fluorescence probes for immunoassay is potentially highly versatile although its practical value has yet to be properly evaluated.

Immunofluorescence. Using fluorescent tagged compounds the distribution of biologically important molecules can be monitored. A widely used technique is to label antibodies to these molecules, thereby enabling their location within tissues to be visualized. This technique of immunofluorescence is normally only studied qualitatively using a fluorescence microscope. It has been very widely applied to the detection of changes in cell surface proteins, location of viruses and bacteria and other cellular antigens. For further information on the methods of antibody labelling and their application the reader is referred to Nairn.[14]

Cell Studies. The increasing availability of microspectrofluorimeters has led to a heightening interest in employing fluorescence to assay cellular enzyme activity and other cellular constituents. β-Glucuronidase, alkaline phosphatase, benzpyrene hydroxylase, ethoxyresorufin deethylase, biogenic amines, DNA and protein have all been estimated fluorimetrically in single cells.

Fluorescence Probes. The fact that the fluorescence of many molecules is dependent on their environment can be exploited to garner information on the binding sites of small molecules to macromolecules. ANS (*see* p. 167) has been widely employed to characterize the hydrophobic binding sites of many proteins[15]. Probes designed to produce more specific interactions are continually being developed. For example, probes are available to assess binding to ATPase and cholinergic receptors, to measure membrane potentials, microviscosity and fluidity and to determine oxygen and solvent accessibility and ΔpH changes across membranes (for further details *see* Azzi[16]).

One interesting practical use of fluorescence probing is as a means of checking possible drug interactions. For example the blood levels of the anticoagulant drug warfarin must be maintained between narrow limits to achieve effective anticoagulant control without undue risk of haemorrhage. Warfarin is very highly bound to serum albumin, therefore only very small amounts of free drug are available to produce the anticoagulant effect. Other drugs may displace the warfarin from albumin thereby causing a sudden increase in free warfarin levels with a concomitant enhanced risk of haemorrhage. It is clearly not possible to check all the possible drugs which might interact with warfarin by *in vivo* methods. Rather a quick *in vitro* system is required. Warfarin fortunately has all the necessary requisites to act as a fluorescence probe in its own right. It undergoes a hypsochromic shift and a spectral intensification on binding to human serum albumin. The warfarin displacing ability of a drug can thus be checked by assessing its ability to reduce the intensity and lengthen the wavelength of warfarin fluorescence.[17]

Tetracycline can be used as a probe to detect calcium-rich centres in the body because tetracycline develops significant fluorescence only when it chelates with calcium. Location of tetracycline binding *in vivo* has been used to diagnose various gastric malignancies. This is normally carried out by feeding tetracycline for several days then lavaging the gastric contents and examining them for the golden fluorescence characteristic of malignant calcium-rich cellular materials.

Acridine has been employed as a nuclear probe. Healthy lung and gastric cells take up only very small amounts of this dye whereas tumour cells may concentrate it, and show a strong acridine fluorescence.

By painting temperature-sensitive phosphors (based on zinc-cadmium sulphide combinations) on the skin, temperature hot spots characteristic of various disease conditions can be visualized.

The potential of fluorescence probing devices is very considerable and many further ingenious applications can be expected in the near future.

REFERENCES

1. Lakowicz J. R. (1983). *Principles of Fluorescence Spectroscopy*. New York: Plenum Press.
2. Parker C. A. (1968). *Photoluminescence of Solutions*. London: Elsevier.
3. Guilbault G. G. (1973). *Practical Fluorescence Theory Methods and Techniques*. New York: Marcel Dekker.
4. White C. E., Argauer R. J. (1970). *Fluorescence Analysis—A Practical Approach*. New York: Marcel Dekker.
5. Bridges J. W. (1974). In *The Poisoned Patient—the Role of the Laboratory*. CIBA Foundation Symposium 26. London: Elsevier.
6. Vo Dinh T. (1984). *Room Temperature Phosphorimetry for Chemical Analysis*. New York: Wiley Interscience.
7. Schulman S. G. (1985). *Molecular Luminescence Spectroscopy: Methods and Applications, Part 1*. New York: Wiley Interscience.

8. Udenfriend S. S. (1963 and 1969). *Fluorescence Assay in Biology and Medicine*, Vol. 1 and Vol. 2. New York, London: Academic Press.
9. Miller J. N. (1974). In *Progress in Biophysics and Molecular Biology*, Vol. 28 (Butler A. J. V., Noble, D. eds) Oxford and New York: Pergamon Press.
10. De Ment J. (1945). *Fluorochemistry*. New York: Chemical Publishing Co.
11. Bridges J. W. (1969). In *CRC Handbook of Clinical Toxicology* (Sunshine I., ed.) Cleveland, Ohio: CRC Press.
12. Bartos J., Pesez M. (1972). *Talanta*; **19**: 93.
13. Leabach D. H. (1976). *An Introduction to the Fluorimetric Estimation of Enzyme Activities*. Koch–Light Laboratories Ltd.
14. Nairn R. C. (1962). *Fluorescent Protein Tracing*. London: Livingstone.
15. Serentz M., Thaer A. (1972). *Analyt. Biochem*; **50**: 98.
16. Azzi A. (1975). *Quart. Rev. Biophys*; **8**: 238.
17. Bridges J. W. (1977). In *Drug Interactions* (Graham-Smith, D. G., ed.) pp. 101–108. London: Macmillan.

12. NMR—*In Vivo* and *In Vitro*

Daphne F. Jackson, J. B. Green and David G. Taylor

Introduction
Basic theory
  NMR imaging
Imaging
  The measurement of NMR parameters
  Contrast agents
  Applications of NMR imaging
NMR Spectroscopy
  ^{31}P NMR spectroscopy
  ^{31}P NMR of organs
  Malignancies
  Enzyme kinetics
  NMR spectroscopy using other nuclei
Future prospects

INTRODUCTION

The phenomenon of nuclear magnetic resonance (NMR) provides the possibility of producing high quality images of the whole body or selected regions and of carrying out spectroscopy in selected regions. Studies may be made both *in vitro* and *in vivo*. The ability of the method to reveal both the distribution of certain elements and the influence of the chemical environment implies that a wide range of studies of normal physiology, the biochemistry of normal and diseased states, tissue architecture, and influence and behaviour of moving body constituents may be undertaken.

The technique is non-invasive, is believed to be without hazard to the patient, and will not cause damage to an excised sample. The absence of damage means that repeated measurements can be made on the same sample and the absence of hazard to the patient means that it is possible to monitor, on a regular basis, the progress of disease or response to therapy.

The principal disadvantages of the method are low sensitivity, which limits the range of elements which may be studied, and high cost.

Many atomic nuclei possess a magnetic property arising from the spin of the nucleus. If these nuclei are placed in a constant magnetic field, the nuclei are distributed in a number of different energy states. However, if energy is supplied in the form of a quantum of electromagnetic radiation, whose energy just matches the gap between one energy state and another, this energy can be absorbed by a nucleus which jumps to the higher energy state. The nucleus subsequently returns to the lower state with a corresponding loss in energy. This energy is transferred to the other degrees of freedom within the material, termed the 'lattice'. The most common isotopes of carbon and oxygen, ^{12}C and ^{16}O, both have zero spin and do not exhibit NMR. The isotopes ^{1}H, ^{13}C, ^{19}F and ^{31}P all have spin $1/2$ and give the simplest pattern of only two energy states. The resonant frequency is directly proportional to the strength of the magnetic field. For typical magnetic fields of $0 \cdot 1$–$4 \cdot 0$T, the frequency is in MHz and can be provided by a radiofrequency transmitter coil. At those frequencies, electromagnetic radiation can penetrate 10–100 cm of tissue.

In the conventional NMR spectrum for a constant magnetic field the position of each resonant line associated with a particular nucleus depends on the chemical environment, whose effect is indicated by a *chemical shift*. The chemical shift depends on nuclear species (see Table 1) and on molecular structure; it

TABLE 1
PROPERTIES OF ISOTOPES

Isotope	Rel. sensitivity (const. field)	Frequency at 1T (MHz)	Detection sensitivity in tissue*	Chemical shift (ppm)
^{1}H	1	42·6	1	10
^{19}F	0·83	40·0		10
^{23}Na	0·093	11·3	$\sim 9 \times 10^{-5}$	10
^{31}P	0·066	17·2	$\sim 4 \times 10^{-5}$	40
^{13}C	0·016	10·7		200
^{39}K	0·00005	2·0		

* These values depend strongly on the nature of the tissue and the size of the region considered.

also varies with pH. Topical NMR (TMR) is a high field, high frequency method which gives high resolution spectra from a small localized volume within a larger specimen.

When a small, linear, magnetic-field gradient is applied, the frequency of the radiation absorbed by each nucleus depends on its position, since frequency ∝ field ∝ position. The intensity of absorption depends on the number of nuclei present. Hence, the absorption spectrum is a projection of the nuclear spin density perpendicular to the magnetic-field gradient. A series of projections may be collected by rotating the field gradient. An image of nuclear spin density may then be reconstructed in a manner exactly analogous to x-ray CT. NMR imaging is, however, much more flexible than x-ray CT and reveals more information. NMR images are not restricted to transverse sections. Multiplanar techniques can be used to give faster throughput. The amplitude of the NMR output signal decays, usually exponentially with time, with a time constant T_2 which is known as the *transverse* or *spin–spin relaxation time*. Equilibrium magnetization is restored with a time constant T_1, which is known as the *longitudinal* or *spin–lattice relaxation time*. Both relaxation effects represent an interaction between the nucleus and its surroundings.

By combinations of measurements it is possible to present images which, to an accuracy of a few per cent, display separately the spatial distribution of T_1 and T_2 relaxation times. These quantities are the key to tissue differentiation in NMR imaging. The extent to which it is possible to interpret them in terms of fundamental biophysical conditions is a matter for further research.

The emphasis in NMR imaging to date has been on hydrogen because of its large magnetic moment and high abundance in most tissues of interest which leads to high detection sensitivity compared with other elements (see Table 1). To an accuracy of a few per cent, the NMR response of tissue arises from hydrogen in water. The presence of fat and blood also has an influence on the images.

The possible hazards of NMR imaging include (1) tissue heating by the radiofrequency radiation and (2) production of eddy currents in the tissue due to pulses or rapid switching of field gradients. The magnitudes of these effects can be calculated and safe limits determined.[1] The effect of (3) static magnetic fields, at the levels used in imaging is not thought to be significant.[1] It is not yet known whether there are additional hazards involved in TMR. Hazards to operating staff should not present problems.

The magnets used in NMR imaging may be superconducting or resistive. TMR magnets are superconducting. Superconducting magnets are operated at very low temperatures and must be continuously cooled with liquid nitrogen and liquid helium. These liquid gases, especially helium, represent a major running cost. Water cooling and electricity represent the major running cost of resistive systems. For stabi-

lity, all NMR magnets should be run continuously. If they are switched off at night to save running costs and staff costs, several hours are lost at the beginning of each day during a stabilizing period. A large fraction of the capital cost arises from the electromagnet, since whole body magnets require good field homogeneity and r.f. electronics capable of handling large volume objects. This, in turn, leads to a requirement for powerful computing facilities to handle the very large quantity of data generated.

BASIC THEORY

Nuclei having a non-zero angular momentum possess a magnetic moment. In the presence of a static magnetic field B_0, the vector μ defining the direction and magnitude of the magnetic moment can assume only certain discrete orientations with respect to B_0. The number of such orientations depends on the value of the angular momentum quantum number I, and in the case of a proton, ^1H, is two. These two orientations correspond to two different energy states. The lower energy state is defined as the one in which the measurable component of μ aligns parallel to the field B_0. In thermal equilibrium, the relative population of the two energy states is governed by the Boltzmann Distribution Law. This ensures a greater population in the lower energy state.

A nucleus residing in the low energy state can be excited into the higher one by supplying the nucleus with an energy exactly equal to the energy difference between the two states. The amount of energy required is directly proportional to the field B_0 and is provided by electromagnetic radiation of angular frequency ω_0 given in equation (1).

$$\omega_0 = \gamma B_0 \qquad (1)$$

where γ, the gyromagnetic ratio, characterizes the species of nuclei (e.g. for ^1H $\gamma/2\pi = 42 \cdot 6\,MHz/T$).

When a whole ensemble of nuclei is considered, we may define a net macroscopic vector quantity called the magnetization M. This is simply the vector sum of all the individual magnetic moments within a sample. In the absence of a static field B_0, the magnetic moments are oriented at random. However, when B_0 is applied more of the magnetic moments orient with the field than against it. Therefore, a net magnetization of amplitude M_0 may be assigned along the z-axis co-axial with B_0. Furthermore, since the orientation of the xy component of each magnetic moment is uncorrelated at equilibrium the average xy component of the resultant magnetization M (M_{xy}) is zero (Fig. 1).

If M is perturbed away from the z-axis it precesses around B_0, with angular frequency ω_0 as seen in a laboratory frame of reference. This rotating magnetization induces an electromotive force (e.m.f.) in a conductive coil, if the axis of the coil is in the xy plane. The e.m.f. is characterized by frequency ω_0, phase ϕ with respect to some arbitrary reference

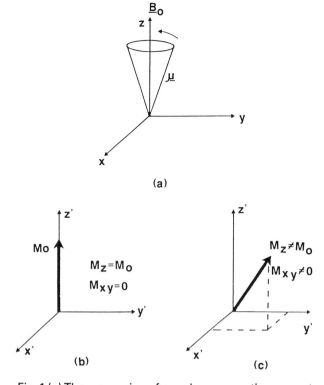

(a)

(b)

(c)

Fig. 1 (a) The precession of a nuclear magnetic moment μ in the laboratory frame of reference when subjected to a static magnetic field B_0. (b) A vector sum of all the nuclear moments produces a net magnetization M which under conditions of equilibrium has a magnitude M_0 along the direction of the field. (c) A perturbation of the magnetization M by the application of an r.f. pulse in general gives rise to components in all three directions x', y', z'.

behaviour, fluid flow velocities etc., are deduced by comparison of the precessing magnetization under a number of different conditions.

To perturb M away from the z-axis a magnetic field B_1 is applied which rotates in the xy plane at the same frequency as ω_0. To see the effect of this field we have to use a frame of reference (x', y', z') which itself rotates around B_0. In the rotating frame of reference the only effective field is B_1. Again M moves under the action of a torque, but this time in a direction perpendicular to the plane containing M and B_1. The magnetization M therefore tilts away from the z' axis towards the y' axis. The angle θ by which M tilts away from z' under the action of a field B_1 of duration t is

$$\theta = \gamma^{B_1} t \qquad (2)$$

A short application of a B_1 field (a radiofrequency pulse) which tilts M exactly by 90° or 180° is referred to as a 90° or a 180° pulse, respectively. Thus a 90° pulse applied along x' rotates M onto the y' axis (Fig. 2).

NMR Imaging

NMR offers numerous ways in which a sample may be imaged, but of these only one is in common use as far as general clinical applications are concerned. This is the 2-dimensional Fourier transform (2DFT) technique which is often referred to as Spin-Warp. Virtually no hardware changes are required in going from one technique to another and a recent article by Taylor and Inamdar[2] has reviewed the required instrumentation. A brief outline of the 2DFT technique, as applied to the planar case, is given in this

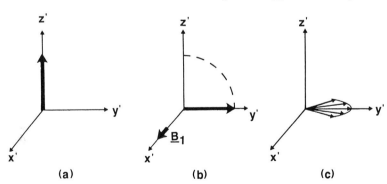

(a)

(b)

(c)

Fig. 2 A schematic diagram showing spin–spin relaxation in the rotating frame of reference. (a) M under conditions of equilibrium. (b) An application of a 90° pulse along x' nutates M on to the y' axis. (c) The spins begin to lose phase coherence as they precess at angular frequencies slightly different from that of the rotating frame.

and an amplitude whose value reflects the component of M in the xy plane. This is the NMR signal. It is important to emphasize that in the NMR technique the physical quantity measured is an e.m.f. induced by a precessing nuclear magnetization. All other quantities such as hydrogen density, relaxation

section to show how different parameters may be mapped, and to provide an awareness of several fundamental factors that affect the quality of NMR images.

Intrinsically NMR imaging is a 3-dimensional technique and though 3D images may be obtained, in most cases imaging is restricted to the planar or multiplanar case, i.e. to thin slices within the patient. To see briefly how this is achieved consider an extended cylindrical sample within which we wish to excite a thin cross-sectional region transverse to the z-axis as shown in Fig. 3.

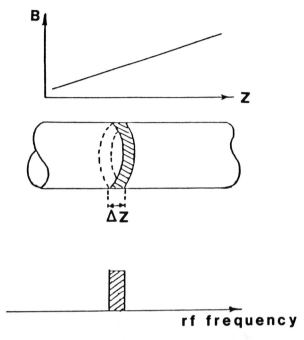

Fig. 3 Selective excitation of the sample in the presence of a field gradient in the z direction. A thin slab of spins Δz is excited by means of a tailored r.f. pulse which has a finite, well-defined frequency bandwidth Δω.

If a linear magnetic field gradient is applied along the z-axis it is clear that the frequency at which the nuclei will absorb energy becomes a function of position along z. Irradiation with an r.f. pulse containing a very narrow rectangular envelope of frequencies (Δω) will then excite only the desired cross-section Δz.

A consideration of the Fourier transform process shows that in order to produce a rectangular envelope of frequencies we need to modulate the r.f. signal with a specially shaped envelope in the time domain. Application of this shaped r.f. pulse in the presence of a gradient results in rapid phase incoherence which for 90° pulses may be recovered by a momentary reversal of the gradient.

The Projection Reconstruction (PR) Method. The earliest technique by which NMR images were acquired relied on reconstruction from a given set of projections of the sample. A typical pulse and gradient timing diagram is shown in Fig. 4.

Here the r.f. pulse is shown to be a modulated, selective, 90° pulse applied in the presence of a gradient along the z direction G_z. The reversal of G_z is intended to achieve the recovery of the phase coher-

ence of the nuclear spins. At the end of this portion of the sequence we have isolated a thin slab of spins transverse to the z-axis. The net magnetization within the slice is rotated through 90° and lies in the xy plane. Its precession induces an e.m.f. into a suitably designed r.f. coil wrapped around the

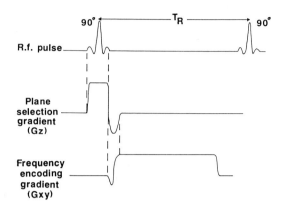

Fig. 4 A saturation recovery sequence in the projection reconstruction technique. The sequence consists of a repeated application of selective 90° pulses at intervals of T_R. The signal is acquired under the influence of gradient G_{xy}.

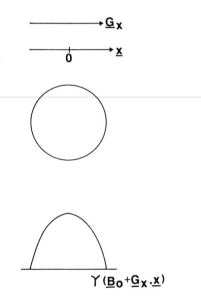

Fig. 5 The application of a gradient G_x produces a projection of the sample onto an axis parallel to the direction of the gradient.

sample. The resulting free induction decay (f.i.d.) is acquired in the presence of gradients G_x and G_y (G_{xy}) in order to encode spatial information within the xy plane. To see this clearly consider the gradient in the x direction alone. From Fig. 5 it can be seen that each vertical element in the slice will have its field modified to $(B_0 + G_x . x)$. Therefore, elements at different points along x will have different precessional frequencies.

The resulting f.i.d. is a sum of all these frequencies and a simple one-dimensional Fourier transform of this composite time signal yields a broadened frequency spectrum. The frequency is directly proportional to distance along x. The amplitude at a given frequency is directly proportional to the magnetization present in an element corresponding to that frequency. This is, in effect, a projection of the magnetization of the sample onto the x axis. Projections along different directions are obtained by altering the magnitude and direction of current flow within the x and y gradient coils. The set of projections obtained by this method may be reconstructed using standard analytical or iterative reconstruction techniques as used in x-ray CT scanning.

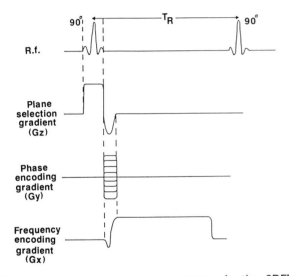

Fig. 6 A saturation recovery sequence in the 2DFT imaging technique. Following each application of a selective 90° pulse only the amplitude of the phase encoding gradient (G_y) changes.

The Two-Dimensional Fourier Transformation (2DFT) Method. The general form of the 2DFT method was first proposed by Kumar *et al*. However, it is the variation on this theme as developed by Edelstein *et al*.[3] that is in common use now. The latter is depicted in Fig. 6 which shows a typical pulse and gradient timing sequence. The slice selection procedure is exactly the same as for the projection reconstruction method. The acquisition period is also very similar since the f.i.d. is acquired in the presence of a gradient G_x. However, here this particular gradient changes neither in magnitude nor in direction, i.e. the projection is always onto the same axis. To see how spatial encoding is achieved in the y direction we have to look at the effect of the gradient G_y prior to the acquisition period.

During the time G_y is on, each spin-voxel along the y direction precesses with a frequency $\omega(y) = \gamma(B_0 + G_y \cdot y)$. When G_y is switched off, all spin-voxels along the y direction precess again at the same value ω_0 (ignoring G_x at present), but each voxel now has

a specific phase relationship with respect to other voxels along y. This is true for a single column parallel to the y direction even in the presence of G_x. The phase that each voxel accumulates during the time G_y is on, t_y, is

$$\theta(y) = w(t) \cdot t_y \tag{3}$$

assuming a rectangular G_y gradient pulse.

Following the G_y gradient pulse the phase of the precessing magnetization varies linearly along the y-axis. A spatial frequency has been imposed in the y-direction. This process is repeated for a number of different y gradient pulse amplitudes corresponding to a set of spatial frequencies.

In the presence of a static gradient in the x direction G_x, each column of spin parallel to the y-axis is uniquely characterized by a frequency of precession. The complete imaging sequence consists of collecting N data points for each of N amplitudes of G_y. This $N \times N$ data set is then Fourier transformed in two dimensions to yield the final image.

The 2DFT technique has advantages over the projection reconstruction method. The distortions caused by magnet inhomogeneity are minimized in the 2DFT method, since all the projections are acquired onto this same axis. Inhomogeneity merely produces a geometric distortion along this direction. In projection reconstruction, on the other hand, as the projection direction changes so does the direction of distortion resulting in an angular smearing of the data. Further, there is greater flexibility in choice of matrix size as 2DFT allows the use of rectangular matrices. These may optimize resolution in a given direction and are particularly useful for body images where overall sample shape is ellipsoidal rather than circular.

IMAGING

The Measurement of NMR Parameters

Density The steady-state, equilibrium value of the magnetization present in a sample in a field B_0 is given by equation (4).

$$M_0 = \frac{\rho \gamma^2 h^2 (I + 1) B_0}{3k T_s} \tag{4}$$

where ρ is the concentration of spins within the sample and T_s is the temperature. If both B_0 and T_s are held constant we see that the measured steady state value of M is solely proportional to spin-concentration or proton density specifically. In order to image the proton density in the human body all we need to do, in principle, is to acquire the f.i.d.'s using a 90° pulse as shown in Fig. 6. A sufficient time must elapse between each f.i.d. to allow M to achieve equilibrium. This time is dependent on sample T_1 and in general the repetition time T_R between each f.i.d. should be greater than $5T_1$. The imaging technique discriminates against nuclei with a $T_2 \lesssim$ ms. In consequence the signal observed in the imaging sequence is that due to the more mobile nuclei, i.e. those whose $T>_2 \gtrsim 1$ ms. Thus in biological tissue only the protons in water and lipid molecules are, in general, observed.

In biological systems the concentration of water varies between different tissues and a repeated 90° sequence as mentioned above may be used to obtain anatomical images of the human body that resemble x-ray CT scans. For instance, there is a 10% difference in the water content between kidney and the liver. There is a similar water concentration difference between grey and white matter in the brain. However, this difference is largely compensated for by the lipid contribution in the white matter.

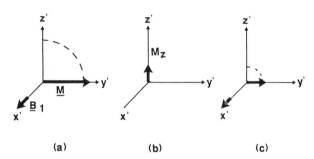

(a) **(b)** **(c)**

Fig. 7 A schematic diagram showing the motion of M in the saturation recovery sequence. (a) M is directed along the y' axis following a 90° pulse. (b) At a time T_R a finite component of M_z has developed along the z' axis. (c) By the application of a second 90° pulse, M_z is nutated onto the y' axis and its amplitude measured.

Spin–Lattice Relaxation Time (T_1) It has been shown that differences in T_1 may be up to ten times those present in proton-density, e.g. the T_1 difference between the kidney and liver is as much as 100%. In order to weight the detected signal with T_1, we have to probe the dynamic behaviour of the magnetization as opposed to the equilibrium magnitude as for proton density. Since T_1 governs the rate at which M_z approaches M_0 we need to measure the z component of the magnetization in the interval $t = 0$–$5T_1$. This may be done by using two 90° pulses with a varying interval between them. Since we measure the component of magnetization in the xy plane, the magnetization that has recovered along the z axis, has to be rotated into the xy plane prior to measurement. This is the function of the second 90° pulse. At the end of the first pulse M is along say the y' axis (Fig. 7). If we assume total dephasing in the xy plane after a time $T_R \gtrsim 5T_2$, we have no detectable signal. At time T_R, the partially recovered component M_z is flipped over onto the y' axis by the second 90° pulse. This generates the signal acquired under the influence of the imaging gradients. If T_R is varied the complete recovery with time of M_z towards M_0 may be plotted. The sequence is generally extended to $90° - T_R - 90° - T_R \dots$ and is usually referred to as Saturation Recovery (SR). The recovery curve

is fitted to the expression in equation (5) to yield a spin–lattice relaxation time constant T_1.

$$M_z = M_0\left(1 - \exp\left(-\frac{T_R}{T_1}\right)\right) \qquad (5)$$

If two tissue types with equal proton densities but different T_1 are present their respective recovery in M_z will be as depicted in Fig. 8.

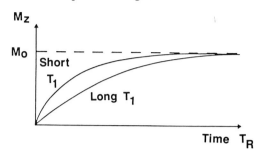

Fig. 8 Diagram showing the growth of the z component of the magnetization with time T_R for two tissues with different spin–lattice relaxation times.

From this we see that provided we choose T_R sensibly we can maximize the difference between the magnetizations within these two tissues, thus maximizing the contrast. Note that the tissue with the short T_1 will appear more intense on SR images as its magnetization is greater than those with a long T_1.

A second pulse sequence that may be used to weight an image with T_1 is the Inversion Recovery (IR) sequence. Figure 9 shows the pulse and gradient timing diagram using the 2DFT method. The first

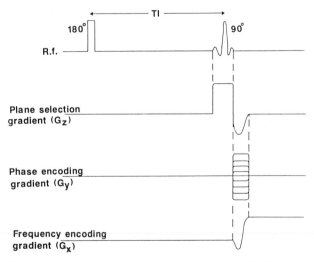

Fig. 9 An inversion recovery sequency in the 2DFT technique. Each selective 90° pulse is preceded by an inverting 180° pulse.

pulse is a 180° non-selective pulse. After its application M_0 has been completely inverted, i.e. its instantaneous value is $M_z = -M_0$. The pulse sequence may be written as $(180 - TI - 90 - T_R)_n$ where TI, the inversion time, is the interval between the 180° and the 90° pulse. For $TI \gtrsim 5T_2$, and $T_R \gtrsim 5T_1$, the recovery is given by equation (6).

$$M_z = M_0\left(1-2\exp\left(-\frac{TI}{T_1}\right)\right) \qquad (6)$$

In practical use, it is unacceptable to wait $5T_1$ as this would result in imaging times of the order of 15–30 min. For $T_R < 5T_1$ the equation above has to be modified to

$$M_z = M_0\left(1-2\exp\left(-\frac{TI}{T_1}\right)+\exp\left(-\frac{T_R}{T_1}\right)\right) \qquad (7)$$

Figure 10 shows the growth of M_z with TI using the IR sequence. By rearranging equation (6) and equating M_z to zero, we see that for $TI < 0{\cdot}69T_1$ M_z is

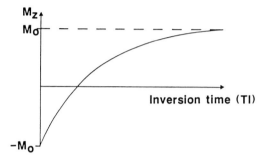

Fig. 10 Diagram showing the growth of the M_z component with time TI in the inversion recovery sequence.

negative. Typical values for TI and T_R generally used in practice are 400 ms and 1 s respectively. Certain tissue types in the human body have a relatively long T_1 (e.g. blood, kidney medulla and tumours). These tissues will display negative signals when TI is short. On the other hand fat, which has a relatively short T_1, appears intense. In general, therefore, the IR sequence produces images that display large contrast differentiation when the sign information regarding M_z is preserved. The T_1 values on a tissue cross-section may be evaluated by running the imaging sequence with different TI values. Recovery curves may then be plotted pixel by pixel to produce T_1 maps, but the use of T_1 weighted density images is more common.

Spin–Spin Relaxation Time (T_2). We have seen that T_2 relaxation is sensitive to slower molecular motion. The density image weighted with T_2 produces images which are quite different from T_1 weighted images (Fig. 11). T_2 values in biological tissues are approximately 10 times shorter than T_1. Where a pathology is accompanied by fluid retention the T_2 contrast differentiation is generally large.

Since T_2 characterizes the irreversible fall of M_{xy} to zero, in order to weight the detected signal with spin–spin relaxation, we have to chart the free induction decay. However, as pointed out earlier, other

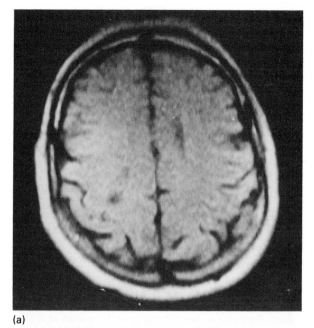

(a)

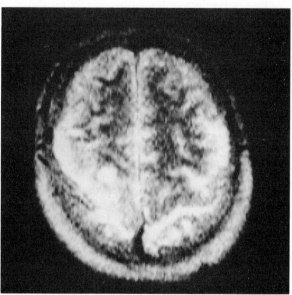

(b)

Fig. 11 ^{1}H NMR images of the head (a) weighted with T_1 and (b) weighted with T_2.

external factors also affect the f.i.d. and pure T_2 effects can be studied only by the use of the spin-echo (SE) sequence. The pulse-train may be written as $(90°-T_{E/2}-180°-T_R)_n$. A typical pulse and gradient timing diagram is shown in Fig. 12.

An echo signal is formed at T_E. To see why, consider the point in the spin-echo sequence where having applied the 90° pulse the spins have already dephased by a certain amount (Fig. 13). If, at time $T_{E/2}$, a 180° pulse is applied along x', the y' component of each spin vector rotates by 180°.

However, since the x' component remains the same, the continuing motion of the spins is such as

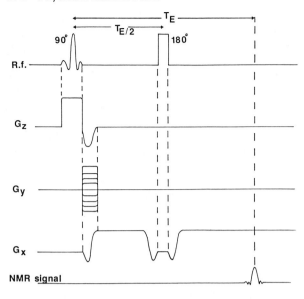

Fig. 12 A spin-echo pulse sequence in the 2DFT technique. Each selective 90° pulse is followed at a time $T_{E/2}$ by a non-selective 180° pulse.

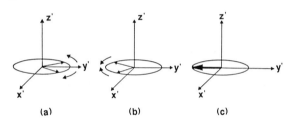

Fig. 13 A schematic diagram showing the formation of an echo signal in the spin-echo sequence. (a) Following a 90° pulse the spins develop a phase incoherence at time $T_{E/2}$. (b) Immediately following the 180° pulse along the x' axis the y' component of each spin is nutated through 180°. (c) At time T_E the spins reform along the y' axis.

to result in a coalescence at time T_E. The variation of the echo amplitude with T_E is given by:

$$M = M_0\left(1 - \exp\left(-\frac{T_R}{T_1}\right)\right)\exp\left(-\frac{T_E}{T_2}\right) \qquad (8)$$

Most commercial machines acquire all signals in spin-echo form and so the equation for the saturation recovery sequence (equation (5)) modified to the one given above for the spin-echo sequence.

An efficient variation on the spin-echo sequence is the Carr Purcell sequence with a Meiboom Gill modification (CPMG). This is essentially a $90°-T_{E/2}-180°$ pulse sequence followed by a train of 180° pulses every T_E seconds later. The r.f. phase of the 180° pulses is 90° relative to the initial 90° pulse. A train of spin echoes is produced at time T_E, $2T_E$, $3T_E$. An image may be generated for each of these echoes or alternatively T_2 may be evaluated for each pixel and plotted as a T_2 map. Further, the method is tolerant of imperfect 180° pulses.

Contrast Agents

One of the limitations of NMR imaging is difficulty in distinguishing between histologically dissimilar but magnetically similar tissues. This can be resolved by increasing signal intensity, either by altering the hydrogen concentration of the tissue or by shortening spin–lattice relaxation times. A decrease in signal intensity from the kidneys following dehydration in human subjects has been demonstrated. However, the apparent change in intensity was small, with a relatively marked alteration in hydration. Emphasis is being placed on research into the use of paramagnetic contrast agents to enhance the small differences in signal observed between isointense tissues.[4]

Paramagnetism. By definition, a paramagnetic substance is one that contains one or more unpaired electrons. These substances possess permanent magnetic moments that are approximately 700 times greater than those of protons and neutrons, and that, in the absence of an applied magnetic field, are randomly orientated. Alignment with an extremely applied field results in the production of a local magnetic field. This causes proton relaxation enhancement (PRE) by shortening the relaxation times of neighbouring nuclei. The resulting decrease in T_1 increases image intensity, while a reduction in T_2 decreases image intensity. Experimental conditions (e.g. pulse sequence and dose of contrast agent given) must be selected to ensure optimization of these changes.

Paramagnetic Substances. Paramagnetic substances potentially useful as contrast agents are shown in Table 2. Limited solubility in biological tissues and toxicity in relatively low doses, make nitric oxide and nitrogen dioxide unsuitable for use.

TABLE 2
PARAMAGNETIC SUBSTANCES POTENTIALLY USEFUL AS CONTRAST AGENTS (FROM BRASCH[5])

Substance	Chemical character
Nitric oxide (NO)	Unpaired electron spins
Nitrogen dioxide (NO_2)	
Molecular oxygen (O_2)	Paired electrons with parallel spins
Transition metal series:	Ions containing unpaired electrons
Mn^{2+}, Mn^{3+}	
Fe^{2+}, Fe^{3+}	
Ni^{2+}	
Cr^{2+}	
Cu^{2+}	
Lathanide series:	
Gd^{3+}	
Eu^{2+}	
Actinide series:	
Pa^{4+}	
Nitroxides	Stable free radicals
Triphenylmethyl	

Molecular oxygen has been little used as a contrast agent. Inhalation of 100% O_2 decreases the spin–lattice relaxation time of blood within the left ventricular cavity (higher O_2) as compared with the right ventricle in human subjects. However, several factors make this molecule unsuitable for use as a contrast agent. These include the inability to chemically complex oxygen with carrier molecules without loss of paramagnetism. There are, therefore, two remaining categories of potentially useful paramagnetic substances; free radicals and metal ions.

Nitroxide stable free radicals (NSFR). Two major subgroups of the NSFR class of compounds that have been investigated for use as contrast agents are piperidine and pyrrolidine derivatives. Paramagnetism in these molecules is due to an unpaired electron that is delocalized between the nitrogen and hydrogen atoms (Fig. 14).

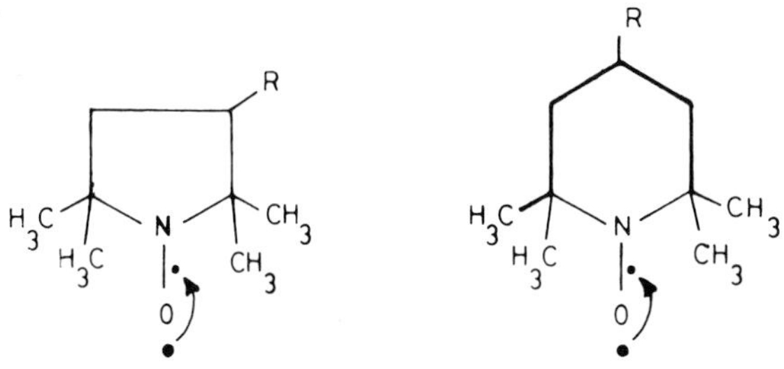

PYRROLIDINE-N-OXYL   PIPERIDINE-N-OXYL

Fig. 14 Chemical structure of pyrrolidine-*N*-oxyl and piperidine-*N*-oxyl. (Reproduced by kind permission of R. Brasch.)

Advantages in using NSFR derivatives include chemical versatility permitting conjugation to molecules to make them tissue specific, and chemical stability over a broad range of pH. However, NSFR derivatives also have a lower paramagnetic effect than metal ions and have a short half-life, undergoing degradation *in vivo* by enzyme systems and antioxidants.

Metal ions. Metal ions currently comprise the majority of research and clinical interest, due to their greater paramagnetic effect. In the ionic form these metals are toxic, and cannot be used clinically. Chelation of metals reduces toxicity. However, it also prevents close contacts of water molecules with the ion, and thus lessens the paramagnetic effect.

(i) *Gadolinium.* Gadolinium has the strongest influence on proton relaxation times of all elements for a variety of reasons, including long electron-spin relaxation time and strong magnetic moment.

Gadolinium is toxic to liver, spleen and bone marrow and is most commonly used as a contrast agent when bound to the chelate diethylene-triamine pentaacetic acid (DTPA).[6] Gd-DTPA has a short half-life in blood and urine (20 min) and is excreted primarily by glomerular filtration, with 90% recovery in the urine in 24 h. A small dose (1/100 of the LD_{50} dose) is sufficient to cause contrast enhancement.

Enhancement obtained using Gd-DTPA is claimed to be superior to iodinated enhancement of CT images and in the separation of tumour and oedema studies indicate an efficacy at least equal to x-ray CT.

Relaxation rate $(1/T_1)$ varies linearly with dose, the kidney having the greatest tissue response. Sensitivity to the effect of this contrast agent then decreases in the order serum, lung, heart, liver, spleen.

Gd-DTPA can only cross the blood–brain barrier when this has been disrupted, and so has great potential as a contrast agent for certain brain pathology.

(ii) *Manganese.* Although manganese is a powerful paramagnetic material it has been little used as a contrast agent. Manganese has two advantageous features; it alters spin–lattice and spin–spin relaxation rates differentially, and its relaxation effect can be enhanced by binding to a macromolecule. The effect of manganese as a contrast agent is dose dependent, and has been demonstrated in the liver, kidneys and heart. Colloidal manganese has produced contrast enhancement of rat livers and manganese chloride has enabled the differentiation of acutely ischaemic kidneys from the normal. However, these compounds are too toxic to be considered for human use.

(iii) *Iron.* Dilute ferric chloride has been used orally in humans to reduce the spin–lattice relaxation time in the fundus of the stomach and the use of iron particles, e.g. magnetite, as orally administered contrast agents is being investigated. Most research using iron as a contrast agent is now being conducted using chelated compounds administered intravenously, such as ferrous-EDTA and iron-EHPG. Contrast enhancement by hepatic iron overload is documented, as is the paramagnetic effect of iron dextran in NMR.

(iv) *Chromium.* Chromium-EDTA has been used to provide enhancement of the kidneys, ureter and bladder, and to differentiate between the renal cortex, medulla and pyramids.

Intravenous contrast agents which are excreted by glomerular filtration, such as Cr-EDTA, Gd-DTPA and Gd-EDTA, may also permit assessment of kidney function. In the normal kidney signal intensity is greatest immediately following administration of the contrast material. This intensity diminishes as the agent is cleared from the kidneys. In the obstructed or diseased kidney continued accumulation of the contrast agent occurs.

(v) *Metalloporphyrins.* Preliminary research is being conducted into the use of metalloporphyrins as contrast agents. These compounds form very stable complexes with paramagnetic metals, tend to concentrate in tumour tissues and are stable *in vivo* for long periods of time. Iron (III) TSPP (*meso* tetra-(*p*-sulphonatophenyl)porphine) has provided good enhancement of the relaxation of bulk water in tumours and manganese TPPS (tetrakis(*p*-sulpho-phenyl)-porphyrin) has been used as a contrast agent for imaging atherosclerotic vascular disease.

Applications of NMR Imaging

Biophysical and Biochemical Considerations. The extensive application of NMR in chemistry and *in vitro* biochemistry is based on NMR spectroscopy, i.e. on investigation of chemical shifts. *In vivo* NMR spectroscopy and tomography are now established as non-invasive methods for studying the physiological and pathological properties of tissues and organs.

TABLE 3

FACTORS AFFECTING NMR RELAXATION TIMES
(AFTER MATHUR-DE VRÉ[9])

Inherent biological factors	Extrinsic physical factors	Data treatment
Biological factors affecting water balance	Temperature	Multi-exponential behaviour
	Resonant frequency	
		Choice of model
Normal and pathological processes	Sample preparation	
Protein dynamics	Storage	
	Instrument settings	

The variation of the relaxation properties provides the opportunity for identification and characterization of tissues. The proton (^{1}H) relaxation times for various tissues obtained from both *in vitro* and *in vivo* measurements have been tabulated[7] but considerable care is needed in the interpretation of data for excised tissue.[8] Factors affecting relaxation times in tissue are listed in Table 3. The effect of the extrinsic physical parameters, instrumental variation and data treatment must be appreciated, and if possible also understood, if investigation of the distribution of T_1 and T_2 by NMR imaging is to provide meaningful diagnostic information. The inherent biological factors have been listed as: (1) the total water content, (2) macroscopic and microscopic distribution of water in different sites, and (3) macromolecular-water interactions. The inhomogeneous distribution of water content contributes to heterogeneity of tissue under normal conditions. In pathological states, heterogeneity can appear in localized form, such as oedema, cysts, necrosis, metastases, etc., or in induced changes in tissues not directly affected by the disease.

Heterogeneity may be investigated by means of the proton signal, and also by measurements of ^{23}Na and ^{19}F. In this situation, it is unlikely that the relaxation is characterized by a single parameter but instead

a multi-exponential model is required. Additional information, such as that obtained from biochemical sampling of compartments, must be combined with NMR measurements to yield information on the micro-environment within a compartment.

Because of heterogeneities, measured values of proton spin–lattice relaxation times may represent average results which may be difficult to relate to underlying biochemical behaviour. For this reason, some workers have concentrated on *in vitro* and *in situ* studies of human physiological fluids, such as amniotic fluid, blood, saliva, urine, pleural and peritoneal fluid.[10] These studies have been carried out at low fields (0·2–1·0 mT).

The relaxation times of normal tissues are influenced by many processes, including age and maturation, metabolism, phase of cell cycle intake of alcohol, stress, menstrual cycle and use of contraceptive drugs. Mathur-De Vre[9] considers that these processes primarily affect the water balance of the tissues. It has been argued, however, that variation in water content does not fully explain the observed effects on T_1 and, in particular, does not account for their specificity. Winter and Kimmich[11] have proposed that the final relaxation process at MHz frequencies is provided by relaxation sinks formed by the ^{14}N^{1}H amide groups in protein backbones. Evidence has been obtained *in vitro* and more recently *in vivo* by observing the ^{14}N^{1}H quadrupole dips in the graphs of T_1 against frequency. These results indicate that the dynamics of proteins, in addition to water content, may determine proton relaxation in water in biological cells.

Investigation of microscopic details of tissues and histological studies require spatial resolution of the order of microns. This can be achieved for small volumes. In whole-body systems, spatial resolution is of the order of millimetres.

Medical Imaging. NMR imaging has a number of features which make it attractive for diagnostic use. The absence of hazard permits repeated examination of the same patient and offers the opportunity to observe progress of disease and treatment. It is possible to obtain coronal and sagittal scans as well as transaxial. Because the water content of bone is very low, bone is effectively not seen in NMR so that bone artefacts do not occur and examination of soft tissue in the the vicinity of bone is possible.

The principal characteristic of NMR imaging is sensitivity to pathological changes in tissue due to changes in T_1 and T_2. The nature of these changes in various conditions and their influence on the NMR image has been discussed in detail by Taylor and Inamdar.[12] Comparisons with other imaging modalities have been given by Budinger[13] and by Jackson and Kouris.[14]

In this section, we list some of the present and potential medical applications of proton NMR imaging. Some images of ^{23}Na have been achieved but with poor spatial resolution and long imaging times. The conventional proton NMR images correspond to combined resonance signals from water and from methylene (CH_2) in lipids, if the macromolecules are sufficiently mobile to be detectable in the time scale of the experiment. This is another effect leading to multicomponent T_1 values. In some techniques, the signal from fat can be suppressed but in high fields ($\leqslant 1 \cdot 5T$) the chemical shift dispersion can be used to separate the two signals and allow construction of an image of water or fat.

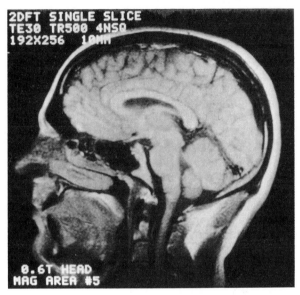

Fig. 15 ^{1}H NMR image of a sagittal section of the head and neck.

Neurology. The absence of bone artefacts leads to exceptionally good images of the brain, with clear separation of grey and white matter (Fig. 15). There has been considerable emphasis on multiple sclerosis and other demyelinating disease but cerebrovascular disease, hydrocephalus, diseases of the basal ganglia, and congenital and inherent diseases and dementia are being studied. Lack of hazard facilitates NMR imaging of the brain in children. The brain stem, spinal cord, and cerebrospinal fluid (CSF) are also accessible in NMR imaging.

Vascular disease. Infarcts, bleeding, and deposits on diseased walls can be observed in NMR imaging. NMR should offer considerable advantages over other modalities in the investigation of deep vein thrombosis.

Neoplastic disease. The original observation of variations in relaxation times in normal, benign and malignant tissues stimulated interest in the application of NMR imaging of neoplastic disease. Calcifications are more readily observed in x-ray CT and separation of tumour and oedema is not straightforward but NMR is an important tool in the diagnosis and control

of intracranial and orbital tumours. It is feasible to undertake *in vivo* studies of tissue response to radiotherapy, following *in vitro* studies in mice.

Heart and cardiac function. A variety of techniques are available, including fast imaging techniques and ECG gating.[15] The presence of infarction, scar tissue, ischaemia, and atheroma can be observed as well as coronary artery anatomy.

Breast. Imaging of the breast presents problems due to variations with age, hormonal activity, lactation, etc. Nevertheless, benign and malignant growths have been detected using standard whole-body coils. The use of surface coils yields better signals and a dedicated coil that images both breasts simultaneously offers considerable diagnostic advantages.

Spine and joints. Sagittal images are particularly valuable for studying the spinal column and intervertebral discs. It appears that pathological changes in degenerate discs may be detected by NMR imaging before biochemical damage becomes clinically evident. Congenital abnormalities, syringomyelia, arteriovenous malformation and changes due to rheumatoid arthritis may be observed.

Liver and kidney disease. Cirrhosis, hepatitis, abscesses and cysts, as well as metastatic growths may be observed and distinguished in the liver. Haemochromatosis and Wilson's disease, which lead to iron and copper deposition, respectively, can also be examined.

The cortex and medulla of the kidney are well separated in NMR imaging. Cysts and tumours can be identified but renal calculi are not well identified. The non-invasive diagnosis of chemically induced renal lesions is difficult, but NMR imaging can be used to identify site-specific renal lesions and to monitor their development.

Forensic medicine. Differences between living and excised tissue have been noted. It is therefore possible in principle to use NMR imaging to investigate the processes of dying and *rigor mortis*.

Non-medical Applications

Pharmaceutical and chemical industries. The sensitivity of NMR response to uptake of various kinds of drugs has already been noted, as has the ability to make repeated measurements on the same subject. Hence, the application of NMR imaging in the pharmaceutical industry could dramatically reduce the number of laboratory animals sacrificed. NMR imaging and TMR could be combined to provide a powerful research tool in drug development.

The excellence of NMR images of fruit, vegetables, and seeds, *in vitro*, has already been established.[15] The effect of horticultural conditions, nutrients, and fertilizers could be studied using growing plants in pots or trays. NMR images of brick, wood and similar materials can be readily achieved, and hence the effect of wood preservatives, fungicides, etc. can be studied.

Food industry. NMR imaging is being used to examine both the raw materials and finished products in the food industry. It is useful to map the distribution of water and to determine its state, as water seems to play a key role in production and shelf life, e.g. in food grains, bread and cake, fruit and vegetables. The filling of pies, uniformity of fish fingers and chocolate bars, fat/meat ratio of carcases, etc., can be

because restricted flow may give an earlier indication of disease than observation of tissue damage due to poor blood supply. Cerebrovascular disease affects blood movement in the brain whereas other vascular diseases occur primarily in the limbs, especially in the legs, and blood flow in the region of the heart reflects heart disease in various forms. Carotid blood-flow is interesting because it involves both laminar and turbulent flow.

Much of the earlier work involved non-imaging NMR observation of blood flow. The applications of these measurements have been reviewed.[16]

NMR images are influenced by flow. Most measurements of flow are made by a time-of-flight technique

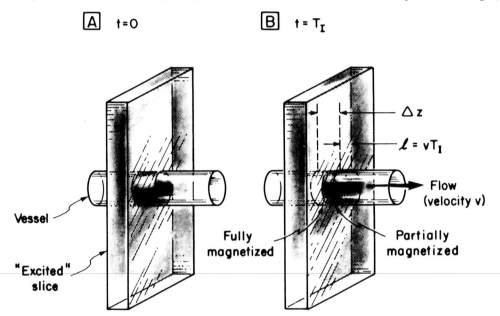

Fig. 16 Principle of flow in slice-selective imaging. (a) At time $t = 0$, an inversion pulse 'tags' the nuclei in the imaging slice. (b) A 90° detection pulse applied at $t = T$, creates transverse magnetization that reflects both the tagged and untagged nuclei in the imaging slice. (Reproduced by kind permission of F. W. Wehrli.)

examined, but not yet with the speed required to monitor products on a conveyor-belt.

Oil industry. It is known that NMR imaging can be used to monitor oil/water interfaces in porous rock. There is already an oil-well logging tool based on NMR.

Flow Measurements. The rapid and accurate measurement of flow rate in fluids is of considerable importance in industry, in large-scale production processes, in on-line control of chemical and other reactions, and in detection of obstructions. Some measurements may be required in hostile environments, e.g. fuel flow in satellite rocket engines. An advantage of NMR, as with ultrasound methods, is that the flow is unaffected by the measurement process.

Non-invasive measurement of blood flow is of particular value in the diagnosis of major diseases,

in which a well-defined active volume is created in one position and time and re-examined at a later time. In a saturation-recovery sequence, the initial r.f. pulse 'tags' the magnetization of the nuclei in the imaging slice. During the waiting time, the spins partially recover but these nuclei also advance with the velocity of the flow. The detection pulse yields an increase in signal strength compared to the absence of flow because new, fully magnetized, nuclei have entered the imaging slice (*see* Fig. 16). As the flow velocity increases, the NMR signal reaches a maximum when the velocity is equal to the ratio of the width of the imaging slice to the waiting time. In the spin-echo sequence, both the repetition rate and the waiting time influence the extent to which the nuclei in the imaging slice are replaced by untagged nuclei. This leads to an increase in the NMR intensity with velocity, followed by a decrease, as shown in Fig. 17. This method has been used to study water flow in plant stems as well as blood flow.

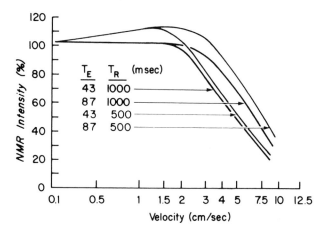

Fig. 17 Experimentally observed NMR signal intensity plotted as a function of flow in a spin-echo sequence. The fluid used is doped water mimicking the relaxation times of blood. Note that the signal intensities are enhanced at the shorter repetition times. Whereas T_E = 43 ms corresponds to a single echo signal, the data recorded at T_E = 87 ms resulted from a second refocusing pulse. (Adapted from Crooks *et al.*, *Radiology*; **144**: 843–52, 1981.)

A second method makes use of a velocity-dependent phase shift, analogous to the Doppler shift in ultrasound measurements. This method does not depend on selective excitation of an active volume. Cardiac gating is necessary for studies of the heart.

Taylor and Bushell[17] have shown that it is possible to image the molecular diffusion coefficient in the absence or presence of flow. This parameter may be useful in monitoring blood perfusion in tissue or seepage in other materials.

NMR SPECTROSCOPY

In biology and chemistry analytical applications have been studied using high-resolution NMR spectroscopy to identify and monitor the state of various chemical species. The detailed information that has been derived from ^1H, ^{13}C and ^{31}P studies on isolated but intact living systems have now established the importance and value of NMR spectroscopy in the study of metabolism. These investigations have culminated in *in vivo* studies of whole animals and humans.

The spectral position of the resonance line (equation 1) depends not only on the magnitude of B_0 but also on the immediate chemical environment of the nucleus. The presence of small electronic currents in molecules produces a very small additional field at the nucleus so that the total field B_{tot}, experienced by the nucleus is in fact

$$B_{tot} = (1 - \sigma)B_0 \qquad (9)$$

where σ is called the shielding factor of the nucleus. This shielding gives rise to a small shift in the resonant frequency of the nucleus termed the chemical shift. The size of σ depends on the type of molecule and

so can be used to recognize the presence of particular molecules in a sample. The chemical shift, δ, is usually expressed in parts per million.

^{31}P NMR Spectroscopy

^{31}P is one of the most widely used nuclei for biological investigation for a number of reasons. Resonance peaks are narrow and well defined, no isotopic enrichment is required, since ^{31}P is a naturally occurring isotope, and many of the metabolites involved in cellular chemical energy transfer contain phosphorus. These compounds are present in free solution in living systems in large enough concentrations to be detectable by NMR (>0·5 mmol). The chemical shift range of biological phosphates is approximately 30 p.p.m.— larger than that of protons. This facilitates the resolution of individual resonance peaks on the NMR spectra. One of the greatest advantages of NMR spectroscopy is that it is non-destructive, and tissue can be rapidly resampled. Thus, as well as detecting individual metabolites and measuring pH, ^{31}P NMR may be used to observe the kinetics of energy exchange.[18]

^{31}P NMR Spectrum of Resting Muscle. Three parameters can be determined from the NMR spectrum; the intensity of the signal, the resonance frequency and the relaxation time.

There are ten well-defined resonance peaks in the ^{31}P spectrum of resting frog gastrocnemius muscle (Fig. 18). Peak A represents the β-phosphate of ATP and peak B corresponds to the α-phosphate of ATP and ADP, and the two phosphate nuclei of NAD. Peak C has been identified as the γ-phosphate of ATP and the β-phosphate of ADP. The chemical shifts of these resonance peaks indicate that ATP, as detected by this technique, is more than 95% bound to magnesium.

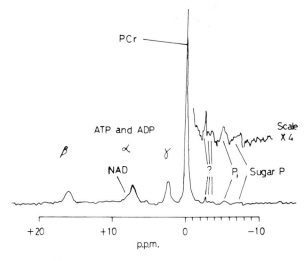

Fig. 18 ^{31}P NMR spectrum of resting frog gastrocnemius muscle. (Reproduced by kind permission of D. R. Wilkie.)

The most prominent peak in this spectrum (D) is assigned to phosphoryl creatine (Pcr). Inorganic orthosphosphate (P_i) is represented by peak F, and sugar phosphates (sugar P) by G. This latter resonance peak is also partly attributable to phospholipids.

Between Pcr and P_i there are three previously unidentified resonance peaks (E). These have now been assigned to phosphodiesters, including glycerophosphorylcholine, glycerophosphorylethanolamine and related compounds. Blood contains little ATP and no Pcr relative to its major NMR-visible metabolite, 2,3-disphosphoglycerate. Thus, it makes no significant contribution to the NMR signal from skeletal muscle.[19]

Concentration of metabolites. The number of phosphate nuclei present in the metabolites is proportional to the areas of the resonance peaks. The quantitative estimates of the concentrations of phosphate-containing compounds by NMR are in close agreement with results obtained from chemical analysis.

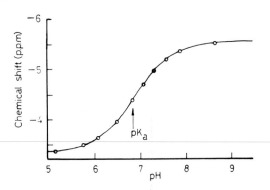

Fig. 19 The chemical shift of P_i as a function of pH. (Reproduced by kind permission of D. R. Wilkie.)

pH measurement. The chemical shift of the single resonance peak obtained for P_i is determined by the relative amounts of H_2PO_4 and HPO_4^{2-} present in the sample. Since P_i has a pK close to neutrality the proportions of these species is pH sensitive. The resonance frequency of P_i is, therefore, pH dependent (Fig. 19).

It is observed that pH, as measured by this technique, alters under a variety of conditions. Muscle becomes more acidic during exercise, ischaemia and with senescence. An increase in pH has been detected in the muscles of patients with Duchenne dystrophy.

Compartmentation of metabolites. Within skeletal muscle the intracellular distribution of sugar P and P_i is dissimilar to that of ATP and Pcr. This has been supported by observations made using ^{31}P NMR spectroscopy. The P_i resonance peak from skeletal muscle is broader than that of ATP and Pcr (although these metabolites have the same line-width in free aqueous solution) and its resonance frequency is pH depen-

dent. A differing distribution of P_i within the muscle cell (compartmentation) may account for this.[20]

Muscle Contraction. ^{31}P NMR spectroscopy has been used to observe changes in the phosphate energy cycle following muscle contraction both *in vitro* and *in vivo*.

Changes in the proportions of high energy phosphates are observed during prolonged muscle contraction *in vitro*,[19] and *in vivo* following repeated contraction of the flexor digitorum superficialis muscle in man. These include a fall in Pcr and an increase in P_i concentration. ATP concentration remains constant until Pcr sources are almost exhausted.

Muscular Pathology. Diseased states of the muscle studied *in vitro* and *in vivo* include Duchenne and Becker dystrophies. Concentrations of phosphorus metabolites observed by NMR are lower in dystrophic muscle that in healthy tissue, although the proportion of total phosphate signal due to ATP is not significantly different. Following excision of the muscle, levels of high energy phosphates alter most rapidly in the diseased tissue.

^{31}P NMR spectroscopy has also been used to localize regions of ischaemia. These are characterized by a reduction or loss of the Pcr peak and a decrease in ATP concentration. P_i concentration is increased and the ischaemic region becomes more acidic.

^{31}P NMR of Organs

The ^{31}P NMR spectrum of liver, kidney, heart and other organs differs from that of skeletal muscle due to an absence of a Pcr resonance peak. However, in most other respects the liver spectrum is similar to that of muscle.

^{31}P NMR studies of the liver have been conducted both *in vitro* and *in vivo*, employing isolated hepatocytes, the perfused organ, and the organ *in situ*. To ensure that a signal free from contamination by other tissues is being received from the liver *in vivo* a coil was surgically implanted. This was used to compare spectra between fed and fasted animals and, hence to investigate changes in the spectra arising from alterations in metabolism.[21]

Changes in the proportions of high energy phosphates have also been observed following infusion of insulin, glycerol and fructose and the induction of ischaemia. It was observed that cyanide intoxication caused a transient loss of ATP resonance peaks, and an increase in P_i concentration which was terminated by perfusion with a cyanide-free buffer. Hepatoxicity has been further investigated using ^{31}P NMR by monitoring the energy status of a liver *in vivo* following ingestion of carbon tetrachloride and recovery of the organ when challenged with fructose.

^{31}P NMR spectroscopy has been used to study a variety of renal preparations, including mitochondria, isolated tubules, the perfused organ and the kidney *in vivo*.[22] Spectra from the tubules isolated from the cortex, medulla, and papillary tip are distinguishable. The morphological, functional and magnetic heterogeneity of the kidney is of particular relevance when attempting to assign and interpret spectra obtained from the whole organ, either *in vitro* or *in vivo*.

Renal pathology that has been studied using NMR includes respiratory and metabolic acidosis, infection, hypovolaemic shock, ischaemia and acute renal failure. In cases of candidal pyelonephritis a polyphosphate peak (not apparent in the control) has been detected. This is considered to be indicative of yeast infection, which, otherwise, can only be diagnosed by renal biopsy.

Observations made following ischaemia and recovery from ischaemic injury are of particular relevance when assessing kidney viability for transplantation. Ischaemia has been characterized by a reversible loss of ATP from the spectra, and a parallel fall in pH. The reduced pH may inhibit renal function, and it has been suggested that a relationship may exist between tissue acidification and the occurrence of irreversible renal damage.

^{31}P NMR spectroscopy may be of value in the assessment of the quality of organ preservation prior to transplantation. The monophosphate to P_i peak ratio has been used to assess renal viability and ischaemic damage and longer spin–lattice relaxation times have been observed in a poorly preserved liver.

Malignancies

^{31}P NMR spectroscopy has been used to characterize malignancies and to follow and assess regression after treatment. It has even been suggested that due to its position in nucleic acids ^{31}P may have value as a probe for the mechanisms of carcinogenesis.[23] Malignancies have been characterized by significantly longer spin–lattice relaxation rates than the healthy tissues from which they were derived.

Rat gliomas have been characterized by increased P_i and decreased Pcr concentrations and it has also been noted that the ^{31}P spectra of tumour cells frequently have 'conspicuous' phospho-monoester and -diester peaks.

The efficacy of radioimmunotherapy of human B cell lymphoma has been assessed using ^{31}P NMR spectroscopy. A transient fall in Pcr and ATP concentrations, and an increase in P_i and sugar P was associated with successful treatment of the cancer. In a case in which there was no regression, but growth was arrested, there was a continued fall in Pcr levels. Other methods of treatment that have been studied using this technique include hypothermia and ovariectomy. In the latter case a rapid change in the proportion of phosphate metabolites occurred in oestrogen-sensitive mammary tumours following surgery.

Enzyme Kinetics

^{31}P NMR spectroscopy has important biochemical applications, including the *in vivo* observation of the roles of enzymes and the measurement of reaction rates.[6]

The enzyme kinetics of creatine and adenylate kinase have been studied using this technique. ATP utilized during muscle contraction is replenished using Pcr and this is catalysed by creatine kinase. Monitoring of this enzymatic reaction has enabled the non-destructive calculation of ADP concentration which, otherwise, cannot be derived from the NMR spectra, and has also led to a theory of cellular compartmentation of ATP. Similarly, the enzyme kinetics of adenylate kinase, which catalyses the reaction:

$$2ADP \rightarrow ATP + AMP$$

have also been observed using ^{31}P NMR spectroscopy.

NMR Spectroscopy Using Other Nuclei

^{13}C NMR spectroscopy has principally been used to study metabolic rates and elucidate pathways by the detection of ^{13}C-labelled intermediates and end-products. The NMR sensitivity to ^{13}C is not as good as that of ^{1}H or ^{31}P, and the analysis of the spectra is not as easy. Work involving ^{13}C NMR spectroscopy includes the study of glucose and amino acid metabolism ketogenesis, hepatic metabolism and the composition of adipose tissue.[20]

As well as observing the pathways of natural metabolites NMR spectroscopy can also be used to follow the metabolic fate of a drug. There is negligible ^{19}F present in biological systems so spectra received from a drug or its metabolites is free of background 'noise', thus facilitating interpretation. ^{19}F has a large spectral dispersion and reasonable sensitivity relative to that of ^{1}H.

Many fluorinated drugs are in clinical use including anaesthetics, anti-cancer drugs and neuroleptics. The potential applications of ^{19}F NMR spectroscopy have been illustrated by the work of Stevens *et al.*[24] in which the metabolism of the anti-cancer drug 5-fluorouracil was followed. Preliminary work has suggested that this technique may be used to assess the metabolism of fluorinated anti-cancer drugs, and so assist with patient management.

The distribution of halothane (a fluorinated anaesthetic), and its metabolites has also been investigated using ^{19}F NMR spectroscopy, and other applications include the use of an analogue of glucose—radioactive ^{19}F-labelled 2-deoxy-glucose—to measure regional glucose metabolism.

^{1}H NMR spectroscopy of biological samples initially developed less rapidly than that of ^{31}P and ^{13}C since the ^{1}H spectrum has a small chemical shift, and a technique for the suppression of the large ^{1}H signal received from water and fat contained within biological samples is needed in order that other ^{1}H containing metabolites may be NMR visible. Applications include the study of human amniotic fluid, serum, dystrophic muscle, cerebrospinal fluid, erythrocyte metabolism, the pathophysiology of cerebral metabolism, and the metabolism of cancers during growth and regression.

Most recently, ^{1}H NMR spectroscopy has been used in preliminary studies to determine the metastatic potential of cancerous tissue and membrane transport.

FUTURE PROSPECTS

Developments in the biochemical and medical applications of NMR spectroscopy and imaging are closely associated with technical progress in instrumentation and computation. Such developments include imaging at higher resolutions for greater sensitivity (of the order of 10 μm), improved imaging techniques to reduce scanning time (e.g. FLASH, and echoplanar), the use of 3-D displays, and the separation of fat and water images.

In ^{1}H NMR imaging there is a persistent need for greater tissue specificity to enable the quantitative characterization of healthy and pathological states. This may be achieved by various methods, including multi-point T_2 analysis using the Carr-Purcell-Meiboom-Gill sequence to obtain full relaxation curves. The use of perfusion and diffusion as NMR parameters, in addition to spin–spin and spin–lattice relocation times, and ^{1}H density, will add further dimensions to quantitative analysis. Greater tissue specificity may also be achieved through further development of targeting contrast agents and their applications.

There is potential for the development of a wide range of applications of NMR spectroscopy. Briefly, these may include further use of various nuclei in the study of drug metabolism and toxicity *in vitro* and *in vivo*, improved resolution of resonance peaks, and the prospect of routine human spectroscopy *in vivo*.

REFERENCES

1. Saunders R. D., Smith H. (1984). Safety aspects of NMR clinical imaging. *Br. Med. Bull*; **40**: 148.
2. Taylor D. G., Inamdar R. (1985). Instrumentation for NMR imaging. In *Physical Principles and Clinical Applications of Nuclear Magnetic Resonance* (Lerski R. A., ed.) London: Hospital Physicists' Association.
3. Edelstein W. A., Hutchinson J. M. S., Johnson G., Redpath T. (1980). Spin warp NMR imaging and applications to human whole-body imaging. *Phys. Med. Biol*; **25**: 751.
4. Runge V. M., Clantar J. A., Lukehart C. M. *et al.* (1983). Paramagnetic agents for contrast-enhanced NMR imaging: A review. *Am. J. Roentgenology*; **141**: 1209.
5. Brasch R. C. (1983). Work in progress: methods of contrast enhancement for NMR imaging and potential applications. *Radiology*; **147**: 773, 781.
6. Gadian D. G., Payne J. A., Bryant D. J. *et al.* (1985). Gd-DTPA as a contrast agent in MR imaging—theoretical projections and practical observations. *J. Comput. Assist. Tomogr*; **9** (2): 242.
7. Bottomley P. A., Foster T. H., Argersinger R. E., Pfeifer L. M. (1984). A review of normal tissue hydrogen NMR relaxation times and relaxation mechanisms from 1–100 MHz dependence on tissue type, NMR frequency, temperature, species, excision and age. *Med. Phys*; **11**: 425.
8. Taylor D. G., Bore C. F. (1981). A review of the magnetic resonance response of biological tissue and its applicability to the diagnosis of cancer by NMR radiology. *J. Comput Tomogr*; **5**: 122.
9. Mathur-De Vré R. (1984). Biomedical implications of the relaxation behaviour of water related to NMR imaging. *Br. J. Radiol*; **57**: 955.
10. Bené G. J. (1983). The NMR proton relaxation in biological fluids: A good way to identify precisely healthy or pathological states. *Ann 1st Super Sanita*; **19**: 121.
11. Winter F., Kimmich R. (1982). NMR field-cycling relaxation spectroscopy of bovine serum albumin, muscle tissues, micrococcus luteus and yeast. *Biochim. Biophys. Acta*; **719**: 292.
12. Taylor D. G., Inamdar R. NMR imaging in theory and in practice. *Phys. Med. Biol*; in press.
13. Budinger T. F. (1981). Medical applications of NMR scanning: some perspectives in relation to other techniques. *Proc. Int. Sym. NMR Imaging*, Carolina, pp. 51–64.
14. Jackson D. F., Kouris K. (1983). The role and potential of new imaging methods. *Prog. Med. Env. Phys*; **2**: 1.
15. Mansfield P., Morris P. G. (1982). *NMR Imaging in Biomedicine*, London: Academic Press.
16. Salles-Cunha S. X., Halbach R. E., Battocletti J. H., Sances A. (1981). The NMR blood flowmeter–applications. *Med. Phys*; **8**: 452.
17. Taylor D. G., Bushell M. C. (1985). The spatial mapping of translational diffusion coefficients by the NMR imaging technique. *Phys. Med. Biol*; **30**: 345.
18. Gadian D. G. (1982). Nuclear magnetic resonance and its applications to living systems. Oxford: Oxford Science Publications.
19. Dawson M. J., Gadian D. G., Wilkie D. R. (1977). Contraction and recovery of living muscles studied by phosphorus-31 NMR. *J. Physiol*; **267**: 703.
20. Gadian D. G., Radda G. K., Richards R. E., Seeley P. J. (1979). Phosphorus-31 NMR in living tissue. The road from a promising to an important tool in biology. In *Biological Applications of Magnetic Resonance* (Shulman R. G., ed.) 463–536. New York: Academic Press.
21. Malloy C. R., Cunningham C. C., Radda G. K. (1986). The metabolic state of the rat liver *in vivo* measured by ^{31}P-NMR spectroscopy. *Biochimica et Biophysica Acta*; **885**: 1.
22. Ross B., Freeman D., Chan L. (1986). Contributions of nuclear magnetic resonance to renal biochemistry. *Kidney Int*; **29**: 131.
23. Zaner K. S., Damadian R. (1975). Phosphorus-31 as a nuclear probe for malignant tumours. *Science*; **189**: 729.
24. Stevens A. N., Morris P. G., Iles R. A. *et al.* (1984). 5-fluorouracil metabolism monitored *in vivo* by ^{19}F NMR. *Br. J. Cancer*; **50**: 113.

13. The Use and Measurement of Radioisotopes

R. P. Parker* revised and updated by D. V. Mabbs

INTRODUCTION

Since the early days of biochemistry it has been desirable to label organic compounds in such a way that their passage through the body and subsequent excretion may be followed in a quantitative manner. This may be achieved by 'labelling' the molecule in question in some manner so that it can be identified but not altered in function.

The biochemical behaviour of a molecule is primarily determined by its electronic structure. If the number of neutrons within the nuclei is altered then the chemical properties are not normally affected, even though the physical behaviour of the molecule (e.g. diffusibility) may be slightly modified. Thus substitution by other isotopes of the same element can provide a suitable means of labelling.

This is sometimes possible by using enriched stable isotopes, such as deuterium ($^2_1$H) as a label for hydrogen, but many isotopes are unstable and their nuclei undergo spontaneous changes with the emission of various radiations. These are called *radioactive iso-*topes and the radiations emitted can provide a convenient means of detection.

The earliest work on this subject was carried out by von Hevesy in 1923, using naturally occurring radioisotopes of heavy elements such as lead, radium and thorium. In 1932 the Curies discovered that artificial radioactive materials could be made, thus widening their use to encompass all the elements. Research workers in the life sciences quickly took advantage of the many possibilities thus provided, and in the late 1930s considerable interest was shown in the application of these techniques, particularly in the United States. World War II, with its atomic energy project and the invention of the nuclear reactor, permitted artificial radioisotope production on an unprecedented scale and now over 1500 radioisotopes are known, covering all the elements.

When designing an experiment or test in which radioactive labels are to be used it is first necessary to decide on the element to be labelled. Normally it is undesirable to use an element which is foreign to the molecule under consideration, although the halogens in particular are often used as label without seriously affecting the biochemical behaviour. For example, ^{125}I can be used as a label for insulin. For the purposes of the particular investigation the labelled compound must follow the appropriate metabolic pathway (or whatever else is being studied) and the labelled atom must not become dissociated. This is frequently a restriction, and behaviour *in vitro*—or even in animals—is not always borne out by behaviour in humans.

Attention must be paid to the radioactive properties of the isotope to be used and this may influence the choice if more than one label is possible. In particular the radiations emitted should be easy to measure quantitatively.

Clinical applications are normally divided into *in vitro* and *in vivo* studies. The biochemist is primarily concerned with *in vitro* tests, in which samples, such as blood or urine, are taken from the body and assayed in a sample counter. The radioactive material may be administered to the patient (as in some saturation analysis techniques) or to the sample (as in radioimmunoassay methods). These are fast-growing fields which are described in Chapter 31). The alternative *in vivo* examinations are primarily concerned with organ imaging (or 'scanning') and functional tests of a physiological nature (such as organ blood flow).

RADIOACTIVITY

A radioactive atom is one whose nucleus contains an unstable ratio of neutrons to protons. A consideration of all the known stable isotopes indicates that, in general, the lighter elements have approximately equal numbers of neutrons and protons whilst the heavier ones have an excess of neutrons. Isotopes having an unfavourable n/p ratio will seek a stable ratio by the process of radioactive decay. The energy

* Deceased

Corrections in liquid scintillation counting represent a special case and are considered on p. 193.

Dead Time. Radiation detector systems will normally take a significant time, τ, to detect and process an event. During this period, which is called the dead time, they will not respond to any new events and so a number of pulses will not be recorded. If N_o = observed count-rate, and N_c = corrected count-rate, then $N_c = N_o/(1 - N_o\tau)$. This correction should be applied before the background correction.

Background. The count-rate due to the background must be subtracted from that due to the (source + background). Since both are subject to statistical fluctuations, the variance of the difference between them will be the sum of the variances of the two quantities. The minimum variance in an estimate of sample counting-rate corrected for background is obtained when the available total counting time, T, is divided between measuring the combined counting-rate, c, and the background counting-rate, b, according to the relations

$$t_c = \frac{T\sqrt{c}}{\sqrt{c} + \sqrt{b}} \quad \text{and} \quad t_b = \frac{T\sqrt{b}}{\sqrt{c} + \sqrt{b}}$$

where $T = t_c + t_b$.

Radioactive Decay. This can be an important correction since many short-lived nuclides are now used clinically. It is normally sufficient to correct decay to the mid-point of the counting period for any one sample. Note that when samples are compared with an aliquot or with others measured at the same time decay corrections may cancel out.

Dilution and Chemical Losses. These need to be corrected for in the usual manner and errors estimated, if necessary by means of a separate tracer experiment. Certain radionuclides (e.g. ^{32}P) are particularly prone to preferential adsorption on the walls of vessels and inactive carriers need to be added.

Geometry, Self-absorption and Detector Efficiency. As discussed earlier, it is important that all samples and reference standards be measured under identical conditions.

Combination of Errors. Since many tracer procedures involve comparison of sample activity with that of a standard, the rules for the combination of errors for products and quotients are given below.

If two quantities, x and y, are measured, their relative standard error being v_x and v_y then the relative standard error of their quotient x/y is

$$v_{x/y} = \sqrt{v_x^2 + v_y^2}$$

which is also the relative standard error of the product $x \times y$.

SPECIAL SAMPLE COUNTING TECHNIQUES

Liquid Scintillation Counting

This is the method of choice for counting low energy β-emitters such as ^3H, ^{14}C and ^{35}S, and is therefore widely used in biochemical laboratories. It can also be used for measuring low energy x- and γ-ray emitters such as ^{55}Fe and ^{125}I and high energy β-emitters such as ^{32}P. A full description of the technique is given by Horrocks.[6]

Method. The counting sample contains three components: the radioactive material, an organic solvent or solvent mixture, and one or more organic scintillators. The sample is therefore intimately mixed with the scintillator, providing excellent geometrical efficiency and virtually no self-absorption. This mixture is contained in a transparent counting vial made of glass or plastic, normally 20–25 ml capacity. The vial itself is coupled to two photomultipliers by means of light pipes and/or reflectors. Low energy pulses are generated by the random thermal emission of electrons from the photocathodes; their effect is considerably reduced by operating the phototubes in coincidence and is often diminished still further by cooling to about 4 °C. Figure 7 gives a block diagram of a typical liquid scintillation counter employing two counting channels, one of which is often adjusted to measure ^{14}C and the other ^3H (together with a small contribution of ^{14}C). The method is very suitable for the automatic processing of large numbers of samples and many machines commercially available are capable of measuring in excess of 400 samples.

Liquid Scintillation Solvents and Solutes. The purpose of the solvent is to ensure intimate contact between the sample and the scintillator and also to aid in energy transfer. Good solvents are to be found in the aromatic hydrocarbon group, toluene being the most widely used together with xylene and dioxane. The solvent forms the largest components of the scintillator mix and is chosen for a particular type of sample.

Scintillation solutes are classified into primary and secondary. The primary solute accepts transferred energy from the solvent and emits a proportion of this energy as scintillations of visible light (usually around 350–400 nm wavelength); if necessary a secondary solute is added which acts as a 'wavelength shifter', absorbing the light and re-emitting it at a longer wavelength more suited to the maximum response of the phototube. In modern equipment the secondary solute may be unnecessary. Table 5 gives details of solutes in common use.

Ready-to-use liquid scintillator 'cocktails' are now available from the large chemical manufacturers.

A number of substances may absorb the energy before it is transferred to the scintillator. This is known as *chemical quenching* and is particularly important with aqueous samples. In addition *colour quenching* can occur, in which the visible light pho-

it is kept in solid form. Only a very brief description can be given here, and the serious user of liquid scintillation equipment is strongly advised to consult a monograph on the subject, such as that by Horrocks listed at the end of the chapter.[6]

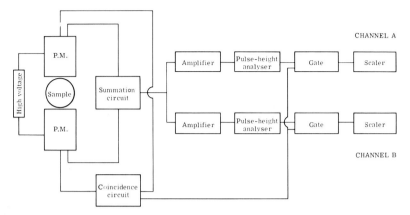

Fig. 7 Schematic diagram of a liquid scintillation counter.

TABLE 5
SCINTILLATION SOLUTES

Solute	Abbreviation	Type	Fluorescence max. nm
2,5-diphenyloxazole	PPO	Primary	363
p-terphenyl	TP	Primary	344
2-(4-biphenyl)-5-phenyl-1,3,4-oxadiazole	PBD	Primary	361
2-(4'-*t*-butylphenyl)-5-(4''-biphenyl)-1,3,4-oxadiazole	Butyl-PBD	Primary	366
1,4-bis-(5-phenyloxazol-2-yl)benzene	POPOP	Secondary	430
1,4-bis-(4-methyl-5-phenyloxazol-2-yl)benzene	DM-POPOP	Secondary	430

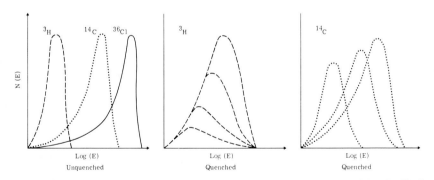

Fig. 8 Quenched and unquenched β-spectra as detected in a liquid scintillation counter.

tons are absorbed by the solution before they reach the photocathodes. In both cases there is a reduction in the observed pulse height causing an apparent downwards shift in the pulse height spectrum or, in the case of ^3H, an actual reduction in the number of β-particles detected (*see* Fig. 8).

Sample Preparation. The source may be introduced into the scintillator in various forms. Ideally it should be dissolved, either directly or with the aid of a solubilizing agent such as methanolic hyamine. Alternatively, a variety of methods are available by which

(a) *Water and aqueous solutions.* Until recently these were prepared by diluting toluene-based scintillants with more polar solvents such as dioxane, the choice depending on both the sample material and the operating temperature of the equipment. Emulsion counting has now become commonplace, in which the water is introduced after the detergent Triton-X100 has been mixed with the scintillator. Up to 40% of water by volume can be incorporated.

High energy β-emitters (about 0·26 MeV, and preferably above 1 MeV) can be assayed by using the liquid scintillation counter to detect the Cerenkov light which is emitted when an electron of sufficient energy passes through a substance such as water. In this case no scintillator is required and sample preparation is particularly easy. Phosphorus-32 can be counted in this way.

(b) *Biological materials.* Solubilizers may be used to facilitate the incorporation in toluene of samples which are normally insoluble in the liquid scintillator solvent. Hyamine has been widely used; recently proprietary materials have become available which are better, and can cope with a wide range of substances such as amino acids, RNA and dried fibrinogen.

(c) *Combustion.* A reproducible and accurate technique of widespread application is to oxidize the sample either directly with oxygen or by wet oxidation, the products being collected. For example, $^{14}CO_2$ and HTO can be collected separately and subsequently measured efficiently with complete isotope separation.

(d) *Coloured samples.* These are best oxidized as in (c) above, but the addition of bleaching agents to the sample preparation can achieve useful results, although problems may be encountered due to chemical quenching and chemiluminescence.

(e) *Solid samples.* The material, in powdered form, form, may be suspended in a suitable gel. Chromatography or filter papers can be measured directly by placing them within the scintillator solution.

Quench Corrections. Reference has been made earlier to the likelihood of chemical and colour quenching occurring. Since quenching affects the counting efficiency it is most important to estimate and correct the amount of quenching, which may even vary between samples in the same batch.

Many methods of quench correction have been devised, the two most common being the channels ratio and external standard techniques. In the first the measured spectrum is divided in two counting channels, covering different ranges of pulse-height. Quenching which causes a shift towards lower energies (*see* Fig. 8) will alter the ratio of the counts in the two channels. Calibration curves need to be prepared using samples of known activity.

The external standard method uses a γ-emitting source such as ^{137}Cs which can be placed close to the sample vial. Gamma-rays interacting within the scintillator will cause scintillations, and the count-rate obtained will depend on the degree of quenching. Thus the correction factor can be estimated after this additional measurement is carried out.

Facilities for these methods are usually provided in commercial equipment and data-processing equipment can be used to apply the corrections automatically to each sample. It must be pointed out that quench correction methods are not necessarily applicable to all samples under all conditions and care must be taken in their application.

Radiochromatography

Chromatographic measurements are of increasing importance in clinical biochemistry, and it is often necessary to determine not only the components of a mixture but the amount of activity associated with each component. In this way the efficiency of a labelling procedure can be studied and any dissociation detected. Liquid fractions are easily assayed by γ- and liquid-scintillation counting techniques, and lend themselves to automatic methods. Chromatography paper may be cut out and measured as separate samples in a similar way. Alternatively the paper may be automatically moved past a slit-shaped β- or γ-detector and the count-rate displayed as a function of the position of the paper. For γ-rays a NaI(Tl) crystal with a slit-shaped lead collimator is used, whilst for β-emitters either a suitable scintillator, such as anthracene, or a Geiger counter is acceptable.

IN VIVO MEASUREMENTS

So far this chapter has been concerned with the measurement of samples, since these are the prime concern of the biochemist. There are, however, a wide range of clinical tests based on *in vivo* measurements using γ-emitters since these are readily detected outside the body. Table 6 lists some of the nuclides used and the type of tests undertaken. These are not in general likely to be the responsibility of a clinical biochemist and therefore only brief reference is made here. Details can be found in Belcher and Vetter.[7]

TABLE 6
SOME RADIONUCLIDES IN MEDICAL USE

Nuclide	Half-life	Typical application
^3H	12·6 y	Metabolic studies
^{14}C	5730 y	Metabolic studies
^{13}N	10 m	Cardiac studies using $^{13}NH_4$
^{15}O	2 m	Respiratory studies
^{51}Cr	28 d	Haematological investigations
^{58}Co	71 d	Vitamin B_{12} uptake
^{52}Fe	8·3 h	Haematological investigations
^{67}Ga	80 h	Tumour localization
^{75}Se	120 d	Pancreas visualization using ^{75}Se-methionine
$^{99}Tc^m$	6 h	Tumour investigation
^{125}I	60 d	Radioimmunoassay
^{131}I	8 d	Thyroid function and therapy
^{133}Xe	5·3 d	Pulmonary function
^{137}Cs	30 y	Therapeutic implants
^{198}An	2·7 d	Therapeutic implants

RADIATION PROTECTION

The biochemist will be well used to dealing with materials which are a potential hazard to the health of the laboratory worker and the patient. The ability of ionizing radiations to cause severe biological damage was recognized many years ago. In consequence Codes of Practice, International Recommendations and, more recently, statutory legislation, have been drawn up to control the use of radioactive materials, with the result that serious radiation injury is an extremely rare event.

Anyone proposing to use radioactive materials must be aware of the inherent dangers and of any statutory requirements which apply. Attention must be paid to laboratory facilities and design, storage, transport and handling arrangements, waste disposal, and exposure of staff and patients. The user should consult the relevant regulations such as the Ionising Radiations Regulations for the UK[10] and the recommendations of the International Commission on Radiological Protection (ICRP), some of which are given in the References below.[8]

REFERENCES AND FURTHER READING

1. Evans R. D. (1955). *The Atomic Nucleus*. New York: McGraw-Hill.
2. Lederer C. M., Shirley V. S. (1978). *Table of Isotopes*. New York: Wiley.
3. Crouthamel C. E. ed. (1970). *Applied Gamma-ray Spectrometry*. Oxford: Pergamon Press.
4. Hine, G. J. (1974). *Instrumentation in Nuclear Medicine*. New York: Academic Press.
5. Parker R. P., Smith P. H. S., Taylor D. M. (1984). *The Basic Science of Nuclear Medicine*. Churchill Livingstone.
6. Horrocks D. L. (1974). *Applications of Liquid Scintillation Counting*. New York: Academic Press.
7. Belcher E. H., Vetter H. ed. (1971). *Radioisotopes in Medical Diagnosis*. London: Butterworths.
8. International Commission on Radiological Protection (ICRP). Various Reports. London: HMSO.
9. International Commission on Radiological Units (ICRU), Report No. 22 (1972). London: HMSO.
10. The Ionising Radiations Regulations (1985). London: HMSO.

14. Ion-selective Electrodes
Leslie J. Russell and B. M. Buckley

INTRODUCTION

Ion-selective electrodes (ISEs) are now widely used in clinical chemistry and, in many cases, have displaced previous methods of analysis through their ease of use and speed in obtaining results. In this chapter, we will describe the general principles and theory behind the use of ISEs; the technologies that are currently applicable in clinical chemistry and some of the problems that have arisen with their use. We shall be concerned only with direct potentiometric ISEs i.e. those that do not entail pre-dilution of the sample prior to measurement, since diluted ISE technology should give results that closely relate to those obtained by more traditional methods. However, the general principles and application of the Nernst equation still apply. Technologies such as ion-selective field effect transistors (ISFETs) and coated-wire electrodes which have been used for *in vivo* and *ex vivo* monitoring, but which are not in current routine use, will be discussed elsewhere in this volume.

General Descriptions

An ion-selective electrode basically consists of an assembly in which an electrically conducting membrane separates two solutions—the sample and an internal filling solution of constant composition. An electrochemical gradient develops across this membrane reflecting the composition of the two solutions and gives rise to a potential difference. The construction of the electrode is completed by the inclusion of an internal reference electrode (IRE), usually a silver wire coated with silver chloride, immersed in the internal filling solution. Any change in potential at this electrode is then determined with respect to an external reference electrode (ERE), which is also in contact with the sample solution (Fig. 1), forming a cell with the ISE.

Types of Membrane

Membranes for ISEs may be generally divided into four categories according to the nature of the membrane material.

TABLE 3

COMPARISON OF SEVERAL COMMERCIAL IONIZED CALCIUM ANALYSERS

Manufacturer/ instrument	Sensing electrodes/ type		Reference electrode junction and salt bridge solution		Calibrant matrix
AVL 980	Na$^+$ K$^+$ Ca^{2+}	– Glass – Neutral carrier/PVC – Neutral carrier/PVC	Open static Calomel	1.2M KCl	Triethanolamine
CORNING 634	Ca^{2+} H$^+$	– Neutral carrier/PVC – Glass	Dialysis membrane Ag/AgCl	Sat. KCl	Mops/Bes
KONE Microlyte	Na$^+$ K$^+$ Ca^{2+}	} Neutral carriers/PVC	Passive porous plug Ag/AgCl	3M KCl	Tris/acetate
NOVA 2	Ca^{2+}	– Liquid ion exchanger/ PVC Ca^{2+} polyphosphate	Open flowing junction Ag/AgCl	2M KCl	CaCl$_2$/NaCl
NOVA 6	Na$^+$ K$^+$ Ca^{2+}	– Glass } Neutral carriers/PVC	Open flowing junction Ag/AgCl	2M KCl	Hepes
NOVA 7	Ca^{2+} H$^+$ t-Ca^{2+}	– Neutral carrier/PVC – Glass – Modified neutral carrier/ PVC	Open flowing junction Ag/AgCl	2M NH$_4$Cl 0·3M Na formate 0·15M Formic acid 0·55M Sodium chloroacetate	Hepes
NOVA 8	Ca^{2+} H$^+$	– Neutral carrier/PVC – Glass	Open flowing junction Ag/AgCl	2M KCl	Hepes
ORION SS20	Ca^{2+}	– Liquid ion exchange/PVC – Ca^{2+} polyphosphate	Open pumped Ag/AgCl	2M KCl	Tris
RADIOMETER ICAl	Ca^{2+} H$^+$	– Liquid exchanger/PVC – Ca^{2+} bis (di-n-octylphenylphos- phate) – Glass	Open static calomel	4·6M Na formate	Tes/Bes

quently, enthusiasm for ionized calcium measurement in clinical chemistry waned and scepticism has arisen about its practical application. However, the recent major improvements in the design both of electrodes and of instruments has enabled routine and reliable measurements of ionized calcium in body fluids.

Plasma Total Calcium Concentration. As the total concentration of calcium in plasma is relatively easy to measure, most clinical chemistry laboratories have measured it in preference to ionized calcium. Although calcium fractions of little biological activity constitute a significant proportion of the quantity measured, plasma total calcium concentration reflects calcium status with reasonable accuracy in most subjects. Even when plasma protein concentrations are abnormal, total calcium concentration can be 'corrected' by any of a number of algorithms, provided the patient is in acid–base balance and does not have excess plasma concentrations of anions such as citrate. As total calcium measurement is both convenient for the laboratory and familiar to clinicians it retains its place in the laboratory repertoire because of a consideration of logistics rather than of patho-

physiology. However, the advent of reliable ISE measurements now prompts a reassessment of this measurement in patient investigation and monitoring. Indeed, it could be argued that had ionized calcium measurement been as convenient in the past, total calcium measurement would not now be commonly performed.

Clinical Use of Ionized Calcium Measurement. Measurement of ionized calcium concentration is most useful when abnormalities of plasma protein concentration, acid–base status or plasma anion composition confound the interpretation of total calcium measurement.

Infusion of large quantities of blood products, for instance during surgery, subjects the patient to a considerable citrate load. The resultant complexation of calcium decreases ionized calcium concentrations although, in general, adults metabolize citrate rapidly, preventing a decrease in ionized calcium concentrations to levels causing myocardial depression. However, citrate clearance may be impaired in hypothermia and liver disease, resulting in extreme decreases in plasma ionized calcium concentration with consequent failure of cardiac excitation and contraction. Ionized calcium monitoring in these circumstances allows rational calcium supplementation and correction of hypocalcaemia. Intra-operative monitoring of ionized calcium is of special value in paediatric cardiopulmonary bypass surgery and in liver transplantation, resulting in improved patient management. Frequent ionized calcium measurement has also been reported to be useful in monitoring exchange transfusion in neonates and plasmapheresis in adults. In these situations it is clearly an advantage that ionized calcium measurement can readily be performed in emergency situations near the patient.

In general clinical chemistry, measurement of ionized calcium will usually be performed when a calcium disorder is suspected either on clinical grounds or because of abnormal total calcium concentrations. The reference range for ionized calcium is much narrower than that for total calcium as the latter also reflects variation in concentrations of calcium binding proteins. Accordingly, ionized calcium has been shown in several studies to be the best indicator of calcium status in hyperparathyroidism and in myeloma. In chronic renal failure, where patients are commonly acidotic and hypoalbuminaemic and have seriously disordered calcium homeostasis, ionized calcium concentration in conjunction with pH is the most physiological index of status.

When ionized calcium analysis is used in this kind of problem-orientated role and where clinicians are familiar with its interpretation, it is logical to extend its use to provide emergency and out-of-hours calcium determinations. Typical of this situation is the investigation of neonatal tetany, where modern ionized calcium analysers usually provide results within two minutes, require as little as 35 μl of whole blood and above all provide a physiologically relevant result.

Factors Influencing Ionized Calcium Measurement. Ionized calcium measurements are influenced both by electrochemical and by pre-analytical factors.

Electrochemical effects. The electrochemical factors which influence sodium and potassium measurements by ISEs detailed on p. 207 also affect ionized calcium measurement. Table 2 shows a comparison of several different commercial analysers illustrating how they differ with respect to ion-selective membrane, reference electrode and bridge design. Calibrant matrix effects are very important in ionized calcium measurement as the buffers used to stabilize pH bind calcium ions. In addition, the calibrant must be kept free of bicarbonate and carbonate to prevent calcium binding. It is recommended that calibrant ionic strength should be maintained at 0·160 mol/kg.[20] At this ionic strength, the activity coefficient of calcium ions in aqueous solution is about 0·36, which approximates that in normal plasma, allowing results of ionized calcium measurement to be expressed in terms of its concentration

in plasma water. A proposed reference method is under discussion to enable results of ionized calcium measurement in plasma to be standardized since there is no definitive *a priori* method with which to establish their true values.[20]

Pre-analytical effects. Hydrogen ions compete with calcium ions for binding to plasma proteins, therefore in a given sample, the ionized calcium concentration decreases as the pH increases. When plasma is exposed to air it loses CO_2 and pH increases. Blood for ionized calcium determination should be collected and handled anaerobically before analysis and because of the close relationship between the two quantities, it is now generally held that pH must be measured and reported simultaneously with ionized calcium concentration. However, where, for convenience, samples are taken and handled without special anaerobic precautions prior to analyses, the ionized calcium concentration must be corrected either to a standard pH (usually 7·4) or to the arterial pH of the patient. This is possible from the known relationship between pH and ionized calcium, as long as the pH change is due to loss of CO_2. However, when the arterial pH of a patient differs significantly from pH 7·4 due to factors other than CO_2 such a correction will mislead and blood must be sampled anaerobically.

When sampling blood, venous stasis in the absence of muscle activity causes only minimal changes in ionized calcium concentration. A delay of up to 4 h between sampling and analysis is acceptable for anaerobic specimens as long as they are kept at 0–4°C. Longer delays and higher temperatures cause lactic acid, a calcium binding ligand, to be evolved from the erythrocytes with a resulting change in pH.

Ionized calcium can be measured in whole blood, plasma or serum, but when whole blood or plasma are used it is important to avoid the use of anticoagulants which chelate calcium. As well as the obvious compounds such as citrate and EDTA, heparin also binds calcium and may significantly decrease measured ionized calcium concentrations although calcium heparin itself contains an excess of calcium ions. This problem can be minimized by the use of calcium-titrated heparins, especially if blood is sampled into capillary tubes where higher concentrations of heparin are needed to prevent coagulation. Because of the difficulty of making up suitable heparin preparations, most users will find it best to purchase purpose-made syringes or capillary sampling tubes. Haemolysis must be avoided during sample collection, otherwise low calcium values are obtained because of dilution with intracellular fluids which contain only micromolar levels of ionized calcium.

Measurement of Other Ions

Measurement of sodium, potassium and calcium ions by direct potentiometry is now routine in clinical chemistry, but measurement of the major remaining ions in blood plasma—the anions chloride and bicarbonate and the cation magnesium—is not commonplace. Indeed, only chloride with its high concentration can be measured with relative ease. Progress to measure these and other physiologically relevant ions will now be briefly described. It is also possible to use potentiometric sensors to measure non-ionic species which produce ions in their reactions (e.g. enzymic reactions which may produce H^+, NH_4^+ or F^-); these will be discussed elsewhere.

Chloride. Conventional, robust chloride electrodes (solid-state electrodes formed from compressed pellets of $AgCl/Ag_2S$) have proved unsuitable for the direct monitoring of chloride ions in plasma due to interference caused by absorption of proteins. However, some systems have been developed for chloride estimation in sweat in the screening of infants for cystic fibrosis. In such systems, the test area is first cleaned and then sweat production induced by pilocarpine iontophoresis; the electrode is placed on the test area and the chloride concentration measured. (Sweat may also be absorbed onto filter paper and the sodium concentration measured indirectly after dilution in a suitable buffer.)

Alternative sensors based on liquid ion exchangers, usually either methyltricaprylammonium chloride (Aliquat 336) or methyltridodecylamine, immobilized in PVC have also been used for chloride ion measurements. It has recently been claimed that by drastically increasing the ion-exchanger/PVC ratio, electrodes of high selectivity, shorter response times, low membrane resistances and longer lifetimes have been achieved.[21] There have been few comparisons of direct potentiometric chloride measurements with the traditional coulometric or colorimetric techniques because of the relatively few instruments available.

Bicarbonate. It has been the practice in some centres to augment the assessment of acid–base status by measurement of either the bicarbonate or total CO_2 content of serum. For practical purposes, the total CO_2 content (mmol/l) may be assumed to equal the bicarbonate level since the dissolved CO_2 varies only between 0·6 and 1·8 mmol/l for a P_{CO_2} of between 20 and 60 mm Hg, although for an accurate conversion either the pH or P_{CO_2} should be known. Thus in clinical practice most methods for estimating blood bicarbonate concentration make use of measured pH and P_{CO_2} values and approximation from the Henderson–Hasselbalch equation.

$$pH = pK + \log \frac{(HCO_3^-)}{(CO_2) \text{ dissolved}}$$

Simon and his group have developed a bicarbonate sensor based on ethanolamine compounds immobilized in PVC which are actually pH electrodes responding to bicarbonate changes in a pH 8 buffer.[22]

Background levels of CO_2 in the buffered bicarbonate samples diffuse through the PVC membrane into the unbuffered internal reference solution. This results in a steady-state change of hydrogen-ion activity at the internal interface of the PVC membrane and the electrode behaves like a bicarbonate electrode because there is no change in the outer membrane potential. However, current typical response times are 5–15 min and although this may be made shorter through using materials such as silicone rubber the sensor is fundamentally more suited to blood gas analysis systems rather than stat electrolyte analysers.

Magnesium. Although the body contains about 1 mole (24 g) magnesium, most of this is distributed intracellularly and only about 1% (0·9 mmol/l) is present in blood plasma. However, as with calcium, this is essential for normal neuromuscular and renal function. Magnesium ions, also like calcium ions, exhibit substantial binding to proteins (32%) and complexation to anions (13%) with only about 55% as free magnesium ions in the plasma. Currently, no ISE membrane is available which is sufficiently selective for magnesium to the exclusion of sodium and calcium in the concentrations encountered in plasma or extracellular fluid. Although no suitable sensor exists for measuring magnesium in plasma, electrodes which should be capable of measuring intracellular magnesium have been prepared.[5]

Lithium. An advantage that flame photometers have had over ISE instruments is their ability to measure lithium ions in plasma. Now, however, several ISE instruments are available for the measurement of lithium, although no sensor has sufficient selectivity to permit the measurement without extensive chemometric calibration routines. Some of these sensors are based on neutral carriers[6] while the remaining instruments use proprietary formulations. Although systems of this type will be useful in the therapeutic drug monitoring of lithium ions in blood, their performance has not been fully described.

APPENDIX

Variation of Activity Coefficient with Ionic Strength

The activity of an ion a_i is related to its concentration c_i by the relationship $a_i = \gamma_i c_i$ where γ_i is the activity coefficient. As anions must coexist in solution with cations, it is not possible to measure the individual activity coefficient of ions a_i but only their mean activity coefficients.

For a solution such as potassium chloride the mean activity coefficient is defined by the relationship.

$$\bar{\gamma}^2_{KCl} = \gamma_{K^+} \gamma_{Cl^-}$$

The mean activity coefficient $\bar{\gamma}^2_{KCl}$ is dependent on the ionic strength and one particular relationship, according to the Debye-Huckel equation, has been illustrated in Fig. 5. In general terms the mean activity coefficient γ_{MN} may be given, in terms of the concentration of all ions present, by the relationship:

$$\log \gamma_{MN} = \frac{-A \, |z_M z_N| \, I^{\frac{1}{2}}}{1 + BdI^{\frac{1}{2}}}$$

where I is the ionic strength, A, B are constants associated with the solvent, z_M, z_N are the charges on the ions, and d is the effective average diameter of the ions.

A number of different approaches have been used by Covington et al.[14] to calculate mean molar activity coefficients of physiologically important cations, using the theories of Debye-Huckel, Pitzer and Bates and Robinson with good accordance of the results of the different approaches.

Selectivity

Since a cation ion-selective electrode does not respond exclusively to the cation it is designed to measure, interfering ions will also contribute to the potentials generated. The extent to which an interfering cation affects the primary electrode response is described by the Nicolsky-Eisenman extension to the Nernst equation.

$$E = E_0 + \frac{RT}{z_M F} \ln \left[a_M + \sum_N K_{MN} (a_N) z_M / z_N \right]$$

K_{MN}, the selectivity constant, describes the degree of selectivity of the electrode for the primary cation, M, over the interfering cation, N, and z_M and z_N are the respective charges on the ions.

If $K_{MN} < 1$ then the electrode is more selective to M than N

$K_{MN} = 1$ then the electrode is equally responsive to both cations

$K_{MN} > 1$ then the electrode is more responsive to the interfering cation N

e.g. $K_{KNa} = 1.43 \times 10^{-4}$ i.e. the electrode is 7000 times more responsive to potassium than to sodium ions

(For calculations of selectivity constants, see reference 9.)

Liquid Junction Potentials

The liquid junction potential between two solutions 1 and 2 is given by the Planck equation:

$$E_j = \frac{-RT}{F} \int_1^2 \sum \frac{t_i}{z_i} d(\ln a_i)$$

where the integration limits relate to the composition of the two solutions and t_i, z_i and a_i are the transference number, the ionic charge and activity of the ith ion respectively.

This equation is valid for any type of junction, but since it contains individual ion activities which are indeterminable the precise value for E_j is unobtainable. To overcome this problem, assumptions are usually made, the most common of which is to assume linear concentration gradients which gives rise to the Henderson equation. Thus, the junction potential E_j at the junction test solution (1) KCl salt bridge (2) becomes

$$E_j = \frac{-RT}{F} \frac{U_1 - U_2}{V_1 - V_2} \cdot \ln \frac{V_1}{V_2}$$

where

$$U = \Sigma C_+ \cdot \lambda_+ - \Sigma C_- \cdot \lambda_-$$
$$V = \Sigma C_+ \cdot \lambda_+ \cdot z_+ + \Sigma C_- \cdot \lambda_- \cdot |z_-|$$

and C_+, C_- are the substance concentrations of both cations and anions of solutions (1) and (2), z_+, z_- are the ionic charges, and λ_+, λ_- are the limiting molar conductances. (For a more detailed account see reference 8.)

REFERENCES

1. Wipf H. K., Simon W. (1969). Selective K^+ transport through synthetic membranes using antibiotics in a potential gradient. *Biochem. Biophys. Res. Commun*; **34**: 707.
2. Simon W. (1971). Cation-specific electrode system. United States Patent 3 562 129.
3. Morf W. E., Simon W. (1978). Ion selective electrodes based on neutral carriers. In *Ion Selective Electrodes in Analytical Chemistry* (Freiser H., ed.) Vol. 1, pp. 211–86. New York: Plenum Press.
4. Eisenman G. (1969). Theory of membrane electrode potentials: an examination of the parameters determining the selectivity of solid and liquid ion exchangers and of neutral ion-sequestering molecules. In *Ion-Selective Electrodes* (National Bureau of Standards, Special Publication 314). (Durst R. ed.) pp. 1–56.
5. Ammann D., Erne D., Jenny H. B., Lanter F., Simon W. (1981). New ion-selective membranes. In *Progress in Enzyme and Ion-Selective Electrodes* (Lubbers D. W., Acker H., Buck R. P., Eisenman G., Kessler M., Simon W., eds) pp. 9–14. Berlin: Springer-Verlag.
6. Metzger E., Ammann D., Asper R., Simon W. (1986). Ion selective electrode membrane for the assay of lithium in blood serum. *Anal. Chem*; **58**: 132.
7. Simpson R. J. (1979). Practical techniques for ion-selective electrodes. In *Ion Selective Electrode Methodology* (Covington A K., ed.) Vol. 1, pp. 58–62. Boca Raton: CRC Press.
8. Covington A. K. (1969). Reference electrodes. In *Ion-Selective Electrodes* (National Bureau of Standards, Special Publication 314). (Durst R., ed.) pp. 107–41.
9. Bailey P. L. (1976). In *Analysis with Ion-Selective Electrodes* pp. 11–34. London: Heyden.
10. Waugh W. H. (1969). Utility of expressing serum sodium per unit of water in assessing hyponatraemia. *Metabolism*; **18**: 706.
11. Apple F. S., Koch D. D., Graves S., Ladenson J. H. (1982). Relationship between direct potentiometric and flame-photometric measurement of sodium in blood. *Clin. Chem*; **28**: 1931.

12. Forrest A. R. W., Shenkin A. (1980). Dangerous pseudohyponatraemia. *Lancet*; **ii**: 1256.
13. Czaban J. D., Cormier A. D., Legg K. D. (1982). The apparent suppression of Na/K data obtained with ion-selective electrodes is due to junction potential and activity coefficient effects, not bicarbonate binding. *Clin. Chem*; **28**: 1703 (and references quoted therein).
14. Draft recommendations on the direct potentiometric measurement of sodium and potassium ions in blood, plasma and serum (1985). European Working Group on Ion Selective Electrodes. Helsinki.
15. Mostert I. A., Anker P., Jenny H. B., Oesch U., Morf W. E., Ammann D., Simon W. (1985). Neutral carrier based silicone rubber membranes for H_3O^+, K^+, NH_4^+ and Ca^{2+} selective electrodes. *Mikrochimi. Acta*; **1**: 33.
16. Siggaard-Andersen O., Thode J., Wandrup J. (1981). The concentration of free calcium ions in the blood-plasma 'ionised calcium'. In *Blood pH, Carbon Dioxide, Oxygen and Calcium Ion* (Siggaard-Andersen O., ed.) pp. 163–90. Copenhagen: Private Press.
17. McLean F. C., Hastings A. B. (1934). A biological-method for the estimation of calcium ion concentration. *J. Biol. Chem*; **107**: 337.
18. Ross J. W. (1967). Calcium selective electrode with liquid ion exchanger. *Science*; **156**: 1378.
19. Tjell J. C., Ruzicka J. (1976). Calcium electrode and membrane and composition for use therein. British patent 1 437 091.
20. Draft recommendations on the measurement of ionised calcium in blood, serum and plasma (1985). European Working Group on Ion Selective Electrodes (Helsinki).
21. Marsoner H. J., Ritter C., Ghahramani M. (1986). Results with a new type of chloride sensitive liquid membrane electrode. Paper presented at 4th European Working Group on Ion-Selective Electrodes meeting. Helsinki.
22. Funck R. J. J., Morf W. E., Schulthess P., Ammann D., Simon W. (1982). Bicarbonate-sensitive liquid membrane electrodes based on neutral carriers for hydrogen ions. *Anal. Chem*; **54**: 423.

15. The Measurement of Blood-gases and pH

D. W. Hill

INTRODUCTION

A knowledge of the hydrogen ion concentration and of the oxygen and carbon dioxide tensions in the arterial blood is of considerable importance in the management of patients with respiratory problems and those in intensive care units (ICUs). In ICUs this information is required quickly and at regular intervals. In many cases such a unit may have its own equipment for the measurement of blood pH and gas tensions and there may be special requirements for small sample volumes if it is a Special Care Baby Unit. In other cases, reliance is placed upon the prompt service provided by a central hospital laboratory. Since, under either system, accurate results will be required at any hour of the day or night, the apparatus must be reliable as possible, easy to use and capable of being calibrated in a rapid and simple manner. There is much to be said for a system which flushes itself after each measurement cycle and is then ready to receive the next sample. However, even if the equipment fulfils these conditions, care must still be exercised in the drawing of the blood sample and its subsequent handling and storing prior to analysis. It is easy to contaminate the sample, to blow off high gas tensions or to allow a significant alteration in the values to occur as a result of metabolic action within the sample.

The electrode systems for pH, P_{O_2} and P_{CO_2}[1,2] measurements are mounted within a housing which contains the associated electronic circuitry and either a water bath for perfusing the outer jackets of the electrodes with circulating water at body temperature or the electrodes are mounted in a metal block whose temperature is thermostatically controlled. Provision is usually made for passing blood samples and calibration buffer solutions of known pH through metal tubing at the electrode temperature and for bubbling calibration gas mixtures through heat exchanger and humidifier coils at the electrode temperature.

The blood pH/blood gas analyser may be mounted on a mobile trolley complete with calibration mixtures for bedside use or it may be located on a laboratory bench.

Earlier forms of apparatus were quite compact and had an analogue indication of the sample's pH, P_{O_2} or P_{CO_2} on a meter which could be switched manually to the appropriate scale. These earlier instruments required a considerable amount of skill on behalf of the operator to calibrate them, load the sample and check that each electrode was functioning properly. The situation has changed dramatically in recent years with the advent of 'smart' systems having an on-board microcomputer. The program for the microcomputer ensures that the analyser is relatively foolproof in operation. An automatic cycle of calibration, introduction of the blood sample, rinsing, checking for correct operation and the calculation of derived variables is provided. By this means a relatively unskilled operator can handle a large number of blood samples with accurate results. These instruments are provided with a digital display and a printout of the results which can be obtained for reference. A further copy can be returned to the clinician.

THE MEASUREMENT OF pH

The Glass Electrode

The essential components of a pH meter are shown in Fig. 1. The solution whose pH is to be measured is placed in a cuvette connected with a measuring electrode and a reference electrode. These electrodes together with the solution can be considered as forming a battery whose EMF is proportional to the pH of the solution. In practice this battery has a high internal resistance, so that its EMF must be measured by means of an electrometer circuit. The output signal of the electrometer can then be calibrated in pH units. The measuring electrode is designed to be responsive to the hydrogen ion concentration of the sample, that is to its pH. The reference electrode is chosen to provide a constant reference potential against which changes in the potential developed by the measuring electrode can be recorded.

tration of H^+ ions in each solution. The glass wall of the bulb acts as a pH-sensitive membrane. The membrane does not have to be in the form of a bulb, it can be flat or in the form of a capillary tube.

A linear relationship exists between the output voltage of the glass-electrode:reference-electrode system and the pH of the blood sample, the line having a slope of approximately 60 mV per pH unit change. The slope is dependent upon the absolute temperature of the sample and increases by approximately 0·34% per °C, in practice, the sensitivity of a pH electrode should be checked at regular intervals

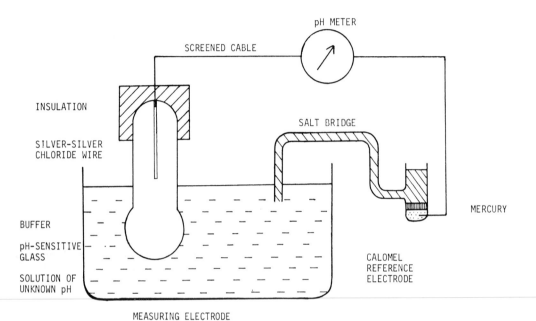

Fig. 1 Schematic diagram of a pH meter.

Laboratory pH meters now always employ a glass electrode as the measuring electrode.[3] The glass electrode is a membrane in which current transfer between the two solutions separated by the membrane is dominated by the hydrogen ions, the membrane acting as if it was permeable only to hydrogen ions. The tubular glass electrode has a thin-walled bulb at one end (Fig. 1). The bulb contains a buffer solution having a known, stable, pH value. A platinum wire dips into the buffer and is connected via a well-insulated, low-leakage, screened cable to the input active terminal of the pH meter. The upper end of the glass electrode is sealed to prevent leakage of the buffer. When the glass electrode is in contact with the sample solution, a DC potential arises between the inside and the outside surfaces of the bulb. The magnitude of the potential is proportional to the difference in pH between the buffer solution inside the bulb and the sample solution outside. It is assumed that this potential difference arises from an ion exchange occurring at the surfaces of the glass bulb, the exchange being controlled by the concen-

with buffer solutions of known value. If the sensitivity has become markedly reduced, the electrode should be etched according to the manufacturer's instructions or discarded. When a glass electrode has been in use for some time, its sensitivity and speed of response may diminish because its surface has become inactive as a result of a depletion of metal ions. A screen is thus formed which partly covers an active layer of the glass.

The effect is more noticeable when the electrode is used in solutions which contain protein, e.g. blood. Etching can partially restore the surface of the glass electrode. The electrode must be carefully rinsed between use with different samples or buffers to prevent cross-contamination.

Reference Electrodes

The function of the reference electrode is to provide a stable potential against which can be measured the changing EMF produced by the glass electrode in response to solutions of different pH values. Currently, some commercial pH meters for use with blood utilize calomel and some silver–silver chloride reference electrodes.

The Calomel Reference Electrode. The lower end of the calomel electrode is formed by an asbestos fibre or ceramic plug (Fig. 2). This acts as a liquid junction between the saturated KCl solution contained within

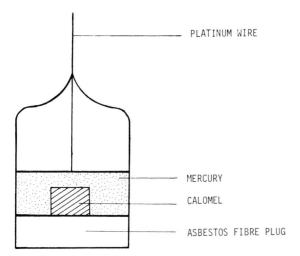

Fig. 2 A calomel reference electrode.

the body of the electrode and the sample. The tubular body of the electrode holds a reservoir of saturated KCl solution. Into this is immersed a cylinder of calomel (HgCl). Contact is made with the calomel by means of a blob of mercury and a platinum wire. The wire is joined to a lead connecting with the reference electrode terminal of the pH meter. The pores of the ceramic plug or of the asbestos fibre must not be allowed to become blocked and the calomel electrode should be thermostatted in order that it maintains a constant potential.

The Silver–Silver Chloride Reference Electrode. A silver–silver chloride reference electrode is shown in Fig. 3. A platinum wire makes contact with a layer of silver–silver chloride crystals held in place by a cotton filler in a saturated potassium chloride solution. A 'donut' of potassium chloride completes the circuit via a membrane to the sample. The sample is also in contact with the glass electrode. The potassium chloride forms a salt bridge as shown in Fig. 1. The silver–silver chloride electrode must also be thermostatted to maintain a constant potential.

The Liquid-junction Potential

The glass and reference electrodes are joined via the sample and the salt bridge. A 'liquid-junction potential' is generated at the junction of the sample and the salt bridge. If a reproducible liquid-junction potential exists together with a stable reference electrode potential, then the only variable EMF in the

pH electrode system is that due to the glass electrode. The response of a pH electrode to buffers may differ from its response to solutions which have markedly different physicochemical properties, e.g. whole blood. Kater et al.[4] have shown that differences in the residual junction potential can be a significant factor in the dependence of the measured pH on the nature of the sample. A reference sample of blood

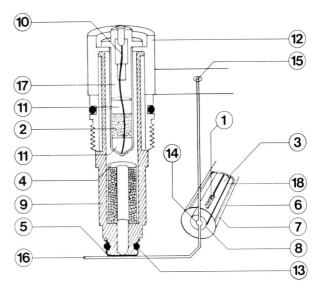

Fig. 3 A silver–silver chloride reference electrode. 1, AgCl bead; 2, Ag/AgCl crystals; 3, filling solution; 4, KCl donut; 5, membrane; 6, pH electrode; 7, plastic electrode body; 8, pH sensitive glass; 9, plastic reference shell; 10, platinum wire; 11, cotton filler; 12, reference electrode; 13, membrane O-ring; 14, sample chamber; 15, sample chamber exit fitting; 16, sample path; 17, saturated KCl solution; 18, silver wire. (Courtesy of Corning Medical.)

serum or plasma overcomes the stability problems of whole blood and has a composition more akin to whole blood than does a buffer. Bird and Henderson[5] have described the use of frozen serum as a reference material for whole blood pH measurement. An aliquot of the serum is thawed and equilibrated with a gas of known P_{CO_2}.

pH Meters

The output voltage from a glass electrode–reference electrode combination is normally zero when the solution in which the glass electrode is immersed is nearly neutral, i.e. the pH is in the region of 7. For acid solutions a positive output is obtained and this changes to negative when the solution is alkaline. The output changes by about 60 mV for each pH unit change. The internal resistance of a glass electrode is in the range of 100–1000 meg-ohms. Hence the millivoltmeter used to measure the potential difference produced by the electrode combination requires an input resistance of the order of 100 000 meg-ohms in order to reduce the loading effect of the circuit to less than 1%. A field effect transistor electrometer circuit is employed for this purpose. A typical range for a blood pH meter would be 6·000 to 8·000 ±0·005 pH units with the blood sample, glass electrode and reference electrode being thermostatted at 37°C ±0·15°C in a water bath or metal block. The pH meter must be able to detect changes of 0·001 pH units (60 μV). The meter is provided with balance and slope controls. The balance control adds a voltage in series with the pH electrode system and allows the operator to adjust the output indication to agree with the known pH value of a standard buffer. The slope control is an amplifier gain control which adjusts the sensitivity of the pH meter, i.e. the mV per pH unit.

Buffer Solutions for Use with Blood pH Meters. All pH measurements made with a glass electrode–reference electrode combination are relative, the unknown pH of the sample being compared with the accurately known pH values of the standard buffer solutions.

Suitable buffers for calibrating blood pH meters are: 6·840 pH buffer containing potassium dihydrogen phosphate, 25 mmol/l and sodium dihydrogen phosphate, 24·89 mmol/l plus 10 ml/l of mould inhibitor. A 7·384 pH buffer would contain potassium dihydrogen phosphate, 8·87 mmol/l and sodium dihydrogen phosphate, 30·3 mmol/l and sodium bicarbonate, 0·23 mmol/l plus 10 ml/l of mould inhibitor. Once buffers have been poured from their storage container they should never be returned. After pouring, the top of the container should be dried immediately and the cap replaced in order to prevent contamination. In some blood pH measurement systems, the pH output signal is arranged to be zero when the electrode is immersed in the pH 6·840 buffer. Any small potential difference existing in practice can be nulled by means of the meter's balance control. Theoretically, the sensitivity of a glass electrode at 37°C should be 61·5 mV per pH unit change. Hence when the pH meter's zero has been set with the pH 6·840 buffer, an output of 33·46 mV should occur with the pH 7·384 buffer. If this is not achieved exactly, the reading of the meter can be corrected by means of the slope control.

The Corning Model 178 Automated pH/Blood Gas System is illustrated in Fig. 4. The control panel is of a pressure-sensitive wipe-down construction. At a push-button command the blood sample is drawn into the analyser through a pre-heater into a common measuring cuvette (sample chamber) and the blood pH, Po_2 and Pco_2 measured. The path taken by the blood sample in passing between the reference electrode and the pH glass electrode is illustrated in Fig. 3. For pH, Po_2 and Pco_2 determinations a syringe blood sample of 200 μl is required. For capillary samples a volume of 85 μl is needed. Split capillary samples of 40 μl each can be handled. A thermostatted

stainless-steel block maintains the electrode set at 37°C ±0·2°C.

The model 178 is fitted with a narrow-bore sample port which stops clots entering the sample cuvette. The port can be quickly twisted free and cleaned off with gauze or water. The cuvette is transparent so that all the sample tubing and the electrode tips can be observed, enabling any air bubbles to be observed and cleared. Transparent gravity-fed containers feed reagents directly into the system without the need for pumps. An on-board internal system-diagnostics capability monitors all the system variables and constantly checks electrode performance, calibration drift, sample chamber condition and rotary sample port alignment.

Temperature Correction for Blood and Plasma pH

The temperature at which blood is stored *in vitro* will produce a reversible change in the acid–base state of the blood. Rosenthal[6] described a linear relationship between the temperature and the pH of a blood sample over the temperature range of 18°–38°C. The temperature coefficient of blood was 0·0147 pH units per °C. Burton[7] measured values of the temperature coefficients of blood pH in patients subjected to profound hypothermia during cardiac surgery. These values differed significantly from Rosenthal's mean value. He also discovered a linear relationship between the blood pH temperature coefficient and the logarithm of the blood Pco_2. Adamson et al.[8] also showed that the temperature coefficient of blood pH depends upon both the value of the blood pH measured at 38°C and the metabolic state of the blood.

The variation of plasma pH with temperature is less than that for whole blood, and is approximately 0·011 pH units per °C. This difference between whole blood and plasma will cause an alkaline error in the pH of plasma which is separated at temperatures of less than 37°C or in the pH of whole blood which is not completely mixed prior to measurement.

The Handling of Blood Samples for pH Measurement

Arterial blood is to be preferred for studies on the acid–base balance of patients and is essential if the sample is required for information on the adequacy of oxygenation. Fletcher[9] makes the point that samples from other sources are useful only as adjuncts or second-best substitutes in the assessment of ventilation and circulation. He indicates that peripheral venous blood, even if arterialized by warming the tissue, is useless for this purpose due to the variations in flow and oxygen uptake of peripheral tissues. 'Arterialized' capillary blood obtained after thoroughly warming the earlobe of adults or the foot of infants may be used as a substitute for arterial blood for the measurement of pH, Pco_2 and HCO_3. Capillary blood does not yield accurate results when the circulation is impaired and it is not usually suitable for the determination of arterial P_{O_2}.

For accurate studies, glass syringes which have been acid washed, thoroughly rinsed and autoclaved should be employed. Although disposable plastic syringes are convenient, they are likely to lead to errors in the measurement of the P_{O_2}. However, Laver and Seiflow[10] found plastic syringes to be satisfactory if no delay is foreseen in the measurement; 2 or 5 ml

sealed with plasticine. Before the capillary tube is offered up to the analyser a magnet is moved up and down the outside of the capillary to move the wire and thus mix the sample. Capillaries should be drilled as soon as they are sealed.

After calibrating the pH meter with the buffer solutions, the cuvette should be purged with air and the first aliquot of the blood sample introduced. When the pH meter reading has steadied, a second aliquot is introduced and the meter reading noted. Finally,

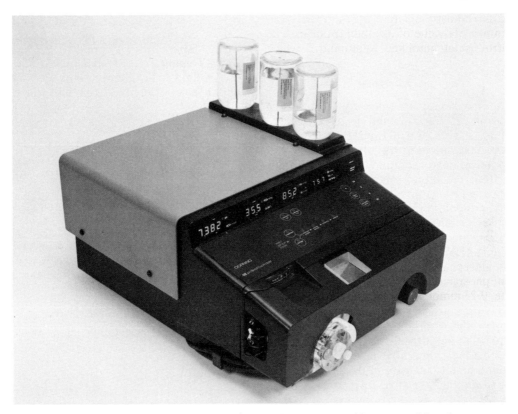

Fig. 4 Model 178 Automatic Blood pH/Blood Gas Analyser. (Courtesy of Corning Medical.)

syringes are suitable. The interior of the syringe should have been thoroughly wetted with heparin solution which should remain only in the dead space of the syringe and needle. The blood sample should be carefully drawn in an anaerobic fashion and the syringe quickly capped with a metal cap containing clean mercury. This both prevents air from remaining in contact with the sample and assists in obtaining a thorough mixing with the blood. The mercury should not be allowed to come into contact with the measuring electrodes or it will 'poison' them. The filled syringe should be stored in iced water to reduce metabolic changes in the blood if the measurement has to be delayed. It must be remembered that oxygen may be lost from samples with a high oxygen tension through metabolism and contact with room air. Capillary samples should be drawn into clean, glass capillary tubes containing dried heparin. A steel wire is then introduced and the ends of the capillary

a third aliquot is introduced and the average of the readings for the second and third aliquots taken. Hill and Tilsley[11] found that the use of 2 ml syringes for blood samples leads to a considerably higher degree of accuracy than is possible with capillary samples. The larger volume of blood allows the cuvette and inlet tubing to be thoroughly washed out. After use with blood samples, the pH electrode should immediately be rinsed out with saline and left filled with a solution – either saline or a buffer. In fully automatic blood-gas analysers, a rinse cycle follows on completion of the readings, the rinsing solution containing detergent.

THE MEASUREMENT OF BLOOD CARBON DIOXIDE TENSION

P_{CO_2} stands for the partial pressure of carbon dioxide. From Dalton's Law of Partial Pressures, the partial pressure of CO_2 in a sample of dry gas at 760 mmHg pressure with a CO_2 concentration of 6% by volume is $(6/100) \times 760 = 45 \cdot 6$ mmHg. If the gas is fully saturated with water vapour at 37 °C, at which temperature the water vapour pressure is 47 mmHg, the partial pressure of CO_2 in the mixture becomes $(6/100) \times (760 - 47) = 42 \cdot 8$ mmHg. If this mixture is in equilibrium with blood, the partial pressures of CO_2 in the gas and blood will be equal. Instead of referring to the partial pressure, it is customary to speak of the carbon dioxide tension in the blood, i.e. the blood P_{CO_2} is $42 \cdot 8$ mmHg. Normal values of CO_2 tension would be 35–45 mmHg for arterial blood and 41–51 mmHg for venous blood.

The P_{CO_2} Electrode

Blood P_{CO_2} is now measured directly by means of a CO_2 electrode.[12,13] Basically, the electrode for P_{CO_2} measurement consists of a pH-sensitive glass electrode arranged to measure the pH of a thin layer of sodium bicarbonate solution. This solution is separated from the blood sample by a polytetrafluoroethylene (Teflon) membrane which is permeable to CO_2 molecules in the blood, but not to other ions which might affect the pH of the bicarbonate solution. In practice, a combination of a glass pH electrode and a reference electrode is in contact with the bicarbonate solution. Carbon dioxide diffuses across the membrane in either direction depending upon the difference between its partial pressures on each side. Hydration of CO_2 in the water of bicarbonate solution produces carbonic acid and changes the solution's pH. The output millivoltage of the pH electrode system is logarithmically related to the pH of the solution, a tenfold increase in the P_{CO_2} is nearly equivalent to a reduction of one pH unit. Because of the slowness of the gas diffusion process relative to the speed of response, the glass electrode must be located as close as possible to the Teflon membrane. A second membrane is placed beneath the outer Teflon membrane. It acts as a wick to contain a thin layer of bicarbonate solution between the outer membrane and the electrodes. This wets the electrodes and serves as a junction between the outer membrane and the electrodes. The inner membrane may be made of Cellophane or Nylon. In one design, the inner membrane is attached to the combined glass and reference electrode by means of an O-ring, a second O-ring attaches the outer membrane to the end of the cuvette into which slide the combined electrodes. In later designs, the Teflon outer membrane has been replaced by one made from silicone rubber and this change enables a 95% response time of 60 s to be achieved.

The Corning Model 178 Automated pH/Blood Gas System covers a P_{CO_2} range of $5 \cdot 0$–$250 \cdot 0$ mmHg with a resolution of $0 \cdot 1$ mmHg. On the SI system of units, P_{CO_2} is quoted in terms of kilopascals where 1 mmHg = $0 \cdot 133$ kPa. The range quoted thus

becomes $0 \cdot 67$–$33 \cdot 33$ kPa with a resolution of $0 \cdot 01$ kPa.

When a silicone rubber membrane is fitted to a Corning P_{CO_2} electrode, the response time is 98 s for a 98% response. This is equivalent to four time constants, so that the time constant is approximately 25 s. The measurement is made at 37 °C, time having been allowed for the blood sample to come into thermal equilibrium with the thermostatted cuvette. For a cold sample initially at $0 \cdot 4$ °C the time to achieve equilibrium with the cuvette at 37 °C is 30 s.

Calibrating a P_{CO_2} Electrode

Using Tonometered Blood Samples. The most accurate method for calibrating both P_{CO_2} and P_{O_2} electrodes is to use blood samples which have been

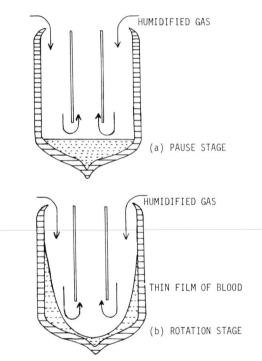

Fig. 5 Cross-section of a thin film tonometer Type 237. (Courtesy of Instrumentation Laboratory.)

tonometered with gas mixtures having known partial pressures of carbon dioxide and oxygen. Although this procedure is more time consuming than merely passing a known gas mixture through the cuvette containing the electrodes, it does remove any discrepancies which may arise when an electrode calibrated with known partial pressures is then used to measure blood-gas tensions. The compact tonometer Type 237 by Instrumentation Laboratory Inc. (Fig. 5), rotates the sample vessel, rather than oscillates it, in the thermostatted water bath. An even thin film of blood is thus formed on the wall of the vessel. The blood sample volume can lie in the range $0 \cdot 1$–10 ml. The speed of equilibration is further enhanced by segmenting the rotation cycle with brief interruptions.

The use of intermittent rotation, rather than continuous oscillation is claimed to prevent the possibility of the occurrence of a significant degree of haemolysis.

The Use of Standard Gas Mixtures for the Calibration of a P_{CO_2} Electrode. When a P_{CO_2} or P_{O_2} electrode is calibrated with standard gas mixtures, these should first have been passed through a pre-heating spiral in the water bath or heated metal block housing the electrodes and then through a humidifier. The passage of dry gas through the cuvette for extended periods will dry out the electrodes. It is important that the gas mixture should not run through a length of rubber or plastic tubing at a slow rate or CO_2 may be lost by diffusion. If an extensive calibration is being performed, the cuvette should periodically be flushed to keep the electrode membrane moist.

Since the P_{CO_2} electrode is basically a pH electrode, the principles of establishing the isoelectric point and the slope of the calibration line are essentially the same. The gas mixture which is employed to simulate the P_{CO_2} of normal blood is usually 5% CO_2, 12% O_2 and 83% N_2. The second gas mixture used to adjust the slope of the calibration is 10% CO_2, 90% N_2. In one commercial P_{CO_2} electrode it is arranged that the isoelectric point occurs at a P_{CO_2} of approximately 35 mmHg (5% CO_2). If x% by volume is the percentage of CO_2 in a calibration mixture which has been humidified at 37 °C, then the corresponding tension in mmHg is given by

$$\frac{(b - 47)x}{100}$$

where b is the barometric pressure in mmHg.

The Temperature Sensitivity of a P_{CO_2} Electrode

The combination of the effects of temperature changes upon the sensitivity of the pH electrode and the P_{CO_2} of the blood sample produce a total temperature sensitivity coefficient for the P_{CO_2} electrode of approximately 8% per °C. Thus a P_{CO_2} electrode should be thermostatted to within at least ± 0.1 °C by means of a circulating-water bath or heated metal block.

The Handling of Blood Samples for a P_{CO_2} Electrode

The cuvette containing the electrode should first be purged with a gas mixture which has a P_{CO_2} value close to that expected in the blood sample. When a large difference exists between the partial pressure in the cuvette and the tension in the blood sample, it may be necessary to pass additional blood through the cuvette in order to obtain a true meter reading for the P_{CO_2}. If pure CO_2 has been used to check the sensitivity of the electrode, the cuvette should be washed out with saline to remove dissolved CO_2 from the membrane and the walls.

Teisseire[14] recommends the use of an arterial blood sample of 3 ml volume drawn into a luer-lock glass syringe, free of air bubbles. He points out that heparin must only remain in the syringe's 'dead' space. Too small a volume of blood (less than 1 ml) when diluted with a similar volume of heparin will lead to a decrease in the pH, P_{CO_2} and total CO_2.

After drawing the sample, the syringe should immediately be capped, agitated and unless it is to be analysed in the near future, it should be stored in ice–water in a vacuum flask. Teisseire states that the person taking the blood sample should carry it personally to the laboratory together with a request form giving the ventilatory conditions for the patient (FIO_2, minute volume, ventilatory frequency, and details of any positive end-expiratory pressure) and the patient's temperature. He says that not more than 20 min should elapse between sampling and analysis.

Freshly drawn blood at body temperature continues to use oxygen and produce carbon dioxide. Hence its oxygen tension falls and its CO_2 tension rises. Lunn and Mapleson[15] found that the P_{CO_2} of blood samples stored in ice–water will change by less than 2.5% of the initial tension during periods of up to at least 2 h and possibly up to 4 h. After storage on ice, the cells and plasma must be mixed again. This can be accomplished by rolling the syringe between the hands.

There is no difference in the calibration of a P_{CO_2} electrode with gas or blood, unlike the polarographic oxygen electrode.

THE MEASUREMENT OF BLOOD OXYGEN TENSION

P_{O_2} stands for the partial pressure of oxygen. From Dalton's Law of Partial Pressures, the partial pressure of oxygen in a sample of dry gas at 760 mmHg pressure with an oxygen concentration of 20% is $(20/100) \times 760 = 152$ mmHg. If the gas is fully saturated with water vapour at 37 °C, the partial pressure of oxygen in the mixture becomes $(20/100) \times (760 - 47) = 142.6$ mmHg. If this gas mixture is in equilibrium with blood, the resulting oxygen tension is 142.6 mmHg (19 kPa).

Polarographic Electrodes for the Measurement of the Oxygen Tension of Whole Blood

Whereas the pH and P_{CO_2} electrodes both make use of a glass electrode, the polarographic oxygen electrode works on a different principle. The glass electrode–reference electrode combination generates an EMF, but the polarographic electrode is supplied with a constant voltage and generates a current which is proportional to the oxygen tension surrounding the cathode.

The polarographic oxygen electrode is supplied with a constant polarizing voltage of the order of 0.6 V and produces a current whose magnitude is proportional to the oxygen tension diffusing to the cathode surface of the electrode. This current arises from the reduction of oxygen at the electrode's cathode according to the equation $O_2 + 2H_2O + 4e^- = 4OH^-$. In Fig. 6, the potentiometer R placed across the mercury battery B taps off about $0.6\,V$ and applies this across the polarographic cell consisting of a platinum cathode and a silver–silver chloride anode. The anode functions as a reference electrode. In simple arrangements with large area electrodes the cell current can be measured with a sensitive galvanometer.

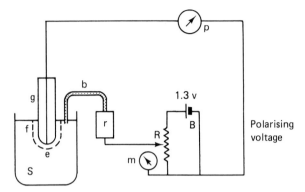

Fig. 6 Basic polarographic arrangement for the measurement of blood oxygen tension: b, salt bridge; r, silver–silver chloride reference electrode; e, platinum cathode; f, membrane; g, glass sheath; s, solution of unknown Po_2; m, millivoltmeter; p, Po_2 meter; B, mercury battery; R, potentiometer.

Each molecule of oxygen reaching the cathode reacts with four electrons and the resulting flow of electrons is measured with a current amplifier. Electrons for this reaction are provided by the silver–silver chloride electrode as silver is oxidized at the anode according to: $Ag + Cl^- = AgCl + e^-$. With this arrangement, each molecule of oxygen reaching the surface of the cathode will be almost immediately reduced. The reduction current is proportional to the amount of oxygen reaching the electrode per unit time. The current is proportional to the oxygen available to the electrode while it is in contact with the sample and not directly to the oxygen tension of the sample. To ensure that the output current from the electrode is a measure of the oxygen tension of the sample, the oxygen must be transported to the cathode only by diffusion. For a correctly functioning polarographic electrode the oxygen tension at the cathode surface will be zero and the amount of oxygen transported to the cathode by diffusion will depend on the difference in the oxygen tensions between the cathode and the sample, i.e. to the oxygen tension of the sample.

The operation of the polarographic electrode removes oxygen from the sample and thus the tension would decrease. In earlier models of polarographic electrodes, it was necessary to agitate the blood sample, for example by continuous shaking, to bring up fresh blood to prevent a decrease in the oxygen tension reading. However, modern blood-gas analysers

utilize a small area cathode working in conjunction with a sensitive current amplifier and agitation is no longer required. In principle, the use of a bare oxygen electrode is attractive, since it can be made sufficiently small to pass down the lumen of a hypodermic needle. In practice a bare electrode requires frequent cleaning when used in tissue or whole blood to remove deposits of protein which 'poison' the electrode. Clark[16] overcame this problem by placing both the platinum cathode and the reference electrode behind a membrane which completely separates them from the blood sample. The membrane is usually made of polytetrafluoroethylene (Teflon).

The oxygen electrode in the Instrumentation Laboratory Inc. Model 1306 Automatic pH/Blood Gas Analyser provides an oxygen tension range of 0–800 mmHg (0–106.6 kPa). The measurement is available 70 s after the sample is introduced into the cuvette and for the Corning Model 178 the range is 0–999 mmHg (0–100 kPa). Mapleson et al.[17] have shown that the response time of a Clark-type polarographic electrode can vary from day to day, and that on average the response is considerably slower than would have been suspected. For their electrode and membranes a 100% response time exceeded 10 min and varied with the Po_2 value of the blood. Rhodes and Moser[18] have discussed possible sources of error which can arise in Po_2 measurements. Evans and Cameron[19] found that nitrous oxide could significantly affect the oxygen tension reading given by some Corning Model 165 blood-gas analyser oxygen electrodes. For example, blood equilibrated at 37 °C with a mixture of 90% nitrous oxide and 10% oxygen gave an apparent oxygen tension reading of 117–130 mmHg instead of the expected 76 mmHg. They make the point that a severe arterial hypoxaemia may go undetected in the presence of nitrous oxide. Severinghaus et al.[12] show that oxygen electrodes can also be affected by the anaesthetic agent halothane.

Oxygen electrodes of small diameter have been designed for intravascular oxygen tension measurements. Scott et al.[20] found that pulsing the polarizing voltage of 0.65 V for 1 s on, 1 s off, diminishes the under-reading which occurs at low blood-flow rates with a constant polarization voltage. The combination of thin membranes and pulsed polarography produces a Po_2 electrode with a fast response time without under-reading the true in vivo Po_2. They covered the blood velocity range of 6–20 cm/s.

Parker et al.[21] described a new approach to in-line gas monitoring using a disposable Clark-type oxygen sensor. This sensor has been utilized by Claremont et al.[22] to monitor continuously the oxygen tension of the circulating blood in an extracorporeal circulation.

Calibrating a Po_2 Electrode

Preferably, tonometered blood samples should be used to eliminate the difference which may exist for a given oxygen electrode between a true blood and a gas calibration. Bird et al.[23] have compared the blood:gas factor for three different oxygen electrodes. For the IL Model 313 there was no significant blood-gas difference for oxygen tensions of less than 150 mmHg, but for the Radiometer Model E 5046 electrode the mean blood:gas difference ranged from 1·8 to 5·7%. Beetham[24] states that the blood:gas difference arises from the fact that oxygen diffusion is hindered in liquids and that liquids will indicate lower oxygen tension values. He quotes differences of the order of 2–6% at normal oxygen tension levels but this figure may increase to as much as 12% at very high oxygen tension values. The tonometer design must allow for anaerobic sampling of blood. Accurate Po_2 measurements are based upon accurately known calibration gases whose oxygen partial pressure has been determined with a precision paramagnetic oxygen analyser or a Lloyd–Haldane chemical analyser. Beetham[24] reminds users that microbial contamination may give rise to falsely low oxygen tension readings and that flushing the cuvette with a bacteriostatic agent (as recommended by the manufacturer) should be performed at regular intervals. The cathode may enlarge during use due to the deposition of silver and this will alter the electrode's response time. The silver deposit may be removed periodically by mechanical abrasion or by the use of concentrated nitric acid.

A truly zero oxygen tension is difficult to obtain merely by bubbling nitrogen through blood and it may be necessary to use a reducing agent such as sodium bisulphite. Heitmann et al.[25] analysed the performance of commercial Po_2 electrodes in terms of their residual current, sensitivity, response time and linearity. They used a glycerine–water mixture for calibration which gave identical readings to blood with a 40% haematocrit. Hulands et al.[26] employed a 30% glycerol in water solution equilibrated with a gas of known oxygen tension to calibrate the oxygen electrode response. However in some blood-gas analysers the blood:gas factor is small and the use of glycerol solutions may not be worthwhile.[23] For the calibration of the Po_2 electrode it is convenient to utilize the two gas mixtures employed to calibrate the Pco_2 electrode, i.e. 10% CO_2 + 90% N_2; 5% CO_2 + 12% O_2 + 83% N_2. The first mixture serves for setting the zero reading and the second for adjusting the analyser to read 12% oxygen.

The Correction of the Blood Oxygen Tension Value for the Patient's Body Temperature

Modern automatic blood-gas and pH analysers are fitted with on-board computers which can calculate the correction of the values for pH, Pco_2 and Po_2 measured at 37 °C for the patient's actual temperature. Kelman and Nunn[27] derived a set of nomograms for the conversion of blood Po_2, Pco_2, pH and base excess for time and temperature.

Teisseire[14] states that the formulae used for the correction of pH and Pco_2 are nearly identical on a number of analysers; this is not the case for the correction of oxygen tension according to the results in the literature. Some formulae use a saturation value calculated from the pH and Po_2 measurements and others only take into account the value of the measured Po_2. Teisseire cites the correction of an oxygen tension of 100 mmHg at 37 °C–25 °C where the corrected values range from 46–62·5 mmHg depending on the correction formula used. The variation found was significant and far greater than the measurement error. He points out that the problem of the temperature correction for Po_2 is complicated due to the action of different haemoglobin ligands; depending on the temperature, the interactions of these different ligands, and especially on changes in the effects of pH, CO_2, 2,3-diphosphoglycerate and temperature as functions of the oxygenation level of the haemoglobin molecule.

QUALITY CONTROL IN BLOOD pH AND BLOOD-GAS MEASUREMENTS

A number of studies have been reported of the comparative performance of commercial blood-gas analysers, such as those of Hill and Tilsley[11] and Burnett et al.[28] It is important to stress the need for continual vigilance in handling the standards. Buffers should be stored in a manner which prevents the absorption of atmospheric carbon dioxide and the growth of moulds. They should not be left open to the air or stored in a refrigerator since this will accelerate CO_2 absorption.

Calibration gases should be purchased from a reputable manufacturer who will provide a certificate of analysis. If suitable compressors are available calibration gas mixtures can be prepared on the spot in the laboratory. When filled the cylinders should be stored for not less than 24 h in a horizontal position to ensure that the contents are thoroughly mixed. Neoprene tubing is recommended for the connection of the cylinder to the blood-gas analyser since gas exchange can occur through thin-walled polyvinyl tubing.

Burnett et al.[28] describe the use of seven different types of commercial quality control materials for the quality assessment of pH and blood-gas analysers. In a comparison of four commercial quality control materials equilibrated in sealed ampoules at 21 °C or 26 °C there were maximum differences for an aqueous mixture with haemoglobin (PRIME) and smaller differences for two aqueous buffers without haemoglobin (GAS and Contril) and none for a fluorocarbon-containing emulsion (ABC).[29] These observations exemplified the difficulties encountered with the influence of ambient temperature on Po_2 in PRIME and the stability of abc.

Care must be taken when collecting blood samples from patients. The sample should be drawn from the required site from the correct patient and must be properly labelled. It must be drawn without coming into contact with the air; an anticoagulant should be used; and provision should be made for mixing the sample prior to analysis. For accurate results it is best to use glass syringes. The analysis should be performed as soon as possible and at most within 20 min unless the sample is cooled to 0–4 °C in which case it may be stored for up to 2 h.[13]

Samples must be mixed and warmed to the temperature of the electrodes before measurements are taken. Care must be taken to avoid the introduction of air bubbles into the sample pathway of the analyser. The sample path, including the electrode cuvette, should be visible to the operator to avoid the presence of air bubbles passing unnoticed. If the membrane of a Pco_2 or Po_2 electrode becomes punctured, large errors in the reading will result. Modern analysers therefore provide a continuous monitoring of electrode integrity. The electrodes are normally thermostatted at 37 °C: it should be remembered that a change in temperature of 1 °C will produce changes of about 0·015 pH units, 4% in Pco_2 and 7% in Po_2. Sufficient time must be allowed for calibration or sample readings to have equilibrated. Analysers now have a 'Data Ready' circuit to alert the operator to the fact that a reliable set of readings is now available.

Tris (hydroxymethylaminomethane) buffer has a higher temperature coefficient than the two phosphate buffers normally used for the pH electrode calibration and Ladenson and Davis[30] have made use of this property to detect errors in blood pH measurements arising from variations occurring in the temperature of measurement.

A simple daily check procedure on the performance of a blood pH/blood-gas analyser is to tonometer an aliquot of whole pooled serum with a gas mixture having a known Pco_2 and to measure the pH of the serum. Then an aliquot of whole blood is tonometered with a gas mixture which has a known Po_2 and Pco_2 and these values are measured with the analyser. The deviation is plotted on a daily basis. Any marked divergence in the plots can then be promptly investigated.

Veefkind et al.[31] used carbon dioxide and oxygen tonometered phosphate–bicarbonate–glycerol–water mixture for the calibration and control of pH, Pco_2 and Po_2.

AUTOMATION

The original manually operated blood pH/blood-gas analyser demanded a considerable amount of skill on behalf of the operator in calibrating the electrodes and in checking blood-gas factors, as well as in the handling of the blood samples. However, the availability of direct-reading electrodes for blood oxygen and carbon dioxide tensions opened up possibilities of improved therapy for patients in intensive care situations. The setting-up of the analyser could be

a distinct problem, particularly for junior medical staff working at night in intensive therapy units. If the analyser was not, in the heat of the moment, thoroughly rinsed out following use, blood clots could put the analyser out of action until the pathways were cleared out. The need in intensive therapy units to have measurements available on a 24 h basis, has led to the development of analysers such as the Instrumentation Laboratories IL 1306, Corning 178 (Fig. 4) and Radiometer ABL4. These operate under onboard microcomputer control and are naturally more expensive than the simpler manual instruments, but as far as possible they render the measurements independent of the operator.

With the Corning 178 analyser, a one-point calibration is automatically performed every 30 min and a two-point calibration every 24 h. Additional calibrations are immediately available at a touch of the control panel. The Model 178 automatically adjusts all values to correspond with the ambient atmospheric pressure. The sample pathway is emptied and the calibration buffer is fed into the system from a gravity-fed glass container. Slope and calibration gas mixtures at a controlled flow are passed in turn into the analyser to be warmed, humidified and passed over the Po_2 and Pco_2 electrodes. During the equilibration period, the Model 178 simultaneously monitors the response of each electrode and will not display end-point values until electrode stability has been achieved.

A 'select sample mode' display informs the operator that the sample chamber has automatically been cleared of the previous specimen and that the next sample may be introduced after selection of the syringe or capillary tube inlet ports. On initiating the sample routine, a sample volume of either 200 µl (syringe) or 85 µl (capillary) is aspirated into the analyser. Sampling is prevented if a successful calibration has not been performed. The narrow bore sample port is designed to prevent clots from entering the sample cuvette. When stable pH, Po_2 and Pco_2 values have been displayed, a vigorous automatic flushing of the analyser's internal pathways is initiated with a gas-equilibrated flushing solution to remove all traces of the blood sample so that protein contamination of the pH glass electrode cannot occur.

A compact desk-top computer such as the Hewlett Packard Model 85 can be connected to the Model 178 analyser to provide print-out of the results and the computer's keyboard can be used to enter details of the patient's identification and with the data management software package the computer can also print up a 24-hour calibration history, a cumulative quality control history and a 31-day plot of the quality control results. Approximately 40 blood samples can be handled per hour with intermediate autocalibration. Corning market their own range of 'Confirm' quality-control reagents which are injected directly from their pressurized cannister into the analyser's sample port to eliminate the chance of room air contamination. Known values corresponding with conditions of alkalosis, normal and acidosis are available. Leary et al.[32] have compared commercial blood-gas quality control material with tonometered blood.

Another automatic blood pH/blood-gas analyser is the Radiometer Model ABL3. This automatically produces two fluids of known pH, Po_2 and Pco_2 by equilibrating two calibrating solutions with two gas mixtures. The gas mixtures having 5·61% and 11·29% CO_2 in air are obtained by mixing pure carbon dioxide and room air by means of a gas-mixing unit which contains no moving parts and uses viscosity-dependent pneumatic resistors to determine the relative proportions of the gas mixtures. Any changes in the gas concentrations arising from either a blocked air filter or an insufficient carbon dioxide supply are indicated by a warning lamp. Under operator control, two-point calibrations may be performed every 2, 4, 6 or 8 h and one-point calibrations every 1 or 2 h.

The ABL3 measures the barometric pressure and also the haemoglobin content of the sample by measuring the transmission of 505 nm wavelength light through the sample contained in a 0·15 mm pathlength cuvette. Approximately 20 samples can be handled per hour. The sample volume of blood required is 125 μl. The versatility of the ABL range has been extended in the latest ABL4 analyser by including an ion-selective electrode to measure the potassium concentration in the blood sample.

Use of Telephone Data Links with Blood pH/Blood-Gas Analysers

The availability of satisfactory blood pH/blood-gas analysers has led to their use in departments such as intensive therapy units, special care baby units and respiratory function laboratories. Burnett et al.[28] found that analysers associated with hospital clinical biochemistry departments gave a better performance than those located outside such laboratories. Corning cite the case of one of their blood pH/blood-gas analysers located in the major injuries unit but operating under the oversight of the technical staff in the biochemistry laboratory some four miles distant.

A control interface card in the analyser links to a standard modem unit enabling tones to be sent via the telephone line to a microcomputer and modem in the biochemistry laboratory. This approach allows remote control of the functions of the analyser and immediate access to the data file even when the analyser is unattended. The data files consist of calibration, diagnostics, quality control data and a maintenance file. The laboratory staff can thus inspect a performance summary before they leave to carry out a scheduled maintenance visit or to effect a repair. It can also be arranged that data stored in blood pH/blood-gas analysers can be captured by the main laboratory or hospital computer to update patients' records.

Corning also quote a situation where local cables in a hospital are used to link blood pH/blood-gas analysers in the intensive therapy and special care baby units with the biochemistry laboratory respectively 200 and 300 m distant.

Derived Variables

A number of blood pH/blood-gas analysers make use of their internal microcomputer to calculate derived variables from the measured pH, Po_2 and Pco_2 data. The Corning Model 178 calculates Actual Bicarbonate, Base Excess and Oxygen Saturation. Details of the patient's body temperature and haemoglobin values are input via the control panel of the analyser. The ABL3 measures the patient's haemoglobin and is fed with details of the patient's temperature in order to calculate plasma bicarbonate, total CO_2, base excess, oxygen saturation, standard bicarbonate and oxygen content. In the case of the calculation of the percentage oxygen saturation, consideration must be given to the patient's condition to ensure that a normal oxygen dissociation curve obtains in order to calculate oxygen saturation from tension.

Beetham[24] discusses the derivation of results from the primary set of measurements taken by a blood pH/blood-gas analyser. Plasma bicarbonate is calculated from the measured pH and Pco_2 values fed into the Henderson–Hasselbalch equation. Beetham says that the derivation assumes a constant value of pK′ and the solubility coefficient, α, which are generally taken to be 6·104 and 0·23 mmol/J respectively. Both values are affected slightly by changes in ionic strength, temperature and pH. Any or all these may be altered in the very ill.

Base excess is obtained from the calculated bicarbonate, measured pH and haemoglobin concentration values. Beetham concludes that in practice marked changes in the haemoglobin concentration do not appear to produce much effect on the calculated value for the base excess. This may be a reflection of the weighting factor placed on the haemoglobin concentration in the particular algorithm used to calculate base excess rather than a true reflection on the contribution of haemoglobin to base excess.

A knowledge of the oxygen content (volume %) of oxygen carried by the blood is important, in addition to a knowledge of the oxygen and carbon dioxide tension since the availability of a satisfactory flux of oxygen is essential for the wellbeing of any tissue. The oxygen carried by the blood expressed in terms of total ml of oxygen per 100 ml of blood consists of a major portion which is oxygen chemically combined with haemoglobin and a minor portion which is oxygen physically dissolved in the plasma. In patients having a low haemoglobin concentration, the oxygen tension and saturation values may indicate an adequate oxygenation, but when there is little haemoglobin available for the transport of oxygen, there may in reality be a deficiency of oxygen in the tissues.

It is usually considered that 1 g of haemoglobin completely saturated with oxygen can transport 1·39 ml of oxygen. Thus the amount of oxygen combined with haemoglobin is given by the haemoglobin content in grams per 100 ml $\times$ 1·39 $\times$ percentage oxyhaemoglobin. The volume of oxygen in ml dissolved in 100 ml of plasma is given by 100 $\times$ 0·003 where 0·003 is the Bunsen solubility coefficient for oxygen in plasma, i.e. for each 1 mmHg Po_2, 0·003 ml of oxygen can be dissolved in 100 ml of blood at 37 °C.

For a patient having a haemoglobin concentration of 15 g/100 ml, Po_2 = 50 mmHg and HbO_2 = 85%, the oxygen content = 15 $\times$ 1·39 $\times$ 0·85 + 50 $\times$ 0·003 = 17·8 ml/100 ml.

The haemoglobin content and the percentage oxyhaemoglobin in a 350 μl blood sample can both be measured with an oximeter such as the Model 282 by Instrumentation Laboratory. This can be interfaced directly to Instrumentation Laboratory blood pH/blood-gas analysers. A number of other parameters can also be calculated such as the alveolar–arterial oxygen gradient, the respiratory index, arterial–mixed venous oxygen gradient, and if the cardiac output is known, the physiological shunt.

The availability of on-board computing power and reliable electrodes and oximeters is making possible the production of as many values of respiratory and acid–base parameters as the management of the patient and a study of his physiology requires.

TRANSCUTANEOUS OXYGEN AND CARBON DIOXIDE TENSION ELECTRODES

The most accurate method of measuring arterial blood oxygen and carbon dioxide tensions is to use a conventional blood-gas analyser with samples of the patient's arterial blood as previously described. However, this 'direct' method requires access to arterial blood and is discontinuous. With infants, there is also the added problem of the limited amount of blood which can be withdrawn. In a number of clinical circumstances there is a requirement to be able to monitor continuously and 'indirectly' without puncturing an artery. A major application of this approach has evolved in the transcutaneous monitoring of oxygen tension in neonates and during anaesthesia.

Transcutaneous Oxygen Electrodes

Baumberger and Goodfriend[33] first reported that oxygen diffusion through warmed skin was sufficient to provide an estimate of the arterial oxygen tension. In their experiments a finger was placed in warm water and the oxygen tension was measured. In practice, the oxygen tension of heated skin is measured with a membrane-covered polarographic electrode.

To enhance the diffusion of oxygen through the skin, the skin circulation must be 'arterialized'. This can be accomplished by heating the skin to a temperature in the range of 43–44 °C

A Clark-type polarographic oxygen electrode is located inside a plastic housing some 1·5 cm in diameter and attached to the skin by means of a double-sided adhesive ring. There is also an electrical heating element and a temperature measuring thermistor. By means of a temperature control circuit, the temperature of the skin beneath the housing can be maintained at a pre-set temperature. For neonates this might be 43 °C and for adults 44 °C; at 45 °C there is a serious danger of burning the skin. The electrode is polarized with a voltage in the range 400–850 mV so it operates on the plateau of its voltage-current characteristic.

The active surface of the electrode's platinum cathode is isolated from the skin by a membrane which can be of polytetrafluoroethylene or polypropylene. Rafferty et al.[34] used a transcutaneous oxygen electrode having a 15 μm thick polypropylene membrane operating at 45 °C with an electrolyte consisting of 95% ethylene glycol and 5% Type II purified water. They placed the electrode in the third or fourth intercostal space close to the sternum, and allowed 20 min for the electrode to stabilize. Al-Diaidy et al.[35] placed the transcutaneous ($tcPo_2$) electrode on the abdomen in neonates and on the anterior chest wall below the clavicle in adults; these positions were selected as having a good cutaneous blood supply.

Transcutaneous oxygen electrodes can be pre-calibrated by immersing them in water at the operating temperature equilibrated with air and with corrections made for the barometric pressure and the partial pressure of water vapour. The zero can be set with water bubbled through with pure nitrogen or a sodium bisulphite solution may be employed. Rafferty et al.[34] set 0% oxygen by bubbling through with a mixture of 5% carbon dioxide, 95% nitrogen and calibrated with a mixture of (12% O_2, 78% N_2, 10% CO_2).

Particularly in the case of monitoring neonates with delicate skins, the site of the electrode should be changed every 2–3 h to avoid excessive skin irritation. The accuracy of the $tcPo_2$ readings depends upon the presence of an adequate peripheral circulation. If this falls, the $tcPo_2$ reading is low. Hugh et al.[36] provide a good review of $tcPo_2$ monitoring. They used the heating power needed to maintain the pre-set temperature as a crude index of the degree of peripheral circulation beneath the electrode. Continuous $tcPo_2$ monitoring has been used for example, in sick children, in normal anaesthetized adults and during cardiopulmonary bypass surgery and bronchoscopy for cystic fibrosis.

Rozkovec[37] states that there is a better correlation of $tcPo_2$ with arterial Po_2 in neonates than adults and in well rather than sick subjects. In seriously ill patients $tcPo_2$ tends to underestimate Pao_2, there is a wide range of error and thus reliance on the transcutaneous oxygen electrode reading alone for a warning of impending hypoxia can be both misleading and potentially dangerous. The main application of tcP_{O_2} monitoring can be to alert the clinician to rapid changes rather than the provision of absolute values.

A number of factors affect the value of the transcutaneous oxygen tension such as the properties of the patient's skin, the adequacy of the peripheral circulation and the patient's core temperature. Underreading occurs with the patient in shock or hypothermic, and may suggest that the patient is hypoxic. The administration of oxygen can be dangerous to

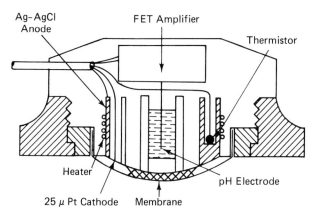

Fig. 7 Schematic diagram of a combined O_2/CO_2 transcutaneous sensor. (Reproduced with permission from Parker and Delpy[39].)

the patient under some circumstances. Commercial versions of tcP_{O_2} electrodes incorporate two thermistors for safety reasons and thermal cut-outs to guard against excess electrode temperatures. A schematic diagram of the construction of one form of tcP_{O_2} electrode is shown in Fig. 7.

Transcutaneous P_{CO_2} Electrodes

Severinghaus *et al.*[38] have described the construction, calibration and temperature-gradient problems of a transcutaneous carbon dioxide electrode. They showed that the carbon dioxide tension of the blood in the capillary loops of the skin dermis lying beneath the heated electrode was higher than the true arterial carbon dioxide tension by a factor of approximately 1·3.

Parker and Delpy[39] ascribe the over-reading of a heated tcP_{CO_2} electrode to three factors.

1. Heating decreases the solubility of CO_2 thus increasing P_{CO_2}.
2. Heating increases the tissue metabolism beneath the sensor and causes an increase in CO_2 production.
3. Heating increases the diffusion of CO_2 through the stratum corneum.

The tcP_{CO_2} electrode is also heated to 44 °C.

Combined Transcutaneous Oxygen and Carbon Dioxide Electrodes

A combined tcP_{O_2} and tcP_{CO_2} electrode operating behind a single membrane with a common electrolyte is an attractive possibility for physiological monitoring. Hahn[40] points out that a problem in the design of a combined electrode arises from the production of OH^- ions at the polarographic oxygen electrode which change the pH of the electrolyte layer close to the membrane and hence affect the operation of the P_{CO_2} electrode. This has led to the use of very small oxygen cathodes or the pulsing of the cathode potential. A combined tcP_{O_2} and tcP_{CO_2} electrode is described in Fig. 8.[41]

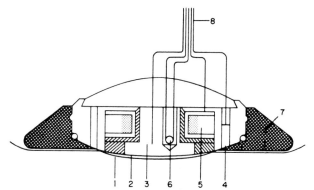

Fig. 8 Schematic diagram of the Roche tcP_{O_2} electrode. 1, skin; 2, membrane; 3, cathode; 4, anode; 5, heating coil; 6, thermistor; 7, fixing ring; 8, cable. (Reproduced with permission from Hill D. W., Dolan A. M. 1982. *Intensive Care Instrumentation*. New York: Academic Press.)

Transcutaneous Gas Monitoring by Mass Spectrometer

A quadruple mass spectrometer can be used to measure gases from a heated sampling inlet chamber connected to the mass spectrometer by a stainless-steel capillary tube. A gas-permeable membrane is supported on a block of porous stainless steel or ceramic contained in a housing heated to 44 °C and held on to the skin by double-sided sticky tape. A small chamber behind the porous material is connected via the capillary tubing to the inlet system of the mass spectrometer.

The advantage of this arrangement is that gases such as oxygen, nitrogen, carbon dioxide and argon can all be monitored. However, the rigidity of the sampling chamber and capillary tubing makes it difficult to ensure an air-tight seal of the chamber to the skin. There is only a small throughput of gas from the sampler, perhaps $10^{-7}-10^{-8}$ ml of oxygen/cm^2/s and small leaks can be troublesome.

REFERENCES

1. Hahn C. E. W. (1981). Techniques for measuring the partial pressures of gases in blood. Part I – In vitro measurements. *J. Phys. 'E', Sci. Inst*; **13**: 470.

2. Hahn C. E. W. (1981). Techniques for measuring the partial pressure of gases in blood. Part II – In vitro measurements. *J. Phys. 'E', Sci. Inst*; **14**: 783.

3. Eisenman G., Mattock G., Bates R., Friedman S. M. (1966). *The Glass Electrode*. London: Wiley.

4. Kater J. A. R., Leonard J. E., Matsuyama G. (1968). Junction potential variations in blood pH measurements. *Ann. NY Acad. Sci*; **148**: 54.

5. Bird B., Henderson F. A. (1971). The use of serum as a control in acid-base determination. *Br. J. Anaesth*; **43**: 592.

6. Rosenthal T. B. (1948). The effect of temperature on the pH of blood and plasma *in vitro. J. Biol. Chem*; **173**: 25.

7. Burton G. W. (1965). Effects of the acid-base state upon the temperature coefficient of pH of blood. *Br. J. Anaesth*; **37**: 89.

8. Adamson K. Jr, Daniel S. S., Gandy G., James L. S. (1964). Influence of temperature on blood pH of the human adult and newborn. *J. Appl. Physiol*; **19**: 897.

9. Fletcher G. (1969). Blood gas analysis. In *Techniques in Clinical Physiology* (Belville J. W., Weaver C. S., eds). London: Collier-Macmillan.

10. Laver M. B., Seiflow A. (1965). Measurement of blood oxygen tension and anesthesiology. *Anesthesiology*; **26**: 73.

11. Hill D. W., Tilsley C. (1973). A comparative study of the performance of five commercial blood-gas and pH analysers. *Br. J. Anaesth*; **45**: 647.

12. Severinghaus J. W., Weiskopf R. B., Nishimura M., Bradley A. F. (1971). Oxygen electrode errors due to polarographic reduction of halothane. *J. Appl. Physiol*; **31**: 640.

13. Stow R. W., Baer R. F., Randall B. F. (1957). Rapid measurement of the tension of carbon dioxide. *Arch. Phys. Med. Rehabil*; **38**: 646.

14. Teisseire B. (1983). Blood Gas analysis. In *Care of the Critically Ill Patient* (Tinker J., Rapin M., eds). pp. 1005–10. Heidelberg: Springer.

15. Lunn J. N., Mapleson W. W. (1963). The Severinghaus P_{CO_2} electrode: a theoretical and experimental assessment. *Br. J. Anaesth*; **35**: 666.

16. Clark L. C. (1956). Monitor and control of blood and tissue oxygen tensions. *Trans. Am. Soc. Artif. Int. Org*; **2**: 41.

17. Mapleson W. W., Horton J. N., Ng W. S., Imrie D. D. (1970). The response pattern of polarographic oxygen electrodes and its influence on linearity and hysteresis. *Med. Biol. Engng*; **8**: 585.

18. Rhodes P. G., Moser K. M. (1966). Sources of error in oxygen tension measurement. *J. Appl. Physiol*; **21**: 729.

19. Evans M. C., Cameron I. R. (1978). Oxygen electrodes sensitive to nitrous oxide. *Lancet*; **11**: 1371.

20. Scott I. L., Black A. M. S., Mayneord P., Hahn C. E. W. (1983). Pulse polarography and intravascular oxygen electrodes. *Br. J. Anaesth*; **55**: 559.

21. Parker D., Delpy D. T., Halsall D. N. (1983). A new approach to in-line gas monitoring. Developments of an oxygen sensor. *Med. Biol. Engng. Comput*; **21**: 134.

22. Claremont D. J., Pagdin T. M., Walton N. (1984). Continuous monitoring of blood P_{O_2} in extracorporeal systems. *Anaesthesia*; **39**: 362.

23. Bird B., Williams J., Whitwam J. G. (1974). The blood-gas factor: a comparison of three different oxygen electrodes. *Br. J. Anaesth*; **46**: 249.

24. Beetham R. (1982). A review of blood pH and blood-gas analysis. *Ann. Clin. Biochem*; **19**: 198.

25. Heitmann H., Buckles H. G., Laver M. B. (1967). Blood P_{O_2} measurements: performance of microelectrodes. *Resp. Physiol. Neth*; **3**: 380.

26. Hulands G. H., Nunn J. F., Paterson G. M. (1970). Calibration of polarographic electrodes with glycerol/water mixtures. *Br. J. Anaesth*; **42**: 9.

27. Kelman G. R., Nunn J. F. (1966). Nomograms for conversion of blood P_{O_2}, P_{CO_2}, pH and base excess for time and temperature. *J. Appl. Physiol*; **21**: 1484.

28. Burnett D., Henfrey R. D., Woods T. F., Fyffe J. A. (1986). Regional quality assessment of pH and blood gas analysis. *Ann. Clin. Biochem*; **23**: 26.

29. Ong S. T., David D., Snow M. (1983). Effect of variations in room temperature on measured values of blood gas quality control materials. *Clin. Chem*; **29**: 502.

30. Ladenson J. G., Davis J. E. (1973). Use of Tris buffers for the quality control of blood pH measurements. *Clin. Chem*; **19**: 651.

31. Veefkind A. H., Van den Camp R. A. M., Maas A. H. J. (1979). Liquid-filled ampoules for pH and blood-gas quality control. In *Blood pH and Gases* (Maas A. H. J., ed.). pp. 96–101. Utrecht: University Press.

32. Leary E. T., Graham G., Kenny M. A. (1980). Commercially available blood-gas quality controls compared with tonometered blood. *Clin. Chem*; **26**: 1309.

33. Baumberger J. P., Goodfriend R. B. (1951). Determination of arterial oxygen tension in man by equilibrium through intact skin. *Fed. Proc. Fed. Am. Soc. Exp. Biol*; **10**: 10.

34. Rafferty T. D., Marenko O., Nardi D., Shalter E. N., Mentelus R., Ngeon Y. F. (1982). Transcutaneous P_{O_2} as a trend indicator of arterial P_{O_2} in normal anesthetized adults. *Anesth. Analg*; **61**: 252.

35. Al-Diaidy W., Skeates S. J., Hill D. W., Tinker J. (1977). The use of transcutaneous oxygen electrodes in intensive therapy. *Intens. Care Med*; **3**: 35.

36. Hugh R., Hugh A., Lubbers D. W. (1973). Transcutaneous measurement of blood P_{O_2} (tcP_{O_2}) method and application in perinatal medicine. *J. Perinatal Med*; **1**: 183.

37. Rozkovec A. (1980). Transcutaneous oxygen electrodes in clinical use. *Intens. Care Med*; **6**: 205.

38. Severinghaus J. W., Stafford M., Bradley A. F. (1978). tcP_{O_2} electrode design, calibration and temperature gradient problems. *Acta Anaesth. Scand*. Suppl; **68**: 118.

39. Parker D., Delpy D. T. (1983). Blood-gas analysis by invasive and non-invasive techniques. In *Measurement in Clinical Respiratory Physiology* (Lazo G., Sudlow M. F., eds). pp. 75–112. London: Academic Press.

40. Hahn C. E. W. (1985). Techniques for measuring the partial pressure of gases in the blood Part II – In vivo measurements. In *Instrument Science and Technology*, Vol. 3 (Jones B. E., ed.). pp. 113–29. Bristol: Adam Hilger.

41. Parker D., Delpy D. T., Reynolds E. O. R. (1979). In *Continuous Transcutaneous Blood Gas Monitoring*. Birth Defects: Original article series. Vol. **15**, no. 4, pp. 109–16. New York: A. R. Liss.

16. Biosensors
P. Vadgama

INTRODUCTION

Spectrophotometric techniques have hitherto played the dominant role in assay procedures in clinical biochemistry. Only for the measurement of ions and gases have sensors become a recognized part of the clinical biochemist's analytical repertoire. The lack of any substantial impact of sensors stems mainly from the failure of most direct-responding devices to function reliably in biological fluids. This is in complete contrast to the generally impressive performance of sensors in simple aqueous solution. As a result, the perception of sensors by analytical chemists is an altogether more optimistic one than that of biochemists engaged in practical assays. The high level of interest now shown in sensors by analysts within biological fields, however, may well improve the outlook for application-orientated sensor technology. A particularly promising approach has been to incorporate a biologically derived species with well-developed solute-recognition properties into a sensor; this juxtaposition of a detector with a biological entity embodies the essential principle of a biosensor.

Early amperometric and potentiometric probes failed to provide the selectivity necessary for the clinical assay of organic solutes and macromolecules. The idea of a biochemical transducer remained attractive, nevertheless, and stimulated the search for suitable alternatives. The major likely advantages which motivated these investigations can be summarized as (1) simple operation, (2) minimum sample preparation, (3) potential for reagentless assay, (4) access to coloured, turbid or otherwise optically opaque samples (notably whole blood), (5) continuous transduction, for *in vivo* monitoring, (6) direct electrical signal output, (7) ready miniaturization for portable analysers, and (8) cheap fabrication for manufacture of disposable devices. The trend towards decentralized biochemical analysis has further highlighted the benefits of sensor-based measurement, and has served as a powerful incentive to research efforts. Indeed, while it is unlikely that biosensors will ever match the speed of operation of large-batch analysers within the central laboratory, their role in providing simplified analysis in the ward or clinic is likely to be unrivalled.

The most commonly used format for a biosensor is a device with a biochemically reactive external coating which converts the analyte to a product detectable at the underlying sensor (Fig. 1). Attempts have been made to use inorganic catalysts for this analyte conversion, but significant success has only been achieved with enzyme coatings. In principle, a variety

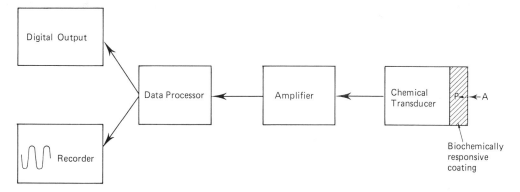

Fig. 1 Signal generation by a biosensor. The biochemically responsive coating here converts the analyte (A) into a product (P) detectable at the underlying transducer.

of underlying detectors could be utilized, and a range of physicochemical parameters followed (Table 1), but in practice electrochemical detectors have proved the most convenient and have received the greatest

TABLE 1

TRANSDUCER TYPES

Detector	Measured parameter
Ion-selective electrode	Potential
Gas sensing electrode	Potential/current
Chemical sensing electrode*	Current
Field effect transistor (FET)	Potential
Conductimeter	Conductance
Capacitor	Potential
Thermistor	Temperature
Piezoelectric crystal	Mass
Optical sensor	Light intensity

* Amperometric electrode responsive to organic redox species.

attention. This chapter will deal primarily with the group of electrochemical biosensors known as enzyme electrodes; these are the only type of biosensor to have so far made a contribution to clinical biochemistry. An enzyme electrode produced from an ion-selective electrode is shown in Fig. 2. Other biosensor systems to be described are, in large part, laboratory curiosities, but commercial interest in their development has increased, and they could provide the basis for specialized laboratory analysers of the future.

IMMOBILIZED ENZYMES

Methods of Immobilization

The high specificity and catalytic power of enzymes makes them attractive reagents for biochemical analysis. However, because they are labile and expensive, considerable efforts have gone into

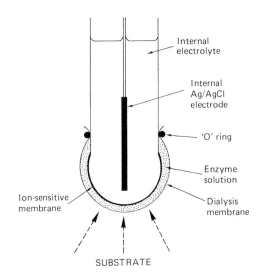

Fig. 2 Potentiometric enzyme electrode made from an ion-selective electrode mounted with a liquid enzyme membrane.

reconstituting them in more stable, reusable forms (Fig. 3). A specialist branch of biotechnology has emerged which concerns itself with enzyme immobilization procedures; solid phase enzymes are of value not only in analysis, but for industrial conversion processes. As with their soluble counterparts, enzymes in immobilized form have proved to be well suited to the task of selective, efficient catalysis on the surface of biosensors.

Adsorption. By far the easiest immobilization technique involves the mixing of an enzyme with a solid that has a high surface area. Provided there are sufficient non-covalent interactions between the enzyme and the solid carrier, adsorption occurs under mild conditions, with a minimum of disturbance to the active enzyme conformation. Charge, hydrophobic

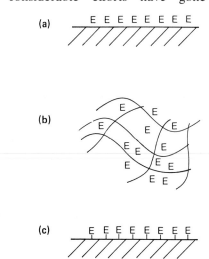

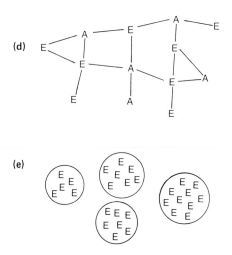

Fig. 3 Immobilized enzymes: (a) physically adsorbed, (b) gel-entrapped, (c) covalently attached, (d) chemically crosslinked and (e) microencapsulated (E = enzyme, A = inert protein).

and Van der Waals forces constitute the chemical basis for the adsorption process. The supports used include activated charcoal, alumina, collagen, ion-exchange resins and controlled-pore glass. The disadvantage of physical adsorption is that there is difficulty in getting a high enzyme loading, with a tendency for desorption to occur, particularly at high ionic strength.

Gel Entrapment. Physical entrapment of an enzyme within a gel provides another mild method for immobilization. Here, low-molecular-weight substrates can have access to the enzyme which itself diffuses only slowly through the gel lattice. Not only can a gel readily take up the geometry of an electrode surface, but its flexibility and permeability may be controlled by varying the gelling conditions. In the case of polyacrylamide, for example, changing the relative concentrations of the acrylamide monomer and the N,N'-methylene bisacrylamide crosslinker permits fine control over gel pore size. One disadvantage of polyacrylamide, though, is the tendency for enzyme denaturation by free radicals (singlet O_2, $SO_4^{\cdot-}$) employed in the polymerization. Other commonly used gel materials are gelatin, carrageenan, starch, polyvinyl alcohol and silicone rubber. These are used unmodified, and their selection is largely empirical at present, but more precisely engineered polymers and copolymers with preselected permeability properties will undoubtedly take their place in future.

Covalent binding. A host of methods have been developed to enable the covalent attachment of an enzyme to an insoluble support. The key step is the chemical derivatization of the support; the conditions employed for this can be quite harsh, but mild conditions are vital for subsequent attachment of the enzyme if denaturation is to be avoided. Inorganic supports chosen are similar to those used for physical adsorption. Glass has been derivatized with dual-function silane coupling agents such as γ-aminopropyltriethoxysilane; silanol groups condense with hydroxyl groups on glass:

$$\text{Si—OH} + (\text{H}_5\text{C}_2\text{O})_3\,\text{Si—(CH}_2)_3\text{—NH}_2 \rightarrow$$

$$\text{Si—O—Si—(CH}_2)_3\text{—NH}_2 \quad (1)$$

and the amino group can then be derivatized (e.g. with glutaraldehyde) and finally coupled to the enzyme. On carbon, surface carboxylic groups can be generated by oxidation; derivatization with thionyl chloride can then produce reactive chloroanhydrides:

$$\text{—COOH} + \text{SOCl}_2 \rightarrow \text{—COCl} \quad (2)$$

Organic supports such as nylon, agarose, cellulose and styrene have been used. Nylon has been activated

by hydrolysis of its amide groups to free amino and carboxylic groups, and by O-alkylation of its amides with triethyloxonium tetrafluoroborate (TOTFB) to give reactive imidates. Hydroxyl groups on cellulose can be utilized for attachment of transition metal salts (*viz.* $TiCl_4$, $SnCl_4$, $FeCl_3$) which can act as a link to enzyme molecules.

Crosslinked Enzyme. Chemical crosslinking of an enzyme with a bifunctional reagent ensures total retention of the enzyme protein. Crosslinked enzyme layers can either be formed directly over an electrode surface, or prefabricated and stored dry before use. High enzyme loadings are possible because a solid support does not have to be included. Glutaraldehyde is the most popular bifunctional reagent; others range from the bisdiazobenzidines which react predominantly with basic amino acid and cysteine residues (diazo coupling) and iodoacetamides which react only with cysteine residues (alkylation). Simple Schiff base formation between glutaraldehyde and amino groups on the enzyme (E) seems improbable and a more likely mechanism is an addition reaction involving α, β-unsaturated oligomeric forms:

$$(3)$$

Distortion of the active enzyme conformation is inevitable; the active site may also be involved itself in the crosslinking. Very large losses of activity may be sustained and the method is not satisfactory for less robust enzymes. Denaturation from intramolecular crosslinking is a particular problem, and one which is only partially resolved by inclusion of an inert protein such as albumin in the crosslinking mixture. Control over the crosslinking process is poor, but may be improved by employing a heterobifunctional crosslinking reagent for sequential binding and addition of free amino acid to terminate the reaction.

Microencapsulation. The encapsulation of enzymes within small ($\sim$100 μm diameter) semipermeable or porous polymeric spheres allows dispersion of catalytic activity throughout a reactor system without a direct, external exposure of the enzyme protein. Interest here stems mainly from the therapeutic use of enzyme microvesicles for the replacement of enzyme activity *in vivo*. Nylon and cellulose microvesicles, as well as red cell 'ghosts' and liposomes, may be used for encapsulation. Good recovery of enzyme activity can be expected since the enzyme is present in soluble form. However, the additional, multiple diffusion barriers presented by the microspheres is a drawback to their use in biosensors where rapid diffusion is at a premium.

Stability

The denaturation of an enzyme in solution remains a poorly understood process involving multiple equilibria between different conformational forms. The increase in stability observed with immobilized enzymes can be attributed to the anchoring of active conformations which are then better able to resist the molecular unfolding occurring during denaturation. For a given enzyme, stability generally increases in the order soluble < physically entrapped < chemically immobilized. However, even a soluble enzyme used in a liquid membrane over a sensor may show increased stability because of the protective effects of a high local enzyme concentration.

Within gels, steric hindrance is well recognized as playing an important part in reducing translational and rotational mobility of an enzyme, but the enzyme molecule is also less likely to uncoil and so will resist thermal denaturation to a greater extent. Stability will further improve if there are other non-covalent (e.g. ionic) interactions between the enzyme and the gel polymer. Additionally, when a charged matrix is used, there is partitioning of hydrogen ions and local pH will be different from that in the bulk solution. In the case of a positively charged polymer, protons are electrostatically repelled and the enzyme is protected from the effects of a low pH; conversely, negatively charged polymers improve stability under alkaline conditions.

A declining enzyme membrane activity can be due to a true loss of enzyme protein. Thus an enzyme may leach out from a gel or diffuse across covering semipermeable membranes. In some instances even covalently attached enzymes have been eluted, as has been reported for enzyme linked to CNBr-activated Sepharose. With strongly immobilized enzyme, a decay in activity could be due to oxidation of constituent amino acids, degradation by microorganisms and co-immobilized proteases, loss of a prosthetic group (e.g. FAD from amino acid oxidase) or repeated exposure to toxic reagents and reaction products (e.g. H_2O_2). The implication for an enzyme electrode is that any instability in the base sensor is further compounded by the metastable covering enzyme layer. Without exception, repeated electrode calibration is needed during use. Also, even with the most carefully worked out immobilization procedure, electrode operational lifetime can be conditioned more by intrinsic enzyme stability than by the immobilization method used; thus, electrodes using oxi-

dases usually function for much longer periods than those employing dehydrogenases. Guilbault[1] has, however, attempted to relate electrode lifetime to the immobilization technique; in his scheme an electrode with a liquid membrane would be expected to last for 1 week, one with gel-entrapped enzyme for 3–4 weeks and a device with chemically crosslinked enzyme for 4–14 months. It needs to be emphasized, though, that electrode stability in aqueous solution may bear little relation to that which is observed in a biological fluid, where the biocompatibility of an electrode is an important additional determinant.

Kinetics

Changes in conformation short of denaturation will alter the true Michaelis constant (K_m) of an enzyme on immobilization. The measured, or apparent K_m, however, may also undergo change. Thus, if solute partitioning occurs, then the equilibrium concentration of a substrate, or co-substrate, will be different from that in the bulk solution. This effect has been studied in greatest detail where a charged support has been used, and where one of the substrates is also charged. Charged groups on the enzyme itself may also affect local concentrations of ionic species, and the effect is most marked in low ionic strength solutions where electrostatic charges are less shielded. Selective partitioning of uncharged substrates, e.g. through hydrophobic interactions, can also occur and may in future provide a general means of adjusting enzyme K_m for analytical purposes.

Perhaps the most important consequence of immobilization is that the substrate has to diffuse to the active site of the enzyme, and mass transfer may then

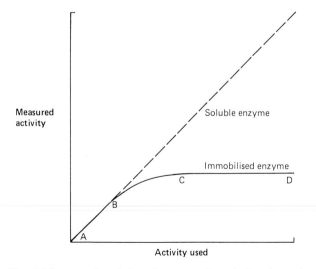

Fig. 4 Measured activity of enzyme in solution (–––) and enzyme immobilized in a membrane (——) related to the amount of activity used. For the immobilized enzyme A–B is the kinetic-dependent region, B–C is the region of mixed dependence and C–D is the diffusion-dependent region; membrane geometry and external stirring are assumed to be constant.

become rate-limiting for the reaction. The more active the enzyme membrane, the more important the limiting effects of diffusion. Thus, in Fig. 4, as enzyme loading is increased the reaction switches from being kinetically controlled (A–B), as for a soluble enzyme, to being diffusion controlled (C–D); both internal and external diffusion resistances contribute to the latter. The implication of such a limit on catalysis is that the size of the signal obtained with an enzyme electrode cannot be increased indefinitely with enzyme loading. Both internal (membrane) and external (bulk) diffusion contribute to mass transfer; for a given electrode internal diffusion can be varied by altering the density of the enzyme layer, and external diffusion by varying the stirring rate. At very high concentrations of enzyme in a membrane, the barrier due to the enzyme protein

kinetics and by Fick's laws of diffusion. The rate of change of product can be described by

$$\frac{\partial[P]}{\partial t} = \left(\frac{\partial[P]}{\partial t}\right)_{diffusion} + \left(\frac{\partial[P]}{\partial t}\right)_{reaction} \quad (4)$$

and by using Fick's second law of diffusion together with the Michaelis–Menten relation:

$$\frac{\partial[P]}{\partial t} = D_p \frac{\partial^2[P]}{\partial x^2} + \frac{k_2[E][S]}{K_m + [S]} \quad (5)$$

where D_p is the product diffusion coefficient, x is the distance from the underlying sensor, k_2 is the second forward rate constant of the Michaelis–Menten equation, E is the enzyme and S the substrate. At the steady state, despite a continuing enzyme reaction, $\partial[P]/\partial t = 0$ and a stable electrode response is

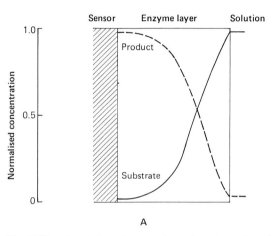

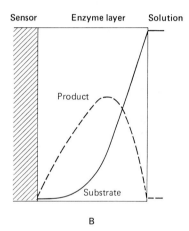

Fig. 5 Steady-state substrate (——) and product (– – – –) concentration profiles through an enzyme layer held over (A) a potentiometric and (B) an amperometric sensor. Diffusion gradients in the bulk solution and partitioning effects have been ignored. Here product is the electrochemically consumed entity at the amperometric sensor.

may actually lead to a lowered diffusion rate and a smaller electrode signal. The advantage of a high enzyme loading, though, is that the reserve of enzyme in a membrane is increased and large losses in activity may be sustained without an appreciable loss in response. Substrate response is, furthermore, 'buffered' against changes in pH, temperature and ionic strength, as well as against the presence of activators and inhibitors in solution.

ENZYME ELECTRODES

Principles of Operation

Product release into the bulk solution from an immobilized enzyme membrane is mainly of interest to the process engineer. With regard to enzyme electrodes, it is the level of product attained inside the membrane which is of main interest. Within a given volume element of an enzyme membrane, the concentration of product (P) is governed both by Michaelis–Menten

obtained. The exact product concentration profile in the enzyme membrane is a complicated function of diffusion and reaction, but only a single plane at the interface with the underlying sensor needs to be considered for signal transduction. The model can be further simplified by neglecting external mass transfer and assuming a high enzyme loading. With an underlying potentiometric sensor, which does not consume the product, the highest product concentrations are reached at the sensor interface (Fig. 5A). With an amperometric sensor, which does consume product, the interfacial concentration is zero (Fig. 5B), but the size of the signal is now determined by product flux and therefore the product concentration gradient at the sensor surface.

For a potentiometric enzyme electrode exposed to bulk substrate concentration $[S]_b \ll K_m$ a simple relation obtains between $[S]_b$ and the product concentration at the sensor interface $[P]_i$:

$$[P]_i = k \frac{D_s}{D_p} \cdot [S]_b \quad (6)$$

where D_s is the substrate diffusion coefficient and k is a constant which depends on K_m, solute diffusion coefficients and enzyme loading. A simple log-linear relation, corresponding to the Nernst equation, should therefore hold between electrode response and substrate concentration giving a slope at 25 °C of 59 mV/decade for a monovalent ionic product (Chapter 14). The limit of detection cannot be better than that of the basic sensor for the product ion ($\sim 10^{-5}$ mol/l) and in many cases it is a good deal worse, especially at low enzyme loading. One useful index of enzyme loading, which allows inter-enzyme comparison, condenses all the relevant parameters into a single dimensionless term; this is the enzyme loading factor, R, given as

$$R = k_2[E]L^2/K_mD_s \qquad (7)$$

where L is enzyme membrane thickness. A loading factor of <25 is associated with a submaximal response. Electrode output is also affected by reaction stoichiometry, and for 2:1 stoichiometry, with monovalent product, the calibration curve is shifted upwards by 59.ln2 mV.

The upper limit of linearity is restricted by enzyme K_m. At $[S]_b \gg K_m$ the enzyme reaction is zero order with respect to $[S]_b$ and the electrode is then no longer analytically useful. However, a mitigating factor is that the operational (apparent) K_m of an enzyme generally increases on immobilization. This is because, as substrate diffuses into the enzyme matrix, it is progressively consumed and its local, effective concentration then becomes lower than that in the bulk solution (Fig. 5).

An ion-selective electrode completes a response within seconds; the presence of an enzyme diffusion barrier over such an electrode increases response times to several minutes. The rate of substrate conversion within an enzyme membrane is also important, and, overall, high enzyme loadings ($R > 10$) give faster responses. It is best to increase loading by increasing the concentration of the enzyme and not the thickness of the enzyme membrane, as response times are a function of L^2.

The basis of amperometric detection is that a current is generated when an electrochemically active species is oxidized or reduced at an electrode surface. The size of response is given by the Cottrell equation

$$i = nFAf \qquad (8)$$

where i is the current, n the number of electrons transferred per molecule, F is Faraday's constant, A is the area of the electrode and f the flux of the electroactive species. For an enzyme-coated amperometric device with high enzyme loading

$$i = \frac{nFAD_s}{L} \cdot [S]_b \qquad (9)$$

The current output is, in fact, equivalent to that of a non-enzyme sensor responding to substrate, but

with an overlying diffusion-controlling membrane of thickness L. The comparison serves to indicate that while an amperometric enzyme electrode signal may be increased with a thinner enzyme membrane it cannot exceed that of an uncoated sensor responding directly to product in free solution. As with a potentiometric electrode, linearity can extend beyond enzyme K_m. Stable responses are obtained within a time interval of $1 \cdot 5\, L^2/D$ seconds, with D a common value for substrate and product diffusion coefficients.

Practical Strategies

Of the many sensors for ions, gases and redox species that have become commercially available in recent years, only a handful are capable of responding directly to species involved in enzymic reactions (Table 2). This limited sensor group has been the main determinant of the various enzyme-sensor configurations

TABLE 2
ELECTROCHEMICAL SENSORS FOR ENZYME ELECTRODES

H^+	O_2	H_2O_2
NH_4^+	CO_2	NADH
$Fe(CN)_6^{4-}$	NH_3	Hydroquinone
I^-		
CN^-		

which have been devised for substrate analysis. In principle, all that is necessary is to choose an enzyme, or sequence of enzymes in which a co-substrate, by-product or end-product of a reaction is detected by one of the sensors listed.

The oxidoreductases are the enzyme group to have been studied most closely, and of these the subclass of oxidases catalysing the reaction:

$$\text{Substrate} + O_2 \rightarrow \text{Product} + H_2O_2 \qquad (10)$$

have proved an especially successful route to substrate analysis. This is not least because of their intrinsic robustness and ability to furnish essentially reagent-free analysis. In nearly all cases, an amperometric sensor is used to monitor the consumption of O_2 or the generation of H_2O_2, but potentiometric I^- sensors have also been utilized to follow H_2O_2 via the indicator reaction:

$$H_2O_2 + 2I^- + 2H^+ \xrightarrow{\text{Peroxidase}} I_2 + 2H_2O \qquad (11)$$

Potentiometric combinations have been produced mainly with decarboxylases and hydrolases.

The overriding consideration during construction is to achieve a high enzyme loading. Preferably, this is done with an enzyme of high specific activity such that a thin, permeable enzyme layer can be applied. The benefits of using a high specific activity are greater than for any other analytical or process application of enzymes and may justify an extensive purification of commercial preparations despite the large losses which might be incurred; the total requirement of enzyme for an enzyme electrode is, in any case, small, amounting to a fraction of a unit for miniature devices. The diffusional resistance of the enzyme membrane gains additional importance, since product and substrate species traverse the full thickness of a membrane to be measured; in many enzyme reactor systems a superficially generated product is monitored within the bulk solution. There have been insufficient studies of the activity and permeability of enzyme membranes for electrodes, and often an empirical approach to fabrication has to be taken.

Once an enzyme membrane has been applied to a sensor surface it needs to be protected by an outer, preferably biocompatible membrane. Haemodialysis and ultrafiltration membranes are commonly used, with the laminate held in position by an O-ring (Fig. 2). If an enzyme gel or liquid film is used, then a spacer needs to be included in the enzyme layer; a 50 μm thick nylon mesh would suffice for this. Thicker enzyme layers can be tolerated with dilute gels or liquid films, as these offer less diffusional resistance than a protein-loaded matrix, especially if it has been crosslinked.

Once an enzyme electrode has achieved a stable baseline in buffer, it can be used much like a laboratory pH electrode; the time needed for stabilization is a matter of minutes rather than the 12 h recommended by some authorities. For most clinical purposes an electrode can be used at ambient room temperature; this applies particularly to electrodes under diffusion control, as these have less temperature dependence. Thermostatting will of course eliminate temperature effects on parameters such as sample pH, Nernst coefficient, reference electrode EMF and glass electrode asymmetry potential, but the importance of this in the clinical context has been overemphasized in recent years. At the very least it is worthwhile checking on the temperature-dependence of an electrode before a thermostatted, and more cumbersome, system is employed. Admittedly, use of an elevated temperature can provide a means of increasing electrode sensitivity, but the danger of thermal denaturation of an enzyme then also increases.

For many enzyme electrodes, reliable measurements are only achieved in stirred solution, where reproducible mass transfer is obtained through the thin, stationary (Nernst) solution layer at the electrode surface. Provided stirring is fast, and external mass transfer rapid, the precise rate of stirring has little influence on the steady-state signal.

Glucose Electrodes

Since Clark and Lyons proposed the concept of an enzyme-coated electrochemical sensor for glucose, a host of publications have concentrated on the characterization and optimization of glucose enzyme electrodes. In virtually all instances glucose oxidase is employed:

$$\text{glucose} + O_2 + H_2O \xrightarrow{\text{glucose oxidase}} \text{gluconic acid} + H_2O_2$$
$$(12)$$

and the three major possibilities of employing O_2, H_2O_2 and pH sensors have been investigated thoroughly. The continued attention given to glucose electrodes by biosensor groups, however, can be taken as some indication of the failure of many systems to satisfy clinical needs.

Glucose–O_2 Electrodes. The Clark O_2 sensor with its covering gas-permeable membrane is blood-compatible and highly selective for O_2. In early studies glucose oxidase was immobilized over O_2 sensors. While this gave selective devices, correction was necessary for background Po_2 variation, and some even considered it necessary to allow for non-enzymic O_2 reduction by ascorbate and urate. Dual-cathode electrode systems were devised where one O_2 sensor had a covering layer of denatured enzyme. In this way it was hoped that the dynamic responses of the enzyme and compensating electrodes to O_2 could be matched; in practice an exact correspondence is difficult to achieve. Also, errors may be quite large at low glucose levels when a subtraction between two large oxygen currents has to be made. In one dual oxygen system designed for implantation, and employing galvanic sensors to attain a self-generated polarizing voltage, responses took over 10 min to complete. This was most likely due to the thick nylon cloth-immobilized enzyme layer used. Readings in blood were consistently lower than those in aqueous standards; altered external mass transfer resulting from viscosity differences in blood may have accounted for this. The electrode was never used in implanted form. Electrode geometry can influence performance, and a reduced enzyme membrane surface area has helped to diminish the dependence on external mass transfer.

In an alternative approach, air-equilibrated samples have been assayed with single O_2-based electrodes. One elaborate system for extracorporeal monitoring has a 2·5 min analytical cycle during which 0·26 ml blood is sampled, diluted in buffer, air-equilibrated and then delivered to a measuring chamber where the initial slope of the glucose electrode response (kinetic mode) is measured. In a novel attempt at escaping dependence on background Po_2, glucose oxidase has been immobilized in gelatin; the solubility of oxygen in a gelatin matrix is 20-fold greater than in water, and provided only a short exposure to blood is used, there is sufficient oxygen in the enzyme layer for the enzyme reaction. The electrode needs regenerating in air between analysis and cannot be envisaged for continuous monitoring.

The electrochemical consumption of the O_2 co-substrate is an undoubted drawback which contributes to a loss of linearity at substrate concentrations well below the K_m. One way of improving the situation is to use an O_2 cathode with a smaller surface area than the outer diffusion surface of the electrode. Curvature has also been reduced by means of external nylon membranes which lower glucose diffusion relative to that of O_2, and in a more recent attempt an oxygen-permeable silicone rubber sleeve around the electrode has been used to improve the O_2 supply to the enzyme membrane.

Glucose–H_2O_2 Electrodes. Measurement of the H_2O_2 product of the glucose oxidase reaction avoids the need to correct for background Po_2 variation. H_2O_2 can be detected simply by reversing the polarizing voltage of an O_2 sensor:

$$H_2O_2 \xrightarrow[\text{(versus s.c.e.)}]{+0.6\,\text{V}} O_2 + 2H^+ + 2e \qquad (13)$$

and replacing the gas-permeable membrane with one allowing H_2O_2 diffusion. For blood measurements, a dialysis membrane is inappropriate, unless a very

for continuous extracorporeal monitoring (Biostator®, Miles Laboratories).[2] To avoid the need for systemic anticoagulation, blood for this system is withdrawn through a double-lumen cannula into which heparin is infused (Fig. 7); the sampling rate (~3 ml/l) exceeds the infusion rate (~1.8 ml/l), and so blood is removed along with the heparin. A continuous-flow system then dilutes the blood (1 in 11) in pH 7.0 phosphate buffer before pumping it through the electrode flow cell. An equilibrium glucose response is produced in 1.5 min, and this compares favourably with the 5 min required for extracorporeal analysers employing a spectrophotometric assay. A monitoring trace with another extracorporeal glucose electrode system is shown in Fig. 8, and demonstrates the short-term fluctuations of glucose which can be

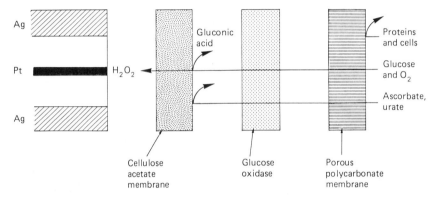

Fig. 6 Enzyme laminate of electrode for Yellow Springs Instrument glucose analyser.

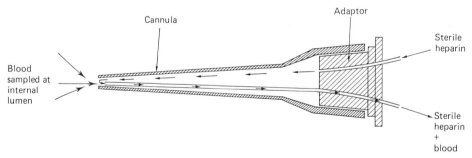

Fig. 7 Double-lumen cannula for continuous sampling and *in situ* anticoagulation of venous blood.

large glucose signal can be generated, as such a membrane allows access to electrochemically active interferents such as ascorbate, urate and tyrosine. By far the most successful approach has been to employ a cellulose acetate membrane with a low-molecular weight cut-off (~250 Daltons) to block off organic interferents. A further refinement, utilized in a commercial instrument (Yellow Springs Instrument glucose analyser), is the inclusion of an outer, parallel-pore ultrafiltration membrane; the low pore size (~0.03 μm) of this membrane prevents cells and proteins from reaching the enzyme layer (Fig. 6). A similar laminate has been used in an electrode designed

detected if response is fast. In the commercial system, the measured glucose level and its rate of change serves to modulate computer-controlled delivery of insulin and dextrose. The result is an artificial biofeedback system, the so-called artificial pancreas, which has provided a powerful means of stabilizing blood glucose levels in selected categories of diabetic patients.

A serious drawback to clinical monitoring has been the short life-times of electrodes in whole blood. The main cause has been platelet and red cell deposition on to electrode membranes. The additional 'biolayer' lowers substrate permeability and electrode sensitivity in an unpredictable fashion, and frequent recalibration is needed during use. This problem of biocompatibility far outweighs any instability due to enzyme denaturation or temperature drift. Anticoagulants have no significant effect on the blood–surface interaction, and even with antiplatelet agents, the average electrode life-time of the commercial electrode (25–50 h) is only appropriate for short-term

a low permeability to glucose is dip-coated on to the enzyme. The polyurethane has the additional effects of preventing contact between the enzyme and tissue, and of presenting a more biocompatible surface. By making the polyurethane membrane the controlling element in mass transfer, responses can be obtained which are independent of external diffusion; this is crucial in enabling the electrode to operate in tissue.

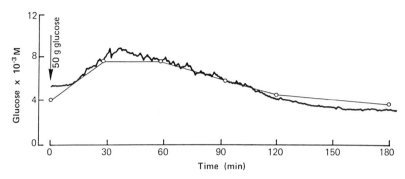

Fig. 8 Oral glucose tolerance test monitored with an extracorporeal glucose electrode. Albumin crosslinked glucose oxidase was used in the enzyme layer; electrode response time was 2 min. (o) blood samples analysed by a routine spectrophotometric method.

use. A key factor which can contribute to improved electrode stability is the design of the flow cell. Turbulent conditions stimulate platelet adhesiveness and increase platelet–surface contact times, therefore, to reduce fouling, laminar flow is preferable. One solution to the problem is to convert a conventional electrode cell (Fig. 9A) into one which has a narrow, uniform flow channel (Fig. 9B) and provided sample flow over the working electrode is maintained, there need not be a loss in sensitivity.

Biocompatible membranes permeable to species other than gas molecules are difficult to engineer. One alternative approach has been to treat the outer electrode membrane with an organosilane (viz. dimethyldichlorosilane). Silane treatment is a standard means of increasing the haemocompatibility of non-permeable surfaces, notably glass, and now shows promise for membranes used in enzyme-electrode construction. With certain types of membrane, an additional benefit is that a substantial decrease in glucose permeability can be obtained relative to that of O_2. The net result is an increased electrode linearity, typically from 5 mmol/l glucose to 50 mmol/l glucose, enabling the electrode to be operated in undiluted blood. Advantages over existing dry reagent chemistries, based on reflectance, is that timed incubation is not necessary, and whole blood does not have to be washed off or separated in some way prior to a reading.

Re-design of the glucose–H_2O_2 electrode in needle form has permitted invasive *in vivo* monitoring.[3] The basic sensor is a silver-coated needle cathode housing a glass-insulated platinum wire anode to detect H_2O_2. In order to extend linearity, a polyurethane layer with

There is only minor dependence on Po_2 down to 3·3 kPa, and despite the presence of the polyurethane layer a 90% response is obtained within 16 s. A less linear electrode has been made to complete a response in 1 s and is appropriate for use in an Auto-Analyzer (Fig. 10). The advantages of invasive monitoring are that tissue and vascular sites can be

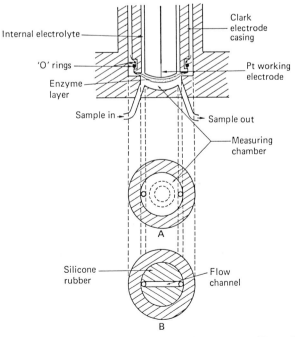

Fig. 9 Enzyme electrode based on a Radiometer (E5046) Clark sensor in (A) an unmodified measuring cell (B) a measuring cell with a narrow (1 mm diameter) flow channel.

sampled selectively and that the long period associated with transfer of sample to an extracorporeal electrode is avoided. A portable artificial biofeedback system has been produced based on the needle

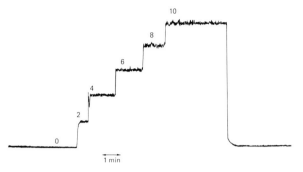

Fig. 10 Needle glucose electrode response to aqueous glucose standards (indicated in mmol/l). This rapid-response device has a thin covering polyurethane layer.

have been used to demonstrate delayed and lower peak glucose levels, in relation to those encountered in blood, following an oral glucose load.

Glucose-pH Electrodes. The gluconic acid from the glucose oxidase reaction, initially liberated as a lactone, induces a local fall in pH in weakly buffered solution. pH sensors coated with glucose oxidase have been used in aqueous solutions, but the strong influence of sample pH and buffer capacity on measurements has, hitherto, prevented use of these devices in biological fluids. Interest in pH-based measurement is, nevertheless, sustained by the possibility of exploiting the large number of other enzymes which can effect a change in H^+ concentration, either directly, or by altering the concentrations of hydrolysable species. A further motivating factor has been the advent of miniature microelectronic devices for ion measurement: ion-selective field effective transistors (ISFETs).[4] These were a natural progression of

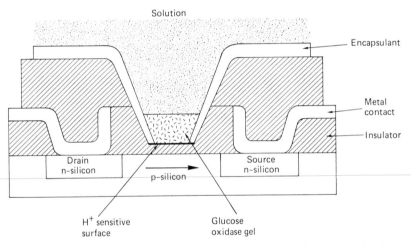

Fig. 11 Schematic diagram showing cross-section of an ion-selective field effect transistor with a glucose oxidase coating (ENFET). An H^+ responsive gate is employed (e.g. Si_3N_4). The direction of current flow between the drain and source is arrowed.

glucose electrode. Prior to use electrodes are conditioned in albumin solution; this leads to ~20% loss in response, with similar subsequent losses after three days continuous operation in tissue. Electrodes have been used for up to 7 days, and this represents the best performance to date of an enzyme electrode within a biological matrix. However, long-term glucose monitoring remains a far-off goal, and considerably more research effort is needed to understand cumulative membrane fouling processes and the functional effects of fibrous tissue formation around implanted electrodes. In this context, the continuing emphasis that is given to glucose electrode stability in aqueous solution seems somewhat misplaced. For the present, short-term *in vivo* use would be a valuable adjunct to intensive care monitoring. Also, basic understanding of dynamic glucose changes would improve, for example, tissue-implanted electrodes

semiconductor fabrication techniques, and enzyme-coated forms, as shown in Fig. 11, have now been produced (ENFETs). The device is, in essence, a transistor with its metal gate replaced by an ion-sensitive layer, which for pH is silicon dioxide or silicon nitride. Current is made to flow between two n-type silicon elements (source and drain) separated by p-type silicon. From the solution side, proton-induced charge build up in the p-type region, transmitted through the insulator, modifies electron flow and gives a measure of pH. Valid readings are only obtained with the ISFET used against a stable reference electrode. A multiple sensor array is possible on a single silicon wafer, and so a second pH detector can be readily located close to the ENFET to enable compensation for solution pH change; it is not yet possible to allow for buffer capacity variations. However, one recent, ingenious suggestion for gauging local buffer capacity has been to incorporate bacteriorhodopsin, a light-driven proton pump, and to relate local pH changes created by the proton pump to fixed levels of illumination.

At sufficiently high benzoquinone concentrations, oxygen was not a significant competing reaction, but a high, variable, background signal was generated in serum by non-enzymic reduction reactions of ben-

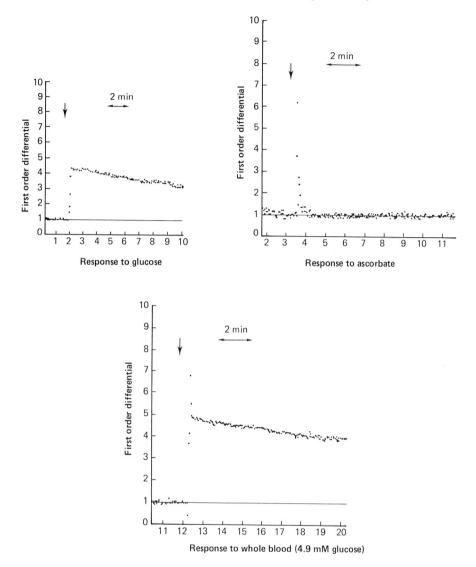

Fig. 12 First order derivative signal for a slow-response amperometric glucose electrode which employed glucose dehydrogenase. Electrochemical interference from ascorbate decays rapidly to leave a residual enzyme-mediated glucose signal. (Divisions on axes are in arbitrary units.)

Use of Artificial Electron Mediators. One way of eliminating the need for O_2 with glucose oxidase is to employ an alternative electron acceptor. Benzoquinone was the first to be utilized in this way:

$$\text{glucose} + \text{benzoquinone} + H_2O \rightarrow \text{gluconic acid} + \text{hydroquinone} \quad (14)$$

The hydroquinone product was measured amperometrically at a polarized platinum electrode ($0.4V$ vs s.c.e.):

$$\text{hydroquinone} \rightarrow \text{benzoquinone} + 2H^+ + 2e \quad (15)$$

zoquinone. Alternative electron acceptors which have been suggested include 2,6-dichlorophenol indophenol (DCPIP) and methylene blue, but a practical, discrete analyser (Hoffman-La Roche) has been produced using hexacyanoferrate (III) in solution.[5] In the absence of a membrane which is permselective for the hexacyanoferrate (II) product, an auxiliary electrode is required to compensate for the electrochemically active reducing species in blood. A general advantage of artificial electron mediators is that their concentration in solution can be more easily controlled than that of oxygen, and more importantly a high mediator concentration can be used to improve electrode linearity.

Co-entrapment of the electron mediator is feasible provided its efficient electrochemical regeneration can be guaranteed. One such arrangement uses ferricinium ion as a mediator incorporated into a graphite electrode.[6] The device permits reagentless assay of glucose with a linearity to 30 mmol/l. The low electrode polarizing voltage (160 mV vs s.c.e.) used to recycle the ferricinium ion and generate the current reduces electrochemical interference, which can be further diminished for anionic species by an external anionic membrane.

An NAD^+-independent, quinoprotein dehydrogenase for glucose (EC 1.1.99.17) has recently been tested for whole blood measurements using DCPIP as the electron mediator. The electrode has long (>30 min) response times, but when the first order derivative of the signal is followed, a steady-state reading is obtained within 30 s. The system illustrates another way of avoiding electrochemical interference; the derivative signal from interferents rapidly decays to zero, allowing selective sampling of the enzyme-mediated response over 15–30 s (Fig. 12).

Urea Electrodes

The urease-catalysed hydrolysis of urea:

$$\text{urea} + 2H_2O + H^+ \rightarrow 2NH_4^+ + HCO_3^- \quad (16)$$

allows several approaches to measurement, involving predominantly the detection of ionic or ionizable species with potentiometric electrodes (Table 3). Early workers concentrated on NH_4^+ glass sensors, but

TABLE 3

UREA ENZYME ELECTRODES

Device	Response time (min)	Log linear range (mmol/l)
NH_4^+ glass	1–2	0·1–10
NH_4^+ nonactin	1–3	0·1–10
NH_3 gas	4–5	0·5–70
NH_3 air gap	1–4	0·1–20
CO_2 gas	1–6	0·1–20
pH glass	1–3	0–0·5*
Ir/Pd MOS capacitor	3	non-linear†

* In 0·002 mol/l phosphate buffer, pH 6·86, signal directly proportional to [urea].
† Measurement range 0·01–5 mmol/l.

despite excellent dynamic responses, use in plasma had to be abandoned because of serious interference from monovalent cations in blood; the effect of Na^+ and buffer on urea measurement is shown in Fig. 13. It is possible to reduce Na^+/K^+ interference by sample pretreatment with cation exchangers, but this hardly constitutes the analytical simplification warranting construction of a biosensor. Clinical use in an instrument (Photovolt Analyser, Photovolt Corp.) had to await more selective NH_4^+ sensors; there has

been improved selectivity with the antibiotic nonactin as the electrochemically active component, which has given selectivity ratios of 6·5 and 750 for NH_4^+/K^+ and NH_4^+/Na^+ respectively. Almost total selectivity is obtained with an NH_3 gas sensor, as the gas-permeable membrane of the device blocks out all interferences except low-molecular-weight amines, which in any case are present at low concentrations in blood.

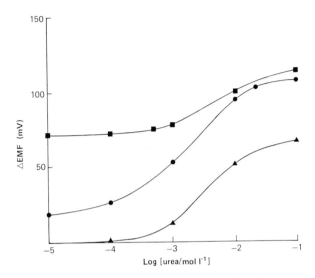

Fig. 13 Urea-NH_4^+ electrode made with 54 U/ml acrylamide gel-entrapped urease held over a Beckman NH_4^+ glass sensor. Calibration curves are in (▲) distilled water, slope 39 mV/dec; (●) 0·05 M tris buffer at pH 7·1, slope 42 mV/dec; (■) 0·05 M Tris buffer at pH 7·1 containing 0·1 M NaCl, slope 22 mV/dec. The curve shift in distilled water is due to liquid-junction effects at the reference electrode.

The principle of operation is similar to that of the Severinghaus CO_2 sensor in that an internal pH electrode registers changes in pH resulting from the diffusion of an analyte into a reservoir solution; in this instance NH_4Cl solution is used and the electrode reaction is:

$$NH_3 + H^+ \rightleftharpoons NH_4^+ \quad (17)$$

The drawback, is that the gas-permeable membrane makes for sluggish (~5 min) responses. Also, a compromise pH is necessary between the optimum for the enzyme (pH 6) and that required for quantitative conversion of NH_4^+ into NH_3 (NH_4^+ pKa = 9·25). Since the NH_4Cl solution acts as a sink for NH_3, the enzyme electrode shows somewhat more complicated behaviour than classical enzyme electrodes; super-Nernstian calibration slopes may be obtained, and response times have a dependence on the composition of the reservoir solution. In the air gap electrode, the gas membrane is, in effect, replaced by an air space, and there is no longer direct contact between the sample and sensing element. Assay involves conversion of urea within the bulk solution by either soluble or immobilized enzyme, with detection of liberated NH_3 after alkalinization. This is not a true enzyme electrode; substantial degradation of the analyte is involved, a steady-state response is not obtained and continuous flow operation is not possible. Complete separation of the components responsible for reaction and detection has been brought about in a commercial analyser (Kimble BUN Analyser, Owens-Illinois Inc.). Here a porous alumina urease column hydrolyses urea at pH 7·5, and after sample alkalinization to pH 11, NH_3 is measured at a gas membrane electrode operating under flow conditions.

The HCO_3^- from the urease reaction can be measured as CO_2 using a Severinghaus electrode. The enzyme electrode can be used at pH 7·0 (HCO_3^- pKa ≈6·1), but background $P\text{co}_2$ changes have to be allowed for. As with glucose-pH electrodes, practical assays with pH sensors have proved to be difficult, but in a study where a thinly coated pH sensor was used with an auxiliary pH sensor, it was found possible to obtain reliable measurements in plasma,[7] provided samples were diluted (1 in 100) to overcome the effects of variable sample buffer capacity. The thin enzyme layer which was employed generated linear, rather than log-linear, responses to urea in selected weak buffers. Reports on the penicillin enzyme electrode, where H^+ is the monitored species, also indicate that proton generation and solution buffering can be balanced so as to give a linear signal output.

More recent techniques have employed conductivity and capacitance measurement. Conductivity change arises from the net change in ion concentration during urease hydrolysis; the background conductivity variation has to be allowed for and high ionic strength solutions are a problem, but sensors are amenable to microfabrication.[8] The capacitance principle has been applied to NH_3 detection with a gas membrane over an iridium-coated palladium metal-oxide semiconductor (Pd MOS) made of p-type silicon. A steady-state reading is obtained according to

$$\Delta V = K \, (P\text{NH}_3)^x \qquad (18)$$

where ΔV is the voltage drop across the capacitor, $P\text{NH}_3$ is the partial pressure of NH_3 and K and x are constants for the system; transient responses to NH_3 are governed by a single constant without the exponential term.

Lactate Electrodes

The reaction catalysed by cytochrome b₂:

$$\begin{aligned} \text{lactate} + 2Fe(CN)_6^{3-} &\rightarrow \text{pyruvate} \\ &+ 2Fe(CN)_6^{4-} + 2H^+ \end{aligned} \qquad (19)$$

has been successfully exploited in various amperometric enzyme electrode configurations:

$$2Fe(CN)_6^{4-} \xrightarrow[\text{(vs s.c.e.)}]{+0\cdot4V} 2Fe(CN)_6^{3-} + 2e \qquad (20)$$

and now forms the basis of a lactate analyser designed for bedside analysis (Lactate Analyser 640, Kontron-Roche). The enzyme is retained as a liquid film over a platinum sensor, and there is an Ag/AgCl reference electrode, in contact with the assay solution via a glass frit and semipermeable membrane, to complete the electrochemical circuit. Samples need to be diluted for analysis, and this can give rise to errors in whole blood; the electrode responds to lactate only in the plasma fraction, and red cell lactate, which does not leak out sufficiently rapidly to participate in the enzyme reaction, is not measured. As a consequence of this a haematocrit-related dilution error is produced for which a correction has to be applied. One way round the problem is to haemolyse the sample; cetyltrimethylammonium bromide (Cetrimide) has been employed, and its use found to be compatible with the electrode.

Hexacyanoferrate (III) in solution has been replaced with ferricytochrome C in the enzyme layer to obtain a reagentless electrode, and currents have even been obtained by direct electron transfer between cytochrome b₂ and the electrode metal. The practicability of these alternative approaches needs to be evaluated.

Lactate 2-monooxygenase (EC 1.13.12.4) which catalyses the reaction:

$$\text{lactate} + O_2 \rightarrow \text{acetate} + CO_2 + H_2O \qquad (21)$$

has allowed the assay of blood lactate in an AutoAnalyzer flow system. Air segmentation of the sample and use of mixing coils in series enabled sufficient air-equilibration to permit measurement without an auxiliary O_2 sensor (Fig. 14). Lactate has also been assayed with lactate oxidase (EC 1.1.3.2):

$$\text{lactate} + O_2 \rightarrow \text{pyruvate} + H_2O_2 \qquad (22)$$

held in the kind of enzyme laminate employed for glucose (Fig. 6). By monitoring the forward reaction (pyruvate to lactate) of the lactate dehydrogenase-catalysed reaction:

$$\text{pyruvate} + NADH + H^+ \rightleftharpoons \text{lactate} + NAD^+ \qquad (23)$$

with this lactate electrode it has been found possible to estimate lactate dehydrogenase in serum.

Lactate dehydrogenase can itself form the catalytic component of an enzyme electrode. In one approach, the soluble mediator dye, phenazine ethosulphate (PES^+), was used to couple NADH production to oxygen reduction:

$$NADH + PES^+ \rightleftharpoons NAD^+ + PESH \qquad (24)$$

$$PESH + O_2 \rightleftharpoons PES^+ + H_2O_2 \qquad (25)$$

Non-enzymic reduction of O_2 by the dye is rapid, and a simple unmodified sensor is used in the enzyme electrode. The dye is unstable under extreme alkaline conditions, but provided pH is carefully controlled and a carbonate buffer employed, assay of blood is feasible. Phenazine methosulphate is less stable, and though its use is exemplified in aqueous lactate solutions, practical clinical exploitation is unlikely. It should be pointed out that direct reoxidation of reduced phenazine dyes can take place at platinum electrodes to generate responses at very low polarizing voltages. Flavine mononucleotide has also been tried as a mediator, and rapid reoxidation of the

mately 5% of that obtained with soluble coenzyme. The electrode also had a short lifetime resulting from incomplete electrochemical regeneration of NAD⁺. Studies have been carried out using platinum anodes, but recycling is less efficient due to further non-specific electrode side reactions, and also higher voltages are necessary for NADH reoxidation. Simpler

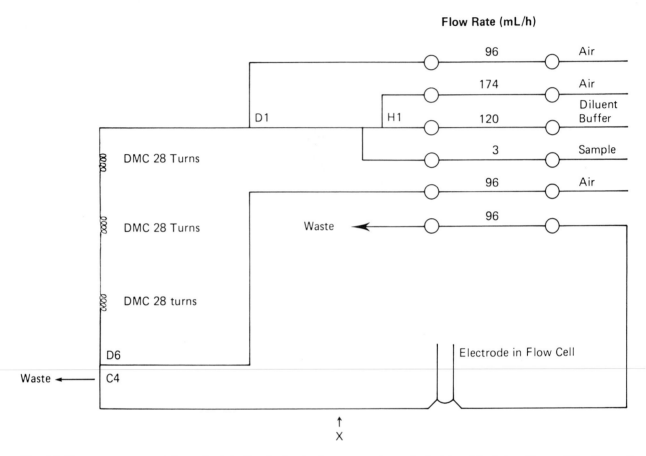

Fig. 14 Flow arrangement for a lactate-O_2 electrode for measuring whole blood lactate. Air equilibration of samples here eliminates the need for a background Po_2 correction. A three-way tap would be inserted at 'X' to permit standardization during extracorporeal monitoring. (DMC is a double mixing coil; D1, D6 and H1 are Technicon AutoAnalyzer glass connectors; C4 is a debubbler.)

reduced form apparently produces high current densities. Enzymic oxidation of NADH is possible with a diaphorase; H_2O_2 can be a product, but mostly O_2-based electrodes have been constructed. There is the added need here to satisfy the assay conditions for two enzymes. A reagentless lactate electrode has been reported where agarose-bound NAD⁺ is retained over a glassy carbon anode and the NADH reoxidized electrochemically.[9] Immobilized coenzyme close to the anode is apparently more easily reoxidized than soluble coenzyme and quite low polarizing voltages (~0·45V vs Ag/AgCl) were usable with this electrode. However, the diffusional constraints on the immobilized coenzyme meant that the NADH formed at sites remote from the anode surface was not available for electrochemical reoxidation and the electrode signal was small, approxi-

NAD⁺ immobilization has been obtained by retention of the cofactor behind an acetylated dialysis membrane.

Other Substrate Electrodes

Oxidase-coated amperometric sensors have been described for a host of substrates; of these, the biochemically relevant species include cholesterol, creatinine, urate, ethanol, pyruvate, galactose and amino acids. In all instances the transition to clinically usable devices has been substantially more difficult than with glucose and lactate electrodes.

Cholesterol oxidase effects a fast, reliable conversion of cholesterol in homogeneous solution, but the situation changes with an immobilized enzyme. Poor diffusion of cholesterol into an enzyme layer may severely reduce catalytic efficiency; in one assay of free cholesterol in serum, substrate did not penetrate the enzyme matrix and only a surface reaction occurred. Specific solubilizing agents (viz. cholate, Triton) affect both the enzymic reaction and the rate of cholesterol transfer through enzyme and overlying membranes. Cholesterol esterase is required for measurement of total cholesterol and can be either co-immobilized with the oxidase or used in solution.

Creatinine has been determined in serum by following the creatinine–picrate reaction with a picrate electrode, but the creatinine needs to be separated from interferents by passing samples through ion-exchange columns. Creatininase selectively deaminates creatinine to N-methylhydantoin, and the enzyme has been used as a liquid membrane over an NH_3 sensor, but viscosity of serum affects sensitivity and there is background interference from NH_4^+ in urine. The most important electrode for creatinine produced to date[10] exploits a multi-enzyme sequence involving creatinine amidohydrolase (CA), creatine amidinohydrolase (CI) and sarcosine oxidase (SO):

$$\text{creatinine} + H_2O \underset{}{\overset{CA}{\rightleftharpoons}} \text{creatine} \qquad (26)$$

$$\text{creatine} + H_2O \overset{CI}{\longrightarrow} \text{sarcosine} + \text{urea} \qquad (27)$$

$$\text{sarcosine} + O_2 + H_2O \overset{SO}{\longrightarrow} \text{formaldehyde} + \text{glycine} + H_2O_2 \qquad (28)$$

The similar pH optima (pH ~7) of the enzymes is a key factor in successful operation, and a glucose oxidase-type laminate (Fig. 6) has allowed serum assay. A dual electrode system is necessary to enable the creatine response to be subtracted; for this a second enzyme electrode bearing only the amidino-hydrolase and oxidase enzymes is employed. There have been tentative studies with uricase immobilized over O_2 sensors to determine buffered urate solutions according to the reaction:

$$\text{uric acid} + O_2 \overset{\text{uricase}}{\longrightarrow} \text{allantoin } H_2O_2 + CO_2 \qquad (29)$$

Though early work indicated that H_2O_2 was complexed with allantoin, and could not be detected electrochemically, direct-responding urate–H_2O_2 electrodes have recently been produced for serum assay.

Alcohol oxidase is not specific for ethanol; other alcohols, as well as aldehydes and carboxylic acids, are substrates. However, only methanol is a serious interferent for clinical analysis. The enzyme has been successfully combined with an O_2 sensor, but detection of H_2O_2 has been a problem because of the failure of the enzyme to liberate this product after a few days of use, despite continuing activity towards ethanol; it is possible that the enzyme catalyses H_2O_2 degradation. Alcohol dehydrogenase can be employed for analysis in an analogous fashion to lactate dehydrogenase, and has the advantage of being specific.

Pyruvate oxidase can furnish an electrode unit with an H_2O_2 sensor, but inorganic phosphate (P_i) is needed as a co-substrate:

$$\text{pyruvate} + O_2 + P_i \rightarrow \text{acetylphosphate} + CO_2 + H_2O_2 \qquad (30)$$

Also, loss of the prosthetic group (FAD) may occur and catalysis is affected by the presence of divalent cation activators. Background effects are important with galactose oxidase, a copper protein, the activity of which is diminished in blood by reducing species. Therefore an oxidant (viz. hexacyanoferrate (III)) is included in assay buffers, along with cupric ions to counter the deactivating effects of added EDTA. The enzyme can also use dihydroxyacetone, glycerol and lactose as substrates and these species have been monitored extracorporeally with a galactose electrode during loading tests in animals.

Despite the attention given to it by analytical chemists, the least attractive oxidase-based electrode is that employing L-amino acid oxidase. The enzyme is not selective for any particular amino acid, and with regard to the H_2O_2 mode of operation, sensitivity is compromised by a non-enzymic reaction between H_2O_2 and the α-keto acid product of the amino acid oxidation. Improved selectivity has been reported using decarboxylases; the amine released from the decarboxylation reaction is amperometrically monitored via co-immobilized diamine oxidase:

$$R\text{---}CH_2NH_2 + O_2 + H_2O \rightarrow R\text{---}CHO + NH_3 + H_2O_2 \qquad (31)$$

For maximum response, an intermediate pH is chosen between the pH optima for the two enzymes; lysine has been measured in this way.

Selective electrodes for phenylalanine, asparagine and glutamine are possible with deaminating enzymes over NH_3 gas sensors, and for glutamate, lysine and tyrosine with decarboxylating enzymes over CO_2 sensors. Other substrates measured on the basis of decarboxylating reactions are urate, salicylate (salicylate hydroxylase) and oxalate. The oxalate electrode provides a special example of an electrode adapted for urine measurement.[11] The high sulphate and phosphate content of urine leads to significant inhibition of oxalate decarboxylase, and this can be allowed for by increasing enzyme loading so that region C–D is reached in Fig. 4. The high, variable $P\text{CO}_2$ of urine makes it difficult to achieve a stable baseline and samples are therefore pre-equilibrated in air. The enzyme converts only free oxalate, and EDTA is added to sequester divalent cations from oxalate complexes in urine; the rate at which this process occurs can be accelerated by alkalinization of the urine sample.

The principle of coenzyme recycling with a second enzyme is illustrated by an electrode for alanine in which alanine dehydrogenase forms NH_4^+:

$$\text{alanine} + NAD^+ + H_2O \rightleftharpoons \text{pyruvate} + NADH + NH_4^+ \qquad (32)$$

An NH_3 sensor is used to monitor the reaction and immobilized NAD^+ is recycled by lactate dehydrogenase (equation 23) in the enzyme layer. An interesting possibility is shown by a bi-enzyme electrode for ATP where glucose oxidase and hexokinase are co-immobilized; the current generated in a constant background of glucose by the oxidase decreases in a concentration-dependent manner in response to ATP due to diversion of glucose by the kinase:

$$\text{glucose} + \text{ATP} \rightarrow \text{glucose-6-phosphate} \quad (33)$$

Microbial and Tissue-based Electrodes

A thin layer of intact, viable microbial cells, retained over an electrochemical device, can be employed for analysis.[12] The result is functionally an enzyme electrode, but now the enzyme does not have to be purified, activity can be regenerated, multi-step biocatalytic pathways may be exploited and coenzyme is not required. The presence of other microbial enzyme systems, however, can compromise selectivity and hindered diffusion through cell membranes retards equilibration; response times of 20–30 min may be encountered. A selected strain of *Sarcina flava* with glutaminase activity has been used, for example, for serum glutamine using an NH_3 sensor; a 10–15 μl cell suspension was employed, corresponding to approximately 10^9 bacteria. Similarly a *Pseudomonas* sp. strain over an NH_3 sensor has enabled histidine assay. Ethanol has been measured with *Trichosporon brassicae* over an O_2 sensor; utilization of ethanol by the microorganism here produces an increase in respiratory activity. There is no response to methanol or carboxylic acids with this alcohol electrode.

The rationale for tissue-based membrane electrodes[12] is similar to that for microbial sensors except that regeneration is not possible. In particular, labile eukaryote enzymes are considerably more stable when employed in their natural immobilized state. Porcine cortical kidney tissue over an NH_3 sensor has given a glutamine electrode with a detection limit of 2×10^{-5} mol/l and response times of 5–7 min. In one hybrid system, arginine was measured by its conversion into urea by liver tissue followed by a urease hydrolysis. These bioselective electrodes are at an early stage of development, and their future role remains uncertain.

Chemically Modified Electrodes

With amperometric devices, the chemical modification of the polarized electrode surface, followed possibly by some further derivatization or addition of a reactive group, can induce major changes in electrode properties. In the case of enzyme electrodes the main aim is to achieve rapid, direct electron transfer between the enzyme active centre, or coenzyme, and the underlying electrode. Chemical modification therefore often entails deposition of

conducting material. Organic polymeric semiconductors, sometimes derivatized for enzyme binding, are undergoing close study by several groups at present. In early work, glucose oxidase close to a surface comprising the conducting salt of tetracyanoquinodimethanide (TCNQ):

PMS^+ $TCNQ^-$ was found to give a glucose signal without the intervention of oxygen; the conductor was able to reoxidize directly the $FADH_2$ of the reduced enzyme generated by the reaction with glucose. Also, NADH oxidation has been shown to occur at quite low polarizing voltages at these electrodes so a more elegant approach to the assay of dehydrogenase substrates can now be contemplated. Such developments have a possible importance for both clinical analysis and biochemical fuel cell research. However, recent enthusiastic descriptions have tended to ignore the behaviour of interferents at these modified surfaces and the extent to which they are able to escape fouling and passivation in blood. These aspects of performance require special consideration since protective, low-molecular-weight cut-off membranes can no longer be interposed between the enzyme and the conducting layer.

THERMAL SENSORS

A thermistor is a semiconductor resistor sensitive to temperature change. It has, as its detector element, simply a globule of sintered metal oxides with two wire connections. The device is easy to miniaturize and can be readily formed in a variety of shapes. A reliable estimate of temperature is obtained provided low operating currents are used to minimize self heating of the thermoresistor. An enthalpy change will inevitably take place with any enzyme reaction, and the thermistor is therefore uniquely suited to be a universal detector for these reactions; it is primarily for this reason that the principles of classical calorimetry have been applied in the domain of biochemical analysis.

Thermal Enzyme Probes

The immobilization of an enzyme over a thermistor tip produces a thermal enzyme probe (TEP). Substrate analysis by TEP can be undertaken without consideration being given to the choice of detector reaction, so frequently a problem with electrochemical sensing. The key factor is the magnitude of the enthalpy change. As an approximation, in the high enzyme loading limit, at steady state:

$$\Delta T = \Delta H \left(\frac{A K_m D_s}{cV} \right) [S]_b \quad (34)$$

where ΔT is the temperature change, ΔH is the reaction enthalpy, A is the probe area, c is the thermal conductivity of the enzyme layer and V its volume. An uncoated thermistor or one which has an inert coating is required as a reference to correct for background temperature variations; such differential measurements are conveniently made using a Wheatstone bridge arrangement. Temperature responses of the order of only $1\,m^\circ C$ can be expected for $[S]_b = 1\,mmol/l$, and this low signal output is the most important failing of the TEP. Its cause is primarily the high rate of heat dissipation into the bulk solution, which is much faster (by a factor of ~ 100) than the rate of substrate diffusion into the enzyme layer.

mal conductivity and low heat capacity of the mercury helped to direct heat towards the underlying thermistor; this TEP had a response time of 10–60 s with a linear range of 5–30 mmol/l urea. Amplification of the substrate signal may in future be obtained by other more practicable heat-conducting supports. Temperature fluctuations due to stirring have been reduced by obtaining laminar flow in the vicinity of a TEP using a specially designed, isothermal, flow cell. Analysis by TEP has received relatively little attention, but these transducers offer an important alternative to enzyme electrodes and permit analysis of substrates for which an electrochemical detection scheme is not available.

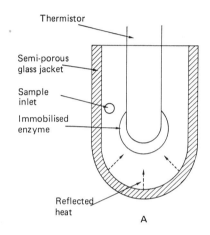
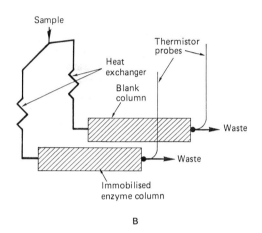

Fig. 15 (A) Thermal enzyme probe (TEP) with a surrounding glass jacket for heat reflection. (B) Split-flow arrangement for an enzyme thermistor; the thermostat jacket is not shown.

It is imperative that a TEP pair is used in a thermally insulated environment. This is because background temperature fluctuations cannot be fully compensated with the reference probe; thermal probes are never exactly matched, and a small apparent difference in temperature between the two probes will be registered if the background temperature alters. For a given thermistor pair, the size of the false signal is defined by the common mode rejection ratio ($CMRR_T$). At a $CMMR_T$ of 100 a background temperature change of 1 °C produces a false signal of 0·01 °C. Thermostatting to $\pm 1\,m^\circ C$ is generally required unless the thermistor pair is well matched, but even this cannot eliminate the random noise associated with local thermal fluctuations in an assay solution.

TEP sensitivity can be improved in several ways. Catalase can be immobilized with an oxidase enzyme; in the case of glucose oxidase ($\Delta H = -80\,kJ/mol$) substantial augmentation of the response would be expected from H_2O_2 decomposition ($\Delta H = -100\,kJ/mol$). Heat loss to the ambient solution can be reduced; a glass jacket around the TEP was used by Tran-Minh and Vallin[13] (Fig. 15A). A urea thermistor has also been reported where urease is adsorbed on a layer of mercury metal; the high ther-

Enzyme Thermistors

Separation of the enzyme and thermistor components produces an enzyme thermistor.[14] While this is not a true biosensor, the system is important in having provided practical assays. An open tubular enzyme reactor or a packed bed enzyme reactor column can be used for enzymic degradation of the analyte. A change in temperature is produced according to

$$\Delta T = \frac{m\Delta H}{C} \qquad (35)$$

where m is the number of moles of analyte converted and C the combined heat capacity of the solution and reaction vessel. There is some loss of heat during transfer of a sample to the thermistor, but sensitivity is, nevertheless, severalfold greater than with TEPs. Thermostatting is still necessary, and a heat exchanger is used to pre-equilibrate the sample with respect to temperature to reduce signal fluctuations during analysis. Temperature change due to the reaction is measured either against a reference thermistor located upstream to the reactor, or at an equivalent site in a blank column with matching flow and thermal properties; such a split-flow thermistor is shown in Fig. 15B. The use of this split-flow arrangement has the advantage of allowing simultaneous compensation for heat changes induced by the sample, and there is then a more precise correspondence between signal fluctuations at the two thermistors. It is necessary during operation to ensure low sample and heat dispersion within the column. Pulsatile flow needs to be dampened, as the signal is sensitive to flow rate changes. Overall flow rates also need to be optimized; at low flow rates there is excessive heat loss to the surroundings, and at high flow rates there is broadening of signal-time curves. It needs to be borne in mind that reactor columns may clog, and that analysis of whole blood necessitates dialysis or filtration. Numerous substrates have been assayed, but other than for glucose, where $0·002$ mmol/l has been measured, detection limits generally allow little room for dilution; in the case of uric acid, the measurement range in one report was $0·5–4$ mmol/l. So far, sample throughput ($\sim$30/h) has been substantially lower than with existing flow analysers, but the low cost and versatility of the technique has some attraction for routine use.

FIBRE OPTIC PROBES

Any changes in the optical property of a solution, during the course of a homogeneous reaction, can be followed with the appropriately positioned fibre optic bundle. As an extension of this approach, a reagent could be immobilized on the tip of an optical fibre and the reaction then monitored within a localized reaction phase. The resulting system has all the attributes of a chemical transducer and is known as a fibre optic probe or optrode.[15] The key requirement is that the optical path between a light source and a detector passes through an immobilized reactor phase. A bifurcated probe (Fig. 16) or a single fibre optic with a beam splitter, can be used, and any optical property (viz. reflectance, fluorescence, luminescence) can be utilized.

Probes for Ions and Gases

In one early device for pH, the fibre optic probe tip held polyacrylamide-bound phenol red bound by a semipermeable cellulose membrane (Fig. 16A). Light from a tungsten source was used to detect the basic forms of phenol red, measured by means of radiation scattered back rather than as an absorbance change. An optically opaque seal is required at the end of such probes to avoid direct interaction between the light source and the ambient solution. The pH probe was capable of reversible sensing, but because of the finite quantity of dye present response was governed by saturation binding and signal output was non-linear. Other, fluorescence sensors for pH have been described based, for example, on cellulose-bound fluoresceinamine. Sensitivity is greater here, and excitation and fluorescence wavelengths can be followed by means of a single optical fibre.

Quenching due to high local concentration of reagent molecules can be a problem. A pH sensor employing the indicator β-methylumbelliferone held at a quartz surface has been used as the internal detector of a CO_2 measuring device. Quenching of light emitted from a fluorophore (perylene dibutyrate) by oxygen has been specifically exploited for oxygen measurement, and a chemiluminescence reaction between oxygen and tetrakis(dimethylaminoethylene) has also been suggested for oxygen measurement.

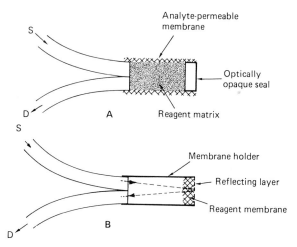

Fig. 16 Fibre optic probe (A) with reagent retained behind a semipermeable membrane, (B) with reagent, e.g. enzyme, immobilized in a membrane disc. (S is the light source, D is the detector.)

Ammonia has been detected with an oxazine indicator dye coated over an optical fibre; change in the colour of the dye due to ammonia affects light transmission by the fibre. None of these devices has a biological component, but in future, biological moieties may be used. A recent illustration of this is in the use of immobilized haemoglobin at a probe tip to measure oxygen.

Glucose Probe

Probably the most important fibre optic probe to have been developed is the glucose affinity sensor. The device has Concanavalin A (Con A) covalently bound to the inner surface of a cellulosic hollow fibre chamber mounted at a fibre tip. Within the chamber is fluorescein-labelled dextran (D*) which binds reversibly to Con A. Glucose which diffuses into the chamber then competes for binding sites on Con A and displaces the bound dextran:

$$\text{glucose} + \text{Con A–D*} \rightleftharpoons \text{Con A} - \text{glucose} + \text{D*} \quad (35)$$

With this exchange there is an increase in the concentration of free labelled dextran in the central, illuminated, portion of the hollow fibre. A glucose-dependent increase in the fluorescence signal is thus generated after a short lag period. The permeability of the cellulosic hollow fibre is such that glucose will diffuse in freely whereas the dextran is fully retained. Photobleaching of the dye is a potential problem, and one which is largely avoided by limited pulsing of the excitation beam. The key advantage for long-term implantation is that this is an equilibrium measurement; there is no net glucose mass transfer at the steady state, and partial membrane fouling does not therefore affect the steady-state signal. Miniaturization of the hollow fibre chamber (to 0.3 mm diameter) has reduced diffusion distances and minimized response times; the time to equilibrium is determined mainly by the rate of binding to Concanavalin.

Enzyme-based Devices

Fibre optic probes have been sensitized with enzyme membranes. In one preliminary report horseradish peroxidase was immobilized in a transparent gel layer at a probe tip to detect H_2O_2. Immersion of the probe in alkaline H_2O_2 solution and luminol gave a chemiluminescence signal. Probe fabrication is simpler here, since a light source is not required, and response is rapid because product diffusion is not involved in signal generation. The probe could, in principle, be used to monitor oxidase-catalysed reactions, but matching the pH requirement of the oxidase with that of the probe is likely to prove a problem.

Immobilization of alkaline phosphatase at the tip of an optical fibre (Fig. 16B) has allowed detection of the *p*-nitrophenol phosphate substrate of the enzyme. The device has two layers of nylon mesh; one which holds the enzyme, and the other is an external limiting layer to reflect light through the enzyme layer from the light source. Diffusion of substrate through the permeable, limiting layer to the enzyme leads to *p*-nitrophenoxide production which is detected by an absorbance change in the reflected light. It may be possible to extend this principle of operation to biochemically relevant enzyme substrates.

IMMUNOSENSORS

Selective recognition of an antigen by an antibody has been exploited in sensor configurations.[16] The simplest approach is to immobilize an antibody on the surface of a transducer and to follow some electrochemical event that emanates from the encounter with antigen. Non-covalent interactions such as Van der Waals forces, hydrogen bonding, change transfer and dipole interaction are responsible for the binding of antigen to antibody. Inevitably, therefore, the charge content of the antibody-loaded surface will undergo some change, and under appropriate circumstances this can be picked up as an electrical signal. In one example, antibody to HCG was immobilized on to titanium wire, and an EMF change, measured against a reference electrode, was generated in the presence of HCG. Analogous responses

to antigen have been shown using ISFETs, and a more conventional potentiometric electrode, mounted with membrane-bound antibody to albumin, has produced a signal in albumin solution. Exposure of such electrodes to high ionic strength or acid solutions removes the antigen and allows their reuse. The flaw in all these devices, however, is that they produce non-specific responses to other adsorbing species, notably proteins, present in biological samples. Furthermore, the magnitude of the signal which is generated is relatively small and assay of trace concentrations is unlikely to be achieved this way. Much attention has therefore been focused on systems where some kind of label is employed.

Enzyme Immunosensors

One successful approach has been to adapt standard enzyme linked immunosorbent assay (ELISA) techniques to sensors. In a typical device an antibody-coated electrode is brought into contact with either a mixture of antigen and enzyme-labelled antigen for competitive binding to the antibody, or sequentially exposed to the antigen and an enzyme-labelled antibody (sandwich assay). The degree of electrode membrane activation by enzyme can be estimated from the electrode signal in substrate. Enzymes which have served as labels include catalase and glucose oxidase, so far only used with O_2 sensors. Also, horseradish peroxidase has been used with an I^- sensor to follow the oxidation of I^- by H_2O_2 (equation 11). Loading by the enzyme has to be in the non-zero region (A–B) in Fig. 4. Species that have been assayed include α-fetoprotein, insulin, albumin, IgG and oestradiol. As antigen/antibody binding is not rapidly reversible, it is difficult to envisage any form of continuous monitoring system at present. With existing technology an on-line electrode undergoing a repeated sample incubation/dissociation cycle seems the best approximation possible.

A variation on the theme of selective binding has been the use of biological molecules with high mutual affinities. Thus, the high binding affinity between avidin and biotin has been exploited for biotin measurement (Fig. 17A). An electrode with a surface-immobilized layer of 2-[(4-hydroxyphenyl)azo] benzoic acid (HABA) is first allowed to develop a coating of enzyme-labelled avidin; HABA has a weak affinity for avidin. Addition of biotin then readily pulls the avidin off and there is an associated drop in the electrode response to substrate. Biotin has been measured in this way in the range 10^{-6}–10^{-4} mg/ml. Analysis is simply based upon the bioaffinity difference between biotin and HABA, and it may be possible to utilize this principle of ligand pair binding to the assay of other low-molecular-weight species where binding differences can be demonstrated, e.g. drugs.

The most elaborate concept for an immunosensor has utilized complement lysis of enzyme loaded lipo-

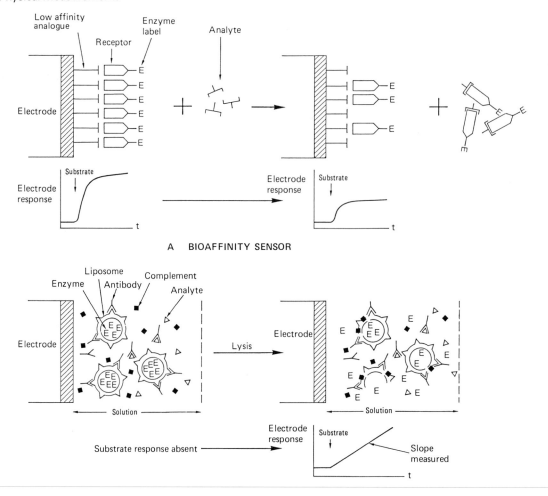

A   BIOAFFINITY SENSOR

B   LIPOSOME IMMUNOSENSOR

Fig. 17 (A) Bioaffinity sensor: displacement of enzyme-labelled receptor molecules by analyte diminishes the steady-state response of the sensor in substrate solution. (B) Liposome immunosensor: antigen and sensitized liposomes compete for antibody binding; subsequent lysis of liposomes by complement, with release of enzyme, provides a measure of antigen concentration. The enzyme-catalysed reaction in bulk solution generates a progressive electrode signal and a steady-state response is not achieved.

somes (Fig. 17B). An antigenic liposome surface is used to compete with free antigen in solution for antibody binding. In the presence of complement, rupture of liposomes occurs and the enzymic contents are released. The quantity of enzyme released is inversely related to the concentration of the free antigen in solution. Theophylline has been assayed in this way using horseradish peroxidase. The method allows for considerable amplification, but as enzyme is released into bulk solution, a steady-state reading is not obtained and the rate of the enzymic reaction is followed using the slope of the electrode response.

Homogeneous Immunoassay

Sensors can be used as detectors for homogeneous immunoassays. An assay for oestradiol has been carried out using competition between oestriol and an amperometrically detectable nitro-derivative of oes-

triol. Morphine has been measured with an electroactive ferrocene-labelled analogue. The retarded translational and rotational diffusion of the antibody-bound labelled compound attenuates its electrochemical activity and enables its ready discrimination from the free form; there is therefore no need for a separation step. Electrochemically active metals can also be used as labels (viz. Pb^{2+}, Zn^{2+}, Co^{2+}) but the more standard use of an enzyme label to furnish an EMIT type assay is more promising. Feasibility has been demonstrated with a glucose-6-phosphate dehydrogenase label for phenytoin; here, NADH formed in the enzyme reaction was monitored at a glassy carbon electrode.

Column Reactors

Antibody immobilized on a chromatography column can provide the site for competitive binding between an enzyme-labelled and an unlabelled antigen or a sandwich assay format can be used. The degree of column activation by bound enzyme is then estimated by introduction of a substrate solution which is passed to a down-stream electrochemical detector; because sample is washed out prior to this step, electrode fouling from protein is not a problem, and background electrochemical interference is avoided. High sensitivity is possible, and in one report IgG has been measured down to 1 fmol. An equivalent procedure has been developed essentially by substituting the reactor column of an enzyme thermistor (Fig. 15B) with one bearing an immobilized antibody. The resulting thermometric enzyme-linked immunosorbent assay (TELISA) has detected antigen concentrations down to 10^{-13} mol/l; albumin, insulin and gentamicin have been analysed to date by the TELISA technique.

Piezoelectric Crystal Immunosensor

The application of a voltage to a quartz crystal produces a physical distortion and a change in the applied voltage can bring a vibration. A piezoelectric crystal oscillator, vibrating at its resonance frequency constitutes a microgravimetric sensor. Adsorption of a species which alters the mass of the crystal leads to a change in the vibration frequency (f) according to

$$f/f_0 = -m/A\rho h \qquad (36)$$

where m is the surface mass, A the area covered by the adsorbate, ρ the crystal density and h the thickness of the layer. It has been difficult to achieve selective adsorption, even for gas phase measurement, however. Recently, a piezoelectric crystal with a silane-derivatized surface has been used as the support for anti-IgG antibody; IgG bound selectively to the surface from solution and the change in crystal vibrational frequency gave a measure of IgG concentration. Non-specific adsorption occurs, but diluted serum can apparently be assayed provided an uncoated reference crystal is used. Piezoelectric crystal devices are robust and could furnish practical assay systems for proteins in the future; sensitivity would not, however, be sufficient for low-molecular-weight solutes.

CONCLUSION

The ingenuity of the analytical chemist is demonstrated by the contrasting types of biosensors described here. From the initial harnessing of electrochemical reactions for analysis, it seems that almost any physicochemical property of a molecule can be exploited for measurement by a biosensor. The recent heightened interest in such probes arises not only from their novel and interesting functional properties, but from the very real need for simple, rapid biochemical profiling of the patient. Admit-

tedly, the majority of biosensors described in this chapter do not satisfy these requirements; the obstacles to success lie, however, not in any specific failing in their basic mode of operation, but in the adverse, complicated interfacial behaviour of biological fluids, with the greatest difficulty arising from the surface activity of macromolecules and cellular elements. Without a recognition of the special needs of 'biological adaptation' for biosensors, the new generation of systems will have little application to clinical practice. With a change in emphasis in research efforts, however, involving the increased participation of the biologist and end-user, there is every possibility that biosensors will make a significant impact on health care in the future.

REFERENCES

1. Guilbault G. G. (1976). *Handbook of Enzymatic Methods of Analysis.* New York: Marcel Dekker.
2. Fogt E. J., Dodd L. M., Jenning E. M., Clemens A. H. (1978). Development and evaluation of a glucose analyser for a glucose-controlled insulin infusion system (Biostator®). *Clin. Chem*; **24**: 1366.
3. Shichiri M., Kawamori R., Yamasaki Y., Hakui N., Abe H. (1982). Wearable artificial endocrine pancreas with a needle-type glucose sensor. *Lancet*; **ii**: 1129.
4. Bergveld P. (1972). Development, operation and application of the ion-sensitive field-effect transistor as a tool for electrophysiology. *IEEE Trans. Biomed. Eng. BME*; **19**: 342.
5. Mor J-R., Guarnaccia R. (1977). Assay of glucose using an electrochemical enzymatic sensor. *Anal. Biochem*; **79**: 319.
6. Cass A. E. G., Davis G., Francis G. D., Hill H. A. O., Aston W. J., Higgins I. J. *et al.* (1984). Ferrocene-mediated enzyme electrode for amperometric determination of glucose. *Anal. Chem*; **56**: 667.
7. Vadgama P., Covington A. K., Alberti K. G. M. M. (1982). Plasma urea determination by enzyme-pH electrode. *Anal. Chim. Acta*; **136**: 403.
8. Winquist F., Spetz A., Lundstrom I., Danielsson B. (1984). Determination of urea with an ammonia gas-sensitive semiconductor device in combination with urease. *Anal. Chim. Acta*; **163**: 143.
9. Blaedel W. J., Jenkins R. A. (1976). Study of a reagentless lactate electrode. *Anal. Chem*; **48**: 1240.
10. Tsuchida T., Yoda K. (1983). Multi-enzyme electrodes for the determination of creatinine and creatine in serum. *Clin. Chem*; **29**: 51.
11. Rechnitz G. A. (1981). Bioselective membrane electrode probes. *Science, NY*; **214**: 287.
12. Vadgama P., Sheldon W., Guy J. M., Covington A. K., Laker M. F. (1984). Simplified urinary oxalate determination using an enzyme electrode. *Clin. Chim. Acta*; **193**.
13. Tran-Minh C., Vallin D. (1978). Enzyme-bound thermistor as an enthalpimetric sensor. *Anal. Chem*; **50**: 1874.
14. Mosbach K., Danielsson B. (1981). Thermal Bio-analyzers in flow streams. Enzyme thermistor devices. *Anal. Chem*; **53**, 83A.
15. Sietz W. R. (1984). Chemical sensors based on fiber optics. *Anal. Chem*; **56**: 16A.

diffuse through the reflective layer into the detection layer where a glucose oxidase-based peroxidase assay is initiated. The rate of colour development is proportional to the free conjugate concentration which, in turn, is proportional to the thyroxine concentration in the sample. Description of elements for immunochemical detection of other analytes have been described by both Eastman Kodak Co.[29] and Fuji Photo Film Company Ltd.[30]

PERFORMANCE

The success of any new technology depends on its performance. Table 4 summarizes the results of comparison studies between reference procedures and the Ames SERALYZER® reagent strip system,[31] Kodak's Ektachem 400 analyser and Ektachem slide chemistries,[32] Boehringer-Mannheim Corp. Reflotron-System and Refloquant-Tests,[22] and Fuji Photo Film Co. Ltd Dry Chem 1000 analyser and Dry Chemslides Flu-P.[20] As can be seen, the dry reagent chemistries correlate well. A brief summary of precision of dry reagent chemistry analyses is presented in Table 5. These results are comparable to the precision obtained from most established methodologies.

UTILITY OF DRY REAGENT CHEMISTRIES

By virtue of their stability and discrete formats, dry reagent chemistry allows cost-effective, low volume

TABLE 5
PRECISION OF DRY REAGENT CHEMISTRIES

System	Analyte	Mean	% CV Within run	% CV Between run	Reference
SERALYZER®	LDH	149 (IU/l)	4·6	6·3	(35)
		251 (IU/l)	4·6	4·1	
		404 (IU/l)	3·4	4·1	
	Creatinine	1·1 (mg/dl)	6·2	5·6	(35)
		2·7 (mg/dl)	3·2	5·6	
		6·0 (mg/dl)	2·6	5·4	
	Cholesterol	286 (mg/dl)	2·9	3·4	(35)
		399 (mg/dl)	3·4	3·1	
	Glucose	103 (mg/dl)	2·9	1·9	(35)
		281 (mg/dl)	2·8	3·0	
	Haemoglobin	8·2 (g/dl)	2·2	1·9	(35)
		14·5 (g/dl)	2·1	1·9	
	AST	34 (IU/l)	2·2	2·7	(20)
		47 (IU/l)	2·7	1·9	
		75 (IU/l)	2·1	1·5	
		193 (IU/l)	2·3	2·0	
	ALT	28 (IU/l)	2·9	3·3	(34)
		59 (IU/l)	2·0	1·3	
		163 (IU/l)	1·8	1·2	
		219 (IU/l)	1·7	2·3	
	Triglyceride	66 (mg/dl)	5·9	6·8	(35)
		252 (mg/dl)	3·3	2·3	
	Theophylline	10 (mg/l)	5·9	5·0	(27)
		15 (mg/l)	3·5	4·6	
		20 (mg/l)	4·3	3·3	
		25 (mg/l)	3·9	4·9	
EKTACHEM® (Eastman Kodak)	Cholesterol	103 (mg/dl)	2·3	2·3	(8)
		168 (mg/dl)	—	1·2	
		364 (mg/dl)	—	1·7	
	Bilirubin (neonatal)	0·64 (mg/dl)	1·9	2·8	(36)
		3·9 (mg/dl)	0·6	0·9	
		9·5 (mg/dl)	0·6	0·8	
		18·4 (mg/dl)	0·4	1·0	
	Glucose	69 (mg/dl)	0·9	1·4	(37)
		100 (mg/dl)	1·0	1·5	
		296 (mg/dl)	0·7	1·3	
	Sodium	110 (mmol)	1·3	2·1	(38)
		130 (mmol)	0·7	1·8	
		149 (mmol)	0·5	1·7	

TABLE 5
PRECISION OF DRY REAGENT CHEMISTRIES

System	Analyte	Mean	% CV		Reference
			Within run	Between run	
	Potassium	2·9 (mmol)	2·2	2·8	(38)
		5·6 (mmol)	1·2	2·7	
		8·5 (mmol)	1·7	2·9	
	Carbon dioxide	14 (mmol)	4·6	6·7	(38)
		23 (mmol)	3·8	5·0	
		34 (mmol)	4·1	5·9	
	Chloride	79 (mmol)	1·6	1·4	(38)
		102 (mmol)	0·8	1·3	
		126 (mmol)	0·9	1·4	
REFLOTRON® (Boehringer-Mannheim Corp.)	Haemoglobin	7·6 (g/dl)	2·2	3·4	(22)
		14·0 (g/dl)	1·8	3·0	
		18·3 (g/dl)	2·0	2·2	
	Cholesterol	162 (mg/dl)	2·0	4·2	(22)
		245 (mg/dl)	1·8	2·4	
		341 (mg/dl)	2·2	2·1	
	γ-GT	26 (U/l)	7·0	8·6	(22)
		129 (U/l)	3·4	7·2	
		320 (U/l)	4·3	2·9	
Dry Chem (Fuji)	Glucose	95 (mg/dl)	1·2	—	(18)
		105 (mg/dl)	1·4	—	
		191 (mg/dl)	—	0.9	
		218 (mg/dl)	1·4	—	

testing, thus providing small clinics or a physician's office with the ability to conduct analyses that otherwise would be sent to a large laboratory. The advantages to the patient and physician include the immediate availability of test results prior to consultation. By the same token, dry reagent chemistries are also well-suited for self-care applications, such as self-monitoring of whole blood glucose by insulin-dependent diabetics. By knowing the blood-glucose level, the patient can adjust insulin dosages, as necessary. At present, 11 dry reagent (Table 6) chemistries are available for whole blood-glucose measurement. All but two can be monitored visually by matching the colour of the developed analytical element with a colour chart. All but two can be monitored with dedicated instruments, thus providing a quantitative measurement. The Ames VISIDEX® reagent strip is an example of a visual method. The patient can easily interpolate glucose concentrations ranging from hypoglycaemic levels to hyperglycaemic levels as high as 800 mg/dl. An example of the effectiveness of visual determination is illustrated in Fig. 19 by a comparison between the results obtained with VISIDEX reagent strips and those obtained by a reference procedure.[33]

Self-monitoring by either instrumental means or by a colour chart should help the diabetic to exercise greater control over his disease and hopefully lead

TABLE 6
DRY REAGENTS AVAILABLE FOR WHOLE BLOOD-GLUCOSE ANALYSIS

Dry reagent	Recommended instrument	Manufacturer
Dextrostix®	Glucometer®, Dextrometer	Ames Co.
Visidex®	—	Ames Co.
Glucostix®	Glucometer II	Ames Co.
Glucopat™	—	Kyoto Daiichi Kagaku Co., Ltd
Stat-tek™	Stat-tek	Boehringer-Mannheim Corp.
Chemstrip® bG	Accu-check™ bG	Boehringer-Mannheim Corp.
Reflocheck®	Reflocheck	Boehringer-Mannheim Corp.
Glucoscan™	Glucoscan II	Lifescan
Beta scan™	Betascan	Orange Medical Instruments
Trend strip™	Trendmeter™	Orange Medical Instruments
Diascan™	Diascan	Home Diagnostics, Inc.

to fewer visits to the doctor and a more normal and productive life-style. The availability of dry reagent chemistries has had a dramatic effect on the field of diabetes and the impact of this testing format on clinical analysis is only beginning to become apparent. They have a tremendous potential for bringing convenient, cost-effective clinical tests much closer to the patient in physicians' offices, hospital wards and emergency rooms and will, hopefully, lead to much more efficient and effective patient care.

analyses into such decentralized settings as the hospital ward, physician's office and even the home.

REFERENCES

1. Comer J. P. (1956). Semiquantitative specific test paper for glucose in urine. *Anal. Chem*; **28**: 1748.
2. Free A. H., Adams E. C., Kercher M. L., Free H. M. (1957). Simple specific test for urine glucose. *Clin. Chem*; **3**: 163.

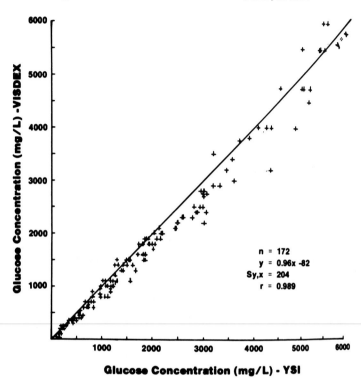

Fig. 19 Comparison results between VISIDEX® reagent strips and Yellow Springs Instruments (YSI) glucose analyser.

SUMMARY

The technology of dry reagent chemistries is sufficiently advanced so that analytical elements can be developed for almost any clinical analyte. Each element contains all the reagents and separation steps necessary to conduct an analysis. This provides the user with several advantages. The ability to obtain several analyses from small sample volumes has already been recognized as desirable with neonatal and geriatric patients. With dry reagent chemistries, usually $10\,\mu l$ of serum or $30\,\mu l$ of whole blood are sufficient per analysis. Hence, a profile of 15 tests can be conducted with $150\,\mu l$ of serum. The waste of reconstituted but unused reagents is eliminated. This provides more efficient and cost-effective use of reagents. The reagents are stable and require little storage space. In addition, they are extremely convenient to use and require only a small amount of technical skill. This allows for expansion of clinical

3. Adams E. C. Jr, Burkhardt L. E., Free A. H. (1957). Specificity of glucose oxidase test for urine glucose. *Science*; **125**: 1082.
4. Free H. M., Collins G. F., Free A. H. (1960). Triple-test strip for urinary glucose, protein and pH. *Clin. Chem*; **6**: 352.
5. Marks V., Dawson A. (1965). Rapid stick method for determining blood-glucose concentration. *Br. Med. J*; **1**: 293.
6. Mazzaferri E. L., Lanese R. R., Skillman T. G., Keller M. P. (1960). Use of test strips with colour meter to measure blood-glucose. *Lancet*; **i**: 331.
7. Walter B. (1983). Dry reagent chemistries in clinical analysis. *Anal. Chem*; **55**: 498A.
8. Dappen G. M., Cumbo P. E., Goodhue C. T. *et al.* (1982). Dry film for the enzymatic determination of total cholesterol in serum. *Clin. Chem*; **28**: 1159.
9. Kortüm G. (1969). *Reflectance Spectroscopy: Principles, Methods, Applications*. New York:Springer.
10. Pesce A. J., Rosen C. G., Pasby T. L. (1971). *Fluorescence Spectroscopy*. New York:Dekker.

11. Kubelka P., Munk F. (1931). Ein Beitrag zur Optik der Farbanstriche. *Z. Tech. Phys*; **12**: 593.

12. Williams F. C., Clapper F. R. (1953). Multiple internal reflections in photographic color prints. *J. Optical Soc. Am*; **43**: 595.

13. Kuan J. C. W., Lau H. K. Y., Guilbault G. G. (1975). Enzymatic determination of serum urea on the surface of silicone-rubber pads. *Clin. Chem*; **21**: 67.

14. Howard W. E. III, Greenquist A., Walter B., Wogoman F. (1983). Automated instrumentation for fluorescence assays on reagent strips. *Anal. Chem*; **55**: 878.

15. Sanderson R. L., Scherer G. W. (1978). EKTACHEM® analyzer instrumentation functions. *Clin. Chem*; **24**: 1008.

16. Stahler F. (1982). Clinical biochemistry: principles and practice. 2nd Asian and Pacific/Congress of Clinical Biochemistry, Singapore, September 19–24, p. 297.

17. Boehringer-Mannheim GMBH (1974). Oxidation indicators containing tetraalkylzenzidines. *Br. Pat.* No 1 464 359. December 21.

18. Kobyashi N., Tuhata M., Akui T., Okuda K. (1982). Evaluation of multilayer film analytical and in plasma and serum by Fuji dry chem slide GLU-P. *Clin. Rep*; **16**: 484.

19. Sunberg M. W., Becker, R. W., Esders T. W., Figueras J., Goodhue C. T. (1983). An enzymatic creatinine assay and a direct ammonia assay in coated thin films. *Clin. Chem*; **29**: 645.

20. Walter B., Berreth L., Co R., Wilcox M. (1983). A solid-phase reagent strip for the colorimetric determination of serum aspartate aminotransferase (AST) on the SERALYZER®. *Clin. Chem*; **29**: 1267.

21. Eikenberry J. N., Erickson W. F., Sandord K. J., Sutherland J. W., Vickers R. S., Weaver M. S. (1982). Clinical enzymes in a dry, thin-film format: Eastman Kodak Co. exhibit presentation. American Association for Clinical Chemistry Annual Meeting, Anaheim, CA. August 8–13.

22. Bush E. W. (1983). Interne Evaluierung von REFLOTRON®. Kongress für Laboratorimsmedizin, Vienna. April 19–23.

23. Charlton S. C., Zipp A., Fleming R. L. (1982). Solid-phase colorimetric determination of potassium. *Clin. Chem*; **28**: 1857.

24. Wong D., Frank G., Charlton S., Hemmes P., Lau A., Fleming R., Atkinson J., Makowski E. (1984). A colorimetric test for serum potassium for use on the SERALYZER® reflectance photometer. *Clin. Chem*; **30**: 962.

25. Walter B., Greenquist A. C., Howard W. E. III (1983). Solid-phase reagent strips for detection of therapeutic drugs in serum by substrate-labeled fluorescent immunoassay. *Anal. Chem*; **55**: 873.

26. Rupchock P. A., Sommer R. G., Greenquist A. C. (1984). A dry reagent ARIS immunoassay for the determination of theophylline with the Ames SERALYZER® reflectance photometer. *Clin. Chem*; **30**: 1014.

27. Rupchock P. A., Sommer R., Greenquist A., Tyhach R., Walter B., Zipp A. (1985). Dry reagent strips for the determination of theophylline. *Clin. Chem*; **31**: 737.

28. Nagatoma S., Yasuda Y., Masuda N., Makiuchi H., Okazzaki M. (1981). Multilayer analysis element utilizing specific binding reaction. *Eur. Pat.* Application No. 81108365.8. October 15.

29. Zon R. S., David S. F. (1979). Particulate structure and element for analysis or transport of a liquid and method of making said element. *Eur. Pat.* Application No. 79303004.8. December 21.

30. Hiratsuka N., Mihara Y., Masuda N., Miyazako T. (1982). Method for immunological assay using multilayer analysis sheet. *US Pat.* No. 4 337 065. June 29.

31. Thomas L., Plischke W., Storz G. (1982). Evaluation of a quantitative solid-phase reagent system for determination of blood analytes. *Ann. Clin. Biochem*; **19**: 214.

32. Kadinyer C. L., O'Kell R. T. (1983). Clinical evaluation of Eastman Kodak's EKTACHEM® 400 analyzer. *Clin. Chem*; **29**: 498.

33. Sherwood M. J., Warchal M. E., Chen S. T. (1983). A new reagent strip (VISIDEX®) for determination of glucose in whole blood. *Clin. Chem*; **29**: 438.

34. Walter B., Co R., Makowski E. (1983). A solid-phase reagent strip for the colorimetric determination of serum alanine aminotransferase (ALT) on the SERALYZER®. *Clin. Chem*; **29**: 1168.

35. SERALYZER® reagent strips package insert. Ames Division, Miles Laboratories.

36. Wu T. W., Dappen G. M., Powers D. M., Lo D. H., Rand R. N., Spayd R. W. (1982). The Kodak EKTACHEM® clinical chemistry slide for measurement of bilirubin in newborns: principles and performance. *Clin. Chem*; **28**: 2366.

37. Curme H. G., Columbus R. L., Dappen G. M. *et al.* (1978). Multilayer elements for clinical analysis: general concepts. *Clin. Chem*; **24**: 1335.

38. Costello P., Kubasik N. P., Brody B. B., Sine H. E., Bertsch J. A., D'Souza J. P. (1983). Multilayer film analysis evaluation of ion-selective electrolyte slides. *Clin. Chem*; **29**: 129.

39. Przyblowicz E. P., Millikan A. G. (1976). *US Pat.* No. 3 992 158.

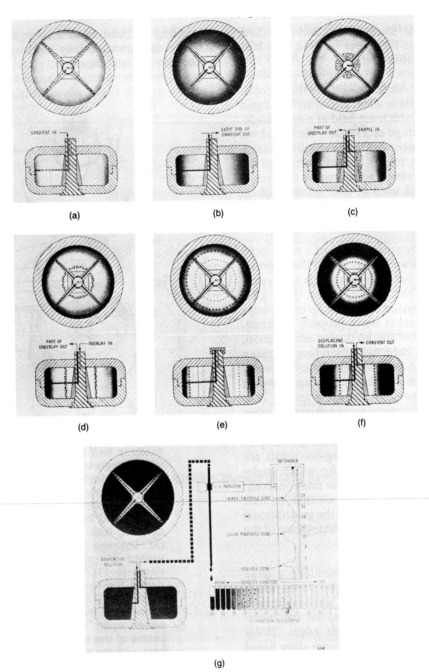

Fig. 10 Loading and unloading of a dynamically loaded zonal rotor. The rotor, viewed in top and side section, is filled and emptied while spinning so that the liquid contents are oriented so that the densest liquid lies at the outside of the rotor. The rotor is shown (a) partially and (b) completely filled with a density gradient which is pumped to the rotor edge with the low density end first. To load the sample (c) the direction of flow is reversed and the sample is introduced through the central line. To move the sample away from the central core an overlay of light liquid is introduced (d). These steps are taken at relatively low speed (5%–10% of the rotor's maximum speed). The rotating seal is next removed and the rotor accelerated to its operating speed to separate the particles present in the sample (e). The rotor is then decelerated to its loading speed and the rotating seal reattached. The gradient is displayed (f) by pumping a dense solution to the edge of the rotor. 'Lifting' the gradient and the separated zones of particles towards the central core and thence out of the rotor. In (g) the liquid displaced from the rotor is monitored and fractions are collected (from Anderson *et al.* (1969) *Anal. Biochem*; **32**: 460).

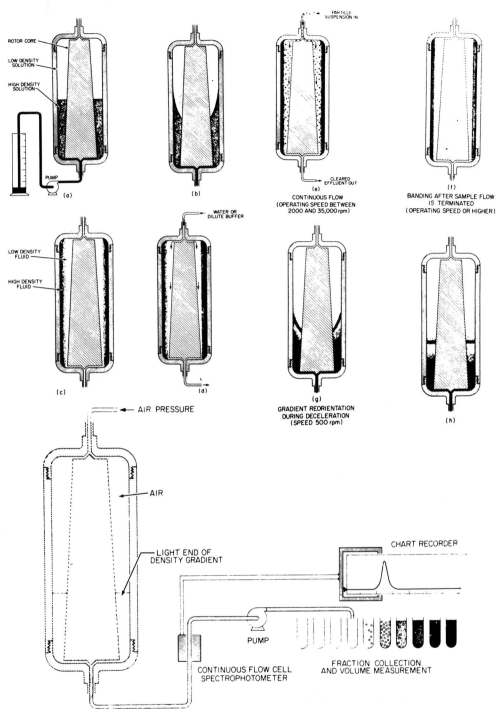

Fig. 11 Operation of a zonal rotor with gradient reorientation. The figure illustrates a continuous flow rotor which is used for harvesting particles (e.g. viruses) from a dilute suspension. When the rotor is used for batch processing, the sample is loaded with the gradient in step (a) and steps (d) and (e) are omitted. (a) The density gradient is introduced with the rotor stationary. If the rotor were operated in batch mode the sample would also be introduced at this time. (b and c) The rotor is slowly accelerated. The gradient reorients so that the densest liquid lies at the outside of the rotor. (d) In a continuous flow rotor, while the rotor is still spinning at a low speed, a dilute buffer is pumped into the centre of the rotor to ensure that the flow channels are free. (e) The rotor is now accelerated to its operating speed and the sample pumped to the centre of the rotor. Particles suspended in the sample fluid sediment into the gradient and band isopycnically. The residual fluid escapes from the base of the rotor. (f) After the sample flow has ceased, the rotor is maintained at its operating speed for sufficient time to ensure isopycnic banding of all the particles present. (g) The rotor is decelerated. Deceleration must be very carefully controlled to prevent mixing as the gradient reorients. (h and i). The gradient, containing the separated bands of particles is recovered from the rotor (from Anderson *et al.* (1969) *Anal. Biochem*; **32**: 460).

should not become a proficient operator. Re-orienting zonal rotors will probably be more simple to use but there is not sufficient published work to be certain that this simplicity will not result in some loss of resolution when these rotors are used for rate separation. Most zonal rotors have a rather large capacity and are used for preparative separations. A small rotor with a capacity of only 80 ml has, however, been used experimentally and seems very valuable in the separation of subcellular particles from needle biopsy samples.

Vertical Tube Rotors. Recently two of the leading centrifuge manufacturers have introduced rotors in which the tubes are held exactly vertical. These rotors are designed for rate or isopycnic zonal separations, not for differential pelleting like angle head rotors. During acceleration and deceleration of the centrifuge the density gradient must re-orient and these rotors may, in many ways, be regarded as the small equivalents of the re-orienting zonal rotors mentioned in the previous section. It is essential that these rotors are used with centrifuges which permit very slow and controlled acceleration and deceleration, or unacceptable mixing will occur. The manufacturers do not claim that these rotors give the same resolution as swing-out rotors but do claim that, for many purposes, the shortened centrifugation time and the increased number of tubes provide compensating advantages.

Preparation of Density Gradients

We have seen that density gradients are essential whether particles are to be separated by rate zonal sedimentation or by isopycnic banding, but the range of densities required in the two cases is different. In the former case, the role of the gradient is simply to stabilize sedimentation; one does not wish any of the particles to reach their isopycnic banding positions. The density of the lightest end of the gradient must be greater than the overall density of the sample. Density gradients are normally prepared by the controlled mixing of two solutions of a density gradient solute. Sucrose is by far the most commonly used compound as it is cheap, causes little damage to biological structures and can form solutions with densities up to 1·3 g/ml. Gradients ranging from 15–30% w/w sucrose, giving a density range of 1·06–1·23 g/ml are widely used for rate sedimentation. Other gradient solutes are used for some purposes, especially when iso-osmotic gradients are required, as in the separation of living cells.

It is not possible, in a short article to give practical details of methods, for preparing density gradients: simple linear gradients can be prepared using simple laboratory-made apparatus which the reader will find described in articles listed at the end of this chapter. More complicated gradients can be made either by use of expensive proprietary gradient makers, or,

providing the experimenter does not mind doing a few calculations, with quite simple 'home-made' equipment. References quoted at the end of this chapter should be consulted for further information.

Fractionation of Density Gradients

We have seen earlier that after centrifugation the gradient containing separated zones of particles is displaced from zonal rotors by pumping a dense solution to the outside of the rotor so that the density gradient flows from the centre lightest end first. A

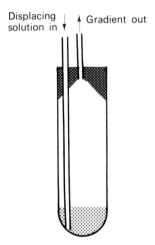

Fig. 12 Displacement of a density gradient from a centrifuge tube. A special cap, shaped inside like an inverted cone, is placed over the top of the tube. Dense liquid is pumped through a probe leading to the base of the tube. This lifts the whole of the density gradient up to the displacing cap, through which it flows with the lightest fractions appearing first.

very similar method is used to fractionate density gradients in the tubes of swing-out rotors. A dense solution is injected to the bottom of the tube. This moves the liquid column upward so that it is funnelled out through a special cap at the top of the tube (Fig. 12). Bands of particles are detected by passing the displaced gradient through a spectrophotometer and fractions are collected for further analysis.

THE USES OF CENTRIFUGATION

Centrifugal methods may be used to separate particles either on the basis of their size or of their density. Clearly the properties of the particles in the mixture to be fractioned will decide which approach will be most useful. For this purpose the simplest method for presenting the properties of the particles is to use what is known as an S-p diagram (Fig. 13). The construction of the diagram is fairly simple.

The choice of density gradient solutes for separation of particles by isopycnic banding is much more difficult than with separations by rate sedimentation. Isopycnic banding normally entails the exposure of the particles to very high concentrations of the gradient solute and, as mentioned earlier, much longer centrifugation is required. Hence the risk of damage to the material being separated is much greater. The

ganelles. There is less risk of damage than with sucrose, but the vicosity of polymer solutions may necessitate prolonged centrifugation. Cells and subcellular structures band at much lower densities in these media than in low molecular weight solutes.

4. Iodinated polycyclic compounds, developed as x-ray contrast media, have proved very useful for isopycnic banding. Solutions of these compounds are not toxic to living cells, cover a wide density range and are less viscous than sucrose

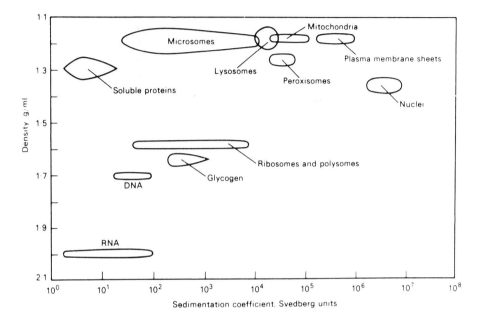

Fig. 13 An S-p diagram indicating the sedimentation coefficients and densities of the particles present in a liver homogenate. The size of the spot gives an estimate of the heterogeneity of the particles. Thus endoplasmic reticulum fragments vary in density from 100 S to about 3000 S and in density from about 1·14–1·22 g/ml (from Prospero, T.D. in Reid (1973)).

choice of solute depends largely on the material which is to be fractionated. Density gradient solutes in common use are divided into four main classes:

1. Salts of alkali metals, notably CsCl and NaBr. These compounds form mobile solutions over a very wide range of densities but tend to damage biological structures, dissociating proteins from each other and from nucleic acids. Salt gradients are very useful for banding macromolecules such as DNA and a limited number of other particles, notably serum lipoproteins, which are stable in solutions of high ionic strength.

2. Sucrose is widely used for the isopycnic banding of cell organelles, but the high osmotic strength of concentrated solutions may damage some structures.

3. High molecular weight hydrophilic polymers such as Ficoll and dextrans may be used for the isopycnic banding of living cells or cell or-

or polymeric solutes. The compounds are, however, rather expensive.

Thus in the example given, which illustrates a liver homogenate, the nuclei are shown to have a density of 1·3 g/ml and a sedimentation coefficient of about 10^7 S. The size of the spot gives a rough idea of the heterogeneity of each type of particle with respect to its size and density.

The rules for deciding what approach will be most useful are fairly simple. If particles differ by a factor of 10 or more in sedimentation coefficient then they may be separated by differential pelleting. Providing that the pellet is washed twice by resuspension and repelleting there will be almost complete separation. With more complicated mixtures such as tissue homogenates it is customary to use differential pelleting to divide the mixture into a series of crude fractions and then to subject each fraction to density gradient centrifugation. Inspection of the S-p diagram will indicate the approach. Thus in the example given in Fig. 13 mitochondria differ in size from lysosomes, microbodies and microsomes, but overlap with these cell fractions in density. Hence rate sedimentation must be used for their separation. Microbodies, on the other hand, are identical in size to lysosomes, but differ in density. Hence these particles must be separated by isopycnic banding. To separate all four types of particle the mixture would first have to be fractioned by rate sedimentation and the zone enriched in microbodies separated and further fractioned by isopycnic banding.

Three factors influence the choice of rotor, the approach to be used, the size of the particles to be separated and the amount of material in the sample. Angle head rotors cannot be used for rate zonal separations, but are to be preferred for differential pelleting because of their simplicity of operation and high capacity. Angle-head rotors can be used very successfully for isopycnic banding, but for most purposes swing-out and zonal rotors will give better results. Swing-out, zonal or vertical tube rotors must be used for rate zonal separations. The resolution obtained with these two types of rotor is almost identical, so that the choice depends on the volume of sample; when particles are to be separated by rate sedimentation the volume of the sample should be less than 5% of the volume of the gradient so that zonal rotors are essential for large-scale fractionations. Vertical tube rotors do not give as good separations as the other two types, but give more rapid separation of very small particles.

Having chosen what type of rotor to use, one must decide on the precise model. The smaller the particle, the higher the speed of centrifugation which will be required. A guide to the suitability of rotors is given in Table 1 which gives the slowest possible speeds for effecting the separation of various sizes of particle. Normally all faster rotors can be used, with some sacrifice in the volume of liquid which can be processed, but one must beware of damage caused by the high hydrostatic pressure which is present in tubes of liquid centrifuged at speeds much in excess of 30 000 rev./min.

Up to this point we have considered the problems of choosing conditions for a centrifugal separation in an abstract way. The principles laid down in the previous paragraph, and other factors which may affect the choice of conditions will be better illustrated by consideration of a number of examples.

Separation of Serum Proteins

First one must consider whether it is worth using centrifugation to separate serum proteins. Normally much more information is obtained by gel electrophoresis. Resolution obtained by centrifugation in an analytical rotor is as good as that obtained by rate sedimentation in a density gradient. More information can, however, be obtained from the former method as the sedimentation rates of individual pro-

TABLE 1

MINIMUM ROTOR SPEEDS REQUIRED FOR THE SEPARATION OF DIFFERENT TYPES OF PARTICLE BY RATE ZONAL SEDIMENTATION. THE SLOWEST ZONAL ROTOR IS ALSO INDICATED. (Note that any faster rotor may be used in any case)

Particle	Approximate diameter (μm)	Speed required (rev./min*)	Zonal rotor
Liver cells	20	1000	A-XII
Nuclei	5	1000	A-XII
Mitochondria	1·5	4000	A-XII
Lysosomes	0·4	8000	HS or Z-15
Microsomes	0·2	20 000	B-XV
Polysomes	0·04	25 000	B-XV
Ribosome sub-units	0·02	27 000	B-XV (Ti) or B-XIV
Large proteins	0·008	40 000	B-XIV

* The speeds mentioned are those which, in the author's experience, will give a reasonable separation within a working day. Slower rotors may be used if overnight running is acceptable. The speeds assume that a normal preparative centrifuge is used. Note that if particles are to be separated by isopycnic banding considerably higher speeds are required.

tein species can be measured. The size distribution of serum proteins in healthy and diseased people has been studied by clinical biochemists but it does not seem that ultracentrifugal analysis can give more information than that obtained more easily by gel electrophoresis. Rate sedimentation can however be used to separate macroglobulins for further study and in this limited field centrifugal methods may be useful.

The 21 S and 27 S globulin fractions are much larger than other serum proteins but do not differ much in their size or density. Hence they are most conveniently separated by rate sedimentation. The small size of the particles (single macromolecules in this case) demands that a high speed rotor, capable of 35 000 rev./min or more should be used. Since centrifugal methods will only be used when one wishes to isolate the macroglobulins for further study, zonal rotors will normally be used for the separation. Hence a reasonable quantity of blood can then be processed in a single step.

The choice of the gradient material for the separation of serum proteins is complicated by the high concentration of protein in serum. Serum may be regarded as a 7% solution of protein in saline of density about 1·006 g/ml. The presence of protein raises the density to about 1·025 g/ml. If sucrose is to be used as the density gradient solute the gradient must start at a sucrose concentration of at least 80 g/l if the sample is not to sink into the gradient. Even when this is done the sample zone will not be completely stable. Molecules of sucrose diffuse much more rapidly than protein molecules. Thus more sucrose molecules will diffuse into the lower part of the sample zone than protein molecules diffuse out. When the concentration of sucrose molecules in the lower part of the sample zone approaches the concentration in the top part of the gradient, the density of the former (containing water, sucrose and protein) will exceed the density of the latter (containing only water and sucrose). The sample zone will thus 'tumble' slightly down the gradient. This increase in the width of the sample band will be reflected in a poorer resolution of the various fractions after centrifugation. The problem can, however, be largely overcome by the use of a high molecular weight gradient solute, such as Ficoll, which will diffuse at the same rate as proteins.

Isopycnic banding is not generally used for the separation of proteins. There is little difference in density among 'simple' proteins, but, as carbohydrates are denser than polypeptides, glycoproteins differ in their density depending on their carbohydrate content. This has been exploited in the fractionation of mucus. The banding density of glycoproteins is so high that it is practically essential to use salts such as CsCl

as the gradient solute. Hence there is little hope that enzyme activities will survive.

Separation of Serum Lipoproteins

In general there is an inverse relationship between the size and the density of different serum lipoproteins; the larger the lipoprotein the greater the percentage of lipid which it contains and the lower its density. The classical methods for separating serum lipoproteins are by stepwise flotation or in the analytical ultracentrifuge. In stepwise flotation the very low-density lipoprotein (VLDL) is separated by centrifuging the sample for 18 h at $150\,000 \times g$. The VLDL, being less dense than serum, floats to the top of the tube and forms a layer which may be removed with a bent pipette. Low density lipoproteins may then be separated from the subnatant by adjusting this to a density of 1·063 by addition of NaBr and recentrifuging for 18 h at $150\,000 \times g$. High-density lipoproteins are separated from the second subnatant by adjusting to a density of 1·21 and centrifuging for 24 h at $150\,000 \times g$. As can be seen this technique

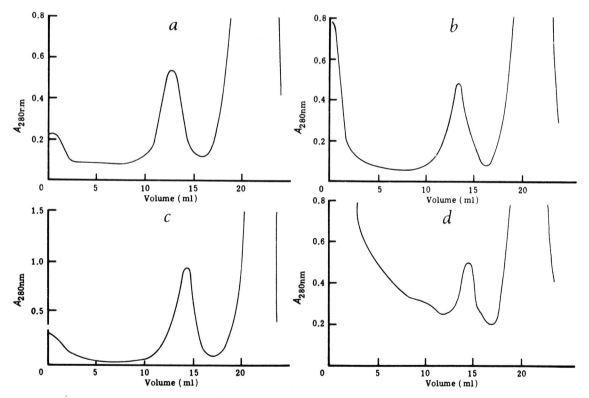

Fig. 14 Preparative separation of serum lipoproteins from hyperlipoproteinaemic subjects. Centrifugation was for 2 h at 30 000 rev./min in a 3 × 23 ml swing out rotor (MSE Scientific Instruments). The gradient was prepared from NaBr and extended from a density of 1·2 g/ml to 1·005 g/ml. All density gradient solutions contained 11·4 g/l NaCl and 0·01 g/l EDTA and were adjusted to pH 7·4. The samples of serum were adjusted to a density of 1·22 with solid NaBr and injected under the gradients. The samples were underlayed with 2 ml of NaBr solution of density 1·5 g/ml to lift them out of the rounded portion at the base of the tube. The samples are as follows. (a) 1·6 ml of serum from a 'normal' subject. (b) 1 ml of serum from a subject with mild Type II hyperlipoproteinaemia. (c) 1·0 ml of serum from a subject with severe Type II hyperlipoproteinaemia. (d) 1·0 ml of serum from a subject with Type III hyperlipoproteinaemia (from Hinton et al. (1974) Clin. Chim. Acta; 53: 355–360).

is simple, yields fractions for further study, but ties up an ultracentrifuge for three days. Much more rapid results can be obtained if the flotation of the lipoproteins from the serum is studied in an analytical rotor, but this rotor is complicated to operate and does not provide fractions for further study.

More rapid separation of lipoprotein subfractions may be obtained by rate flotation. It is essential to use flotation as VLDL and chylomicrons are less dense than water and hence will not sediment in aqueous media. The technique is fairly simple. The sample is adjusted to a density greater than the density of any of the components under investigation and is then injected under a density gradient by use of a syringe with a long needle. On centrifugation, the particles float at a rate chiefly determined by their size. Using this technique VLDL and LDL can be separated from up to 2 ml of serum within 2 h. The gradient material of choice is NaBr. Sucrose is not suitable because the high viscosity of dense sucrose solutions slows the separation of lipoprotein from the sample zone. While different types of hyperlipoproteinaemia show distinctive patterns after rate flotation (Fig. 14) the technique is not really suitable for routine scanning of patient samples, gel electrophoresis is much simpler and more rapid. The real use of centrifugal methods is in the preparation of lipoprotein fractions for further study and here rate flotation offers many advantages over stepwise flotation, providing greater resolution and more rapid separation. If more than 2 ml of serum is to be fractionated at one time zonal rotors should be used; for smaller quantities swing-out rotors give excellent results.

Separation of Lysosomes

As stated at the beginning of this chapter, the major use of centrifugal methods is the separation of cell organelles from tissue homogenates. This is not, at the moment, of direct importance to the clinical biochemist, but fractionation of human tissue has been used, for example in the elucidation of the causes of storage diseases such as glycogen storage disease Type II and the Hunter-Hurler syndrome (gargoylism). Both of these diseases involve a deficiency in a lysosomal enzyme. However, methods have been developed for fractionating very small samples such as are obtained by needle biopsy. These are likely to be complicated for routine laboratories but are of great value in clinical research. The problems involved in determining the activity of a lysosomal enzyme are illustrated by the following examples in which rat liver lysosomes are examined for the presence of an enzyme capable of splitting L-leucyl β-naphthylamide (LNA).

In rat liver, active aryl amidases capable of splitting LNA are found in the plasma membrane and in the cytosol. Activity is found in the 'lysosomal fraction' prepared by differential pelleting, but similar rates

of activity of other enzymes known to be present in the plasma membrane are also found in this fraction. One suspects that the LNAase activity is due to contamination of the lysosomal fraction by plasma membrane fragments. When the 'lysosomal fraction' is further fractionated by rate sedimentation the bulk of the LNAase is indeed found to be present in structures different in size from lysosomes. There does, however, appear to be more activity of LNAase than of other known plasma membrane enzymes in the lysosome-rich region. If material from the central part of the gradient is further fractionated by isopycnic banding, lysosomes are separated from the few remaining plasma membrane fragments and some LNAase activity is shown clearly to be associated with the lysosomes. Thus to prove that some LNAase activity is present in lysosomes it has proved necessary to separate sequentially by three different methods, differential pelleting, rate sedimentation and isopycnic banding. Equally complex procedures are necessary to isolate lysosomes from other tissues and from pathologically altered liver. At all stages in a cell fractionation experiment it is essential to monitor 'markers'* for cell organelles other than the one being studied.

Although most tissue fractionation studies have been carried out with animal tissue, there has recently been much more interest in changes in all organelles in diseased human organs. Disorders of liver lysosomes have been found in several, relatively common, human diseases and in particular enlargement, and consequent fragility of lysosomes may be responsible for the cirrhotic changes in alcoholism and haemochromatosis. The presence of these enlarged and atypical lysosomes has been demonstrated by isopycnic banding in a special low-volume rotor.

Separation of Living Cells

The individual cells which make up a tissue can often be separated from each other by perfusing the tissue with a mixture of a collagenase and of a chelating agent. Such cell suspensions can be fractionated by centrifugal methods. Both rate sedimentation and isopycnic banding may be used, but it appears at the moment that the latter will usually be more useful. However, the situation has been further complicated by the development of specialized elutriator rotors and by the introduction of new gradient materials.

---

* A marker for a cell organelle of any tissue is a chemical constituent or, more usually, an enzyme activity which:

(a) is uniquely associated with a particular cell structure when the tissue is studied by electron microscopic cytochemistry,

(b) shows a distribution, after fractionation of the tissue homogenate by centrifugation, similar to that of fragments of the cell structure identified morphologically.

It should be noted that one cannot confidently predict that an enzyme which is a marker for some cell constituent in one tissue will also be uniquely associated with that structure in other tissues.

A particular problem in the separation of living cells is the selection of the density gradient solute. The organization of the living cell is much more complex and more sensitive to disruption than the individual cell organelles. High concentrations of sucrose or of low-molecular-weight salts are lethal to most cells. The most suitable density gradient media for the separation of living cells are high-molecular-weight polymers such as Ficoll or some of the iodinated polycyclic compounds. Also, when separating intact cells, care must be taken not to subject the cells to very high centrifugal fields or they may be literally torn apart due to the difference in density of various cell structures.

The risk of damage to preparations by high concentrations of the gradient media is most evident when attempting to separate living cells, but one must always guard against damage to any material which is being separated by the density gradient medium. Thus exposure to high concentrations of sucrose damages respiratory control in mitochondria. A further problem which may be encountered is interference by the density gradient material in the assay of separated fractions. Thus many enzymes are inhibited if the assays are carried out in the presence of high concentrations of sucrose, although this inhibition may be completely reversed by dilution. As with all separation methods, centrifugation experiments must be designed in such a way as to check that none of the material which is being studied is lost during the separation.

CONCLUSIONS

At present, centrifugation is a technique of fairly limited interest to most clinical biochemists. Centrifugation and gel electrophoresis are both essentially methods for separating particles on the basis of their size. Experience suggests that particles with a molecular weight of less than one million can be separated more effectively by gel electrophoresis. Centrifugation is more suited to separation of particles varying in size between serum low-density lipoproteins and whole cells. Few of the structures in the body fluids fall into this category, but wider use may be made of the technique as more clinical biochemists embark on studies of tissue chemistry.

Technically, centrifugation methods are quite simple, but the apparatus is expensive. For this reason, if no other, it should be fully used. More than with most techniques, the results obtained in gradient centrifugation depend on the care and skill of the user, especially in applying the sample to a gradient and in fractionating the gradient after centrifugation, rather than on the state of equipment. If possible an experienced worker should be consulted before starting experiments. Care must be taken to choose an appropriate technique for the work in hand. Obviously if the particles to be separated differ only in their density, not in size, isopycnic banding must

be used. However, because of the long centrifugation times and the high concentrations of gradient material to which the particles are exposed, there is more risk of damage in separations by isopycnic banding than by rate sedimentation. When particles are to be separated by sedimentation rate, either differential pelleting or rate zonal sedimentation may be used. The former is used for particles differing considerably in size but, because of the large amount of material which can be handled, is frequently used as a preliminary to a final separation by rate zonal sedimentation. The latter is the most flexible of the centrifugal techniques but one must remember that the capacity of the density gradients used is limited and if too much material is loaded, resolution will suffer.

It is hoped that this chapter will have given the reader some idea of the scope and limitations of centrifugal methods. Although gel electrophoresis may give better resolution, fractions separated by centrifugation are instantly available for further study. In its proper field of large particles, there are usually no alternatives to the use of centrifugal methods.

SUGGESTIONS FOR FURTHER READING

A. General Techniques. (i) Differential pelleting. The technique of differential pelleting is so simple that most writers have concentrated on the presentation and interpretation of results. Among these de Duve C. (1966) in *Enzyme Cytology* (Roodyn D. B., ed.) London: Academic Press, is helpful while the historical review by de Duve (1971). *J. Cell Biol*; **50**: 20D–55D has much interesting material.

(ii) Density gradient centrifugation (rate zonal sedimentation and flotation and isopycnic banding). The article by Hinton R. H. and Dobrota M. (1976) in *Laboratory Techniques in Biochemistry and Molecular Biology* (Work T., Work E., eds), North Holland, Amsterdam discusses the whole field of density gradient centrifugation with especial emphasis on practical methods. A more recent account is given in Price C. A. (1982). *Centrifugation in Density Gradients*, New York: Academic Press.

(iii) Analytical ultracentrifugation. Bowen T. J. (1980). *An Introduction to Centrifugation*, Wiley Interscience, New York, concentrates principally on the use of analytical rotors in measuring the physical properties of macromolecules.

B. The Theory of Centrifugation. The most rigorous account is that of Schumaker V. N. (1967). *Adv. Biol. Med. Phys*; **11**: 245–339.

C. Methods for Particular Separations. Methods for separating particles by centrifugation are scattered widely through the literature. Methods using newer gradient materials such as Percoll or Nycodens (a derivative of triiodobenzoic acid) can often be obtained from the manufacturers and a collection of procedures is to be found in Rickwood D. (ed.) (1983). *Iodinated Density Gradient Media: a Practical Approach*, Oxford: IRL.

The cost of these media is so great that sucrose remains the favourite material for gradient formation. Here, the best approach is via the contents pages of journals specializing in the tissue of interest.

19. Ultrafiltration and Dialysis
A. G. E. Wilson

INTRODUCTION

The analytical techniques of dialysis and ultrafiltration are being increasingly used in biochemistry. Applications of these techniques include; separation and/or concentration of high molecular weight solutes (usually with MW in excess of 10^4, e.g. proteins); investigation of molecular weight, size and shape; solute homogeneity; subunit structure and chemical purity. These techniques have also found extensive application in the investigation of molecular associations, e.g. binding of small ligands to proteins.

The physical processes of dialysis and ultrafiltration form the basis of important physiological and therapeutic functions (e.g. glomerular filtration, haemodialysis, peritoneal dialysis), in the treatment of patients who have taken an overdose of a drug and for the rapid removal of some environmental poisons.

Dialysis refers to the diffusion of a solute species across a semipermeable membrane as a result of a difference in the chemical potential of the solute on either side of the membrane. Differences in the rates of diffusion of different solutes provide the basis for separation. In ultrafiltration the rate of movement of a solute across a semipermeable membrane is enhanced by inducing a flow of solvent through the membrane. The flow of solvent is effected by establishing a pressure gradient across the membrane. Because the application of this pressure tends to reverse the normal process of osmosis, ultrafiltration has been referred to as 'reverse osmosis'. Essentially the only difference between these two terms is the size scale of the particles which are separated. For convenience, the term 'reverse osmosis' is usually reserved for the separation of solutes whose molecular weight is within one order of magnitude of the solvent (e.g. salts, sugars).

An approximate guide to the separation ability of dialysis and ultrafiltration with respect to other commonly used separation techniques is shown in Fig. 1. This figure is an oversimplification and other factors, in addition to those shown, may also effect the separation.

In most separation procedures the solute molecules are subject to two forces acting in opposite directions,

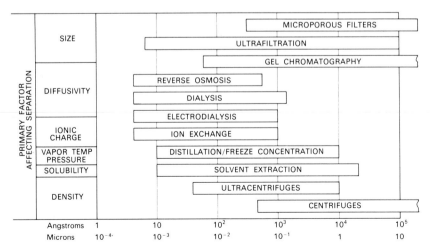

Fig. 1 Spectrum of separation processes (reprinted with the permission of Amicon Corporation).

these two classes of forces may be termed impelling and retarding. The impelling forces include; hydrodynamic (e.g. chromatographic separation), electrostatic or electrokinetic (e.g. electrophoresis), molecular kinetic (diffusion), gravitational and centrifugal (e.g. sedimentation methods). Retarding forces either act on molecules in homogenous solution (molecular frictional effects), or arise from the addition to the system of a stationary phase accessible to the solute molecules.[1] For dialysis and ultrafiltration the impelling forces are osmotic and hydrostatic respectively, whereas retarding forces are mainly molecular sieve effects.

DIALYSIS

Dialysis Membranes

A number of different types of membrane have been used for dialysis including regenerated cellulose, cellulose acetate, cellulose nitrate, polyamide and polyvinyl chloride. The most widely used types are the commercially available cellulose sheet and tube materials. These are prepared from cellulose by various modifications of the cuprammonium process, and may contain traces of copper, nitrogen and sulphur. Such impurities, along with the plasticizer glycerol, can be removed by presoaking in de-ionized water or boiling in water. These cellulose membranes exhibit good reproducibility and minimal adsorption, although the latter is highly dependent on the nature of the solute.

Cellulose membranes consist of pores and cavities of various shapes and sizes. The pores are not uniformly straight holes, but are irregular channels with cross connections, dead ends and widely varying diameters and cross-sections. Because of this heterogeneity in porosity it is possible to separate a mixture of solutes quantitatively only if the components differ greatly in molecular size. In general the cellulose membranes are of low average pore diameter, ranging from about 4 to 8 nm and are impermeable to substances with a molecular weight in excess of about 10 000. It should be stressed that other factors such as solute size and shape are important determinants of permeability. Craig and his co-workers[2-4] have performed extensive studies on the selectivities of cellulose membranes. They have demonstrated that cellulose tubing (e.g. that produced by Visking) of different diameter differs widely in its permeability, presumably due to differences in manufacture. They have also shown that the permeability of such membranes can be altered by both physical and chemical treatments, e.g. acetylation decreases permeability, whereas stretching, or treatment with zinc chloride or sodium hydroxide increases permeability. Mechanical treatment can decrease or increase the porosity depending on whether the tubing is stretched linearly only, or both linearly and circularly.

Dialysis Apparatus and Procedure

A large number of different procedures and apparatus designs have been employed in dialysis studies.[1,3,5-8] The apparatus design and the precautionary measures employed in dialysis studies are to a large extent dependent on the type of separation to be carried out (e.g. desalting by dialysis requires less precautionary measures than does protein–ligand interaction studies). One of the simplest and most widely used apparatus designs is illustrated in Fig. 2.

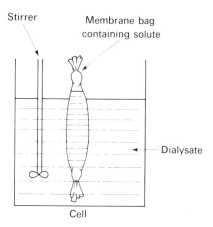

Fig. 2 Simple dialysis cell for laboratory separations.

The most common way of performing dialysis is to make a sac from wet cellulose tubing, although techniques using sheets of membrane are also widely employed. The cellulose membrane is usually presoaked, e.g. in de-ionized or boiling water, to remove the plasticizer glycerol and other solutes. Impurities in the cellulose can be leached out, if desired by repeated soaking in dilute acid (e.g. 0.01 M acetic acid). Metals can also be removed from the membrane, if necessary, by pre-soaking the membrane in EDTA (0.05 M) and then washing with distilled water.

Following pre-soaking, one end of the cellulose tubing is tied and the tube filled with solution to be dialysed. The other end is then tied forming a sac, leaving sufficient air space to allow for fluid expansion and the movement of liquid. This air space usually means that the sac will float in the solvent. This can lead to better mixing, as the sac will spin when the solvent is stirred (see Fig. 2). Alternatively the sac can be connected directly to a magnetic stirrer or stirrer rod; the stirring disturbs the concentration gradients which develop near the surface of the membrane and impede dialysis, until eventually an equilibrium concentration of the diffusible solute between the two solutions is established. The time for the attainment of the equilibrium is variable and depends on the solute, solvent, apparatus, etc. After the establishment of equilibrium, dialysis can be recommenced by repeated replacement of the diffusate with

Ultrafiltration Procedures

In ultrafiltration apparatus the sample is either contained directly above the membrane (the so-called batch method, as in Fig. 4a), or passed across the membrane (i.e. continuous ultrafiltration, Fig. 4b).

ectly through any filter that retains dissolved substances, two detrimental effects may occur:

1. Pores within the membrane may become progressively clogged or plugged.
2. A concentrated gradient of the retained solute

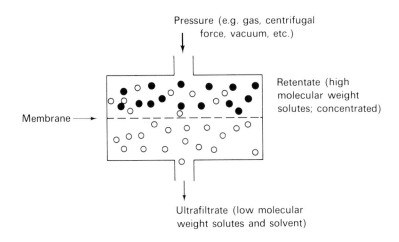

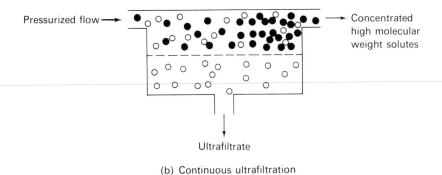

(a) Batch ultrafiltration

(b) Continuous ultrafiltration

Fig. 4 Modes of ultrafiltration.

With ultrafiltration the relatively high molecular weight of the retained solute (usually higher than 500, e.g. proteins, polymers) makes osmotic pressure differences across the membrane negligible, so that low pressures (5–100 p.s.i., 0·4–7 atmos) are adequate to obtain high filtration rates. A positive pressure (e.g. N_2 gas pressure) on the solution side of the membrane is more commonly employed than a negative pressure on the ultrafiltrate side (vacuum). However, a number of other methods of achieving the necessary ultrafiltration pressure have been used and include; centrifugal force (e.g. Fig. 5), mercury columns and even spring tension.

During the process of ultrafiltration retained substances are progressively concentrated upstream whilst the solvent and any membrane-permeating species emerge as ultrafiltrate. When fluid moves directly

may develop above the membrane at the fluid-/membrane interface.[10] Such an effect can occur even in well-mixed systems and may, if left undisturbed, act as a secondary membrane tending to reduce the ultrafiltration rate. This phenomenon is called 'concentration polarization'. The extent of polarization is determined by macrosolute concentration, temperature (a viscosity effect, the more dilute the solution the less likelihood of concentration polarization), and the geometry of the system.

If left undisturbed concentration polarization restricts solvent and solute transport through the membrane. It can also alter the filtration selectivity by forming quasi-gel phases. Therefore to counteract concentration polarization and sustain high ultrafilt-

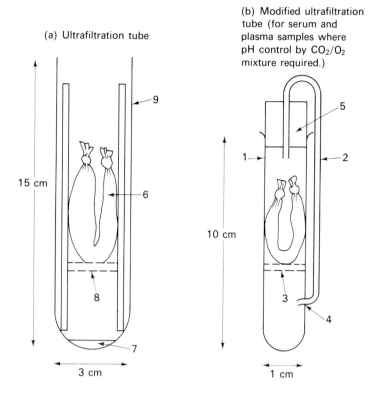

(a) Ultrafiltration tube

(b) Modified ultrafiltration tube (for serum and plasma samples where pH control by CO_2/O_2 mixture required.)

Key

1. Glass tube
2. Polyethylene tube (2 mm O.D.)
3. Glass sinter (porosity grade 1)
4. Adhesive and parafilm seal
5. Rubber bung
6. Dialysis bag
7. Ultrafiltrate
8. Glass sinter incorporated into glass tube
9. Polycarbonate centrifuge tube (50 ml)

Fig. 5 Ultrafiltration apparatus employing centrifugal force.

ration rates, as well as fractionation efficiency, three methods are frequently employed. Two of these, magnetic stirring and vibrational agitation, are employed in batch type systems, obviously systems with no agitation have no polarization control. Continuous ultrafiltration systems depend on the flow of fluid across the membrane to disperse the concentrated layers. Thin-channel ultrafiltration systems, such as that manufactured by Amicon, employ the shear forces generated by the laminar flow in the very thin channels in order that the bulk of the liquid has access to the membrane surface. This proves effective particularly at high concentrations of macromolecule solute. Simple ultrafiltration performed by using centrifugal forces also avoids concentrated layer build up, as the angle of the centrifuge tube produces fluid shear on the membrane surface which promotes high flow through the membrane. Numerous systems for ultrafiltration have been described in the literature.

Diafiltration

A useful application of ultrafiltration is the 'washing of solutions' by the addition of pure solvent at the same rate as ultrafiltrate is produced. Termed 'diafiltration' this procedure offers an alternative to conventional dialysis, but has the important advantage of taking considerably less time than conventional dialysis (e.g. 1/10–1/100 of time). The advantage in efficiency is particularly marked at low salt concentration and for relatively small volumes (less than 20 ml). Diafiltration can also be used in a continuous and discontinuous mode (Fig. 6). Diafiltration systems employ the same type of anisotropic membranes as described above. A commercial diafiltration system is marketed by Amicon. The applications of diafiltration include; desalting, removal of low-molecular-weight organic compounds from sera and for protein binding studies. A significant advantage of diafiltration over both dialysis and ultrafiltration in the study of protein binding is that it has the provision for the maintenance of a fixed volume in the sample compartment.

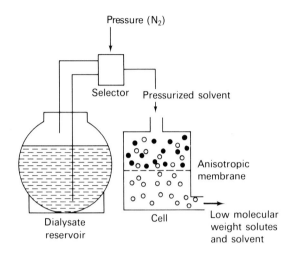

Fig. 6 Diafiltration. Figure depicts diafiltration in the continuous mode, an essential feature is that dialysate enters the cell at the same rate as ultrafiltrate is removed. Diafiltration can also be performed in the discontinuous mode.

ADVANCES IN MEMBRANE TECHNOLOGY

The preceding discussions have emphasized how the success of both dialysis and ultrafiltration is largely dependent upon the membrane. This has been demonstrated by the increased versatility found for these techniques by the introduction of anisotropic polymer membranes. It is evident that the future importance of membrane filtration as a separation technique depends on the development of more versatile and selective membranes. A considerable amount of effort is now being directed towards this end.

One example is Nuclepore®. This membrane is made from a thin sheet of polycarbonate plastic using an irradiation-and-etching process. The manufacturing process consists of two basic steps; the plastic film is first exposed to charged particles that produce sensitized tracks in the film. These tracks are then etched into uniform, cylindrical pores. By controlling the length of the etching process a specified pore size is produced. The pore density (pore/cm²) is controlled by the length of time the plastic film is exposed

to the charged particles in the nuclear reactor. This manufacturing process results in membranes with several advantages:

1. Straight through, cylindrical pores for sieve-like filtration.
2. Very accurate pore sizes, for absolute retention (precise pore size cut-off).
3. High pore densities for maximum flow rate (up to 1×10^9 pores/cm²). Membranes are available in a range of pore sizes from 0·03 to 8 μm.

These membranes are resistant to attack by most acids and organic solvents, except for halogenated hydrocarbons and most strong bases. They withstand high temperatures and are usually hydrophilic in nature, although they can be made either partially or completely hydrophobic. The membranes exhibit good physical uniformity from membrane to membrane and are very thin being either 5 or 10 μm thick depending on pore size. They are very flexible and also have high tensile strength (average 7000 p.s.i.). These membranes are capable of high flow rates and smaller particles will generally pass through the straight-through pores of the Nuclepore membrane more easily than with tortuous path filters. Nuclepore membranes do, of course, become clogged by particles larger than, or approximating to, their rated pore size. Electrostatic charges and secondary valence forces may also cause a build up of particles on the cylindrical walls of the pores. Backwashing with a reverse flow pulse can often unplug the membrane allowing its re-use.

The continued advancement in membrane technology is leading to a greater sophistication and selectivity in the techniques of dialysis and ultrafiltration. Although still in relatively early stages of development, membrane filtration seems likely to become one of the more important unit operations in the field of separation technology.

REFERENCES

1. Morris C. J. O. R., Morris P. (1964). *Separation Methods in Biochemistry*. London: Pitman.
2. Craig L. C. (1967). In *Methods in Enzymology* (Hirs C. H. W., ed.). Vol. XI, 870–905. New York: Academic Press.
3. Craig L. C., King T. P. (1962). In *Methods of Biochemical Analysis* (Glick D., ed.), **10**, 175–199. New York: Interscience.
4. Craig L. C., Konigsberg W. (1961). Dialysis studies III. Modification of pore size and shape in cellophane membranes. *J. Phys. Chem*; **65**: 166.
5. Berg E. W. (1963). *Physical and Chemical Methods of Separation*, Chapter 12, pp. 227–241. New York: McGraw-Hill.
6. Carr C. W. (1961). In *Physical Methods in Chemical Analysis* (Berl W. G., ed.) **4**, 1–43 New York: Academic Press.
7. King T. P. (1974). In *Clinical Biochemistry–Principles*

and Methods (Curtius H. Ch., Roth M., eds), Vol. 1, 195–207. Berlin, New York: de Gruyter.

8. Weder H.-J., Bickel M. H. (1970). Interactions of drugs with proteins II. Experimental methods, treatment of experimental data, and thermodynamics of binding reactions of thymoleptic drugs and model dyes, *J. Pharm. Sci*; **59**: 1563.
9. Craig L. C., Chen H. C. (1972). On a theory for the passive transport of solute through semi-permeable membranes. *Proc. Natl. Acad. Sci*; **69**: 702.
10. Michaels A. S. (1968). In *Progress in Separation and Purification* (Perry E. S., ed.), **1**: 297–334. New York: John Wiley.

FURTHER READING

Other Articles

Blatt W. F. (1971). *Agric. Food Chem*; **19**: 589. Membrane partition chromatography. A tool for fractionation of protein mixtures.
McDonald D. P. (1971). *Manufacturing Chemist and Aerosol News*; November, 73–77: Membrane filtration.
Porter M. C., Michaels A. S. (1971). *Chem. Tech*; January, 56–63: Membrane ultrafiltration.
Schratter P. (1970). *American Laboratory*; October, 53–61: Thin-channel ultrafiltration.

20. Osmosis and Osmometry
P. Garcia-Webb

INTRODUCTION

There are a number of circumstances in clinical medicine in which it is useful to know the solute concentration in extracellular fluid, normally sampled as plasma (or serum) or urine. An example occurs in the investigation of low sodium concentration in plasma. The measurement of solute concentration in samples of plasma and urine help clinicians to decide whether the prime cause is insufficient sodium or excess water.

In the human, water balance is achieved in part by the secretion of antidiuretic hormone (ADH). This small peptide increases the permeability of the renal collecting ducts and descending tubules to water and thus has the effect of decreasing the rate of loss of water in urine. The secretion of ADH is controlled by an osmoreceptor located in the hind brain. It is thought that a difference in concentration of solutes on either side of the osmoreceptor cell membranes results in the transfer of water either into or out of the cells. Water enters the cell when extracellular fluid has become more dilute than the intracellular fluid, i.e. during states of water excess. As a consequence, secretion of ADH is decreased, the collecting ducts become relatively impermeable to water and the excess water is lost from the body as urine. On the other hand, if there is a deficit of extracellular water, water leaves the osmoreceptor cells, ADH secretion increases and water is retained by the kidneys.

In the physiological setting explained briefly above, it would be useful to be able to measure the solute concentration difference between the extracellular and osmoreceptor cell fluid. In practice solute concentration can only be measured in samples of extracellular fluid.

Water transport across membranes resulting from differences in solute concentration on either side of the membrane occurs in other physiological areas. Transfer of water across the renal collecting ducts and the formation of lymphatic fluid are but two examples, although in the latter case other factors are involved as well. This movement of water across cell membranes is a function of the concentration of particles, ions or molecules, dissolved in the water.

There are four properties of particles in solution that could be exploited to provide a measurement of particle concentration. These properties have been called colligative properties (from Latin *con ligare*—to bind together). As will become apparent later, the common factor that binds these properties together is the alteration in the free energy of the solvent that is due to the presence of dissolved particles. The four properties are:

1. Osmosis.
2. Depression of freezing point of the solvent.
3. Depression in vapour pressure of the solvent.
4. Increase in the boiling point of the solvent.

PRINCIPLES OF OSMOSIS

Definition and Explanation

In simple terms osmosis is the word used to describe the passage of a solvent across a membrane. Water passes into or out of the osmoreceptor by osmosis.

The membrane has the important characteristic of being impermeable to one or more of the solutes dissolved in the solvent. It is referred to as a semipermeable membrane. A better description might be selectively permeable, since it is the selectivity against one or more of the solutes in the solution that allows osmosis to occur. Consider the situation

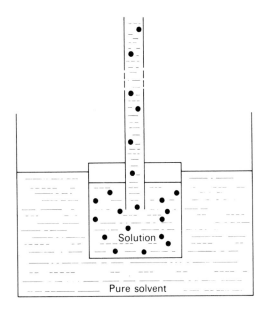

Fig. 1 Conventional diagram illustrating osmotic effects. Note that osmotic pressure is in the solvent outside the porous pot; the pressure inside is hydrostatic. Reproduced with permission from R. R. McSwiney (1978) Osmosis and Osmometry. In *Scientific Foundations of Clinical Biochemistry*, 1st edn, Vol. 1, p. 389.

in which there are different particle concentrations in two solutions separated by a membrane permeable to the solvent but impermeable to the dissolved particles. Under such circumstances solvent will move across the membrane towards the side where the concentration of particles is the greater. This passage of solvent will continue until the particle concentration on either side of the membrane is the same or until some other equilibrium is reached (Fig. 1).

Why does solvent flow across the membrane? A number of explanations have been provided in the past. Perhaps the easiest to understand is that the presence of solute particles decreases the free energy of the solvent. The greater the number of particles in solution, the more the solvent free energy will be reduced. In the example shown in Fig. 1, the free energy of the pure solvent is greater than the free energy of the solvent in the more concentrated solution. Not surprisingly, solvent moves down this energy gradient.

Note that this explanation does not use the word pressure at all. Pressure enters the topic, at least in part, because of the method of measuring osmosis that was used in days gone by. The pressure measured

was the hydrostatic pressure of the column of solvent (usually water) that osmosis gave rise to when the sort of apparatus depicted in Fig. 1 was used. Reflecting the way it was measured, the working description of osmosis then became: the osmotic pressure of a solution is the pressure which must be exerted on it to prevent net movement of solvent through a semipermeable membrane which separates the solution from pure solvent. A pressure exists only so long as there is some resistance to the flow of solvent. This resistance might take the form of the effects of gravity on a column of fluid, be due to the semi-rigidity of cell membranes etc.

In the functional sense, cell membranes act as semipermeable membranes in that they are relatively impermeable to some solutes. Physiologically, the most important of these solutes are sodium and potassium. Urea is a relatively unimportant solute since most cell membranes are freely permeable to urea. Mannitol is used in the treatment of cerebral oedema to increase the particle concentration of extracellular fluid and thus cause water to flow out of the brain cells.

Theoretical Considerations

The average kinetic or free energy of a molecule of a gas is kT where T is temperature in degrees kelvin and k is Boltzmann's constant, $1\cdot3804 \times 10^{-23}$ JK^{-1}. For one mole of gas, the free energy is $N_okT = RT$ where N_o is Avogadro's number ($6\cdot02449 \times 10^{23}$) and R is the universal gas constant (the product of Botzmann's constant and Avogadro's number, i.e. $8\cdot3170$ $Jmol^{-1}K^{-1}$).

For a gas the relationship between free energy and pressure is given by the well-known equation, $PV = nRT$, where P is pressure in pascals ($m^{-1}kgs^{-2}$), n is the number of moles of gas in the volume V in m^3 and RT is as defined above.

For a solution, the equation for calculating osmotic pressure was found empirically by Van't Hoff in 1877 to be similar to the gas equation.

However, account must be taken of the facts that (a) the number of particles that are derived in solution from one mole of solute may not equal Avogadro's number and (b) particles in solution often do not act as ideal particles (see below). Thus one mole of sodium chloride, if completely dissociated in solution would give rise to twice Avogadro's number of particles. In practice the sodium chloride is not completely dissociated and the degree of dissociation may vary.

Particles in an ideal solution have the effect, in the measurement of one of the four colligative properties, that would be expected from the number of particles. For a non-ideal solute the observed effect may be more or less than that which one would expect from the number of particles in solution. The degree to which solute particles act as ideal particles is defined as activity. If the activity is one, each particle exerts the theoretical effect: the activity of a solute may be more or less than one.

More recently it has been shown that the osmotic activity of an ideal solution depends not on the concentration of the solute alone, but on the mole fraction of the solute in the solvent. Mole fraction is equal to $m/(M + m)$ where m and M are the molal concentration (mol/kg) of solute and solvent respectively. The molal concentration of water is 55·5 mol/kg.

Thus for a dilute ideal solution, the osmotic pressure may be calculated:

$$\pi = \frac{nRTm}{V(M + m)}$$

where V is the volume of the solution in m^3 and pressure is expressed in pascals. It is more convenient to express volume as a litre, in which case pressure is measured in kPa, there being 1000 litres in a cubic metre.

For a dilute solution (i.e. m is in the mmol range) the expression $M + m$ is very similar to M, and thus the equation can be simplified to:

$$\pi = \frac{nRTm}{VM}$$

Now for water the number of moles in a litre is very similar to the number of moles in a kilogram. The quantities n and M are therefore essentially equal, thus

$$\pi = \frac{RTm}{V}$$

The concentration of solute is in moles per kilogram of water and so a slight improvement to the equation is to include the density of water d to allow for the fact that the volume V is in litres. The equation is now

$$\pi = \frac{RTmd}{V}$$

For a solution with a solute that has an osmotic activity not equal to one, the formula becomes

$$\pi = \frac{aRTmd}{V}$$

Finally account must be taken of the number of particles in a molecule of solute, p. For example, for sodium chloride $p = 2$. The final formula is

$$\pi = \frac{aRTmdp}{V}$$

There are two points that should be borne in mind. First, the derivation of the formula shown above is a gross simplification of the thermodynamics involved. Those interested in reading further are referred to modern text books of physical chemistry.

Second, in clinical biochemistry the formula is not used in the measurement of osmotic pressure. Nor, as is described below, is it used in the measurement of any of the other colligative properties. Instead the instruments used depend on the fact that colligative properties all vary with m.

Osmotic pressure has often been expressed in terms of atmospheres. Since the standard atmospheric pressure is 101·325 kPa, R becomes 0·082055. At 0°C the pressure exerted by an ideal solute in water at a concentration of 1 mol/kg is $RT = 22·41$ atmospheres.

Units

Clinicians use the word osmolality when requesting information concerning the particle concentration of a sample.

The osmolality of a solution is the number of osmoles of an ideal solute per kilogram of solvent. Similarly, the term osmolarity refers to osmoles per litre. What is an osmole?

Gamble introduced the unit os-millemole in 1934. The name of the unit has since been changed to osmole, or milliosmole at the concentrations encountered in body fluids. An early definition of an osmole was the mass of solute which when dissolved in one litre of water gave a solution which had an osmotic pressure of 22·41 atmospheres at 0°C. Such a definition could be criticized from a number of points of view, not the least of which is that the solvent should be expressed in terms of kilograms. In essence, however, the definition can be rephrased as: an osmole is the mass of a substance which when dissolved in one kilogram of solvent results in a solution that acts as though there were Avogadro's number of particles per kilogram of solvent. It is apparent that an osmole will only equal a mole for an ideal non-dissociated solute in dilute solution. The major problem with the unit from the theoretical point of view is that the actual mass of any one substance that contains Avogadro's number of osmotically active particles varies with the concentration of the solute, the nature of the solvent and, on occasions, the presence of other solutes in the solution.

It is therefore not surprising that the osmole is not accepted as a base unit in the International System of Units.

Most substances of interest in clinical biochemistry do not behave as ideal solutes from the point of view of both degree of dissociation and osmolar activity. The mole is a satisfactory unit only for non-electrolytes with an osmotic activity of one. For all other substances the number of osmotically active particles will not equal the number of particles implied by the use of the unit mole. For example, a solution of sodium chloride at a concentration of 162 mmol/kg has an osmotic effect equivalent to an ideal solute with a concentration of 300 mmol/kg. This raises the question; which unit should be used to express particle concentration in a solution?

Unfortunately, no satisfactory alternative unit has been recommended. The IUPAC/IFCC Committee on Quantities and Units neatly side-stepped the issue in the early 1970s. In the index of their recommendations, the word osmolality is mentioned. The reader is referred to a table listing depression of freezing point (the most common method of measurement of particle concentration) and the units shown are °K (°C would presumably be a satisfactory alternative). The logic behind this was to report the quantity in terms of the actual measurement made. However, as is mentioned below, the modern instrument does not measure temperature.

The unit °K is unsatisfactory, both to the clinicians and to the laboratory. Another unit used nowadays is mmol/kg. This of course is also illogical since no measurement of moles has been made at all. The unit is based on the fact that the sample has behaved in the measuring system in a way comparable with that of an ideal solution containing a single non-dissociating solute at a concentration of so many mmol/kg. Note that it is better to express the quantity of solvent by the unit kg than by the unit litre. The kg refers to the mass of solvent not to the mass of the solution. This contrasts with the term mmol/l used to express concentration, where the l refers to a litre of the resulting solution.

Perhaps a more reasonable approach would be to express the quantity as a ratio of the effect in the measuring system of the sample divided by the effect of a particular standard solution of osmolality similar to that of 'normal' plasma. The quantity would thus have a dimension of zero and the problem of units would disappear. Furthermore the result would still be understandable in the clinical setting. In the meantime I can only advise the reader to adopt a pragmatic approach. Modern text books of medicine use mosm/kg. Clinical biochemists in different countries use either that unit or mmol/kg. One should understand both.

METHODS OF MEASUREMENT

Direct Measurement of Osmotic Effect

Theoretically it is possible to measure osmotic effect directly by applying sufficient pressure to a system just to prevent the flow of pure solvent through a semipermeable membrane. Certainly the pressure changes expected would be large enough for accurate measurement (approximately 100 kPa for a solute concentration of approximately 41·5 mmol/kg).

The difficulty of using this approach for the measurement of osmotic effect of samples of plasma or urine is in the choice of an appropriate semipermeable membrane. The classical membrane for small molecules is a precipitate of cupric ferrocyanide in the supporting porous walls of an earthenware pot; this is satisfactory for non-electrolytes in aqueous solution, but the cupric ferrocyanide is dispersed into colloid form by electrolytes. For large molecules membranes of cellulose, collodion or gelatin are available. However, small particles of the size of electrolyte ions or molecules, or urea or glucose readily pass through such membranes. In the past the approach has been used to estimate the molecular mass of a protein in solution but this has been superseded.

Depression of Freezing Point

Theory. The presence of dissolved particles depresses the freezing point of a solution. For a dilute solution of an ideal solute, the depression of freezing point (Δt) is given by the formula:

$$\Delta t = \frac{RT^2 m}{H(M + m)}$$

where R is the gas constant, T is the freezing temperature of the pure solvent in °K and H is the molar heat of fusion of the solvent, i.e. the heat of fusion per gram of solvent multiplied by the molecular mass of the solvent (see above for m and M).

It is convenient to consider the mole fraction of the solute and solvent as molal concentration $[m]$, i.e. moles of solute per 1000 g solvent.

Thus
$$\frac{m}{(M + m)} = \frac{[m]}{(1000/M_{ws}) + [m]}$$

where M_{ws} is the molecular mass of the solvent. Since, as before, m is small in comparison with M, this equation approximates to

$$\frac{[m]}{(1000/M_{ws})}$$

The formula for the depression of freezing point then becomes

$$\Delta t = \frac{RT^2 M_{ws}[m]}{1000 H}$$

For water, using an ideal solute, the molal depression constant (depression of freezing point by a 1 mol/kg solution) is

$$\frac{RT^2 M_{ws}}{1000 H} = \frac{(8·314)(273·15^2)(18·02)}{(1000)(18·02)(333·5)} = 1·86$$

Thus it follows that the molal concentration of an ideal solution in water can be calculated as $C = \Delta t/1·858$. For non-ideal solutions it is possible to derive an activity coefficient equal to the observed depression of freezing point divided by the theoretical depression.

Measurement of depression of freezing point, therefore, provides similar information about the particle concentration of a solution as does the measurement of osmotic pressure.

Neither sodium chloride solutions nor samples of plasma or urine behave as ideal solutions. For solutions of sodium chloride the activity coefficient varies in a non-linear manner over the concentration range 0·1–1·0 mol/kg, approximately between the limits of 0·93 to 0·91. A solution of sodium chloride at a concentration of 147 mmol/kg (activity coefficient = 0·93, number of particles per molecule = 2) depresses the freezing point of water by 0·51°C and not by the expected 0·55°C.

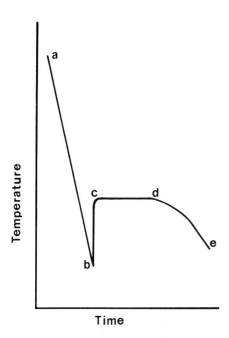

Fig. 2 Temperature curve during measurement of depression of freezing point. The solution is supercooled (a to b) and then agitated (b). The temperature rises as freezing occurs until it reaches a plateau (cd) during which the reading is taken. Once fully frozen the sample temperature falls again (de).

Measurement. If a solution is cooled sufficiently, it will freeze. If the rate of cooling is controlled the temperature of the solution follows a characteristic curve (Fig. 2). The solution initially becomes supercooled. If the solution is then agitated it will quickly freeze, and the temperature of the freezing solution will rise due to release of energy in the form of the latent heat of fusion. Continued slow cooling results in a temperature plateau as more of the solution freezes and more latent heat of fusion is released. During this time there is an equilibrium between the solid and liquid phases of the solution. Finally as all of the solution becomes frozen the temperature will fall again.

Use of this phenomenon is made in instruments that measure depression of freezing point. Note that the actual temperature of the solution in the equili-

brium state will depend on the rate of cooling and on the conductivity of the parts of the apparatus in contact with the sample. Because of this, the instrument does not measure the actual temperature of the freezing solution and the particle concentration of the solution cannot therefore be deduced by first principles. Instead modern instruments use a temperature-sensing thermistor to detect temperature changes. A thermistor is a device in which the resistance to the flow of an electrical current varies with temperature. The change in thermistor resistance that occurs during freezing of a calibrating solution is compared with the thermistor response to the unknown sample using an electronic equivalent of the Wheatstone bridge.

In operation a small sample (sample size varies with instrument, but is in the order of 200 μl) is added to a suitable glass vial. The vial is placed in contact with a cooling bath maintained at approximately −6°C or in contact with some other cooling source. The instrument head is lowered such that a thermistor probe and mechanical agitator are immersed in the sample. The sample is rapidly cooled to about 0°C and then cooled more slowly. At an appropriate moment freezing is induced by activating the agitator. A reading is taken or the instrument is calibrated during the temperature plateau of the equilibrium phase. The result is displayed on an electronic or mechanical digital display. The actual operating sequence varies with the instrument used.

TABLE 1

COMPOSITION OF STANDARDS SUITABLE FOR THE MEASUREMENT OF FREEZING POINT DEPRESSION

Osmolality of standard (mmol/kg)	Sodium chloride (g/kg)	Expected depression of freezing point
100	3·094	0·186
300	9·476	0·557
750	24·03	1·394
1000	32·12	1·86

The instrument is calibrated using standard sodium chloride solutions. The concentration of the standard solutions is chosen so that the display indicates a result that would be expected from an ideal solution (Table 1). Thus a reading of 100 mmol/kg is obtained using a sodium chloride solution at an actual concentration of 55·7 mmol/kg. Similarly a result for a sample of 280 mmol/kg signifies that the sample has depressed the freezing point by an amount equivalent to the amount that would be expected if one were measuring an ideal solution with a concentration of 280 mmol/kg. Such an ideal solution would contain 0·28 times Avogadro's number of particles per kg. Note that for plasma or urine samples a result of 280 mmol/kg in no way implies that the actual substances in solution are at a real substance concentration of 280 mmol/kg.

Vapour Pressure

Theory. Vapour pressure is the pressure exerted when a liquid is in equilibrium with its own vapour. As might be expected vapour pressure varies with temperature. For example the vapour pressure of pure water is 1·81 and 2·33 kPa at 16 and 20 °C respectively.

The presence of particles in a solution will lower the free energy of the solvent. It is thus not surprising that the vapour pressure of the solution will also be lowered.

Providing the solute has an infinitely small vapour pressure, the vapour pressure of a solution, p, will equal the vapour pressure of the solvent.

$$p = \frac{M}{(M+m)}p^{\circ}$$
$$= \left(1 - \frac{m}{M+m}\right)p^{\circ}$$

where p° is the vapour pressure of the pure solvent.

This second equation will apply providing the mole fraction of the solute is small enough not to affect the character of the solvent in any way. The equation can be rearranged

$$\frac{p^{\circ} - p}{p^{\circ}} = \frac{m}{(M+m)}$$

The accurate measurement of the two pressures p and p° is not easy. Instead the difference between the two pressures is measured. However instruments available in modern clinical biochemistry laboratories do not measure vapour pressure. Instead a thermocouple is used to indicate temperature. In this instance the temperature measured is the dew point of the air sealed in a small compartment above the sample.

As a trapped sample of air in contact with water (or any solvent) is cooled, a temperature is reached at which the air is saturated with water vapour. Cooling below this point, the dew point, results in condensation of the water. The dew-point temperature of a trapped sample of air in contact with a solution is the temperature at which the saturated vapour pressure of the mass of air is equal to the vapour pressure of the trapped water vapour (assuming constant air pressure and constant water content of the trapped air). The dew point of air above a solution varies directly with the vapour pressure of the solution. It follows therefore that the presence of solute will depress both the vapour pressure of a solution and the dew point of a mass of air trapped above the solution.

As with depression of freezing point, it is not technologically easy to measure the actual dew-point temperature. Instead the instrument allows the dew point of a sample of plasma or urine to be compared with the dew point of a standard sodium chloride solution.

To appreciate how this instrument works, it is first necessary to understand some properties of a thermocouple. Heating one end of a strip of metal causes a flow of electrons from the hot end towards the cool end. This flow of electrons gives rise to a potential difference between the hot and cool ends of the metal strip which will depend on (a) the temperature difference between the two ends and (b) the actual metal employed. The circuit can be completed by connecting the hot and cool ends of metal strip with another strip of metal. Obviously, the second metal strip must be different metal to the first since otherwise the potential differences will be identical and current flow will be impossible. A potential difference will also exist between the hot and cold ends of the second metal. The final measured voltage difference between the hot and cool ends will vary with the metals used. This effect whereby the heat applied to the one end of a metal strip results in a potential difference is called the Seebeck effect and is the principle of operation of a thermocouple.

The vapour pressure osmometer cools a sample by a process described as the Peltier effect, the antithesis of the Seebeck effect. Passing an electric current through a thermocouple transfers heat from one end to the other. An electric current will therefore cool one end of a thermocouple. When the applied current is turned off, the difference in temperature between the two ends of the thermocouple will again result in a potential difference that is proportional to the temperature difference.

Measurement. To measure depression of vapour pressure a small piece of filter paper saturated with the sample is sealed into a chamber containing a thermocouple. During equilibration some water evaporates, depending on the ambient temperature of the chamber. The end of the thermocouple is then cooled by passing a current through it (Fig. 3). As the temperature falls it passes through the dew point, at which temperature water condenses out onto the end of the thermocouple. The temperature of the end of the thermocouple is monitored electronically. Condensation of water vapour at the end of the thermocouple releases heat, the latent heat of condensation. This heat raises the temperature back towards the dew point. The temperature will not rise above the dew point since in that case the latent heat of evaporation would cool the temperature down to below the dew point again. An equilibrium is thus reached. The voltage that is recorded is the difference between the thermocouple voltage at ambient temperature and the thermocouple voltage at the temperature of equilibrium. It follows therefore that prior to any particular measurement the instrument must be in equilibrium with ambient temperature and that there must be no rapid alteration of ambient temperature during operation.

The instrument is calibrated using a standard. During calibration the gain of the amplifier is adjusted such that the display shows a value appropriate for that standard. Recalibration of the instrument is essential if there is a change in ambient temperature. The concentration of the standard is again chosen such that a result of 300 mmol/kg, for example, reflects an instrument response that would be obtained if particles of an ideal solute were present at a concentration of 300 mmol/kg.

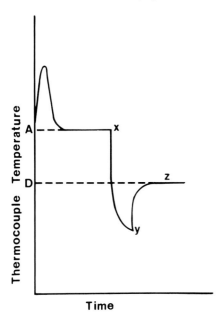

Fig. 3 Thermocouple temperature curve during measurement of depression of vapour pressure (dew point). After an initial increase in temperature as the sample is sealed in the chamber, the thermocouple returns to ambient temperature A. At time point x the sample is cooled by the Peltier effect to below the dew point (xy). Condensation occurs and a temperature plateau is reached (z). This is the dew point temperature D.

Vapour pressure osmometers are not as popular as freezing point osmometers in clinical biochemistry laboratories. This is because the latter are more robust and simpler to use. In general, freezing point instruments are capable of better precision. The small sample size required by the vapour pressure instrument (approximately 7 μl) has advantages when samples are to be taken from small babies.

The presence of a volatile substance, such as ethanol, in a sample of plasma depresses the freezing point roughly in proportion to its molal concentration. (For reasons that are not clear, adding ethanol to plasma results in an increase in the osmolality measured by freezing point that is slightly greater than would be expected from the molal concentration of ethanol in the sample.) In a vapour pressure instrument on the other hand the presence of ethanol or

other volatile substances has little or no effect over the concentration range likely to be encountered in clinical practice. Thus adding ethanol to plasma to give concentrations of 100–350 mg/dl (approx. 22–76 mmol/l) only increased osmolality measured by vapour depression by up to 2 mmol/kg. This may be explained by the fact that the vapour pressure of a solution is the sum of the vapour pressures of solvent and solute. Although the presence of ethanol acting as particles in solution depresses the vapour pressure of the water in which it is dissolved, this effect is counteracted by the increase in total vapour pressure of the resulting solution due to the vapour pressure of the ethanol.

Calculation of Osmolality

It is possible to make an approximate calculation of plasma or serum osmolality given the concentration of the substances in solution and the activity coefficients of these substances. From the practical point of view it is only necessary to take into account those substances that are normally present at concentrations of 4 or more mmol/l. Calculations that have appeared in the literature have been based on the measured concentrations of sodium, potassium, glucose and urea. In the main it is assumed that the two anions will be balanced by cations and that taken together the electrolyte mix will have an activity coefficient similar to that of sodium chloride. Note that the substance concentrations are reported as per litre while measured osmolality is reported as per kilogram. It is better to refer to the calculated variable as osmolality since it is that quantity that the calculation is designed to approximate.

A commonly quoted formula is that of Dowart and Chalmers: calculated osmolality = 1·86 × [sodium] + [glucose] + [urea] + 9 where sodium, glucose and urea are expressed in mmol/l. This formula has been challenged by workers in my laboratory as having a negative bias, i.e. underestimating osmolality. Two new formulae have been suggested. The first formula is slightly less accurate than the second but is easier to calculate. Both formulae were derived using computer based iterative analysis designed to minimize the difference between measured osmolality (depression of freezing point) and calculated osmolality. The two formulae are:

osmolality = 1·86[Na + K] + [glucose] + [urea] + 10
osmolality = 1·89[Na] + 1·38[K] + 1·03[urea] + 1·08[glucose] + 7·45

where all concentrations are expressed in mmol/l.

It is not possible to derive a formula suitable for calculation of osmolality in samples of urine.

Density

The specific gravity (or relative density to use the SI phrase) of urine is often measured on hospital

The main principle of paper chromatography is that of liquid–liquid partition, in which the stationary phase is a liquid, immiscible with the mobile phase, which is trapped in the interstices of the supporting paper matrix.) The mobile phase may be a gas or a liquid. The combination between the possible mobile phases and the possible stationary phases give rise to four major types of chromatographic system, liquid–solid, liquid–liquid, gas–liquid and gas–solid chromatography. In general, adsorption is the basic principle employed where the stationary phase is solid and partition is the basic principle employed where the stationary phase is liquid.

It is difficult to give detailed guidelines on the choice of methods available to effect a particular separation. There are few sound principles for coming to such a decision, and most methods are chosen empirically. In general, however, the following suggestions might be found helpful.

Partition chromatography is usually more effective at separating a number of closely related compounds. If the components are volatile, or can be made into a volatile derivative, GLC usually gives superior separations to those obtained by 'ordinary' liquid–liquid chromatography, and is preferable for quantitative analysis; but HPLC is now able to produce quantitative results and efficient separations comparable with, if not better than, those obtained by GLC. Liquid–liquid chromatography is usually superior to GLC if the purpose of the separation is to isolate and purify the components in a mixture, or if components are heat labile.

Adsorption chromatography is often more appropriately used for separating different classes of com-

pounds from each other or for separating molecules with widely differing physicochemical characteristics. TLC and paper chromatography are widely used to effect rapid qualitative or semiquantitative separations either for routine screening programmes or as a preliminary to further, more-sophisticated separations.

Chromatographic separations can thus be used for the qualitative screening, preparation, identification and quantitative analysis of a wide variety of chemical compounds.

THE THEORY OF CHROMATOGRAPHIC SEPARATION

In the ensuing discussion most of the principles will be relevant to all forms of chromatography, although the details will mainly apply to, and examples will mainly be drawn from adsorption chromatography. Fuller accounts of the principles underlying partition chromatography, ion-exchange chromatography, gel-filtration, affinity chromatography and electrophoresis are given in the following chapters.

Zone Migration

Before discussing the ways in which a mixture of compounds is separated by a chromatographic system, it is necessary to consider the way in which a single, pure substance will migrate through the system.

Let us consider a zone of identical molecules which has been applied at the origin of a chromatographic system (Fig. 1) and migrates through the system when a mobile-phase solvent is applied. In accordance with the basic principles of chromatography the molecules of the solute which make up the migrating zone will spend a proportion of time, t_s, in the stationary phase and for the remainder of the time, t_m, will migrate in the direction of flow of, and with the same speed as, the mobile phase. The total distance, l, travelled in time t by the zone will therefore be smaller than the total distance run by the leading edge of the mobile phase, L. The ratio of the distance moved by the zone to that moved by the mobile phase is a fundamental parameter referred to in thin-layer and paper chromatography as the R_f value, which is related to the variables mentioned above as follows:

$$R_f = \frac{l}{L} = \frac{t_m}{t} = \frac{t - t_s}{t} \qquad (1)$$

In elution chromatography it is not usual to stop the chromatographic run after a fixed time. Under these circumstances it is more appropriate, when considering the kinetics of zone migration, to base the argument upon the time required for the zone to migrate a fixed distance, usually the full length of the chromatographic column. The fundamental parameter in this situation is the retention time, t_R (*see* Chapters 22 and 23). The basic argument is, however, similar.

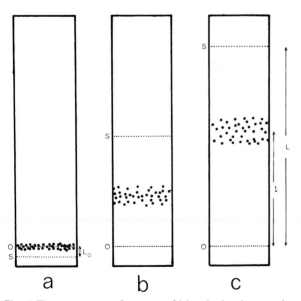

Fig. 1 The progress of a zone of identical solute molecules during the development of a chromatographic run. (a) At the beginning, (b) at the half-way stage, and (c) at the end of the run. The distances L, l, and L_0 are referred to in the text, s is the position of the solvent front at each stage and O is the origin.

Flow Velocity

In elution chromatography the velocity of the solvent flow can be regarded as being constant throughout the chromatographic run, although in practice, even in this system, the flow velocity does tend to decrease with time as the particles of the stationary phase become packed more closely, especially if additional pressure is used to force the solvent through the column. In ascending TLC and paper chromatography, however, the velocity of solvent flow is by no means constant. The major factor causing the solvent to ascend the plate or paper is capillary attraction and this decreases as the solvent front rises above the level of solvent in the tank.

The distance ascended by the solvent front, L, after a certain time, t, is given by:

$$L^2 = kt \qquad (2)$$

where k is directly proportional to the surface tension of the solvent, inversely proportional to the viscosity of the solvent, and dependent on the size of particles and the distribution of pores and channels in the adsorbent bed. k is constant for a given system of stationary and mobile phases at a fixed temperature. By differentiation, the velocity of the solvent front at this time, V_t, is given by:

$$V_t = \frac{dL}{dt} = \frac{1}{2}\sqrt{\frac{k}{t}} \qquad (3)$$

$$V_t = \frac{k}{2L} \qquad (4)$$

The overall velocity (V) of the solvent front between time 0 and time t is given by:

$$V = \frac{L}{t} = \frac{k}{L} \qquad (5)$$

Just as the velocity of the ascending solvent front is dependent upon the length of the chromatographic run, so too is the velocity of a migrating zone of solute molecules. The relationships expressed in equation (1) still hold however and, using them in equations (4) and (5), it is possible to arrive at the following relationship concerning the rate of migration of a zone of solute molecules up a thin-layer plate or paper chromatogram:

$$l = R_f \sqrt{kt} \qquad (6)$$

$$v_t = \frac{R_f^2 \cdot k}{2l} \qquad (7)$$

$$v = \frac{R_f^2 \cdot k}{l}. \qquad (8)$$

where l = distance moved from the origin after time t;
v_t = velocity of the zone at time t; and
v = overall velocity of the zone between time 0 and time t.

In the above discussion no allowance has been made for the distance moved by the solvent front before it reaches the 'origin' of the chromatogram (i.e. the position of the applied sample spots). In order to account for this, equation (6) must be modified as follows:

$$l = R_f \sqrt{kt} - R_f \cdot L_0 \qquad (9)$$

where L_0 is the distance between the initial solvent level and the 'origin' of the chromatogram (see Fig. 1) and t is the time taken from the instant when the plate is placed in the solvent.

Zone Widening

In addition to migrating through the chromatographic system as described above, a zone of identical solute molecules will also become wider and more diffuse as the run proceeds. In order to achieve satisfactory separations it is of primary importance that this effect of zone-widening should be reduced to a minimum. The theoretical treatment of zone-widening discussed below has been developed largely by Giddings.[1]

Factors Responsible for Zone-widening
Simple diffusion. Three main factors lead to zone widening. Of these the simplest to understand is *diffusion.* If a zone of a solution is surrounded by the pure solvent, molecules of solute will move in all directions. The net result of this random motion of the molecules will be a diffusion of the solute from regions of high concentration to those of lower concentration and the zone occupied by the solution will expand spherically. The longer the time allowed for diffusion, the larger and more dilute will be the zone of solute molecules. If the initial concentrated zone of solute molecules is present in a tube and bounded on each side by pure solvent, the solute molecules will quickly distribute themselves evenly across the tube, but random diffusion will continue to occur indefinitely along the length of the tube resulting in a widening of the zone in one dimension. If a zone of solution is introduced into a thin layer of pure solvent, diffusion in two dimensions will take place by similar processes so that the area of the zone will increase with time.

This simple diffusion process will still occur if the solvent, containing the zone of solution, is caused to move. The zone of solute molecules will continue to expand as the molecules migrate from areas of high concentration to those of less concentration, but the entire zone will also be propelled in the direction of flow of the system as a whole; if no other forces are allowed to affect the migrating zone its rate of change of shape will be no different in the moving system than that which is observed in the stationary system. (In practice the walls of the column in which the solvent and zone of solution are flowing impose important variations in the rate of flow of fluid in different regions which distort this ideal system.)

last function. The general relationship expressed mathematically in equation (14) can be expressed graphically (Fig. 3). H is minimum when the slope is zero. This is fulfilled when

$$V^2 = \frac{A}{C} \tag{15}$$

In the above argument it has been assumed that the velocities of the mobile phase and of the zone of solute molecules remain constant throughout the

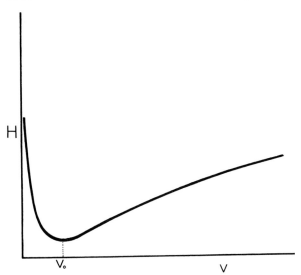

Fig. 3 Graphical representation of the relationship between the velocity flow V, and theoretical plate height, H. The optimum flow velocity, V_0, corresponds to the lowest value of H.

run. As has been indicated earlier, this is usually not the case and is never so in ascending paper and thin-layer chromatography. The value of H varies as the velocity of flow, V, changes. In ascending TLC or paper chromatography an overall value of H, (H'), for a total run time of T, can be derived by first obtaining the expression for H at an intermediate time, t (where $0 < t < T$), and then integrating H between 0 and T. For a zone which has migrated a distance l with average velocity of v,

$$H' = \frac{AR_f}{v} + B + \frac{Cv}{2} \log_e \left(\frac{l}{L_0} \right) \tag{16}$$

In this expression L_0 is the distance that the solvent front must travel at the beginning of the run before it reaches the position on the plate or paper where the solute has been applied. As l will normally be much greater than L_0, H' is not greatly dependent on L_0.

Equation (16) is obviously similar in form to equation (14) and the terms A, B and C are similar constants. Examination of equation (16) shows that at very high flow velocity, as occurs at the very beginning of a run, the third term in the expression, relating to non-equilibrium, will be large; as the run progresses the velocity quickly falls and the signifi-

cance of this third term is reduced. If the run is allowed to continue for a long time the velocity will become very low and the significance of the first term in the expression, the ordinary diffusion term, will increase. Experimental evidence suggests, however, that during a normal TLC run the major factor affecting the value of H' is the second term, B. (In elution chromatography the third term, that relating to non-equilibrium, has the greatest effect on the value of H.)

B is the term representing the contribution of eddy diffusion to the factors responsible for zone-widening. It is a measure of the degree of variation in the length of the paths through the adsorbent bed taken by both solvent and solute molecules. It is dependent upon the mean diameter of the particles of the stationary phase, d_p:

$$B = 2\lambda d_p \tag{17}$$

where λ is a factor dependent on the packing arrangement of the stationary phase particles. Irregularities in the size of the particles and in the way in which they are packed will increase the value of λ and hence of B and H. A stationary phase consisting of evenly packed particles which are of regular, small diameter will achieve a small value of B, thus producing a more efficient TLC plate.

Another useful parameter describing the efficiency of a chromatographic system is that of the 'number of theoretical plates', N, which is a measure of the total equivalent theoretical plates to which a substance is exposed as it moves along the chromatographic system. In elution chromatography all components in the mixture to be separated will pass through the entire bed-length. N is thus relevant to all components and can be simply calculated by dividing the bed-length, L, by the height-equivalent of a theoretical plate, H:

$$N = \frac{L}{H} \tag{18}$$

In development chromatography each component passes only part of the way through the stationary phase and will be exposed to a fraction, N', of the total number of theoretical plates, where:

$$N' = NR_f \tag{19}$$

N is a useful parameter for comparing the efficiency of different chromatographic systems. Thus for a normal 15 cm length of a thin-layer chromatoplate, N will be about 1000 theoretical plates, and most components will be exposed to about 700–800 of these. Capillary GLC columns may, however, have an N value of more than 100 000.

Size of Sample Application Zone. The above theoretical discussion predicts that the dimensions of a zone of a substance migrating through a TLC system will expand both longitudinally (i.e. in the direction of flow of the solvent) and horizontally (i.e. at right angles to the direction of flow). Expansion along this second axis is not of great practical importance as, by applying spots sufficiently spaced from each other, no overlap between the components of adjacent samples need occur. If samples are applied as long or short streaks, expansion of the horizontal dimension is even less important.

Expansion of the zone in the longitudinal dimension, however, is of primary importance and should be kept to a minimum. It is frequently experienced in TLC and paper chromatography that those spots which migrate furthest have a shorter final length than those which follow. This observation is not, as it may seem, a contradiction of the above prediction but is partly a consequence of a factor which has so far been neglected in the discussion, namely the size of the applied sample zone.

Up to now it has been assumed that the sample is applied as a discrete point whose dimensions are so small as to be negligible; in practice such is not the case and samples are often applied so that they initially cover a circle of up to 1 cm diameter.

Consider an extreme situation in which a solution of a pure substance has been applied to a chromato-plate as a circular spot with a 1 cm radius. Assume that the R_f value of the substance is 0·5. When the solvent front has advanced to a position 2 cm above the origin, the lower edge of the spot will have moved a total distance of 1·5 cm (as the R_f value is 0·5). The upper edge of the spot will have moved only a distance of 0·5 cm from its original position. The lower edge of the spot will then be 0·5 cm above the origin and the upper edge 1·5 cm above the origin; the total length of the spot, 1 cm, will thus be only a half of its original length. As the run proceeds there will be no further foreshortening of this dimension. This specific example can be generalized to the following relationship, where w_0 is the initial width and w the final width of the zone in the longitudinal axis:

$$w = w_0(1 - R_f) \qquad (20)$$

This factor thus results in *narrower* zones of those components with greater R_f values. In contrast the factors responsible for zone widening tend to lead to *wider* zones of components with high R_f. In practice both types of factor will play their part and the size of the final separated spots will depend on the result of their opposing actions.

Consideration of the factors involved shows that the smaller the size of initial spot, the smaller will be the separated component spots and the better the separation.

ADSORPTION CHROMATOGRAPHY

Interactions with the Stationary Phase

The second factor needed for good chromatographic separation of a mixture into its components lies in the ability of the stationary phase to interact reversibly with the individual components in the mixture in such a way that the migration of each component is retarded to a different degree from that of each of the other components. The major interaction in TLC is adsorption. This type of interaction is also fundamental to the separations achieved by a number of liquid–solid column systems and by gas–solid chromatography. Partition, the major interaction involved in liquid–liquid and gas–liquid chromatography and more specific interactions involved in ion-exchange chromatography, gel filtration, affinity chromatography and electrophoresis are described in the following chapters.

Adsorption is the fundamental process underlying TLC, liquid–solid and gas–solid chromatography. The stationary phase, or adsorbent, is a particulate matrix containing a number of reactive groups on the surface of each particle. The molecules of the moving solvent phase compete for these reactive groups with molecules of the solute components in the mixture being separated. Each type of molecule will interact with the reactive adsorbent groups to different degrees; those molecules which interact less readily will be carried along more rapidly by the mobile phase.

Theory of Adsorption

The theory of adsorption chromatography has been developed over the past two decades and has been reviewed by Snyder.[2,3] In essence, the kinetics of the reaction between a solute X and an adsorbent A can be summarized by an equilibrium reaction:

$$X_f + A_f \rightleftharpoons XA \qquad (21)$$

where X_f = the free solute molecules;
       A_f = the free binding sites on the adsorbent; and
      XA = the solute molecules bound to adsorbent.

The equilibrium constant, k, is given by

$$k = \frac{(XA)}{(X_f)(A)} \qquad (22)$$

If the solute concentration is small, then the amount of solute bound to the adsorbent is much smaller than the total concentration of the adsorbent, which can therefore be assumed to be constant for a particular system. Thus

$$\frac{(XA)}{(X_f)} \text{ is a constant.}$$

This constant, K, the *adsorption coefficient*, is given by:

$$K = \frac{\text{concentration of adsorbed solute}}{\text{concentration of non-adsorbed solute}} \qquad (23)$$

This relationship between the concentration of adsorbed solute and the concentration of the non-adsorbed solute is called the *adsorption isotherm*; when it is linear the adsorption isotherm is said to be 'ideal' and it will have slope K. In order to effect good chromatographic separation it is necessary to choose conditions such that the adsorption isotherm is as close to linearity as possible. In practice, providing that the concentration of solutes is low, a linear adsorption isotherm can readily be achieved. Under this condition the concentration profile through a migrating zone approximates closely to a Gaussian distribution. As the solute concentrations are increased there is an appreciable decrease in the number of binding sites available for solute molecules, and eventually a point will be reached beyond which any further increase will result in the value of K being reduced. The fall in the value of K at high solute concentration results in a convex adsorption isotherm, which is associated with significant tailing of the migrating zones, leading to poor resolution.

The *linear capacity* of an adsorbent or chromatographic system is defined as the maximum solute concentration which can be achieved without the adsorption isotherm deviating significantly from linearity. It is possible by controlling a number of factors to maximize the linear capacity of a given chromatographic system. This is of practical use as, in order to visualize the components in a mixture or to isolate components in order to carry out further studies, it is often necessary to apply as much of the mixture as possible whilst still maintaining adequate separation.

The main factors affecting the adsorption coefficient and the linear capacity are (*a*) the nature of the adsorbent, (*b*) the properties of the developing solvent and (*c*) the chemical structure of the solute. K is also temperature dependent.

The Adsorbent. The forces which are of importance in determining the adsorption interaction in chromatography are:

(a) hydrogen bonds,
(b) weak covalent bonds,
(c) dipole forces,
(d) dispersion forces.

In addition to these relatively weak forces, stronger interactions may also exist between the adsorbent and the components being separated. These interactions are sometimes referred to as 'chemisorption' and result from strong covalent or ionic bonding. In general chemisorption is not desirable in chromatographic systems as the desorption process is frequently so slow that the length of time required to complete a chromatogram is impractically long. Use is sometimes made of chemisorption in separating some components, which are strongly bound to the adsorbent and which remain at the origin of the chromatogram, from those which are held by weak forces only and which migrate through the adsorbent bed. By changing a property of the eluting solvent, e.g. its oxidation state, pH or ionic strength, it is sometimes possible to break the chemisorption bonds and allow the bound components to pass through the system. The technique is particularly used in column systems, including ion-exchange chromatography, but its success does depend upon changing the nature of the eluting solvent, either by discrete changes or continuously as in gradient elution.

For most chromatographic separations, particularly when only one solvent system is being used, it is necessary to minimize the effects of chemisorption and to rely for separation on the weaker interactions listed above.

Another undesirable property of certain adsorbents is the ability of their active groups to act as catalysts which promote chemical changes in the molecules of solvent or solute.

The characteristic properties of adsorbents which are exploited in adsorption chromatography are:

1. the surface area of the adsorbent, which is directly proportional to the adsorbent volume and inversely proportional to the particle size, and
2. the nature, frequency and distribution of reactive groups—active sites—which should enter into a reversible adsorption reaction with solute and solvent molecules, but which should not bind such molecules irreversibly.

These properties can be modified by deactivation processes, as described below, or by interaction with the solvent or solute or with compounds deliberately added to the adsorbent in order to change its characteristics.

In general, adsorbents can be polar or non-polar; the polar adsorbents can be acidic, e.g. silica, or basic, e.g. alumina. Charcoal is a classical example of a non-polar adsorbent. Polar adsorbents will retain polar compounds relative to non-polar ones; acidic adsorbents will preferentially retain basic solutes and *vice versa*. Non-polar adsorbents tend to retain preferentially compounds of higher molecular weight and compounds with aromatic properties.

The properties of an adsorbent can be deliberately modified in order either to minimize undesirable properties, such as the presence of chemisorptive groups, or to add a desirable property, e.g. changing the pH of silica by adding sodium carbonate to give a basic adsorbent. Polar adsorbents have a variable number of water molecules adsorbed onto the surface of the particles. These tend to deactivate some of the binding groups. For some separations this is an advantage; indeed it may be necessary to deactivate still further by allowing further adsorption of water. For other separations it may be necessary to increase the activity of the adsorbent by heating at between about 100 and 150 °C to drive off some of these adsorbed water molecules. Activity can also be increased by reducing the mean particle size. This has the beneficial effect of increasing the efficiency of the adsorbent. Increasing the activity may, however, have the undesirable effect of decreasing the linear capacity.

Relatively few adsorbents have found widespread use in TLC, silica being by far the most popular. Others which are used include alumina, cellulose powder, Florisil (magnesium silicate), Kieselguhr, starch and Sephadex. The particle size of most commercially available adsorbents is about 20–50 μm.

The adsorptive properties of *silica* depend upon the presence of hydroxyl groups linked to the silicon atoms on the surface of the particles. These groups may be free hydroxyls or may be hydrogen-bonded to each other. Both forms are active and adsorb solvent or solute molecules mainly by hydrogen-bonding. Silica is frequently termed 'silicic acid' in column chromatography' or 'silica gel' in TLC; it has a good linear capacity, shows activity to a wide variety of compounds and does not catalyse decomposition of sample. Silica does not separate well compounds which differ only in their content of double (olefinic) bonds; but it can be used for this purpose if silver nitrate is added to the adsorbent. A separation of fatty acid methyl esters on silica gel impregnated with silver nitrate is shown in Fig. 7 (p. 310).

The structure of *alumina* is similar to that of silica, chromatographic separation probably depending mainly on hydrogen bonding between the solute molecules and hydroxyl groups on the alumina. Some workers have suggested that electrostatic forces also have a significant influence. Alumina is an adsorbent which has a wide range of applications, but also has a tendency to catalyse sample decomposition and to chemisorb acidic compounds.

Details of other adsorbents are given by Snyder.[2,3]

In order to bind the adsorbent particles together and to the supporting glass plate, a binding agent, usually calcium sulphate, is frequently added to the adsorbent when thin-layer plates are being prepared. While inclusion of binder gives some advantages, there is no doubt that some modifications to the properties of the adsorbent layer are introduced, some of which are undesirable. Most commonly used adsorbents can be applied in practice without binder, although if solvents of high strength are used there is a tendency for pure adsorbents to peel off the plate.

As can be seen from the above discussion, a rather small range of adsorbents is normally used in adsorption chromatography and the modifications which can be made to the adsorbents are relatively limited and designed to increase the efficiency of the separation and maximize the linear capacity rather than affect the specificity of the separation. This limited variability of adsorbents cannot account for the wide range of specificity of separation which can be achieved by adsorption chromatography. The adsorbent can therefore be looked at as a reactive but relatively non-specific matrix which will interact with a wide variety of molecules, both of the solvent and of the compo-

nent solutes. The specificity of these interactions will depend on the molecular structure of the solvent and, especially, of the solute.

The Solute. Each compound (solute) in a mixture subjected to chromatographic separation will interact with the adsorbent to a different degree, which is described by a solute parameter, S, termed the 'solute adsorption energy'. The value of S will depend upon the particular chromatographic system used, especially upon the nature of the solvent and the activity and type of adsorbent. It is customary to define a standard solute adsorption energy, S^0, for each solute, with each adsorbent, under defined conditions (usually with pentane as solvent and with an activated form of the adsorbent). The value of S^0 can be estimated experimentally. By determining S^0 for a wide variety of known compounds it has been found, to a first approximation, that the adsorption energy of a solute molecule is equal to the sum of the adsorption energies of each of the constituent groups and atoms in the molecule:

$$S^0 = \Sigma\, Q_i^0$$

where Q_i^0 is the adsorption energy of the ith group.

This primary effect of molecular structure on adsorption energy is modified by the presence and relative positions of other groups in the molecule. The adsorption interaction of one group with an active site on the adsorbent will obviously be affected by interactions of neighbouring groups with the adsorbent. This secondary effect of molecular structure on the adsorption energy is beyond the scope of the present discussion, but is explored by Snyder.[2,3]

The group adsorption energy, Q_i^0, is dependent upon the adsorbent used although, as can be seen from Table 1, Q_i^0 values are generally similar on alumina or silica. The major exceptions to this generalization occur when the group is basic or acidic; acidic groups have larger Q_i^0 values on alumina than on silica; basic have larger values on silica than on alumina.

TABLE 1
Q_i^0 VALUES FOR SOME ALIPHATIC CHEMICAL GROUPS ON ALUMINA AND SILICA

Group		Q_i^0 value	
		Alumina	Silica
methyl	—CH₃	−0·03	0·07
methylene	—CH₂—	0·02	−0·05
methene	—CH=	0·31	0·25
chloro	—Cl	1·82	1·74
thiol	—SH	2·80	1·70
aldehyde	—CHO	4·73	4·97
ester	—COO—	5·00	5·27
hydroxyl	—OH	6·50	5·60
amino	—NH₂	6·24	8·0
amide	—CONH₂	8·90	9·6
carboxylic acid	—COOH	21·0	7·6

The value of assessing the effects of individual groups in a molecule on the adsorption energy, and hence on the chromatographic properties of that molecule, lies in assisting in the identification of unknown compounds and in predicting chromatographic characteristics. The efficiency of TLC systems is not usually sufficient to make accurate predictions of molecular structure, but such considerations can narrow the field and add supplementary evidence to other identification investigations. Similar considerations apply in other fields of chromatography, although the parameters involved in partition chromatography are not strictly the same. The much greater efficiency which can be achieved in GLC, where retention volumes can be measured accurately, enables a more sophisticated interpretation of molecular structure to be made. It is unwise to identify a compound merely on its chromatographic properties, however accurately those properties can be measured.

The Solvent. Before a full assessment of the interaction between solute and adsorbent can be made, the effect of the composition of the mobile solvent on the adsorption process must also be considered.

Although the major factor in determining the chromatographic properties of a compound is its molecular structure, important modifications are brought about by changes in the composition of the solvent system. Discussion about the simplified adsorption reaction between solute and adsorbent, equation (21), must be complemented by consideration of the competition between the solvent and solute molecules for free sites on the adsorbent.

During a chromatographic run, solvent passes through the adsorbent bed ahead of solute molecules. Thus, when the solute reaches a particular zone of adsorbent an equilibrium will already have been set up between the molecules of the solvent and the binding site on the adsorbent:

$$E_f + A_f \rightleftharpoons EA \qquad (24)$$

where E_f = free solvent molecules;
A_f = free binding sites on the adsorbent; and
EA = solvent molecules bound to adsorbent.

As the solute molecules, X, then enter the zone a second equilibrium will be set up between solute molecules and adsorbent:

$$X_f + A_f \rightleftharpoons XA \qquad (25)$$

This equilibrium will be affected by the availability of free binding sites, and hence by the tenacity with which solvent molecules are bound to these sites. The proportion of the solute which is bound, and hence the value of the adsorption coefficient, K, will depend on the relative affinities of solute and solvent molecules for the adsorbent binding sites. This leads to a competitive equilibrium as follows:

$$X_f + EA \rightleftharpoons XA + E_f \qquad (26)$$

A parameter describing the affinity of solvent molecules for absorbent is the 'solvent strength', e^0. A change of eluting solvent which causes an increase in solvent strength will increase the rate of migration of a particular solute by reducing the available number of free binding sites.

If there is a disparity between the size of a relatively large solute molecule and a relatively small solvent molecule it is possible that the above relationship will not be a one-to-one molecular equilibrium. Instead, one molecule of solute might displace more than one molecule of solvent. In the following discussion the molecular area occupied on the adsorbent surface by a solute molecule is represented by A_x.

The total number of binding sites available will also depend on the total volume of adsorbent, V_a, and on its activity, α. The factors described above are related to each other and to the adsorption coefficient, K, as follows:

$$\log K = \log V_a + \alpha (S^0 - A_x e^0) \qquad (27)$$

In the case of a given solute passing through a given adsorbent, V_a, A_x, α, and S^0 will be constant and equation (27) becomes:

$$\log K = M - Pe^0 \qquad (28)$$

where M and P are constants.

This is the equation to a straight line and shows that $\log K$ is inversely proportional to the solvent strength.

The importance of solvent strength in the practical application of chromatographic procedures has led to the listing of solvents in the eluotropic series (*see* Table 2).

TABLE 2

ELUOTROPIC SERIES OF A NUMBER OF COMMON SOLVENTS TOGETHER WITH THEIR SOLVENT STRENGTH VALUES (e^0) FOR A POLAR ADSORBENT

Solvent	e^0
pentane	0·00
hexane	0·01
carbon tetrachloride	0·18
isopropyl ether	0·28
benzene	0·32
chloroform	0·40
ethylene dichloride	0·44
methyl ethyl ketone	0·50
acetone	0·55
diethylamine	0·63
pyridine	0·71
ethanol	0·88
methanol	0·95

The above discussion on solvents is confined to the properties of a single solvent system. In practice multiple solvent systems are frequently used and minor changes in the solvent strength of the system can be achieved by increasing the proportion of one of the solvents of solvent strength e_1^0 at the expense of another of solvent strength e_2^0. Another modification which can be tried is to change the pH of the solvent by adding, for instance, ammonium hydroxide or acetic acid. The object is to change the K values of the components in the mixture so that at the end of the run they will be distributed as separate spots along the whole of the TLC plate, and not congregated near the origin or near the solvent front.

Separation Parameters

The term 'separation' can be used in chromatography to describe the disengagement of the centre of the zone of each component substance from that of each other component. When used in this way it is not intended to give any indication of the degree of dispersion and widening of the zones nor of the degree of overlap between adjacent zones. The correct term to describe these functions is the 'resolution', R.

The main function of a chromatographic system is to effect a satisfactory resolution of two or more substances initially present in a mixture. As discussed above, such resolution is dependent both upon an adequate disengagement of the zone-centre of each substance from every other zone-centre and upon the width of each zone being relatively narrow. A highly efficient chromatographic system, i.e. one with a large number of theoretical plates, will produce a

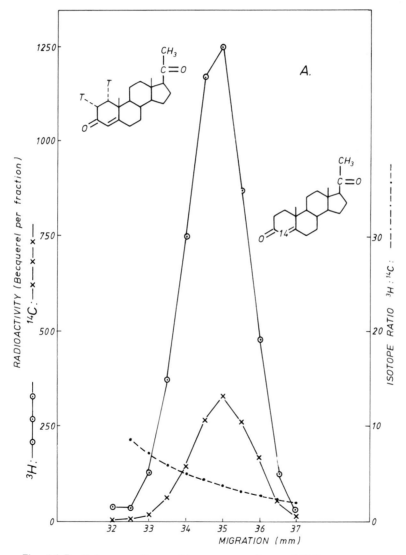

Fig. 4A Partial separations of two preparations of [^{3}H]progesterone and [^{14}C]progesterone on TLC. The stationary phase was silica gel ('HP-TLC', 0·20 mm, Whatman Co.). The solvent was 2% (v/v) isopropanol in dichloromethane. The solvent front migrated to 125 mm above the application spots. Solutions (5 μl) containing mixtures of each radioactive species plus 2 μg of unlabelled progesterone were used as the samples. A shows the partial separation of [1α,2α-^{3}H$_2$(N)]progesterone (Amersham Co.) and [4-^{14}C]progesterone (New England Nuclear Co.).

narrow zone of each substance, but will have little resolving power if it does not also have the capability of significantly retarding the migration of some substances relative to that of others. Likewise a chromatographic system with low efficiency, i.e. a low number of theoretical plates, may have little resolving power however well it might differentiate between substances in terms of their rate of migration; the width of each zone will be so large that the resulting overlap between zones will nullify the separating power.

The main functions of the component substances that enable them to separate from each other are the presence or absence of reactive groups that adsorb onto the stationary phase and their lipophobic or lipophilic nature that determines the force with which they are attracted to the mobile phase. Other physicochemical features such as molecular size and shape and electrical charge also play a less important role. Isotopic difference as well as chemical difference will also affect the migration of components along a TLC plate. This feature is illustrated in Fig. 4, for which the author is grateful to Dr J. J. Pratt, Isotope Laboratory, Groningen, The Netherlands. The figure shows the partial separation of tritiated progesterone from [^{14}C]progesterone. In Fig. 4A, the peak migration distance of the di-tritiated progesterone [1,2-^{3}H(N)]progesterone, is about 0·2 mm less than that of [4-^{14}C]progesterone; when four further tritium atoms are introduced to give [1,2,6,7,16,17-^{3}H$_6$]progesterone (Fig. 4B) the difference in migration distance has increased to about 0·6 mm. The change in the isotope ratio, illustrated in the figure, confirms this partial separation of the isotopes.

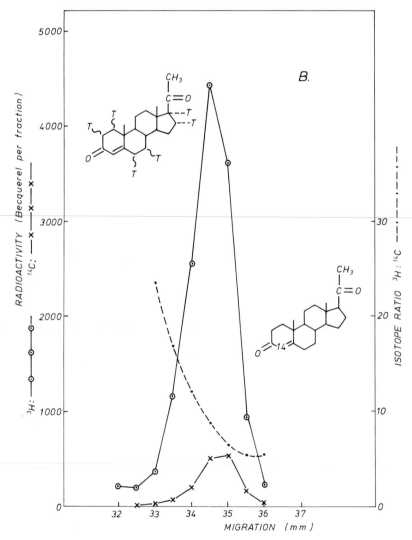

Fig. 4B This shows the partial separation of [1,2,6,7,16,17-^{3}H$_6$(N)]progesterone (Amersham Co.) and [4-^{14}C]progesterone. In the absence of a chromatographic isotope-effect the line representing the isotope ratio would be horizontal. In the structural diagrams T stands for a tritium atom (on the left) and 14 for a carbon-14 atom (on the right in each case). (Reproduced by courtesy of Dr J. J. Pratt.)

Most resolutions achieved by TLC are of course somewhat better than that illustrated in Fig. 4. In order to obtain maximum resolution in a particular chromatographic system it is useful to have a quantifiable measure or resolving power. Changes made in the conditions used can be correlated with changes produced in the resolving power. In this way optimum conditions can be achieved. The conditions for the best resolution of one pair of components may not be identical with those for the best resolution of another pair. In practice therefore it is usual to study the resolution of one particular pair of components, chosen because they have similar R_f values under many conditions or because of the importance which is placed on achieving their separation.

If the distances migrated by these two components, 1 and 2, are l_1 and l_2 and if the standard deviations of spread of their zones are s_1 and s_2, then resolution $R_{1,2}$ is given by:

$$R_{1,2} = \frac{(l_2 - l_1)}{2(s_1 + s_2)} \qquad (29)$$

Resolution is regarded as adequate if $R_{1,2}$ is greater than 1·0. The standard deviation of the zone width is not a directly measurable parameter and, in practice, use is made of the fact that the total width, w, of a zone is approximately equal to $4s$. Thus:

$$R_{1,2} = \frac{(l_2 - l_1)}{8(w_1 + w_2)} \qquad (30)$$

(*see* Fig. 5).

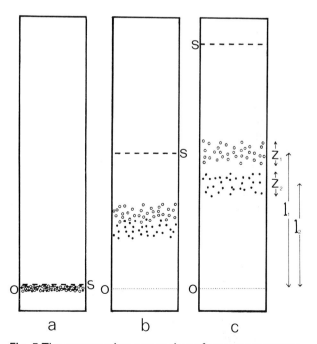

a   b   c

Fig. 5 The progressive separation of two components, z_1 and z_2, during a TLC run (a) soon after the start, (b) at the half-way stage and (c) at the end of the run. S is the position of the solvent front and O is the origin.

The art of TLC is to produce an optimum separation of all the components in a mixture in a reasonable time by judicious modification of particularly the solvent system, and also other factors such as the type and pore size of the adsorbent, the temperature, and the pH of adsorbent and solvent. To some extent this can be achieved empirically and by reference to the extensive literature, but in order to obtain maximum benefit from the technique a planned investigation of the factors involved, based on the theoretical principles outlined above, should be undertaken when each new separation is attempted.

PRACTICAL ASPECTS OF TLC

It is beyond the scope of this chapter to cover comprehensively and in detail the practical applications of TLC and the variety of methods which have been employed to obtain satisfactory separations of specific mixtures. The reader is referred to the excellent and comprehensive standard texts[4-6] which cover wide ranges of applications of the techniques, some of which are concerned particularly with applications of TLC in clinical biochemistry. The following discussion will be confined to a general description of the technique of TLC and of modifications which have been introduced which may be of interest to the clinical biochemist. A selection of the type of apparatus used in TLC is shown in Fig. 6.

Basic TLC Technique

Classically TLC is carried out on 20 cm × 20 cm or 5 cm × 20 cm glass plates covered with a uniform 250 μm thick layer of adsorbent (usually silica gel). Samples are applied as spots about 1–2 cm apart in a line across the lower part of the plate, the 'origin', about 1·5 cm from the bottom edge. The plate is placed into a suitable tank with a close-fitting lid. In the bottom of the tank is a solvent, or mixture of solvents, the 'mobile phase', to a depth of 0·5– 1 cm, so that the lower part of the adsorbent layer is immersed in the solvent, but the applied spots are a short distance above the solvent level. The solvent rises up the plate by capillary attraction and the plate is removed from the tank when the solvent front is 15 cm or so above the origin. This will usually take about 30 min. The solvent is allowed to evaporate from the plate which is then sprayed with a colour reagent to elucidate the positions of the separated components from each applied sample. These are the basic methods introduced by Stahl in the late 1950s, when he was largely responsible for popularizing the general use of a technique which had previously been employed by only a few chromatography experts. Since then many modifications have been introduced to facilitate particular separations and to meet specific needs, but the basic technique remains remarkably similar to that instituted almost three decades ago.

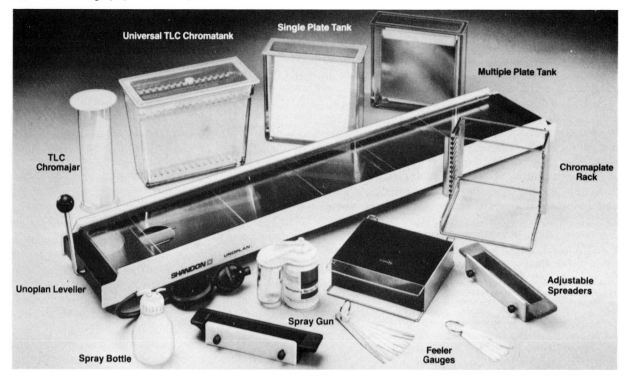

Fig. 6 Typical TLC equipment. (Reproduced by courtesy of Shandon Southern Ltd., Runcorn, Cheshire.)

Preparation of the Chromatoplates. Although the 250 μm thick adsorbent layer has proved to be about the optimum thickness for most separations, thicker layers, up to 2 mm, are frequently used for preparative purposes. A number of manufacturers have produced a variety of 'applicators', for preparing thin-layer plates of standard 250 μm thickness and most can be adjusted to produce the thicker preparative plates. The apparatus usually consists of a rectangular reservoir, slightly longer than the normal 25 cm plate width, along the lower back edge of which is a slit of variable width through which the slurry of adsorbent passes onto the plate beneath. In some methods, the applicator is moved across a line of plates, in others plates are pushed under the applicator. Various types of home-made systems have also proved satisfactory.

The plates initially used were made of glass, although in recent years other more flexible materials such as polyester, cellulose paper, aluminium foil and glass fibre are also used, particularly for commercially prepared plates. The important properties of the plate are that it be planar, scrupulously clean, smooth and without blemish.

The adsorbent is usually prepared as a slurry in water. As an example, 25 g of silica gel with 50 ml distilled water will make sufficient slurry to produce five 25 cm × 25 cm plates on which the adsorbent is 0·25 mm thick.

Additives needed to modify the nature of the gel may be incorporated either by mixing the dry additive

with the dry adsorbent or by dissolving the additive in the water with which the slurry is made (Fig. 7). Also at this stage a dyeing reagent can be incorporated into the gel; the dye should not, of course, be soluble in the developing solvent.

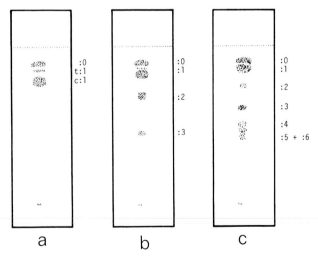

Fig. 7 Separation of fatty acid methylesters by 'argentation' chromatography. Solvent system: light petroleum (b.p. 40–60°C):diethyl ether (85:15, v/v). Stationary phase: Silica Gel G containing silver nitrate at a concentration of (a) 10%, (b) 5%, w/w and (c) 3%, w/w. The number of double bonds in each component is represented by the figure following the colon. c:1 and t:1 represent cis- and trans-isomers of monoenoic acids.

Once the slurry has been mixed it is necessary to make the plates immediately. The wet plates are allowed to dry in the air for about 20 min, and then stored, preferably in a desiccator, and if necessary activated by heating prior to use.

For quick qualitative screening of samples for a limited number of components, microscope slides have been found useful. These need to be run for only about 5 min to give a crude separation which is nevertheless satisfactory for these purposes.

For reproducibility of chromatographic properties it is better to use plates prepared by one of the specially made applicators or by using pre-prepared commercial plates. The manufacturing process can produce regular, homogeneous and flawless adsorption layers and each plate in a batch will have highly reproducible chromatographic properties. These plates are preferred for identification work. Special features are also sometimes incorporated into manufactured plates. Regular channels about 1 cm apart can be scored in the adsorbent layer along the length of the plate. This technique minimizes edge effects and leads to more reproducible R_f values. Another feature of some commercial plates is the inclusion of a pre-adsorbent area in the lower 2 cm of the plate, on to which the sample can be applied more quickly and less painstakingly. The pre-adsorbent area is made of a material which absorbs relatively large volumes of sample, but has minimal adsorptive properties. The solvent front rapidly rises through the pre-adsorbent area taking with it all the component solutes in the sample. By this means, a relatively tight, concentrated band of sample is carried to the interface between the pre-adsorbent band and the adsorbent proper, where the chromatographic process starts.

Application of the Sample. Samples may be applied as discrete spots, as short streaks (about 1 cm long) or as a continuous streak extending across almost the whole width of the TLC plate. This last method is of special value in preparative TLC.

Ideally spots should be applied so that they cover as small an area of adsorbent as possible, and should certainly not be more than 5 mm in diameter. In order to achieve this, it is necessary to use relatively concentrated solutions, preferably in a volatile solvent. Up to about 50 g of a sample mixture can be applied to each spot on a 250 μm thick layer; the volume of the sample should be about 1–10 μl. A 10 μl syringe or a syringe driven by a micrometer are the most acceptable manual instruments for applying samples. Glass capillaries are also useful. Mechanized, multiple-sample applicators are available commercially.

In applying the spot it is necessary that the integrity of the adsorbent layer be maintained. Scratches made by the syringe needle will interfere with the normal chromatographic development of the sample and will lead to abnormally shaped component spots. Removal of the pointed end of the syringe needle

with a file will help prevent inadvertent piercing of the adsorbent layer. Because the layer is fairly fragile it is advisable to use some sort of spotting template which will both protect the surface of the adsorbent and indicate the positions at which to apply the samples; effective templates can readily be made in the laboratory.

Even with the best apparatus and with easily applied samples, it will take some minutes to apply up to 20 samples on one thin-layer plate. The components of those sample spots which are applied first will have to spend a few minutes in a dry state on a finely divided, activated adsorbent, conditions which favour oxidation and other decomposition reactions. It is therefore advisable to apply relatively unstable samples under a continual stream of nitrogen. Shielding from UV light can further prevent sample decomposition.

The application of samples as short streaks helps to reduce diffusion of the sample along the axis in which the chromatogram will be run. In contrast with spot application the sample applied as a short streak is not all applied at the same point. This enables one portion of the sample to dry as another portion is being applied a little distance away. In spot application it is frequently necessary to wait for some seconds in order to allow already applied solvent to evaporate before adding more sample to the spot. Continued application of sample solution to an already moist spot will cause unacceptably large spots, to the perimeter of which much of the sample will be eluted, resulting in rings rather than homogenous spots. One minor disadvantage of applying samples in short streaks is that fewer samples can be run on each plate. Such a degree of care in sample application is not required when using the manufactured plates which have a pre-adsorbent spotting area.

Along with the sample spots a number of standard reference mixtures should also be applied. It is important that these should be applied between unknown samples and not all in one part of the plate or, for instance, at the edge. It is sometimes useful to run two or more different concentrations of reference mixtures in case the R_f values change slightly with increasing concentration.

Running the Plate. Decomposition of sample components is minimized by beginning the chromatographic run as soon as possible after sample application.

The volume of solvent used should be sufficient to immerse the lower 0·5–1·0 cm of the adsorbent layer on the thin-layer plate, but not to reach the level of applied samples. The solvent mixture is allowed to equilibrate with the air in the tank prior to the start of the run. It is important that this equilibration is neither unduly disturbed when the plate is placed in the tank nor subject to change during the run due to leakage of vapour through an ill-fitting lid. As any chromatographic run proceeds the composition of the solvent mixture becomes richer in the less volatile solvents and poorer in the more volatile ones. If the atmosphere within the tank is enclosed and equilibrated with the solvent, this change in composition is minimal and does not cause practical problems. If the system is not totally enclosed, vapour will escape which is particularly rich in the more volatile solvent; in order to maintain equilibrium some of this more volatile liquid will evaporate from the plate and leave a changed composition of the eluting mixture. This will result in abnormal development, non-reproducible R_f values and uneven migration of sample near to the edge of the plate will also be exaggerated. These edge effects can be noticed even in properly enclosed systems, but are minimized by removing narrow strips of adsorbent from each edge of the plate, or by scoring straight lines in the adsorbent along the length of plate, about 0·5–1 cm in from each side edge. Samples should then be applied within the limits of these lines. In order to assist equilibration in relatively large tanks their walls can be lined with sheets of filter paper.

Another way of ensuring that rapid, complete and stable equilibration is achieved is by making the internal volume of the tank as small as possible. This can be done by placing a second plate, which may be either of plain glass or a second chromatoplate, on top of the adsorbent layer but separated from it by a thin spacer of air-tight material placed in between the plates along their side and top edges (Fig. 8). A small gap is left at the lower edge and this extends internally between the plates. The lower edge is then immersed into the solvent mixture, which should also be enclosed within the system. This is the so-called 'sandwich system' of TLC, and can readily be made up in the laboratory or obtained commercially.

Chromatoplates made from microscope slides should be developed in a small tank, such as one of the pots which are used for staining microscopy sections. Flexible plates can be bent into a cylindrical shape with the adsorbent on the inner surface, and developed in cylindrical tanks (thereby reversing the historical evolution of TLC which was initially envisaged as a chromatographic column which had been opened out to form a flat sheet).

A standard chromatographic run is complete when the solvent front has moved about 15 cm above the origin. A line can be scored across the plate through the adsorbent layer at this sort of distance, prior to development; this will arrest further development of the plate and enable the exact length of the chromatographic run to be standardized. Whether or not this technique is adopted it is important not to leave the plate in the tank for long periods after development, otherwise excessive diffusion of spots and abnormal R_f values will be experienced.

Detection of Components. Except under the fortuitous circumstances that all the separated components from each sample are coloured, the next stage in TLC is to detect the positions to which the spots have run. This can be done either by exploiting an inherent property of the component, such as its colour, fluorescence or radioactivity, or to subject the whole or part of the plate to a reagent which will react with the components to produce coloured spots. Ideally such a reagent should be easily applied, produce a distinctive colour with each of the components, from which it should be readily removed leaving them chemically unaltered. Needless to say, no reagent available for this purpose fulfils all these criteria and compromises must usually be made.

A reagent can be applied to the adsorbent layer during the preparation of the chromatoplates, a procedure that has the advantage of producing a homogeneous distribution of reagent throughout the adsorbent, or after development of the chromatogram by spraying or dipping. Spraying is the more widely used method and is satisfactory for most purposes. However, if quantitation of the spots by scanning densitometry is to follow, dipping is preferable as it produces a more even application.

A number of dyeing reagents are available in the form of aerosol sprays; use of them saves time, but limits the operator's choice of conditions. A more generalized method is to use a spray gun consisting of a pressurized propellant gas container to which is fitted a glass bottle containing the reagent in suitable solution.

In order to ascertain the position of spots in conditions when it is not desired to spray the sample spots themselves, it is possible to spray only part of the plate, containing the separation of a known standard mixture, while keeping covered the rest of the plates containing the sample components. The standard 'marker' mixture will direct attention to those unstained areas of the plates where the spots are situated. This technique is particularly useful in preparative TLC.

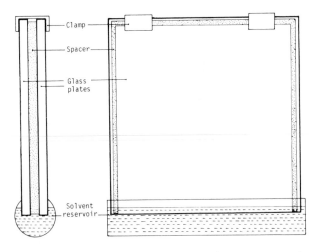

Fig. 8 Side-view (a) and front-view (b) of an example of the 'sandwich' system of thin-layer chromatography.

On all occasions when it is necessary to maintain the chemical integrity of the samples care should be taken to minimize the possibility of oxidation by carrying out the detection process swiftly in a nitrogen environment.

A large number of specific colour reagents have been used in TLC, and are referred to in chromatography textbooks. Three widely used and generally applicable methods of detection are:

1. Charring the components with concentrated sulphuric acid–water (1/1, v/v). This reagent must be used with an all-glass spray-gun and great care. The reagent chars most organic components yielding spots of varying shades of grey which can be measured semiquantitatively by densitometry. With sterols, sterol esters, steroids and bile acids, the sulphuric acid reagent will produce a Liebermann–Burchard reaction yielding a variety of pink, purple or brown spots, the colour being characteristic of the particular compound.
2. Iodine vapour. The plate is placed in an enclosed dry tank at the bottom of which some crystals of iodine are scattered. The spots on the plate take up the vapourized iodine and turn brown; most compounds are not chemically affected by this treatment. The method is widely applicable.
3. Fluorescent reagents, usually a 0·1% solution of 2′,7′-dichlorofluorescein in ethanol–water (95/5, v/v), or a similar solution of Rhodamine G. These are particularly useful in the detection of lipid compounds. Plates sprayed with these reagents are viewed under UV light when the spots fluoresce against a dark background.

Radioactive spots can be detected either by autoradiography or by means of a radioactive scanner.

Identification of Components. The methods of identification available in TLC are by comparison of R_f values and, in a limited number of cases, by the specificity of a colour reaction which can be carried out on the plates. Theoretical considerations (see above) can lead to predictions of chromatographic properties of compounds and give indications of the possible chemical nature of unknown spots. It must be stressed, however, that full identification cannot be made on chromatographic properties alone, particularly if run in only one system. In order to achieve accurate identification the spot or streak containing the compound should be scraped from the plates, the compound eluted from the adsorbent and subjected to further analytical techniques such as infrared spectroscopy or mass spectroscopy. TLC is primarily a separation technique; the R_f value merely provides an indication of the identity of a component.

In clinical biochemistry, however, the range of components in most samples likely to be encountered is now fairly well understood. The past experience of the laboratory staff supplemented by information from the literature will enable reasonable identification of most compounds to be made. Standard mixtures of known composition should be run alongside unknown samples to assist identification and if there is any doubt samples should be run in more than one chromatographic system. Too great a reliance placed upon previous experience may, however, occasionally lead to errors in identification: the clinical biochemist must always be on the lookout for the unexpected.

Quantitation. Quantitation of components separated from a mixture can be carried out either on the plate, or after the spots or streaks containing the components have been scraped from the plate and eluted from the adsorbent.

Quantitation *in situ* is best carried out by use of an instrument specially designed for scanning chromatography spots. A number of instruments are available commercially including some which employ the more preferable 'flying-spot' technique. An even adsorbent background is advantageous. A series of standard samples of the compound being measured should be run on the same plate as the unknowns and scanned similarly. A standard curve can then be drawn from which concentrations of unknown samples can be read. These instruments depend on light reflected from the surface of the plate: the opacity of the layer precludes the use of transmitted light.

The methods of quantitation of components after elution from the thin-layer plate are legion. Providing that a substance can be eluted completely, in sufficient amount and free from contamination there is no reason why the most sophisticated methods of identification and quantitation cannot be applied. It is beyond the scope of this chapter to discuss these methods further.

Non-standard Methods of TLC

During the forty years since TLC was introduced a number of modifications to the standard technique described above have been introduced. Some of the more important of these are described below.

Preparative Chromatography. In order to obtain from a thin-layer plate sufficient of a component to carry out further studies it is often necessary to load the plate with more than is applied in the standard technique. About 30 times the usual maximum load can be separated if the sample is applied as a streak across the whole width of the plate. The loading factor can be further increased by a factor of about 5–10 times by using TLC plates with adsorbent layers of up to 2 mm thick.

Once the separation has occurred strips of adsorbent can be scraped from the plate and the components eluted with a suitable solvent. If two or more components are poorly resolved by this first separation they can be eluted and re-run on a second plate under different conditions of adsorbent thickness or solvent composition.

Commercially made systems for removing adsorbent and for eluting components are available.

Multiple Development Systems

Consecutive one-dimensional separations. It is sometimes advantageous to run the whole or part of a plate in more than one solvent system in order fully to separate a number of components. This type of technique may be used to rid the mixture under investigation of substances which are not required. Thus it may be possible to use one solvent system to remove unwanted components to the top of a plate from where they can be removed and then to run the plate a second time in a second solvent system to effect the desired separation. Multiple one-dimensional development can also be carried out without removing components at an intermediate stage. The plate is simply developed in one solvent system and then re-run in a second system. Up to four systems have been used consecutively to improve certain separations. It should be pointed out that however low their R_f values, those components which do not migrate very far in earlier runs will inevitably move closer to most of the faster-running components in subsequent separations. Also the physical integrity of the adsorbent layer deteriorates with each development, limiting the number of consecutive separations which can be carried out.

Discrete changes in the solvent system can be readily used in a standard TLC apparatus, but it is also possible to adapt standard apparatus, or purchase specially made apparatus, which will enable the solvent system to be changed continuously through the course of a run. This procedure is analogous to gradient elution as practised in column chromatography, although in the author's experience the use of such gradient techniques in TLC does not give the very real benefits which can be achieved by gradient elution in column chromatography.

Two-dimensional separations. Standard one-dimensional TLC methods for biological samples do not allow adequate separation of many more than ten components. Some separations which are routinely carried out in clinical biochemistry are of mixtures containing many more than ten components, e.g. amino acid separations. The technique of two-dimensional TLC has been employed in these cases.

The sample mixture is applied about 1·5–2·0 cm in from the corner of the plate, which is run in one direction by one solvent system and then turned through 90° so that the line of separated components forms the origin for a second run in the second direction by a different solvent system. A 'fingerprint' of the components in such multiple mixtures is sometimes difficult to identify but experience of the separation of a particular group of substances using a standardized two-dimensional technique soon enables the laboratory worker to tell at a glance if a normal component is missing or present in an unusual concentration, or if an abnormal constituent is present. A typical two-dimensional separation of urinary amino acids is shown in Fig. 9.

The disadvantages of this method are that only one sample can be run on one plate, that the time of separation is at least doubled, and that standards have to be run separately. It is usual therefore, in a clinical biochemistry screening programme, to use a simple uni-dimensional run as the primary screen, and to supplement this, where necessary, with a two-dimensional run of any samples which appear abnormal.

Two-dimensional TLC is also useful in the investigation of possible artefacts which may occur during a chromatography run. The sample is run in two dimensions, but the same solvent system is used in each direction. This should result in a single diagonal line of separated components across the plate. Any component not lying on this line can be assumed to be an artefact.

Other Non-standard Techniques

Gradient plates. Just as it is possible to develop a thin-layer chromatogram with a solvent system in which the composition is continually being changed, so too is it possible to change the composition of the adsorbent along the chromatoplate. This change in adsorbent composition can either be as discrete bands of adsorbent each of which is different in composition from the preceding one, or as a continuous gradient. Applicators for producing either of these non-homogeneous layers can be obtained commercially.

It is also possible to produce a 'gradient' layer in which the thickness of the adsorbent increases steadily along the chromatoplate. If such plates are used so that samples are applied to the thicker part of the adsorbent layer, and development begins from this end of the plate, it is possible to apply more concentrated sample spots without the danger of overloading. As the chromatogram develops, the thinner layer is able to produce better resolution. By the time the components reach the thinner part of the layer, with its better resolving properties, overloading is no longer a problem as components will be wholly or partly separated from each other and will also be rather more diffuse.

Horizontal chromatography. A number of advantages can be achieved by running thin-layer plates in the horizontal plane. Chief of these are the increased speed of the run and the ability to allow the solvent to flow off a plate after it has migrated along the total length.

Solvent is admitted to the plate by means of a filter paper wick, as wide as the chromatoplate, which is applied at the lower part of the adsorbent layer and allowed to dip over the lower edge of the plate into a trough of solvent. A similar wick can be applied at the upper end if needed, but this does not dip into a solvent trough; the solvent which drips from this wick can however be collected, and in this way TLC can be carried out in the elution mode rather than the development mode. (In practice, however, TLC is not often used in this way.)

The velocity of the solvent and of the zones of sample components and their respective R_f values are different from those achieved in ascending TLC. Rates of solvent flow are more affected by uneven thickness of the adsorbent and by the positioning of the plate than is the case in ascending TLC and thus, unless very regular and even chromatoplates are used, and unless the plate is positioned accurately in the horizontal plane, R_f values will not be reproducible.

Radial TLC. A further modification of horizontal TLC is that of radial development. In this method a filter paper or cotton wick carries solvent to a central point on the plate. The samples are applied at points equidistant from this central point in a circle about 2 cm diameter. The plates can be run either with the adsorbent facing downwards and the wick rising from the reservoir of solvent, or with the adsorbent uppermost with the wick carrying the solvent from a reservoir above the plate. The former method produces better and more reproducible separation, but the latter method can readily be used for gradient development. The technique is described by Zlatkis and Kaiser.[8]

The R_f value in radial chromatography, $R_{f(rad)}$, is related to the linear R_f value, $R_{f(lin)}$, as follows:

$$R_{f(lin)} = (R_{f(rad)})^2 \qquad (31)$$

High-performance thin-layer chromatography (HPTLC). This name has been applied to a system of TLC in which a number of developments and modifications have been incorporated concurrently. Some workers who have had experience of these techniques claim that:

1. up to 40 different components can be separated in a single run,
2. highly reproducible R_f values can be achieved,
3. the resolving power can be significantly better than that of conventional TLC,
4. the time required for separation can be substantially reduced.

The main improvement introduced into this system is the use of adsorbent with small particle-size and a much narrower particle-size distribution. The beneficial effects of using smaller particles of more regular size could be predicted from equation (17), relating the particle size to the amount of eddy diffusion which, as has been previously shown, is the most important factor leading to zone widening in TLC.

In addition to this modification HPTLC plates have a rather thinner adsorbent layer than is usually employed. Great care is taken in HPTLC to control conditions of the layer and equilibration of the layer with the solvent system, and to ensure accurate sample loading and constant temperature. HPTLC is often, but not invariably, carried out radially.

HPTLC is of special use in separating small amounts of sample (in the nanogram range) for identification purposes, rather than in preparation of microgram or milligram amounts of purified compounds. The technique is described by Zlatkis and Kaiser.[8]

Reverse-phase TLC. This is a form of TLC in which a particulate phase such as silica gel or alumina is not used for its adsorptive properties but as a support for a liquid non-polar phase, such as silicon or paraffin oil, which coats the particles and which itself acts as the stationary phase. An *aqueous* mobile phase is used. The technique has been especially useful in separating aqueous solutes. Partition is the major interaction responsible for such separations.

Combined chromatographic techniques. Considerations so far in this chapter indicate that TLC is usually effected by adsorption processes. However, other types of chromatography such as partition, ion-exchange and affinity chromatography, gel-filtration and electrophoresis can also be carried out on thin-layers of stationary phase using similar techniques to those of thin-layer adsorption chromatography. Also many separations achieved in TLC are not dependent entirely on adsorption, as one or more of the other types of chromatography may also play important, although minor, parts.

Applications of TLC in Clinical Biochemistry

TLC has certain advantages which should make its use attractive to clinical biochemistry laboratories. Separations of families of compounds can theoretically be carried out swiftly, in large numbers and at little expense. It would therefore seem to be an ideal method for screening procedures, e.g. for the detection in the neonatal population of certain abnormal components in a number of inborn errors of metabolism, or for rapid identification of compounds in the emergency investigation of acute poisoning. Despite these attractions, however, TLC has not found general and widespread use in hospital laboratories. Undoubtedly one of the major reasons for the relative under-utilization in clinical biochemistry of this promising technique, which has found favour in other branches of scientific endeavour, is the difficulty in quantitating the results accurately. Methods of quantitation at present available are usually either time-consuming or demand expensive apparatus, thereby nullifying two of the main advantages of the technique. Also in order to obtain samples suitable for chromatography it is sometimes necessary to carry out extensive extraction procedures which cannot readily be 'automated'.

Nevertheless a limited number of TLC separations have proved useful in clinical biochemistry. A few, illustrative methods will be briefly discussed.

Sugars. TLC has been used to detect the presence of abnormal sugars in blood, urine or faeces of patients suffering from some gastrointestinal disease or one of the inborn errors of carbohydrate metabolism. Samples of plasma or serum (2 μl), urine (2 μl of a 50:50 mixture of urine and 2-propanol) or an extract of faeces can be run on Silica Gel G. Developing solvents which have been used include butan-1-ol:propan-2-ol:0·5% aqueous boric acid (30:50:20, by vol.). This single system is suitable for separating glucose, galactose and fructose. More sophisticated separation can be achieved by a two-dimensional run using the above solvent system in the first direction then acetonitrile:water (85:15, v/v) in the second.

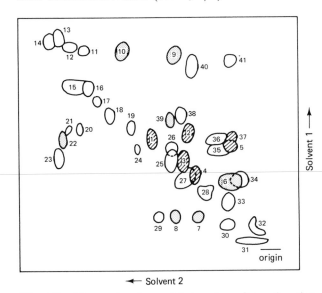

Fig. 9 Positions of amino acids in urine after using the two-dimensional thin-layer chromatography technique described in the text. Amino acids present in urine: ⊘ = normally, ⊙ = sometimes, ○ = occasionally in small amounts. Key, Amino acids detected by two-dimensional TLC of urine. 1, alanine; 2, serine; 3, glycine; 4, glutamine; 5, histidine; 6, lysine/ornithine; 7, aspartic acid; 8, glutamic acid; 9, threonine; 10, ethanolamine; 11, tryptophan; 12, phenylalanine; 13, leucine; 14, isoleucine; 15, valine; 16, methionine; 17, pipecolic acid; 18, tyrosine; 19, proline; 20, α-amino-n-butyric acid; 21, α-amino-iso-butyric acid; 22, β-amino-iso-butyric acid; 23, γ-amino-n-butyric acid (GABA); 24, β-alanine; 25, homocitrulline; 26, hydroxyproline; 27, citrulline; 28, homocystine; 29, α-aminoadipic acid; 30, argininosuccinic acid; 31, phosphoethanolamine; 32, cystine; 33, arginine; 34, asparagine; 35, carnosine; 36, 3-methyl-histidine; 37, l-methyl-histidine; 38, glucosamine; 39, taurine; 40, methionine sulphoxide; 41, methionine sulphone. (Reproduced by courtesy of Edwards, Grant and Green, 1988.)

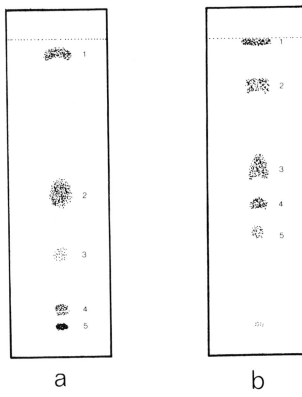

a b

Fig. 10 Separation of plasma lipids on Silica Gel G. (a) using light petroleum (b.p. 40–60 °C):diethyl ether (85:15, v/v): 1, cholesterol ester; 2, triglyceride; 3, free fatty acids; 4, overlapping spots of free cholesterol and diglyceride; 5, phospholipids (+monoglyceride) at origin. (b) using chloroform:methanol:water (65:35:5, by vol.): 1, neutral lipids; 2, overlapping spots of phosphatidyl ethanolamine and phosphatidylserine; 3, phosphatidylcholine (lecithin); 4, sphingomyelin; 5, lyso-lecithin.

Another one-dimensional system employs ethyl acetate:pyridine:acetic acid:water (60:30:5:15, by vol.). Separations achieved by this system can be somewhat improved by running the plate a second time in the same direction in the same solvents. 1,3-naphthalenediol (0·2 g in 95 ml ethanol + 5 ml conc. H_2SO_4) or 4-aminobenzoic acid (1·4 g in 97 ml methanol + 3 ml phosphoric acid) have been used as identification reagents.

Amino Acids. Aminoacidurias can be investigated by running 2 μl of urine:2-propanol (50:50, v/v) in a two-dimensional TLC system. A typical system uses cellulose plates with pyridine:dioxan:ammonium hydroxide:water (35:35:15:15, by vol.) as the first solvent and butan -1-ol:acetone:acetic acid:water (35:35:7:23, by vol.) as the second. Ninhydrin, 0·5 g in 100 ml ethanol:acetic acid (98:2, v/v), is a suitable detecting agent. An alternative two-dimensional system has recently been described by Edwards et al.,[7] in a paper which also covers the important topic of the interpretation of the resulting chromatograms. They use DC-Alufolien Cellulose plates

(Merck/BDH Poole, Dorset) with the following solvent systems: first direction: *t*-butanol:methyl ethyl ketone:25%(aq.) ammonia:water (50:30:10:20, by vol.); second direction: butan-1-ol:acetone:glac. acetic acid:water (35:35:10:20, by vol.) (*see* Fig. 9).

Lipids. Separation of the neutral lipids from an organic extract of plasma can be readily achieved on Silica Gel G with a solvent system of light petroleum (b.p. 40–60):diethyl ether (85:15, v/v). This separation has not found clinical application, but is the simplest method of separating esterified cholesterol from free cholesterol and of obtaining uncontaminated triglyceride (Fig. 10a).

Phospholipid separation can also be achieved readily on Silica Gel G with a solvent system of chloroform:methanol:water (65:25:10, by vol.). This method readily separates phosphatidylcholine (lecithin) and sphingomyelin. A semiquantitative ratio of these compounds in amniotic fluid has been used as an indicator of fetal lung maturity (Fig. 10b).

Drugs. A number of schemes have been described for analysing blood, urine or gastric contents for a wide variety of drugs, one or more of which may have been taken by a patient suffering from acute poisoning. Usually these schemes include TLC used in association with other complementary techniques, such as the production of colour reactions and GLC, in order to obtain as full a picture as possible. Some workers have described schemes of analysis based entirely on TLC,[9] in which several different solvent systems and more than one stationary phase may be used. Probably the most successful of these is that commercially available as the Toxi-Lab system.[10]

This system has provided probably the greatest advance in the practical use of TLC in clinical biochemistry laboratories during the last decade.

REFERENCES

1. Giddings J. C. (1975). In *Chromatography—A Laboratory Handbook for Chromatographic and Electrophoretic Methods*, 3rd edn (Heftmann E., ed.). New York and London: van Nostrand Rheinhold.
2. Snyder L. R. (1975). In *Chromatography—A Laboratory Handbook of Chromatographic and Electrophoretic Methods*, 3rd edn (Heftmann E., ed.). New York and London: van Nostrand Rheinhold.
3. Snyder L. R. (1968). *Principles of Adsorption Chromatography*. New York: Marcel Dekker.
4. Stock R., Rice C. B. F. (1986). *Chromatographic Methods*, 4th edn. London: Chapman and Hall.
5. Touchstone J. C., Rogers D., (eds) (1980). *Thin-layer Chromatography: Quantitative, Environmental and Clinical Applications*. Chichester: Wiley Interscience.
6. Touchstone J. C., Sherma J. (1985). *Techniques and Applications of Thin-layer Chromatography*. Chichester: Wiley Interscience.
7. Edwards M. A., Grant S., Green A. (1988). A practical approach to the investigation of amino acid disorders. *Ann. Clin. Biochem*; **25:** 129–41.
8. Zlatkis A., Kaiser R. E. (eds) (1977). *High-Performance Thin-Layer Chromatography*. Amsterdam and Oxford: Elsevier.
9. Stead A. H., Gill R., Wright T., Gibbs J. P. (1982). Standardised thin-layer chromatographic systems for the identification of drugs and poisons. *Analyst*; **107:** 1106–8.
10. Jarvie D. R., Simpson D. (1986). Drug screening: evaluation of the Toxi-Lab thin-layer chromatography system. *Ann. Clin. Biochem*; **23:** 76–84.

22. Gas Chromatography— Mass Spectrometry

J. Chakraborty and Norman Lynaugh

INTRODUCTION

Gas chromatography (GC) is a form of chromatography which allows separation of volatile materials by using a gaseous instead of a liquid mobile phase. Soon after the initial report by James and Martin in 1952, gas chromatography was available commercially and in the years that followed GC instrumentation and its ancillary components went through vast advances in scope and sophistication. The progress made in the development of column materials and technology, detection devices, sample injection modes and data processing systems led to a widening of the capability of GC and to increases in its specificity, sensitivity and speed of analysis. GC, thus, emerged as a powerful analytical tool with widespread applications in every field of analysis including those related to health and disease. In the biomedical field, although the versatility of GC has made a profound impact on diverse research investigations, in routine clinical biochemistry its role still remains modest to this day because of certain practical limitations.

Among the physicochemical techniques that have been used for confirmation of the chemical identity of analytes eluted from GC columns, mass spectrometry (MS) is the most important. Complete systems, linking gas chromatography to a mass spectrometer (GC-MS), are now to be found in many laboratories concerned with GC, and this combination represents the most powerful means for the qualitative and quantitative analysis of trace amounts of chemical constituents of a complex mixture.

The vast growth in the interest and uses of GC reflected well in the number and range of publications devoted to this technique. Numerous reports of new methods, and modified versions of the old ones, are published every year in scientific journals. Those of particular interest to clinical biochemists are to be found in periodicals such as *Journal of Chromatography, Clinical Chemistry, Annals of Clinical Biochemistry, Journal of Chromatographic Science, Analytical Biochemistry* and *Clinica Chimica Acta.* It is intended in this chapter to present the key features of GC and GC-MS and discuss their uses with particular reference to those relevant to clinical biochemistry. For further and more elaborative treatment, the reader is referred to sources given at the end of the chapter. The application section is by no means exhaustive or up to date; it is expected primarily to convey a true impression of the versatility of GC in the biochemistry laboratory, highlighting some procedures developed in recent years for use in the routine and specialist investigations of patients.

THE CHROMATOGRAM, TERMINOLOGY AND THEORY

In gas chromatography, the sample to be analysed is introduced into a gas stream (carrier gas) and the mixture traverses a specially made column. The separation of the analytes takes place in the column either by differential adsorption on a solid phase (gas–solid chromatography, GSC) or by partition between the gaseous phase and a liquid (stationary phase) held upon an inert solid matrix (gas–liquid chromatography, GLC). Because of its prevalence in practice, GLC is often meant by the term GC, which will hereafter be used in this chapter. At the column outlet the presence of the resolved components in the carrier gas is monitored by a suitable detection device and the response is recorded against time.

In the idealized chromatogram shown in Fig. 1, the horizontal axis represents the time and the vertical axis the detector response in millivolts. The total amount of any component in the separated mixture is proportional to the detector response integrated over the time taken by that component to pass through the detector. The value can be obtained by means of an integrator accessory fitted to the chromatograph or manually by triangulation or multiplication of peak height by peak width at half-height. Thus in Fig. 1, the total detector responses to components 1 and 2 vary directly, as shown below, with C_1 and C_2, the amounts injected.

$C_1 \propto DG$ (peak height) $\times CE$ (peak width at half-height)

$C_2 \propto JM$ (peak height) $\times IK$ (peak width at half-height)

two peaks divided by the average peak width. For components 1 and 2 in Fig. 1 it would be:

$$R = 2(OM - OG)/(BF + HL)$$

R should preferably be greater than 1 and the separation is adequate if $R = 1.5$. Resolution R can also be related to the number of theoretical plates and the retention times concerned. It should, therefore, be possible to find out how many theoretical plates may be required to achieve a given resolution.

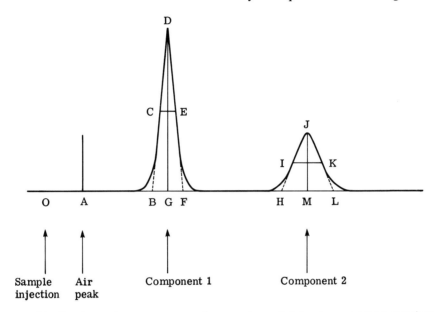

Fig. 1 An idealized gas chromatogram of a sample containing two components 1 and 2.

Retention. The column is chosen so that analytes in question travel at different speeds and emerge at different times, ideally as symmetrical Gaussian peaks. The times taken to reach the peak maxima are called the retention times (t_R), and correspond in Fig. 1 to OG and OM for components 1 and 2 respectively; the equivalent volume is the retention volume (V_R), given by $V_R = t_R \times F_c$, where F_c is the flow rate of the carrier gas at the outlet pressure and temperature of the column. The symbol V_R^0 stands for retention volume when corrected, for the pressure gradient across the column. The retention of a substance in GC is a function of its partition coefficient, β, in the stationary phase-carrier gas system. It is also influenced by several operating variables of the column, such as the dead volume, pressure drop across the column, temperature of the carrier gas and the load of stationary phase in the column. For a given sustance, the equation that relates retention volume with its partition coefficient β is:

$$V_R^0 = L(\alpha + m\beta) \qquad (1)$$

Where L is the length of the column and α and m are the volume of carrier gas and mass of stationary phase per unit length of the column, respectively.

Resolution (R) means the distance between the

In equation (1), the product αL is the total dead volume of the column (V_M^0) and mL is the total weight of the stationary phase in the column (W). Equation (1) then becomes:

$$V_R^0 = V_M^0 + W\beta \qquad (2)$$

Thus the retention volume of a non-retarded substance ($\beta = 0$), such as the solvent in GC, gives directly a value for the dead volume, $V_R^0 = V_M^0$ which corresponds to OA in Fig. 1. The net retention volume (V_N) is obtained by correcting V_R^0 for V_M^0, that is:

$$V_N = V_R^0 - V_M^0 = W\beta \qquad (3)$$

In Fig. 1, net retention volumes for components 1 and 2 correspond to the adjusted retention times (t_R') AG and AM respectively. Often retention time is expressed as a ratio with that of a chosen standard.

Resolution and Efficiency. In GC analysis of a mixture under controlled experimental conditions, the retention of components will be primarily governed by their distribution between the gas and the stationary phases. The shape of the peak, thereby the quality of separation of the components, will also be determined by the longitudinal diffusion of the analyte and axial diffusion through the pores of the packing material.

In practice, the overall column performance is empirically expressed in terms of a number of theoretical plates (N), a concept that originated from the traditional countercurrent separation process. A theoretical plate may be defined as a layer at right angles to the column of such a thickness that the solute at its mean concentration in the stationary phase in this layer is in equilibirum with its vapour in the mobile phase leaving the layer. It can be calculated from knowledge of the retention time and peak width. There are two ways of deriving the value of

in the column effluent. The response is recorded (R) in the form of peaks after necessary amplification (A) of the signal. The detector response may also be integrated and expressed in numerical form. An eluate stream-splitter (S) can be used for diverting part of an analyte for further examination by techniques such as mass spectrometry (M).

Carrier Gas

The carrier gas should be inert and pure. Molecular-sieve filters, to remove traces of water vapour, oxygen and other contaminants from the carrier gas, are

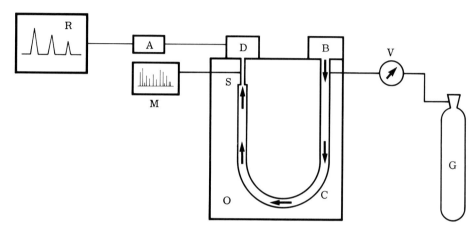

Fig. 2 Schematic representation of a gas chromatograph. A, amplifier; B, injection block; C, column; D, detector; G, gas cylinder; M, mass spectrometer; O, oven; R, recorder; S, stream splitter; V, gas valve.

N as shown below with reference to component 1 in Fig. 1.

$$N = 16(OG/BF)^2 \tag{4}$$
$$N = 8.1n2 . (OG/CE)^2 \tag{5}$$
$$= 5.54 . (OG/CE)^2$$

The number of theoretical plates per metre of column (N/L) or an alternative 'height equivalent to a theoretical plate', HETP (L/N) is often quoted for the purpose of comparison of columns (L is the length of the column in metres) and for a good GC packed column, the number of plates would be around 2000 per metre.

BASIC INSTRUMENTATION

A typical arrangement of the basic components of a gas chromatograph is shown in Fig. 2. The carrier gas is delivered from a pressurized cylinder (G) via a suitable regulatory device (V) and passes through the injection block (B) into which the sample to be analysed can be introduced. The sample is vapourized, and together with the carrier gas travels along the column (C) which is enclosed in a thermostatically controlled oven (O). The detector (D), at the other end, senses the presence of the sample components

commercially available. The gas in common use is nitrogen but for GC-MS and capillary column work helium is preferred. The gas flow is kept constant during the chromatographic run and its rate depends on the type of column and the nature of analysis at hand. For standard (4 mm i.d.) columns the gas flow is usually within the range 20–60 ml/min; a much lower rate is used in capillary columns.

Sample Injection

A sample can be a gas, liquid or solid. The injection block is usually maintained 30°–50 °C above that of column so that a liquid or solid sample is flash-evaporated at introduction. It is important that the analytes remain intact chemically and are flushed into the column as a narrow band.

Gas samples can be used in amounts from under $10 \,\mu l$ to 1 ml or more for packed columns by a gas syringe through one of several types of gas sampling valves. For any type of sample, the choice of injection volume and the amount of analytes depend largely on the linear range of the detector and column characteristics. Liquid samples are generally used in volumes between 1 and $5 \,\mu l$ on standard packed columns. For capillary columns, on the other hand, some form of sample splitting device allows only a small proportion of the injected sample to pass into the column.

Improved chromatographic separation may be obtained by evaporating liquid samples to dryness in needles or capsules which may then be dropped into the injection block area. There are now good automated sampling devices available for handling specimens in large numbers.

Oven

The oven which houses the column is controlled thermostatically. In relatively simple analyses adequate

Columns used in GC vary widely, e.g., in length and internal diameter, tubing material, stationary phase and its solid support. The conventional analytical columns are usually 1–3 m long, 2–6 mm i.d. and made of glass, copper or stainless steel; the micropacked columns can be up to 50 m in length with i.d. of 1 mm or less. In order to avoid sample decomposition, especially for steroids and drugs, glass columns deactivated with dimethylchlorosilane (DMCS) are preferred for chromatography at high temperatures.

One of the major developments in gas chromatography in recent years was the introduction of open tubular columns for analytical work. These are long

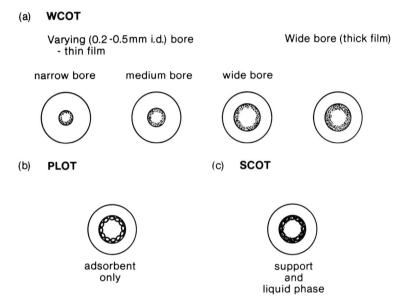

Fig. 3 Types of capillary columns. (a) WCOT: wall-coated open tubular column. (b) PLOT: porous layer open tubular column (adsorbent only). (c) SCOT: support-coated open tubular column (support and Liquid Phase).

separation of components may be obtained under isothermal conditions. For more complex mixtures, temperature programming may be essential; the temperature of the oven is programmed to increase between pre-set low and high temperature limits at a specified rate. It enables better separation of relatively more volatile components of a mixture at the lower temperature; the higher temperatures later in the run prevent too great a delay in the elution of the less volatile components.

Column

GC columns are either packed with uniformly sized particles which support a thin film of the stationary phase or this phase is coated onto the walls of the column; the stationary phase is liquid at the temperature used and plays a key role in the separation of analytes. In gas–solid chromatography the packing consists only of a solid with a high surface area for adsorption and thereby for resolution of analytes.

lengths, up to 50 m, of capillary tubing with internal diameter less than 1 mm. The tubing is made of stainless steel, nickel or more commonly glass. In recent years, fused silica columns are gaining increasing popularity because of their flexibility and inertness. Various types of such columns are shown in Fig. 3. The liquid phase is coated as a thin film (0.1–$1.5 \, \mu m$ and sometimes more) on the inner wall of the tubing in wall-coated open tubular columns (WCOT) which gives them very high permeability. Therefore, long column lengths can be used giving an enormous resolution power. Column life may be prolonged by more permanent chemical bonding of liquid phase to the surface of the inner wall of the tubing. As these columns can be washed with organic solvents to remove interfering agents, they are particularly suitable for splitless and on-column injections. In support-coated open tubular columns (SCOT) small particles of an inert material adhere to the wall and provide enlarged surface area on which thicker films of stationary phase can be deposited. Compared to WCOT columns, SCOT columns have higher sample capacity and retention volumes, but lower efficiency. Another type of capillary column useful for analysis of light hydrocarbons and permanent gases is the porous layer open tubular columns (PLOT) in which the inside wall is coated with a layer of a porous material such as Al_2O_3/KCl and molecular sieves.

In conventional gas chromatography, the function of the solid support is to hold a thin film of the stationary phase. The desirable characteristics of a column support material would be large surface area per unit volume, chemical inertness, thermal stability, low adsorption capacity, favourable pore structure, high mechanical strength and uniformity of particle size. The most commonly used supports originate from diatomite (also known as diatomaceous silica, diatomaceous earth and kieselguhr), which is essentially microamorphous silica with minor amounts of metallic oxides. The structure of support particles is important in achieving the most effective coating with the stationary phase. More directly, the adsorption of analytes on solid support causes peak tailing and shifting of retention times. Such interactions, particu-

larly evident on columns with a stationary phase that is non-polar or low in loading, are generally attributed to surface hydroxyl groups (silanol) or other active sites that take part in forming hydrogen bonds. To eliminate or reduce this problem one needs to modify the support surface as follows: (a) removal of extraneous mineral impurities by acid and/or base washing; (b) silanization with reagents such as hexamethyldisilazane (HMDS) and dimethylchlorosilane (DMCS), or by (c) coating the support particles with a layer of a polar stationary phase. For analytical work, particularly when stationary phase level is under 5%, it is advisable to use acid-washed and silanized solid support. Most diatomite solid supports carry the name Chromosorb[R], which is a registered trademark of Johns-Manville Corporation, USA. There are four basic grades indicated by letters A, G, P and W (Table 1) and each of these materials is further differentiated by additional letters such as NAW (non acid-washed), AW (acid washed), HMDS (treated with hexamethyldisilazane), AW-HMDS and HP (high performance). In fact, the range of these supports is further expanded by many

TABLE 1
PHYSICAL PROPERTIES OF CHROMOSORB SUPPORTS

Material	Free fall density	Packed density g/cc	Surface area m²/g	Surface area m²/cc	Stationary phase loading capacity
Chromosorb A	0·40	0·48	2·7	1·30	25%
Chromosorb G	0·47	0·58	0·5	0·29	5%
Chromosorb P	0·38	0·47	4·0	1·88	30%
Chromosorb W	0·18	0·24	1·0	0·29	15%
Chromosorb T*	0·42	0·49	7·5	—	5%
Chromosorb 750**	0·33	—	0·75	—	7%

* Made from PTFE resin, has a highly inert surface, recommended for analysis of very polar compounds.
** Recommended by manufacturers as the most inert and highly efficient support.
(Source: Catalogue, Chromapack UK Ltd.)

TABLE 2
LIST OF EQUIVALENT COLUMN SUPPORTS

Non-acid washed	Acid washed	Acid washed and DMCS treated	Acid washed and DMCS treated, high performance (B = extra base washed)
Chromosorb W	Chromosorb WAW	Chromosorb W AW DMCS	Chromosorb WAP
Gaschrom S			
Anakrom U	Gaschrom A	Gaschrom Z	Gaschrom Q(B)
Diatomite C	Anakrom A	Anakrom AS	Anakrom ABS(B)
		Anakrom Q	Anakrom SD
Chromosorb G	Supelcon AW	Supelcon AW DMCS	Supelcort
Chromosorb P	Chromosorb GAW		
Gaschrom R	Chromosorb P AW	Chromosorb P AW DMCS	Varaport 30
			Diatoport S
Anakrom C22	Gaschrom RA	Gaschrom RZ	Diatomite CLQ
Diatomite S			Diatomite CQ
Sil-O-Cel			Chromosorb GHP
Firebrick C22			Chromosorb 750

DMCS = dimethylchlorosilane
(Source: Chromapack UK Ltd. Guide, 1981)

brand names and by the introduction of newer and allegedly improved preparations (Table 2). The surface of the support particles and their pore structure are important in gas–solid chromatographic separations. The general categories of these adsorbents are: (a) inorganic materials, e.g. alumina, silica gel, molecular sieves, Carbopack, Porosil and Sperosil; (b) inorganic materials modified with a bonded organic monolayer, e.g. Duropak and Sperosil SIA; and (c) organic porous polymers, e.g. Porapak series (P, PS, Q, QS, R, S, N and T), Chromosorb-100 series (Table 3) and Tenex GC. The particle size of supports is generally expressed in terms of screen openings. Those sizes normally used in GC are 60/80 mesh (250–177 μm) and 80/100 mesh (177–149 μm).

atives of several chemical groups and determined the Kovats Indices on squalane, the least-polar stationary phase standard. When Kovats Indices of these chemical probes on other stationary phases are reduced by corresponding Kovats Indices on squalane, the resultant values are known as McReynolds' constants. The sum of five of these constants (for benzene, 1-butanol, 2-pentanone, nitropropane and pyridine) is chosen as the criterion for the overall polarity of a stationary phase and its comparison with others. Of the numerous chemicals used as stationary phases in GC, polysiloxanes are most popular (Tables 5 and 6). They offer a wide choice of products in terms of chemical composition, selectivity and thermal stability.

TABLE 3

PHYSICAL PROPERTIES OF SOME POROUS POLYMER COLUMN PACKING MATERIALS

Material	Polymer type	Free fall density, g/cc	Surface area, m²/g	Pore diameter, μm	Temperature limit (isothermal) °C
Chromosorb* 101	Styrene-divinyl benzene	0·30	50	0·3–0·4	275
102	Styrene-divinyl benzene	0·29	300–400	0·0085	250
103	Cross-linked polystyrene	0·32	15–25	0·3–0·4	275
104	Acrylonitrile divinyl benzene	0·32	100–200	0·06–0·08	250
105	Polyaromatic	0·34	600–700	0·04–0·06	250
106	Non-polar cross-linked polystyrene	0·28	700–800	0·005	250
107	Acrylic ester	0·30	400–500	0·009	250
108	Acrylic ester	0·30	100–200	0·0235	250

* These cross-linked resins with a uniform rigid structure and distinct pore size are usable without a stationary phase coating. Another range of similar products are known as 'Porapaks'.
(Source: Catalogues, Chromapack UK Ltd and Camlab Ltd, UK).

Column efficiency increases with decreasing particle size up to a point; in the main, 100/120 mesh size is likely to be found most appropriate for most chromatographic separations.

In column packing material for GC, the amount of stationary phase used ranges between 1 and 20% of the total weight. Important among the general requirements of a good stationary phase are purity, consistency of composition from batch to batch, and stability and low viscosity at the operating temperature. The organic chemist's rule of 'like dissolves like' can provide a useful lead in the choice of stationary phase (Table 4). More precise ways of classifying stationary phases have to encompass their polarity, i.e., those physicochemical characteristics which confer selectivity on column performance. The Kovats Index (I) for a certain compound on the liquid phase in question may be obtained as follows:

$$I = \frac{\log t'_R - \log t'_R(n)}{\log t'_R(n+1) - \log t'_R(n)} \times 100 + 100n$$

where t'_R is the net retention time of the compound eluting between normal hydrocarbons C_nH_{2n+2} and $C_{n+1}H_{2n+4}$. McReynolds selected some represent-

TABLE 4

EXAMPLES OF COLUMNS USED IN VARIOUS GC ANALYSES

Analytes	Column
1. Alcohol	Carbowax (20M, 600, 1500), diglycerol, OV-210, Porapak Q
2. Aldehydes and ketones	Carbowax (20M, 1500), Porapak, polysiloxanes (e.g. OV-210, DC-550)
3. Esters	Carbowax 20M, DEGA, EGS, NPGS, polysiloxanes (e.g. SE-30, OV-17, OV-101, Dexil-300)
4. Steroids, sugars and amines (as silyl and other derivatives)	Polysiloxanes (e.g. OV-1, SE-30, OV-17, OV-101, OV-225, QF-1, XE-60, Dexil-300)
5. Hydrocarbons	Squalene, apiezon L, porapak Q, polysiloxanes (e.g. SE-30, Dexil-300)

With MS detectors it is essential to choose stationary phases with minimal bleeding at the operating temperature. SE-30, OV-17, OV-101 are among those used commonly.

The column temperature should be high enough so that an analysis can be completed in a reasonable

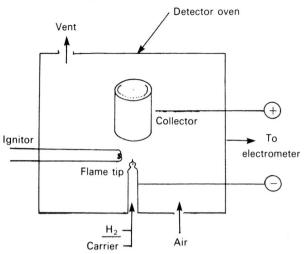

Fig. 4 The basic parts of a flame ionization detector. (Reproduced with permission, C. H. Hartman (1971) *Anal. Chem*; **43**: 113A–35A.)

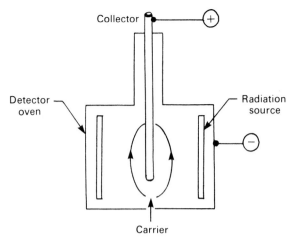

Fig. 5 The basic components of an electron capture detector. (Reproduced with permission, C. H. Hartman (1971) *Anal. Chem*; **43**: 113A–35A.)

a hydrogen flame acts as the ionizing source. The basic design of FID is shown in Fig. 4. Hydrogen is mixed with the effluent gases and is burnt in an atmosphere of air. The jet serves as one electrode, the other being the collector electrode which is polarized by a positive potential of between 200 and 300 volts with respect to the cathode. When only the carrier gas flows into the flame, a very low concentration of charged particles will be produced thereby causing the constant background current. In practice, this is reduced to zero. When an eluted organic solute passes into the flame, its combustion generates charged particles, proportional to the amount of the substance entering the flame in unit time.

The current is passed through a resistor, the voltage across the resistor is amplified and recorded. For optimum performance, the shape and size of the flame is critical and these are determined by the relative proportion of hydrogen, carrier gas and air present in the mixture and by the design of the detector. For each detector it is best to determine the appropriate gas flow rates experimentally. As the sample is destroyed during FID detection, an effluent-splitting device before the detector would be necessary if any additional analysis is to be performed on the resolved sample components. The lack of response to water, universality in response, good sensitivity, wide linear range and robustness make FID the most popular detector in gas chromatography.

Electron Capture Detector (ECD). In ECD (Fig. 5) the column effluent gas, e.g. a mixture of argon and methane (9:1) is exposed to ionizing radiation from a suitable radioactive source, e.g., ^3H or more commonly ^{63}Ni, producing positive ions and free electrons. When a suitable voltage is applied between the two electrodes in the detector, the ions are collected, thus giving a standing current. Substances with high electron affinity, e.g. halogen and nitro-

compounds, conjugated carbonyls, nitrites and organometallics will remove electrons from the ionization chamber and form negatively charged ions which because of their low drift velocity will recombine with the positive ions present. The result will be a reduction in the standing current. The size of the drop in current will not only be a function of the amount of that compound present but also its electronegativity.

ECD is extremely sensitive to certain molecules as mentioned earlier. For halogens, the response increases with atomic weight (F < Cl < Br < I) and multiple substitution enhances the effect. Several reagents are available for converting an analyte into an electron-capturing form thus making it amenable to ECD analysis. One major limitation of ECD is its low range of linearity. The sample size should, therefore, be small. It has to be dry also because traces of water disturb detector response. Other factors which affect detector performance include detector temperature, applied voltage, purity and flow rate of carrier gas. As radiation source ^{63}Ni is preferred to ^3H because it can be heated to 350°C, although the latter provides a wider linear range.

Alkali Flame Ionization Detector (AFID, also known as nitrogen-phosphorus detector, NPD). These detectors are similar in operation to FID discussed earlier except that they have a quantity of an alkali salt, e.g. of Na, K, Rb and Cs placed near the tip of the flame (Fig. 6). The result is enhancement of response to nitrogen and to compounds containing nitrogen or phosphorus and to a lesser extent to halogenated compounds.

The mechanism underlying this selectivity is not fully understood. The sensitivity and selectivity of AFID detectors depend on various factors such as electrode geometry, the detector temperature, the nature, purity and configuration of the alkali salt and

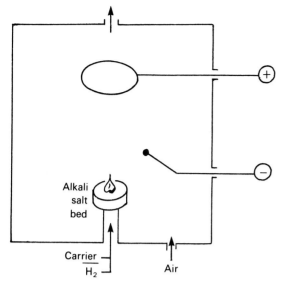

Fig. 6 Diagrammatic representation of an alkali flame ionization detector. (Reproduced with permission, C. H. Hartman (1971) *Anal. Chem*; **43**: 113A–25A.)

the carrier-gas flow rate. Among the detectors of this type, the nitrogen-selective form of AFID has useful applications in clinical biochemistry. It is more sensitive than the FID and its reliability has also improved in recent years.

Mass Spectrometer Detector. When a powerful analytical tool like a mass spectrometer (MS) was linked up for on-line analysis of components resolved on GC columns, the combined GC–MS technique opened up a new era in biomedical applications of gas chromatography. MS detectors can be used in various modes, for definitive characterization of analytes and also for their quantitative measurements. Despite the increasing uses of such systems, they still remain beyond the reach of average gas chromatographers because of the prohibitive cost of a good system and the specialist handling needed for running of the instrument and its maintenance. It is, however,

essential that those concerned with GC are conversant with the principle underlying MS and the integration of this technique with gas chromatographic analysis. GC–MS is described separately in the following section.

GAS CHROMATOGRAPHY–MASS SPECTROMETRY (GC–MS)

Direct Coupling of Gas Chromatograph and Mass Spectrometer

The packed GC columns used initially by chromatographers posed a difficult problem for instrument designers attempting direct coupling with a mass spectrometer. Packed column GC works with carrier gas pressures of 30–40 p.s.i. at the column inlet and atmospheric pressure at the column outlet resulting in a total carrier gas flow rate in the range of 40–80 ml/min. MS, however, operates under high vacuum conditions and many commercial instruments could handle only 0·1–0·5 ml/min total gas flow rate. In order to make the two instruments compatible it was necessary to reduce the carrier gas flow at the MS inlet to 0·5 ml/min preferably without loss of sample. To accomplish this, several ingenious devices, collectively known as 'molecular separators', have been designed. The earliest of these was the Ryhage jet separator, the design of which is shown in Fig. 7. It consists of four in-line small orifice jets, sealed in an evacuated housing. The eluant from the chromatograph enters the left-hand jet and on entering the first low pressure region the light helium gas diffuses rapidly away from the nozzle whereas the heavier sample vapour diffuses less. At the entrance to the second jet therefore the atmosphere is richer in sample vapour than in helium. This process is repeated in a lower pressure second stage such that on exit from the final jet into the MS source the helium concentration is reduced in the eluant by a factor of approximately 100 but that of the sample is reduced by a factor of only 2 or 3.

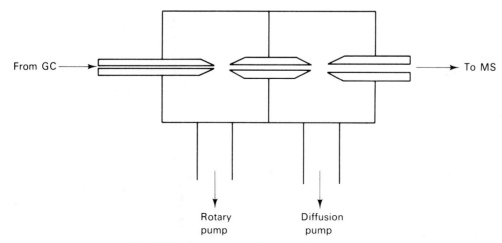

Fig. 7 The Ryhage double-stage jet separator.

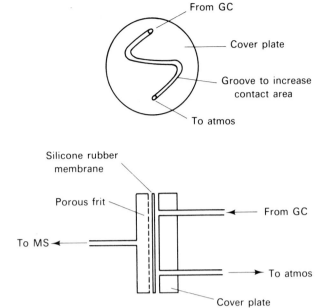

Fig. 8 The Llewellyn membrane separator.

Important among the other types of separator are those based on the semipermeable membrane principle; an example, the Llewellyn membrane separator is shown in Fig. 8. This consists of a thin (0·15 mm) section of silicone rubber laid over a stainless-steel or glass porous frit. The eluant from the GC is allowed to pass over the surface of the membrane whereupon the organic material passes through into the MS whilst the inorganic carrier gas flows out to atmosphere. The membrane is capable of helium depletion by a factor of 200 whilst transmitting 90% of organic material. Several other semipermeable membrane devices based on silver–palladium or Teflon have also been reported. Each particular type of separator has its advantages and disadvantages. Stainless-steel designs all have the disadvantage that the sample may decompose on the hot metal surfaces. Membrane systems (e.g. the silicone rubber system) tend to be temperature dependent and somewhat selective in transmission of organic materials, and contribute to mass spectrometer background. Improvements in mass spectrometer design, particularly in the use of higher capacity pumping systems have reduced the requirements placed on interfaces so that open tubular or capillary GC columns, operating with flow rates up to 10–15 ml/min, require no separator. For packed columns requiring flow rates of up to 80 ml/min only a single-stage jet separator is required. Many manufacturers are now offering these devices, made entirely in glass or with glass jets housed in a stainless-steel envelope. The good transfer (>60%) and chemical inertness of these separators makes them very useful for most materials encountered by the modern organic chemist or biochemist.

Today the majority of GC applications are carried out using high resolution capillary columns with carrier flow rate typically only 1 ml/min, making the use of molecular separators unnecessary except in special applications where high (microgram) sample loading is required. Furthermore the advent of long (up to 50 m) fused silica wall coated capillary columns with internal diameter in the range 0·2–0·4 mm has presented the modern chromatographer with a robust column of small size capable of up to 100 000 theoretical plates. In addition to the obvious advantage of low flow rate, these columns allow total transfer of organic material direct to the mass spectrometer ion source, avoiding any possibility of sample degradation by contact with hot metal surfaces. The high resolution characteristics also mean that the sample is concentrated into a narrow time interval and hence produces a more intense peak leading to increased sensitivity.

The total sample loading allowable with fused silica capillary columns is considerably less than that allowed using packed columns and should not exceed about 100 ng total sample (all components) but is nevertheless well within the detection capability of a modern mass spectrometer.

The GC-MS System

A schematic diagram of the GC-MS system is shown in Fig. 9. The eluant from the GC, containing a suitably low level of carrier gas, passes into the mass spectrometer source. In this region the sample is bombarded by a stream of electrons generated from a hot tungsten filament. The energy of the electrons (usually 70 eV) is sufficient to ionize the sample molecule forming a singly charged, positive radical ion, normally referred to as the 'molecular' or 'parent' ion:

$$M \rightarrow M^{+\cdot} \tag{9}$$
$$M^{+\cdot} \rightarrow A^+ + B^{\cdot} \tag{10}$$
$$M^{+\cdot} \rightarrow C^+ + D \tag{11}$$

There is, however, sufficient energy transferred to the molecule to cause bond cleavage. The original radical ion breaks down to produce a second positive ion of smaller mass together with a radical (equation 10) or in some cases a neutral species (equation 11). The ions produced in this way are extracted from the ion chamber by a potential difference of several kilovolts. This whole process occurs in a time scale of the order of microseconds and the ions emerging from the source consist of 'molecular' ions and fragment ions in a random distribution which is weighted to some extent in favour of one or other by particular structural features of the original molecule. The ion beam thus formed is focused by a series of electrodes into a line image at the entrance to a sector magnetic field. Since the ions emerging from the source are all accelerated through the same potential difference all have essentially the same energy. Some energy

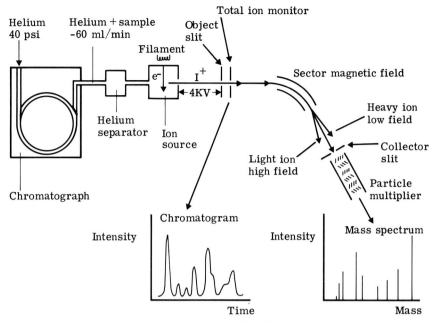

Fig. 9 Schematic diagram of a GC–MS system.

spread is introduced by source parameters and thermal effects. Since, however, the ions have different masses they have different velocities. At low magnetic field strength lighter ions of higher velocity are caused to follow a curved path and are focused as a line image at a small slit at the exit of the magnetic sector whilst heavier ions with lower velocities do not undergo sufficient deflection to pass through the slit. At higher field strength, light ions are deflected through a small radius and are lost whilst heavier ions are focused at the exit slit. As the magnetic field is scanned from a low to a high value therefore, ions of increasing mass are allowed to pass through the exit slit. A plot of ion current arriving at the exit slit against magnetic field strength therefore generates a mass spectrum. Because the ion current at the exit slit is so small (of the order of 10^{-12} amps) a particle multiplier is employed with a gain of 10^6 in order to achieve a current output measurable by a fast-response amplifier. In order to generate a conventional chromatogram, a metal electrode placed in the source region of the instrument intercepts part of the unresolved ion beam. The current arriving at this electrode is amplified and displayed on a chart recorder. The response of this recorder therefore varies in intensity as consecutive components elute from the GC. This electrode is referred to as the 'total ion monitor' and replaces conventional FID or ECD detectors. When used in conjunction with a computerized data recording system the total ion plate monitor is dispensed with and the chromatogram trace is reconstructed in the computer by summing all the recorded intensities of the focused ions reaching the final collector. This technique has several advantages: (1) the recording is made after the particle multiplier and is therefore of higher intensity

overall; (2) the greatest advantage lies in the ability to re-examine the stored data and reconstruct a chromatogram either of total ion current or of recorded ion current at selected mass values. This 'reconstructed ion current chromatogram (RIC)' may be displayed and modified to reveal information difficult to extract by any other means.

In practical terms then, a sample is injected onto the GC column and the magnetic field is scanned rapidly and repetitively. After the retention time of the first component has elapsed the total ion monitor or RIC records an increasing ion current and a mass spectrum of that component is obtained. In order to avoid changing sample concentration in the ion source during the mass scan, the scan time should be small compared with the width of the GC peak. Conventional packed GC columns generally give rise to peak widths in the range 20–60 s and the spectrum may be scanned in 3–10 s. Capillary columns may generate peaks with widths of only 3–5 s and in this case a 1 s (or less) spectrum time is required. Under these conditions a usable spectrum may be obtained from 1 ng of sample injected onto the GC column.

For chromatograph applications the mass spectrometer should have certain minimum performance specifications. The majority of samples with boiling points in the range acceptable for GC analysis have molecular weights up to 500 amu. The mass spectrometer should therefore be capable of detecting ions of mass at least 500. In some cases the volatility of a sample may be increased by derivatization such that it becomes amenable to GC, e.g. silylation of polyhydroxy materials such as sterols or carbohydrates. These derivatization procedures may increase the molecular weight of the sample such that masses of 800–900 amu are not uncommon. A good GC-MS system should therefore have a mass range up to 1000 amu. Since it is important to determine the molecular weight of a component to an accuracy of at least 1 amu the MS should be able to differentiate ions of mass 1000 and 1001. An instrument which can differentiate ions of mass m and m + 1 with a 10% valley between the recorded peaks is said to have a resolving power 'm'. In this case then, the GC-MS system should have a resolving power of 1000. The design of source and electronic recording system should be capable of producing a spectrum from 1 ng of sample in one second with a signal-to-noise ratio on the most intense peak of the order of 50:1 if the spectrum is to be usable.

Mass Spectrum. In qualitative terms the mass spectrum may be considered as a 'fingerprint' of a particular material. In GC applications the parameters, e.g. column type, temperature, carrier-gas flow rate, and retention time provide valuable evidence for the identity of a sample and comparison of the mass spectrum 'fingerprint' with tables of standard mass spectra may be all that is required for confirmation. If the identity of the sample is more obscure and the fingerprint alone is not enough the mass spectrum may be investigated more thoroughly. The methods involved in this case are best illustrated by example. Consider the spectrum of the silyl ether of cholesterol shown in Fig. 10. The most intense peak in the spectrum, termed the 'base peak' is given an arbitrary intensity of 100 units and all other peak intensities are plotted as a percentage of this value. A mass spectrum presented in this form is said to be 'normalized'. The peak at mass 458 corresponds to the molecular ion M^{+}. The next peak with significant intensity appears at mass 443, fifteen mass units below the molecular mass. This corresponds to the elimination of a methyl radical from the molecular ion. The next peak at mass 368 corresponds to loss of the trimethylsilyl ether group from the 'A' ring. The mass difference of 90 mass units cannot have arisen by simple cleavage of the CO bond and is accounted for by invoking a hydrogen atom rearrangement mechanism which is not uncommon in the mass spectra of sterols. The remaining significant peaks in the spectrum, those at 329 (M-129) and 129

arise from cleavage of $(CH_3)_3SiO$—from the molecular ion with charge retention on this group (129) or on the remainder of the molecule (M-129). By relating the masses of fragment ions to the molecular mass in this way a great deal of structural information concerning the original molecule can be obtained. In cases where the relationship between a fragment ion and the parent molecule is ambiguous or obscure the technique of isotopic substitution may be employed.

In the above example, to prove that the peak at mass 129 is indeed the 'A' ring fragment, the sample is prepared using, for example, a deuterated trimethylsilyl derivative and the mass spectrum recorded again. In this case there is no peak at mass 129 but a peak at mass 138 (129 + 9) from the 9 deutero atoms and the molecular ion is shifted to mass 467.

In quantitative terms the mass spectrometer has a dynamic range of at least 10^4, that is from 1 ng to 10 μg in the scanning mode and is linear over the entire range. The reproducibility of GC-MS measurements is therefore as good as that of the GC alone which is better than 1%. In the scanning mode quantitation would normally be carried out using the total ion trace together with an internal standard in the same way as the standard FID trace is used in normal chromatography. The mass spectrum itself may also be used in a quantitative manner by measuring the height of an intense peak in the spectrum. Precise quantitation is then obtained by comparison with a calibration run of a known quantity of the same material. Calibration must be carried out for all components of the chromatogram since ionization efficiencies vary over a small range for different compounds.

Mass Fragmentography. The qualitative and quantitative aspects of GC-MS may be combined in the extremely powerful technique of mass fragmentography. The use of this technique for detecting a very small amount of cholesterol-TMS-ether in a biological specimen is illustrated in Fig. 11. The GC trace may look something like that at the top of the figure. The large number of components in the chromatogram make identification by retention time alone impossible. The low resolution of the chromatogram and the low level of cholesterol-TMS-ether present probably make

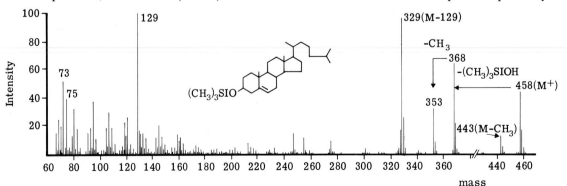

Fig. 10 Mass spectrum of cholesterol TMS ether.

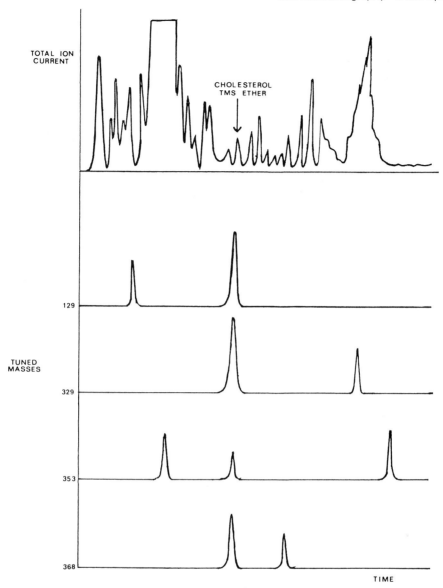

Fig. 11 Mass fragmentography.

identification by mass spectral scanning difficult if not impossible. Examination of the spectrum of cholesterol TMS ether (Fig. 10) shows that the relative ratios of peaks 129, 329, 353 and 368 are probably sufficient to establish the presence of cholesterol-TMS-ether; there is probably no real requirement to see the complete mass spectrum. If now, for example, the mass spectrum has a peak of interest at mass 500 and the mass range from 0–1000 is scanned in 1 s, then from the definition of resolving power given earlier the time spent collecting ions of mass 500 is 0·5 ms.

Since ion generation is essentially a statistical technique the limit of detection is directly related to the number of ions collected at a given mass. If therefore, instead of scanning the mass spectrum in one second, more time is spent collecting ions of mass 500 the detection level will be greatly improved. The time spent at mass m is limited initially by the width, in time, of the GC peak. The time is also limited in the practical case because of the requirement that the intensities of at least four of the ions in the spectrum must be recorded in order to characterize the sample. If the peak is 10 s wide at the base and at least 10 samples of the ion current at each of the four masses are recorded during the time of the GC peak, the time per peak per sample is then 1/40 of 10 seconds i.e. 250 ms. In comparison with the scanning mode, the time spent collecting ions has increased from 0·5 to 250 ms. The detection sensitivity has also increased by a factor of 500. Hence if 1 ng gives a spectrum with 50:1 signal to noise on the base peak in the scanning mode the same signal to noise ratio can be achieved from 2 pg in the mass fragmentography technique. The detection limit (1:1 signal to noise) of this technique is therefore 40 fg.

GC run in the normal full scanning mode a control program interrogates the database for each compound of interest and searches for the listed characteristic mass values at the appropriate retention time.

If the mass values are detected they are then subjected to relative intensity checks as described above to establish that they all relate to the compound of interest. If all identity criteria are passed, reconstructed ion chromatograms are prepared and used to determine quantity via peak area measurement. Incorporation of internal standards and 'spikes' allows precise quantitation together with estimates of recovery levels obtained from the extraction procedure.

Finally the quantitative data are written back to the database and control is passed to a spreadsheet program which generates a report in the style appropriate to the end user.

Such automated analysis techniques are beginning to be applied in clinical biochemistry in screening for inborn metabolic diseases. The power of this technique lies in the speed and wide range of components which can be detected simultaneously.

GC-MS Computer Systems. In the time scale of a capillary GC run (ca 45 min) it is possible to generate some 2000–3000 mass spectra. The enormous amount of data available from only one day of routine operation is beyond manual interpretation and data handling. Mini- and microcomputers with up to 1 megabyte of core storage and up to 100 megabytes of disc storage which are capable of storing and reducing this enormous amount of data are now readily available. Modern data acquisition systems are capable of presenting normalized summaries (eight largest peaks) in real time. Background subtraction, deconvolution of GC multiple peaks, real-time mass fragmentography, element mapping and limited compound identification in chemical terms are now possible. Libraries of standard spectra (e.g. NBS 42 000 and Wiley 69 000) can be stored and searched in comparison with an unknown. In addition to output data handling, the computer can also be used to control the instrument. The computer can load appropriate set points to the GC, initiate data acquisition and search and lock onto a series of mass values for mass fragmentography experiments. The level of sophistication of GC-MS computer systems is virtually unlimited and, as computer systems become less and less expensive, more and more of the possible options are incorporated as standard features of commercial instruments.

QUALITATIVE AND QUANTITATIVE ANALYSIS

Qualitative Analysis

Gas chromatography performed under standardized conditions can provide information useful for qualitative examination of organic analytes. Thus, the retention times of column fractions may be compared with those found with appropriate standards. A retention time is dependent on many operation parameters, correlation of such data from different sources may be difficult. For this reason the use of relative retention time, i.e. retention time calculated with reference to a selected standard substance, is preferred. However, even the most thorough investigation of retention data cannot confirm peak identity beyond all doubts. For this, auxiliary techniques such as MS, NMR and IR may be applied to components collected after separation on the columns. Of the techniques mentioned, MS is most important and its interfacing with the GC system is highly developed (*see* previous section). In the main, the approach to qualitative identification of components separated by gas chromatography may be summarized as follows:

1. determination of retention time or relative retention time on two or more columns with stationary phases of different polarity;
2. 'spiking'—addition of a tiny amount of the pure compound suspected to be present and the observation of augmented detector response at the appropriate retention time;
3. repetition of (1) after chemical modification of the sample prior to GC;
4. positive identification of a portion of the analyte, eluted from the column, by other physicochemical techniques, e.g. MS.

Quantitative Analysis

The uses of gas chromatography in clinical biochemistry are mostly for quantitative analyses. Sample sizes can vary over a range of $10^{-12} - 10^{-6}$ g depending on the type of detector and equipment concerned. One important advantage of gas chromatography over many other analytical techniques lies in its ability to separate and measure simultaneously the multiple components of a mixture. The availability of the retention time data can assist in the validation of an assay procedure from the viewpoint of specificity. Some essential features concerning the uses of gas chromatography for quantitative determinations are listed below:

1. Establishment of the chemical homogeneity of each peak under consideration.
2. Selection of a method for measuring the detector response (peak area).
3. Finding linear range of the detector for any particular analyte.
4. Standardization of the entire procedure—checking for losses prior to and during gas chromatography.
5. Possible interference from other substances that may be present in the sample.

Under constant experimental conditions the peak height should be a direct measure of an analyte within the linear range of a detector. For this, the instrument has to be calibrated by injecting varied amounts of the compound in hand under identical chromatographic conditions. A better means of quantitation which is amenable to automation is the peak area. The use of peak area compensates for variations in sample injection and chromatography features; it is also a little more accurate for asymmetrical peaks. The methods available for measurement of peak include planimetry, cutting out each peak from the chromatrogram and weighing, triangulation (peak height multiplied peak width at half-height) and the use of integrators. Of these, the triangulation method is still most common, although it is being replaced rapidly by the more accurate and reliable automated integrator systems. Present day digital integrators offer various features necessary for automatic operation and handling of a variety of input signals. The read-out consists of a retention time count and several digits of area data.

Prior to any quantitative analysis, it is necessary to establish the linear range of the system, i.e. to check whether the response increases linearly with the amount of the sample injected over the required concentration range. For quantitative work the lowest concentration should give a detector response about five times the noise level. Deviation from linearity can be due to the detector or the column or in some cases both. A common source of such problems is the column. There are various ways of dealing with the column–sample interactions and they include (a) use of glass instead of metal columns, (b) deactivation of the solid support by silylation or similar means, (c) varying the stationary phase content, (d) chemical modification of the sample prior to gas–liquid chromatography. Sometimes error in sampling technique in combination with the column factor can further complicate the measurement.

Internal standardization offers the best method for obtaining acceptable accuracy and precision in GC analysis. This entails the addition of an appropriate internal standard, taking it through the entire procedure and finally plotting the detector response ratio against the mass ratio of the unknown and the added internal standard. The selection of an internal standard must satisfy the following criteria:

1. The internal standard should be as close as possible to the compound(s) of interest in its chemical structure and properties;
2. It should chromatograph well and be separated from the sample components. Ideally the difference in the retention times should not be too large;
3. It should be chemically stable and, especially under the analytical conditions, must not react with the sample or column components.

The attraction of the internal standardization method is that it largely eliminates the factors that affect the reproducibility of an assay. Once the internal standard is added, evaporation, spillage, etc. should not affect the results. The method is not influenced significantly by minor changes in the chromatographic conditions and is independent of the size of the sample injected. Furthermore, unlike the use of a trace amount of the radiolabelled compound for checking the losses during sample preparation, the entire procedure can be quantitated.

SAMPLE PREPARATION

Gas Samples

Depending on the concentration of the volatile components in the gaseous phase and the sensitivity of the detection system GC analysis may be carried out by direct sampling or after concentration of the sample. For each analyte the best experimental conditions such as temperature, pH of the fluid matrix, and duration of heating under which the gas sample is collected have to be established. When sample enrichment is necessary, the volatiles may be trapped with suitable polymeric solid adsorbents followed by thermal desorption of the material onto the column.

Liquid Samples

Despite major developments in detectors, automated sample injection devices, and data processing systems, the application of GC for routine analyses in clinical biochemistry still remains very limited. The reason is that body fluid specimens such as blood, plasma, urine, cerebrospinal fluid and amniotic fluid have to be processed to a varying degree prior to the GC analysis (Table 8). In the main, this entails extraction of the specimen at an appropriate pH with a suitable solvent, removing impurities by some other form of chromatography, e.g. column, paper or thin-layer chromatography, and then concentration of the sample by distillation under reduced pressure or by heating under an atmosphere of nitrogen (Fig. 13). It is essential that the solvent is pure and volatile to facilitate removal during concentration. The need for these somewhat extensive preliminary procedures, which do not lend themselves readily to automation, adds considerably to the time needed for each GC assay. An increasingly useful feature of sample preparation that has extended the scope of GC for clinical analyses is chemical conversion of the compound(s) under consideration into less polar, more volatile or more stable derivatives before chromatography. The derivative chosen depends on the analyte concerned but there are also other considerations such as the rate and yield of the reaction at the appropriate concentration range of the compound, cost of the reagents, complexity of the procedure and the chromatographic behaviour of the reaction products other than the desired derivative.

TABLE 8

TYPICAL EXAMPLES OF GLC PROCEDURES DEVELOPED FOR THE ANALYSIS OF BODY FLUID CONSTITUENTS

Specimen	Analysis	Derivative	Detector and column	Brief outline of the procedure
1. Urine or serum	α-oxo acids	Oxime-TMS	FID, MS; glass, 3% OV-17	Sample saturated with sodium chloride, acidified and extracted with ethyl acetate. Extracts dried and converted into derivatives.
2. Urine	Catecholamines	N-pentafluoro-propionyl	ECD; glass, 10% SE 30	Adsorbed from urine at pH 8·5 on microcolumns of alumina, eluted with acetic acid and derivatized.
3. Bile	Bile acids	Methyl ester trifluoroacetate	FID; glass, 3% QFI	Enzymic hydrolysis of conjugates, acidified, extracted with diethyl ether. Extracts dried and methylated with diazomethane. Solvent removed and the residue acylated.
4. Urine	C_{19} and C_{21} steroids	Methoxime–TMS	FID, MS; open tubular capillar, glass, OV-101 20 m × 0·25 mm i.d.	Enzymic hydrolysis of conjugates, steroids extracted on Amberlite XAD 2 column. Extract dried and chromatographed on LH 20 column. Fraction dried and converted into derivative; selected ion recordings at m/e 466, 474, 271, 273, 287, 436 and 368.
5. Amniotic fluid	Fatty acids	Methyl ester	FID, MS; glass, 10% EGSS-X	Centrifuged, supernant extracted with chloroform–methanol mixture. Chloroform extract evaporated to dryness and methylated with BF_3/methanol. Methyl esters extracted with n-hexane from saturated salt solution.
6. Cerebrospinal fluid	Neutral and acidic metabolites	Methyl ester TMS ether; O,O-dimethyl O-TMS ether	FID, MS; glass, 5% SE 30, 5% OV-25	Specimen saturated with sodium chloride and extracted with ethyl acetate and diethyl ether at pH 1. Extract dried and converted into derivatives.
7. Urine, serum or amniotic fluid	Short chain dicarboxylic acids	Dimethyl ester	FID, MS; glass, 20% EGA	Sample acidified and extracted with chloroform/methanol (2 : 1, v/v). Extract cooled, made alkaline and centrifuged. Upper layer separated, dried, dissolved in water, pH 6·5 and chromatographed on Dowex resin column. Eluted (0·1 M HCl), neutralized to pH 7–8, saturated with NaCl and extracted with ethyl acetate. Extract dried and methylated with diazomethane.

Standard packed colums were used except where indicated otherwise. FID, Flame ionization detector; ECD, electron capture detector; MS, mass spectrometer.

The advantages of the use of derivatives are as follows:

1. Non-volatile compounds can be made volatile enough for gas chromatography.
2. Derivatives can be more stable than the parent compound, reduce column adsorption and improve peak shape and resolution.
3. Chromatographic characteristics of derivatives can provide useful clues to the chemical structures of organic compounds. Certain derivatives, such as N,N-dimethylhydrazones, O-methyloximes, and silyl ethers, by producing recognizable ions, are specially useful in mass spectrometric examination of column effluents.
4. Specific elements, such as nitrogen, sulphur and phosphorus, can be incorporated into a molecule during the preparation of derivatives thus making it possible to make use of the highly sensitive selective detectors for GC work.

Derivatives made with halogenated groups, such as heptafluorobutyrate and chloroacetate, can be detected at picogram levels by the electron capture detector.
5. Radiolabelled derivatives have also been used in GC in combination with the measurement of radioactivity in column eluates.

Some examples of the derivatives that have been found useful in GC are listed in Table 9.

APPLICATIONS OF CLINICAL INTEREST

GC methods exist for almost every class of organic compound of medical and diagnostic interest. Such determinations may be divided broadly into two types: (a) single component analysis, e.g. cholesterol, ethanol, acetaldehyde, acetone, a drug, steroid hormone or prostaglandin, and (b) multicomponent analysis, or 'biochemical/metabolic profiling', mean-

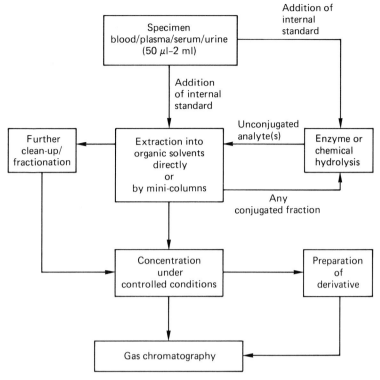

Fig. 13 Processing of biological specimens for gas chromatographic analysis.

TABLE 9

SOME DERIVATIVES USED IN GAS CHROMATOGRAPHY

Functional group	Derivative	Example
1. Hydroxyl group, e.g. alcohols, phenols, hydroxy-acids, sterols, bile acids, carbohydrates	Ester	Acetate, choloroacetate, trifluoroacetate, heptafluorobutyrate.
	Ether	Methyl, trimethylsilyl, chloromethyldimethylsilyl, t-butyldimethylsilyl
2. Carbonyl group, e.g. aldehydes, ketones, oxo-acids, steroids, carbohydrates	Hydrazone	N,N-dimethylhydrazone, 2,4-dinitrophenylhydrazone, 2,4,6-trichlorophenylhydrazone, pentafluorophenylhydrazone.
	Oxime	Oxime, methoxime, ethoxime, pentyloxime, butyloxime
3. Amino group e.g. biogenic amines, amino acids	N-Acyl	Acetyl, monochloroacetyl, trifluoroacetyl, isopropionyl, pentafluoropropionyl
	N-Silyl	Trimethylsilyl
4. Carboxyl group, e.g. fatty acids, hydroxy acids, oxo-acids, amino acids, bile acids	Ester	Methyl, ethyl, trichloroethyl, n-propyl, isopropyl, n-butyl, amyl, hexafluoroisopropyl, heptafluorobutyl, substituted benzyl, trimethylsilyl

ing analyses that describe the patterns of a group of metabolically or analytically related compounds, e.g. organic acids, drugs and metabolites, steroids, sugars and breath volatiles. Some examples of these applications of GC analysis, taken from the recent literature, are discussed in this section. They highlight several areas of clinical biochemistry where GC can be most rewarding and illustrate not just the versatility of this analytical tool but also the varying complexity of GC procedures.

Volatile Substances

Gas chromatography is a powerful technique for the analysis of volatile substances eliminated in the expired air or present in thermodynamic equilibrium with body fluid matrix under standardized experimental conditions (known as 'head space analysis'). More than 200 organic compounds have been detected in human breath and for many of these the metabolic origin or clinical significance is not known. However, the potential of breath analysis as a non-invasive diagnostic technique is evidenced by reported association of increased concentration of some constituents of breath with certain clinical states (Table 10).

Breath analysis is an attractive approach because samples are easy to collect, closely reflect arterial concentrations and do not require processing. It is essential, before diagnostic criteria can be defined for the use of breath analysis as a screening test, that

TABLE 10
ANALYSIS OF VOLATILES BY GC

Patient background	Analyte(s)
Diabetes and patients on low carbohydrate diet	Acetone
Renal diseases	Dimethylamine and trimethyl-amine
Hepatic diseases	Dimethylsulphide, mercaptans, fatty acids, methanediol, ethane-diol, ammonia
Periodontal disease	Volatile sulphur compounds, nitrogen-containing aromatic compounds
Drug therapy	Anaesthetics, e.g., halothane, CS_2 (after disulfiram)
Alcohol ingestion	Ethanol, methanol, acetaldehyde
Environmental pollution and Occupational exposure	Various solvents, e.g. benzene, acetone and toluene, and halo-genated compounds, e.g. chloro-form, dichloromethane and trichloroethylene

further work is done on the standardization of breath-ing, collection and sample enrichment techniques, and that there is greater understanding of the effects of many physiological variables such as diet, sex, exercise, body fat, endocrine status, diurnal variation and microbial interference. It has been recently reported that, with the help of a linear discriminant analysis procedure GCMS profiles of expired air can be used to distinguish between patients with lung cancer and normal subjects, even though a visual inspection of the chromatograms may not reveal any clear difference. In this study three out of the 49 breath volatiles, identified by relative retention index as acetone, methylethyl ketone and n-propane gave a classification accuracy of 93%. Breath analysis may also be suited for the investigation of genetic dis-orders such as aminoacidurias where volatile metabo-lites are formed and in measuring volatile hydrocarbons as an index of lipid peroxidation *in vivo*. Measurement of exogenous low-molecular-weight alcohols, hydrocarbons and their metabolites in exhaled air provided an effective means of moni-toring exposure to toxic chemicals (Fig. 14).

The 'head space analysis' of blood ethanol and ace-taldehyde avoids the problem of protein accumu-lation in the column and the injection of relatively large quantities of water encountered in the direct injection of diluted blood. Analytes that may be mea-sured in body fluids in the same manner include endo-genous ketone bodies and foreign chemicals of toxicological interest (Fig. 15). For the analysis of volatile compounds present in body fluids, sample enrichment by some specialist device is essential before proceeding with chromatography. Too little is known about these naturally occurring volatile products to assess, at this stage, their diagnostic sig-nificance.

Organic Acids

These include dibasic acids, ketoacids, phenolic acids, indole acids, amino acids, prostaglandins and related products. Their determination in body fluids can provide valuable support to the diagnosis of vari-

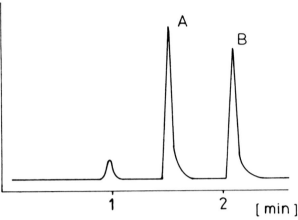

Fig. 14 Gas chromatogram obtained by head space analysis of urine from a worker exposed to trichloro-ethylene. Detector—FID. Column—packed glass, 2·5 m × 3 mm i.d., 10% carbowax 20M on chromosorb WAW 100–120 mesh. Peaks: A = chloroform, B = n-butanol (internal standard). (Reproduced with per-mission, V Senft (1985) *J. Chromatogr;* **337**: 128–30.)

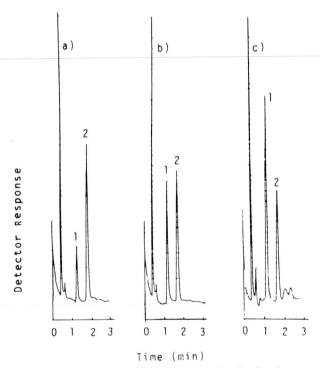

Fig. 15 Head space analysis of ketone bodies in plasma from a patient with diabetes. Plasma was (a) untreated, (b) treated with acetoacetate decarboxylase, and (c) treated with 3-hydroxybutyrate dehydrogenase and acetoacetate decarboxylase. Components: 1, acetone; 2, methylethyl ketone. (Reproduced with permission, M. Kimura *et al.* (1985) *Clin. Chem;* **31**: 596–600.)

ous organic acidaemias that are due to enzymic deficiencies in the catabolism of amino acids, lipids and carbohydrates. Other areas of interest in respect of organic acids include liver diseases (Fig. 16), rheumatoid arthritis, uraemia (Fig. 17) and congenital or acquired disorders, e.g. neural crest tumours, hyperoxaluria.

For organic acid analysis, GC is by far the most effective technique although the procedures tend to be very elaborate. The carboxyl group has to be ester-ified to an alkyl or silyl derivative. Further chemical modification depends on the nature of the other functional groups present in the acids concerned, e.g. oximation of carbonyl group, acylation, allylation or silylation of hydroxyl, sulphydryl and amino groups. A good choice of reagents is now available for preparing derivatives and it is possible to improve the specificity and sensitivity of a method by chemical manipulation such as using halogenated reagents which allows the use of ECD detector. As in most

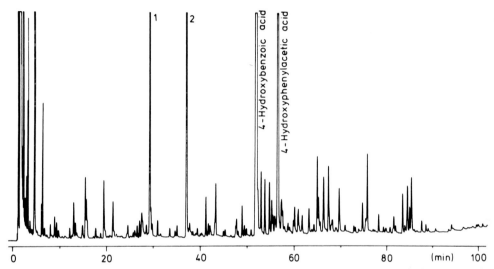

Fig. 16 Some organic acids in the urine of a patient with cirrhosis. Detector—FID. Column—glass capillary 25 m × 0·2 mm i.d. coated with OV-17. Numbered peaks: 1 = benzoic acid, 2 = phenylacetic acid. All acids were methylated at the carboxyl and, if present, at the hydroxyl groups. (Reproduced with permission, H. M. Liebich and A. J. Pickert (1985) *J. Chromatogr*; **338**: 25–82.)

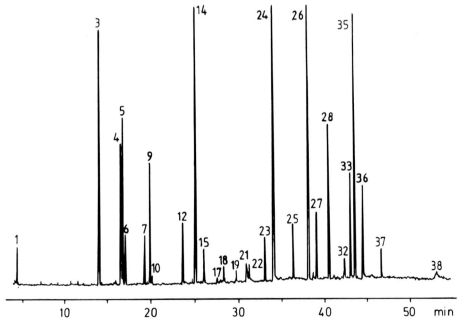

Fig. 17 Amino acid profile from haemofiltrate of a uraemic patient. Detector—FID. Column—fused silica capillary 50 m × 0·22 mm i.d. chemically bonded phase OV-1701. Amino acids were converted to heptafluorobutyric-n-butyl ester. The retention indices of the main peaks correspond to: 3, alanine, 4, valine, 5, glycine, 9, leucine, 14, unknown, 24, creatinine and phenylalanine, 27, tyrosine, 33, internal standard, 35, lysine, and 36, 1-methylhistidine. (Reproduced with permission, K. Schneider *et al.* (1985) *J. Chromatogr*; **345**: 19–31.)

instances organic acids are analysed in groups, the criteria for the choice of derivatives and reaction conditions for preparing them must apply to each analyte. Elaborate separation schemes involving organic solvent extraction, ion-exchange column, high-performance liquid chromatography and thin-layer chromatography have been implemented for isolation of organic acids from body fluid matrix and the removal of interfering substances. The problem of limited resolution of organic acids on standard packed columns has largely been surpassed by the introduction of capillary column. The FID detection profile thus obtained, for example, with urinary organic acids can be exceedingly complex, making identification and quantitation of individual peaks somewhat difficult. These are being resolved by the use of mass spectrometer in conjunction with computer processing of GC-MS data.

Steroid and Related Compounds

Although the GC procedures for serum cholesterol determination are reasonably straightforward and adequate, for routine use they still do not match the ease of colorimetric and enzymic methods. Both the native sterol and its trimethylsilyl derivative chromatograph on standard packed polysiloxane columns. But, for a more detailed analysis of cholesterol and other lipids simultaneously the use of capillary columns is more appropriate. Conjugated bile acids are first extracted by ion-exchange resin, hydrolysed and then transformed to derivatives compatible with GC analysis (Fig. 18). Generally, esterification of the carboxyl group is followed by acylation or silylation of the hydroxyl groups. Electron capture detection gives the extra sensitivity needed for serum bile acid measurement; derivatives such as *O*-trifluoroacetyl hexafluoroisopropyl ester have been used for this purpose.

All GC methods for individual steroid hormones have been replaced by variants of immunoassay procedures. However, of the two chromatographic techniques uniquely suited for 'steroid profiling', as part of the investigation of patients with congenital or acquired abnormalities of steroid biosynthesis, GC is often preferred. Some common features of the procedure are hydrolysis of conjugated steroids, isolation from the biological matrix by solvent extraction or other appropriate means and finally conversion to a chosen derivative (Fig. 19). Among the numerous steroid derivatives used, methoxime trimethylsilyl ether (MO-TMS) is probably the most popular. As with other multi-component analyses, it is essential to establish reaction conditions universal for all steroids under consideration. FID is most widely used for detection although more specific systems such as NPD and ECD are also available as options as long as the derivatives are chosen accordingly. As for other analytes, mass spectrometers are increasingly

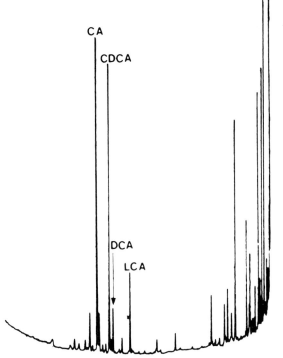

Fig. 18 Taurine-conjugated bile acids in the plasma of a patient with jaundice. Detector—FID. Column—capillary 25 m × 0.32 mm i.d. CPSil 5 (CB) with film thickness of 0·12 μm. Peak retention times of methyl-ester–dimethylethylsilyl ethers correspond to: CA = cholic acid; CDCA = chenodeoxycholic acid; DCA = deoxycholic acid; LCA = lithocholic acid. (Reproduced with permission, J. M. Street *et al.* (1985) *J. Chromatogr*; **343**: 259–70.)

becoming a part of steroid GC methodology (Figs. 20 and 21).

Amines and Metabolites

Catecholamines and metabolites are measured in various clinical conditions, e.g. in patients with hypertension, certain types of tumours and CNS disorders. Their chemical structures do not lend themselves to GC in the parent form. Various ion-exchange resins and ion-paired or other extraction techniques are applied to isolate the amines from body fluid specimens before preparing derivatives for GC. Acylation or a combination of acylation with silylation are aimed at the amino, hydroxyl and the phenolic moieties. Only the use of ECD or MS offers the sensitivity required for serum assay and for this the pentafluoropropionyl derivative is widely used (Fig. 22). GC-MS provides a reference method against which less vigorous procedures such as HPLC assays, amenable to routine use, can be evaluated. GC with FID detection, on the other hand, is adequate for monitoring the urinary metabolities of catecholamines. The NPD detector has been used for head space analysis of urinary methylamines (produced in the gut by bacterial action) and capillary

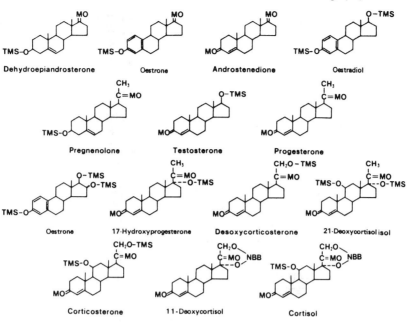

Fig. 19 Examples of some derivatives of steroids used in GC-MS analysis. NBB = B–C$_4$H$_9$; MO = CH$_3$ON; TMS = (CH$_3$)$_3$Si.

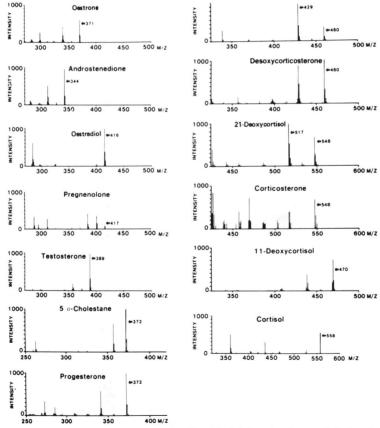

Fig. 20 Mass spectra of steroid derivatives shown in Fig. 19. Molecular ions of derivatives of the steroids are as follows: m/z 371 for oestrone, m/z 344 for androstenedione, m/z 416 for oestradiol, m/z 417 for pregnenolone, m/z 389 for testosterone, m/z 372 for 5α-cholestane, m/z 372 for progesterone, m/z 460 for 17-hydroxyprogesterone, m/z 460 for desoxycorticosterone, m/z 548 for corticosterone and 21-deoxycortisol, m/z 470 for 11-deoxycortisol, and m/z 558 for cortisol. (Reproduced with permission, K. Ichimura *et al.* (1986) *J. Chromatogr;* 374; 5–16.)

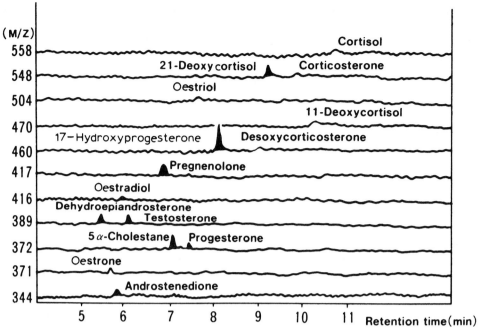

Fig. 21 Plasma steroid mass fragmentogram of a boy with 21-hydroxylase deficiency. Derivatives were as shown in Fig. 19. Column—glass capillary 25 m × 0·2 mm i.d., 0·11 μm thick film of cross-linked methylsilicone. (Reproduced with permission, K. Ichimura *et al.* (1986) *J. Chromatogr*; **374**: 5–16.)

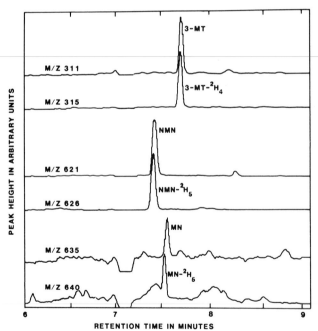

Fig. 22 Ion traces from mass spectrometric assay of human cerebrospinal fluid. Detector—MS in negative ion chemical ionization mode. Column—DB-5 fused silica capillary, 30 m × 0·26 mm i.d., film thickness 0·25 μm. Peaks: 3MT = 3-methoxytyramine, NMN = normetanephrine, MN = metanephrine and their deuterated analogues added as internal standards. (Reproduced with permission, O. Beck and K. F. Faull (1985) *Anal. Biochem*; **149**: 492–500.)

GC of polyamine metabolites in the urine from cancer patients. The latter compounds were analysed as their methyl heptafluorobutyryl derivatives.

Drugs and Allied Substances

The unique applications of GC for the analysis of exogenous volatile substances in breath and head space of body fluid samples has been mentioned earlier. Simple procedures are also available for measuring low-molecular-weight foreign compounds in body fluids and of these the determination of blood ethanol is probably the most common GC assay in routine use. In the field of drug analysis GC was once the dominant analytical technique; during the last ten years the choice has become wider—between GC, HPLC and immunoassay methods. Of course, only the chromatographic methods offer the option of concurrent monitoring of several drugs or the metabolite profile of a drug as may be desired. The drug and/or its metabolite(s) originally present in the specimen or liberated by enzyme/chemical hydrolysis is put through processing steps of varying length and complexity depending on the drug in question. The currently popular practice of using 'mini columns' ('cartridges') packed with various materials such as ion-exchange resins and various silica preparations has simplified sample preparation without compromising analyte purification and its enrichment. Preparation of derivatives more suited to GC is often a feature of procedures for drug analysis. The acidic nitrogen function of barbiturate and hydantoin structures are alkylated with trimethylammonium hydroxide or trimethylanilium hydroxide and this N-adduct can be produced 'on-column'. Amine, alcohol and other functional groups with replaceable hydrogen atoms can be acylated with reagents such as acyl halides, anhydrides and imidazoles. Reagents may be chosen to introduce one of different acyl groups such as acetyl, trifluoroacetyl, isobutyryl, pentafluoropropionyl, pentafluoropropionyl and heptafluorobutyryl. The commonest derivatives, however, would probably be those silylated on the carboxyl, alcohol, phenolic and in some cases amine groups.

Until recent years most GC analysis of drugs had used standard packed glass columns with stationary phase chosen, in the majority of cases, from the range of polysiloxanes and occasionally from polyesters and more polar materials like carbowax. From the published retention-indices data-bank for several stationary phases in packed columns, it would appear that the most reproducible values are found with methyl silicone phases. The current trend, in switching over to capillary columns is also reflected in drug analysis. The high resolution, rapid analysis and reproducible retention data achieved with capillary GC strengthened the role of gas chromatography especially in toxicology screening (Table 11). In routine analyses, detection by FID tends to be tried in the first instance before, for special reasons of specificity and sensitivity, other alternatives such as NPD and ECD are considered. The formidable combination of MS with capillary column GC has now become an integral part of any specialist centre engaged in the identification and measurement of drugs/metabolites in body fluids. The wide scope of GC in the field of drug analysis is reflected in some recently reported applications shown in Table 12 and Fig. 23.

TABLE 11

RELATIVE RETENTION TIMES AND RETENTION INDICES OF SOME DRUGS ON CAPILLARY COLUMN*

Drug	Relative retention	Retention index
Amitriptiline	0·540	2236
Atropine	0·590	2269
Caffeine	0·185	1840
Carbamazepine	0·710	2337
Clonidine	0·386	2113
Cocaine	0·536	2233
Codeine	0·900	2422
Diazepam	1·000	2461
Imipramine	0·580	2262
Lidocaine	0·225	1914
Meperidine	0·155	1775
Nitrazepam	2·050	2740
Nortriptyline	0·570	2256
Pentobarbital	0·150	1763
Phenytoin	0·730	2347
Thiopental	0·224	1912

* Cross-linked methyl silicone, siloxane deactivated fused silica capillary column, 25 m × 0·2 mm, i.d.
(Source: Lora-Tamayo C., Rams M. A., Chacon J. M. R. (1986). *J. Chromatogr*; **374**: 73–85)

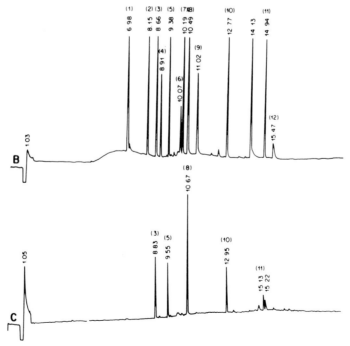

Fig. 23 Capillary gas chromatography of hypnotic-sedative drugs in serum. B = a calibration mixture of drugs; C = a serum extract from a comatose patient. Detector—NPD. Column—fused silica capillary 12 m × 0·2 mm i.d., cross-linked with 50% phenylmethyl silicone, 0·52 μm film thickness. Peak numbers: 1, methylprylon, 2, butabarbital, 3, amobarbital, 4, pentabarbital, 5, secobarbital, 6, glutethimide, 7, carisoprodol, 8, maphobarbital, 9, phenobarbital, 10, methaqualone, 11, diazepam, and 12, nordiazepam. (Reproduced with permission, V. A. Soo *et al.* (1986) *Clin. Chem.*; **32**: 325–8.)

TABLE 12
DRUG ANALYSIS BY GAS CHROMATOGRAPHY

Matrix	Drug	Internal standard	Derivative	Detector/column	Working concentration range
Plasma 1 ml	Cibenzoline	$^{15}N_2$-cibenzoline	Pentafluoro-propionyl	MS; glass, 120 cm × 2 mm i.d., 3% SP2250, 80–100 mesh Supelcort	1–50 ng/ml
Plasma/urine 5 ml	Theophylline	[^{15}N, ^{13}C]-theophylline	7-N-pentyl	MS; 12 m × 0·23 mm i.d., cross-linked dimethylsilicone silica	2–40 µg/ml
Plasma 0·5 ml	Valnoctamide	p-terbutyl-phenol	—	FID, MS; glass 180 cm × 2 mm i.d., 5% FFAP, 80–100 mesh Gaschrome Q	0·3–200 µg/ml
Plasma 1 ml	Nitrendipine	Chemical analogue	—	MS; 10 m × 0·32 mm i.d., WCOT SE 52	0·5–73 ng/ml
Plasma 20–100 µl Urine 2–5 µl	Dixopram	Diazepam	—	NPD and MS; Silica, 9 m × 0·32 mm, i.d., DB-5, film l µm	0·1–50 µg/ml
Plasma 0·5 ml	Tranylcypromine	Phenyl-propanolamine	N-pentofluoro-propionyl	MS; glass, 1·8 m × 2 mm i.d., 3% OV-1, 80–100 mesh Supelcort	35–140 ng/ml
Plasma 1 ml Urine 0·1 ml	Oxypentifylline and metabolites	Chemical analogue	O-trifluoro-acetates (for metabolites)	NPD; fused silica, 23 m × 0·31 mm i.d., cross-linked methylsilicone, film 0·17 µm	1–2500 ng/ml (plasma) 0·1–50 µg/ml (urine)
Plasma/blood 0·5 µl	Bencyclane	Meferamic acid	—	FID/NPD/MS; glass, 2 m × 2 mm i.d., 10% OV-11, 110–120 mesh Supelcort	10–100 ng/ml
Serum 1 ml	Medroxy progesterone acetate	Propionate analogue	Trifluoroacetate	MS; fused silica, 25 m × 0·32 mm i.d., CP Sil-5	10–150 ng/ml
Urine 1 ml	Buprenorphine	Etorphine	Pentofluoro-propionate	EDC; glass, 1·8 × 2 mm i.d., 3% OV-17, 80–100 mesh Gaschrom Q	10–1000 ng/ml
Plasma 1 ml	Phentermine	Amantadine hydrochloride	—	NPD; glass 2 m × 4 mm i.d., 10% Apiezon-L + 20% KOH, 80–100 mesh AW Chromosorb W	20–150 ng/ml
Plasma 0·25–1 ml	Mefloquine	Isomer	Heptafluorobutyl	ECD; glass, 1·5 m × 4 mm i.d., 3% GE-SE 30, 100–120 mesh gaschrome Q	37·5–600 ng/ml
Plasma 0·5 ml	Nitrazepam	Trifluoro-methylnitra-zepam	—	ECD; glass 1·22 × 4 mm i.d., 1% OV 17, 80–100 mesh, Chromosorb WHP	10–100 ng/ml
Urine 1 ml	Pentopril	Chemical analogue	Methyl	FID; glass, 1·83 m × 2 mm i.d., 3% OV-101, 80–100 mesh chromosorb WHP	1–100 µg/ml
Plasma 2 ml	Buspirone	5-Fluoro-buspirone	—	MS; fused silica, 8 m × 0·25 mm i.d., DB-5, film 0·25 µm	0·05–5 ng/ml
Plasma 0·5 ml	Oxcarbazepine	Carbamazepine	Trimethylsilyl	FID; fused silica 30 m × 0·31 mm i.d., cross-linked methyl silicone, 1 µm	0·1–3 ng/ml

GAS CHROMATOGRAPHY IN CLINICAL BIOCHEMISTRY SERVICE

Despite its long history, early promise and subsequent impressive technical advances, gas chromatography fell far short of becoming a key technique in hospital laboratories. This is due to two primarily management considerations: (1) for the most frequently requested tests the specrophotometric and enzymic procedures for measuring the analytes are more convenient, faster and less expensive than those based upon GC; (2) the elaborate sample processing necessary for most GC procedures does not fit easily into the large work throughput of a busy hospital biochemistry laboratory. The cost of accessory components such as automated sampling systems and peak integrators needed for batch analysis may be hard to justify except in centres with substantial daily workload of drug, steroid or some other GC determinations.

Notwithstanding the above apparent limitations, GC is looked upon as an important analytical tool in clinical biochemistry. Because of its inherent versatility and the continuous technological developments associated with this technique, GC is often the technique of first choice when it comes to developing new methods, both qualitative and quantitative, and searching for new biochemical probes which may emerge as the routine diagnostic tests of the future. GC can also provide reference methods which can be used to evaluate alternative procedures being considered for routine use. In the field of therapeutic drug monitoring and toxicological screening, a major proportion of the analyses are carried out by GC or HPLC. GC may be preferred in some cases, because of factors related to sensitivity and selectivity.

One feature of GC is its capability to cope relatively easily with multi-component analyses. In addition to studies on drug metabolism, this approach of associating a pattern of analytes rather than a single substance with metabolic defects and other clinical disorders has been fruitful in several areas such as organic acidaemias and the adrenogenital syndrome. The biochemical profiles reported in recent years particularly those from breath and head space analysis of body fluids may be signposts for future advances in clinical biochemistry. At this stage emphasis appears to have been placed on the analytical aspects, their efficiency, practical feasibility and reproducibility, and on devising effective ways of data-processing and statistical analysis. Rapid progress can be anticipated in the coming years on the standardization of analytical procedures for screening tests and the establishment of normal patterns and their variations in disease. In this most exciting phase of clinical biochemistry high-resolution capillary GC, linked to a mass spectrometer with a computerized data base, will certainly play a central role.

BIBLIOGRAPHY

For general reading
Grob R. L. (ed.) (1985). *Modern Practice of Gas Chromatography*. New York: Wiley.
Heftman E. (ed.) (1983). *Chromatography—Fundamentals and Applications of Chromatographic and Electrophoretic Methods*. Parts A & B. New York: Elsevier.
Mafadden W. (1973). *Techniques of Combined Gas Chromatography/Mass Spectrometry*. New York: Wiley-Interscience.
Perry J. A. (1981). *Introduction to Analytical Gas Chromatography*. New York: Marcel Dekker.
Walker J. Q., Jackson M. T., Maynard J. B. (1977). *Chromatographic Systems*. New York, London: Academic Press.

Special aspects of GC
Blau C., King G. (eds) (1977). *Handbook of Derivatives for Chromatography*. London: Heydon.
Gates S. C., Sweeley C. C. (1978). Quantitative metabolic profiling based on gas chromatography. *Clin. Chem*; **24**: 1663.
Gudzinowicz B., Gudzinowicz M. J. (eds) (1977–80). *Analysis of Drugs and Metabolites by Gas Chromatography—Mass Spectrometry* (in 7 parts). New York: Marcel Dekker.
Hill R. E., Whelan D. T. (1984). Mass spectrometry in clinical chemistry. *Clin. Chim. Acta*; **139**: 231.
Ioffe B. V., Vitenberg A. G. (1984). *Head-space Analysis and Related Methods in Gas Chromatography*. New York: Wiley.
Jack D. B. (1984). *Drug Analysis by Gas Chromatography*. London: Academic Press.
Jennings W. G. (ed.) (1981). *Applications of Glass Capillary Gas Chromatography*. New York: Marcel Dekker.
Lawson A. M. (ed.) (1988) *Mass Spectrometry—Application in Clinical Biochemistry*. Berlin: Walter De Gruyter. (in press).
McLafferly F. W. (1980). *Interpretation of Mass Spectra*. California: University Science Books, Mill Valley.
Tsuji K. (1978–79). *GLC and HPLC Determination of Therapeutic Agents* (in 3 parts). New York: Marcel Dekker.

23. High-performance Liquid Chromatography

R. U. Koenigsberger

INTRODUCTION

Chromatography with a liquid mobile phase is a very gentle and powerful separation technique. From its very beginning, the separation of chlorophylls by Tswett, the method has been applied with spectacular success to the separation of materials of biological origin. Simple equipment and an almost random choice of conditions can give remarkably useful results.

There appeared to be little incentive for the rigorous approach needed to improve performance. The conditions required for fast separations, columns packed with small particles and operated under pressure, were given by Martin and Synge as early as 1941[1] but relatively few advances were made in the practice of liquid chromatography. In contrast, the technical problems posed by using gas as a mobile phase forced the users to pay more attention to operating conditions and to devise sensitive, fast detectors with a linear response to sample concentration.

The advantages of gas-liquid chromatography (GLC) in terms of speed, selectivity, and automatic operation, on its own or combined with mass spectrometry and data handling systems, are so great that GLC became widely used in clinical work, even though many compounds of clinical interest are not sufficiently volatile or stable at elevated temperatures to be subjected to GLC without derivative formation.

The principles discovered in the study of GLC have now been applied to the improvement of the performance of liquid chromatography,[2] and the use of high-performance liquid chromatography (HPLC) is becoming increasingly attractive as an analytical tool in clinical chemistry. It is preferable to use this description of a group of very useful methods rather than the earlier terms 'high pressure liquid chromatography'. The best performance is achieved by making compromises between conflicting requirements for resolution, speed, sensitivity, ease of operation and cost of the equipment, and pressure is only one of many variables to be considered.

The initials HPLC are now in common use, and it is convenient to retain a name to fit them, rather than emphasize the speed or drop the words 'high performance' and thus lose the differentiation from earlier, or alternative, less-sophisticated methods.

The advances made in the speed, flexibility, and sensitivity of these methods have been brought about by the interactions between the study of fundamental principles, the demands of practitioners and advances in instrument design. The advent of microprocessors has made automation easy: clean-up and concentration steps can be integrated with the final analysis, and even the choice of the most appropriate conditions can be automated.

Identification by retention times can be made more reliable by exploiting the specific properties of detectors, post-column reactors, and by combination with mass spectrometry.

The HPLC methods developed in the 1960s were not sufficiently sensitive for clinical work, but a better understanding of all the factors affecting performance has led to the development of procedures which are proving to be very useful in this field. There has been a striking increase in the number of publications which are introduced by the claim that the new HPLC methods are faster, need less sample preparation or derivative formation and are more specific than previous ones. This aspect is often emphasized when it is important to detect and determine drugs together with their metabolites in biological fluids. In many instances metabolites, generally more polar and more difficult to extract than the original drug, had not previously been identified. Reverse-phase chromatography exploiting ion pair equilibria is the most widely used technique in this context.

Retention in reverse-phase liquid chromatography (R-PLC) is a function of the hydrophobic, electronic, and steric properties of the sample, and the study of chromatographic systems can provide useful data for the study of structure–activity relationships,[3] as well as lead to improvements of analytical methods.

INSTRUMENTATION

Safety

R-PLC needs eluents which are soluble in both aqueous and organic systems, and have low viscosites. These features are likely to be associated with toxicity.

There is increasing awareness of the hazards of prolonged exposure to organic solvent vapours, as well as of the possible fire risk. Care must be taken to site the equipment where ventilation is adequate. It should be kept in mind that most solvent vapours are heavier than air, and accordingly the exhaust intake will be more effective below the apparatus.

The high pressures do not constitute an appreciable danger when the apparatus is used correctly. Liquids are not sufficiently compressible to store and release energy under these conditions, and a small leak in the system will merely result in a trickle of liquid. A powerful jet may, however, be produced if pressure is applied to a packed column at one end while it is open at the other. This may result in the penetration of tissues by the solvent and serious toxic effects.

Apparatus

The components of an HPLC system are: a solvent delivery system; an injector; a column; and a detector (Fig. 1). In order to achieve high performance in

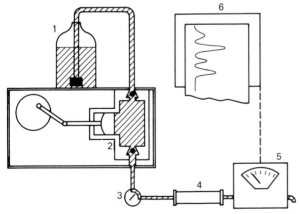

Fig. 1 Diagrammatic representation of a typical HPLC system. Key: 1. Reservoir, 2. Pump, 3. Injector, 4. Column, 5. Detector, 6. Recorder. (Reproduced with permission from Koenigsberger R. (1981). In *Therapeutic Drug Monitoring* (Richens A., Marks V., eds) p. 135. Edinburgh: Churchill Livingstone.)

liquid chromatography it is necessary to design the whole system to minimize peak broadening effects. The primary cause for the high performance of modern LC is the use of small particles. This makes it necessary to apply excess pressure to pump the eluent through the column. The sample must be introduced into the system against this pressure, columns and fittings must be designed to avoid unswept areas and the detection system must be able to 'see' the sample against a background of excess solvent and to work with very small flow-through cells.

Solvent Delivery Systems

Solvent Reservoirs. Solvents for HPLC must be kept free of dust and the feed line to the pump should be fitted with a filter. Dissolved air in the solvent can give rise to bubbles which may cause disturbances in the pump and in the detector, particularly with aqueous systems. Solvents can be degassed by applying a vacuum while stirring or immersing the container in an ultrasonic bath. Alternatively the dissolved gases may be removed by purging with helium. Some commercial systems provide solvent reservoirs with special facilities for degassing, stirring, or sparging, but an ordinary flask is usually adequate. Great care must be taken to avoid accidental changes in eluent composition, which will cause changes in retention behaviour.

Pumps. The range of pressures required for modern analytical work is between 3.5×10^6 and 3.5×10^7 Pa (500–5000 p.s.i.). In the early stages of development of HPLC it was found that simple reciprocating piston pumps gave rise to pulsating flow causing periodic noise which interfered with detection. Other solvent delivery systems such as syringe or gas displacement pumps were designed to overcome this disadvantage but the technical difficulties of operating syringe pumps, and of keeping constant flow rates with gas displacement pumps, has made them unpopular in analytical work.

The new microprocessor controlled multiple head reciprocating pumps meet the exacting requirements for HPLC. Two or three pistons operate to compensate for flow changes, and pulsing is further reduced by flow-feedback devices. Flow rates can be pre-set, and changes in pressure, indicating changes in column conditions, can be monitored.

Specially designed or adapted pumps capable of delivering very low flow rates with minimal noise are needed when working with narrow columns, *microbore* columns, with diameters of about 1 mm. Syringe pumping systems are again being developed in this context.

Provision for Gradient Elution. The continuous change of solvent composition is a powerful method of dealing with mixtures of compounds of widely different properties. Gradients may be generated at high pressures by programming the flow into a mixing chamber from two pumps working in tandem, but this is an expensive system. When pump volumes are low, as with reciprocating pumps, solvent composition gradients can be generated at atmospheric pressure. The flow of the individual components of the solvent system into a mixing chamber is controlled to form a mobile phase of appropriate composition, which is then transferred to the column by the pump. Gradient formers using microprocessors to control solvent flow to give gradients of any desired profile are commercially available.

Injection Systems

Sample volumes in HPLC range from 1 or 2 to about $100 \mu l$. Comparatively large volumes lead to increased sensitivity in trace analysis, and volumes must be kept very low with very small columns.

Claims that direct on-column syringe injection through a septum improves performance are outweighed by the difficulties of manipulation, particularly when volumes greater than $20 \mu l$ are to be injected. Six-port rotary injection valves with standard sample loops are generally used for analytical work. Septumless syringe injectors can be used if small variable injection volumes are required, but they are less precise and may contribute to band broadening. Systems combining loop injection with a by-pass are used in automated equipment.

Care must be taken that the solvent used to dissolve the sample does not have a greater eluting power than the mobile phase. It is generally preferable to dissolve the sample in the mobile phase to avoid alteration of the column conditions, and disturbance of the detector response, particularly when retention volumes are low.

Columns

The internal surface and geometry of the column are important factors in achieving high performance in liquid chromatography. Glass columns can be used up to about 4×10^6 Pa (600 p.s.i.) and occasionally at even higher pressures, but most columns are made of stainless steel, and it is important that the internal surface should be very smooth.

The dimensions of the column will affect resolution, efficiency, sensitivity, and, through their effect on speed and solvent consumption, the cost of analysis. The particle diameter of the packing must be considered in column design.[4]

The most commonly used dimensions are 4–5 mm i.d. × 100–250 mm length. Extra column length is best obtained by joining straight sections with stainless-steel capillary tubing. Long columns have been found to be less efficient than joined sections, probably because it is difficult to pack them uniformly. Lengths of narrow capillary tubing do not contribute

appreciably to band broadening but all fittings must be designed to minimize dead volumes and unswept areas.

Long columns require high inlet pressures, give rise to long analysis times and high eluent consumption, but may be necessary when the highest resolving power is required. In contrast, very short columns, about 30 mm long, packed with 3 μm diameter particles, can be used for fast analysis[5] with high sensitivity and low solvent consumption, but resolution is limited, and the requirements for low dead volumes are stringent (Fig. 2). *Microcolumns* with internal diametres of 2 mm or less have recently been developed.[6] There are three types:

1. packed *microbore* columns, i.d. 1–2 mm
2. packed capillary columns, i.d. 500 μm or less
3. open tubular capillary columns, i.d. 50 μm or less with an internal coating of a layer of liquid, a bonded organic layer, or a fine adsorbent.

(2) and (3) present considerable design problems and need very long retention times. They are still in the research stage, their main practical value is likely to be in combination with a direct inlet for mass spectrometry (see below).

Microbore columns, have a number of important advantages in terms of solvent economy and sensitivity.[7] Reduction in column diameter reduces the volume flow rate in proportion to the square of the diameter. For the same eluent velocity, the volumetric flow rate through a column of 1 mm i.d. will be about 5% of that through a conventional column (4·6 mm i.d.). It follows that consumption of eluent is drastically reduced, with corresponding reductions in cost and hazards due to toxicity and flammability.

This makes it possible to use eluents of a high degree of purity and materials which would be too expensive for use on a larger scale. Deuterated eluents exhibit specific selectivity for deuterated samples, and deuterated or halogenated eluents are potentially useful with detectors based on IR or NMR spectroscopy. The consideration of low volume–low cost applies equally to stationary phases: chiral column packings, liquid crystals, metal salts, crown ethers, cryptands, perfluorinated alkyl groups with extremely low polarity, can be used to solve problems of selectivity.

Fast separations can be obtained by increasing the operating pressure or by raising the temperature. In the case of microbore columns it is easier to control elution time by the control of temperature. Using a temperature gradient reduces analysis time and sharpens late eluting peaks, and makes it possible to carry out fast efficient separations with short microbore columns.[8]

Systems with microbore columns need pumps capable of delivering low flow rates and detectors with very low cell volumes, they are likely to be particularly useful in conjunction with electrochemical

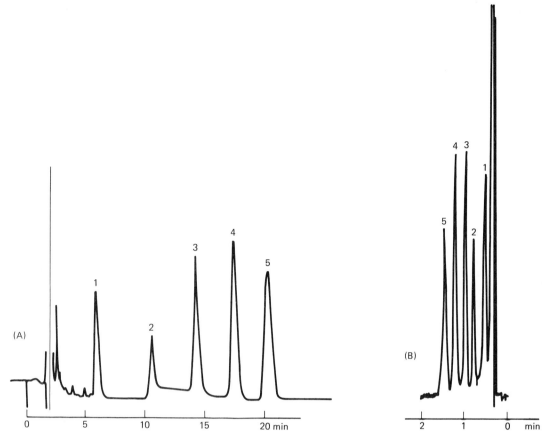

Fig. 2 HPLC profile of prostaglandins. A: on a 30 cm × 4·6 mm i.d. μBondapak column. Sample size: 800 ng of each compound, flow rate 1·5 ml/min, detector attenuation 0·2. AUFS. B: on a 3 cm × 4·6 mm i.d. Brownlee cartridge packed with 5 μm Spherisorb ODS-C$_{18}$. Sample size 1 μg of each compound, flow rate 2 ml/min, detector attenuation 0·4 AUFS. (Reproduced with permission from Freixa R., Casas J., Rosello J., Gelpi E. (1984). *J. High Res. Chromatogr. Chromatogr. Columns*; **7**: 156.)

detectors and specially designed optical detectors using laser light sources (see below).

Column Care, Precolumns and Guard Columns

The packing of efficient columns is still more an art than a science and whether in-house or bought, good columns are precious and should be treated with great care.[9] If pressure is changed rapidly, or the column is dropped or shaken, voids may be formed inside, and this will lead to a dramatic loss in efficiency or the appearance of double peaks.

Columns packed with small particles are easily clogged. To avoid this, a filter should be placed between the pump and the injector, and samples should be filtered before injection to prevent the accumulation of particles at the top of the column.

It has been found that aqueous mobile phases with ionic components dissolve the silica backbone of bonded phases even at pH values near neutrality, but reduce column life very markedly at pH above 9 or 10. The deterioration is more marked with packings with many accessible silanol groups. It can be prevented by placing a precolumn filled with silica (40–50 μm diam.) between the pump and the injector, where it will not affect the efficiency of the separation.

The 'head' of the column—the end nearest the pump—is most exposed to damage from pressure surge from the pump and deposition of sample components which may reduce the permeability and separation characteristics of the packing. This damage can be reduced by placing a guard column between the injector and the column (Fig. 3). This will be part of the analytical system and the connections must be designed to avoid excessive peak broadening. The type of packing must match the column packing in polarity, but it is possible to use pellicular packings with diameters of about 40 μm, which can be conveniently filled, emptied, and repacked by a dry tap-fill method in the laboratory. With reverse-phase systems, the packing of the guard column should be less retaining than that of the main column, and with silica the mobile phase must contain sufficient water to ensure that the guard column cannot be more active than the main column. When used with short

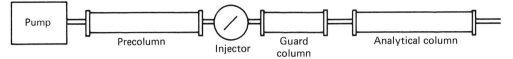

Fig. 3 Column sequence.

main columns, guard columns should have small diameters.

It is advisable to check column performance at regular intervals, using mixtures of stable standard compounds and applying the performance criteria given below.

Solutions of salts, complexing agents and acids used in reverse-phase systems will corrode stainless steel if left in contact for any length of time. At the end of analytical work, they should be removed by first pumping water through the column and following it by an inert solvent such as methanol.

Treatment with 20% nitric acid can be used to passivate stainless steel against organic acids and chlorides.

Chlorinated hydrocarbons may cause corrosion when used with other solvents. Chloroform or dichloromethane are less likely to cause trouble than carbon tetrachloride.

Temperature Control

Many HPLC separations can be carried out at room temperature.

Heats of transfer from one phase to another are smaller in liquid chromatography than in gas chromatography, and small changes in temperature do not have a great effect on peak separation. There are, however, other reasons which may make working at higher and precisely controlled temperatures necessary. Speed and efficiency increase with increasing temperature due to lower viscosity of the mobile phase and faster diffusion rates. Peak heights are increased at higher temperatures, leading to improved sensitivity and better quantitation. These factors, and the increase in solubility of samples which have poor solubility at lower temperatures are of particular importance when dealing with large molecules in exclusion chromatography. Temperature control is important in partition systems and when using refractive index detectors. Temperature is one of the variables which can be used in the optimization of resolution.

Detection Systems

Specifications. A detector can be described as a transducer which translates a concentration profile into a voltage profile. The response should be linear over a wide range of concentration. There is a need both for a general detector which will give a response for every compound present, and for specific detectors which respond selectively to certain compounds of interest. The intensity of the physical property measured, e.g. UV absorption, fluorescence, etc. will vary from one compound to another, and the sensitivity of the detector can only be stated for a given compound under given conditions. Most detectors used in liquid chromatography are concentration sensitive, and *sensitivity* is expressed as the relation between *the instrument output in mV* and the *change in sample concentration (wt/vol) in the detector*. The lower limit of detection will depend on the signal to noise ratio. Acceptable values are 2 : 1 for qualitative analysis and 5 : 1 for quantitative work.

The detection limit of the method will be affected by the conditions of analysis as well as by the sensitivity of the detector. Retention time and efficiency will affect peak shape and therefore the peak height, and thus determine the smallest amount that can be 'seen' by the detector. If a comparatively large volume of sample can be injected, very dilute samples will give a measurable response.

The importance of low extra-column dead volumes has been stressed. If the sample leaving the columns is diluted in the detector, the resultant peaks will be made wider and lower, and both resolution and the sensitivity will be reduced. Under favourable conditions, peak volumes may be as low as 0·05 ml (i.e. a peak is eluted in 3 s at a flow rate of 1 ml/min) and, ideally, the detector volume should be less than one tenth of this, i.e. less than 5 µl. The response time of the detector must be short enough for the speed of analysis to avoid distortion of the signal.

Ultraviolet Photometers and Spectrophotometers (*see* also Chapter 9). By far the most commonly used detectors measure absorption in the UV, either at fixed or variable wavelength. The latter have the advantage that, by choosing the appropriate wavelength, it may be possible to increase sensitivity for a specific compound, and reduce interference from others. Identification can be assisted by measuring absorbance at more than one wavelength and calculating absorbance ratios on either side of the peak maximum. Variation in these ratios will indicate the presence of impurities. Detectors which allow the user to programme automatic wavelength changes to maximize sensitivity, and to plot absorbance ratios at selected wavelengths to detect components which may be hidden by unresolved peaks are now available. Variable wavelength spectrophotometers can thus be used both as a fairly general and as specific detectors.

Peak identification obtained in this way is particularly useful in conjunction with procedures for optimizing mobile phase composition for the separation of complex mixtures, but it should be kept in mind that changes in eluent composition, baseline drift, and unresolved peaks will affect the result. Very specific information can be obtained by using multichannel detectors with an array of photosensing elements. Use of a computer-controlled photodiode array spectrophotometer as an HPLC detector can show the UV spectrum of each peak as it elutes, and makes it possible to produce a three-dimensional representation of the chromatogram relating retention time, wavelength, and absorbance (Fig. 4).

With a spectrophotometer capable of operating at low wavelengths, down to 200 nm, it may be possible to detect compounds not normally considered 'UV absorbers', e.g. sterols. Detection in the low UV range fits in well with the 'UV-transparent' methanol, acetonitrile, and water systems used with reverse-phase packings, but requires solvents of very high purity, and sensitivity at low wavelengths tends to be low.

The obvious limitations of all UV detectors are that they can deal only with compounds which have sufficiently strong absorption bands at a suitable wavelength, and with solvents which do not absorb in this region. The advantages are sensitivity, a wide linear range, and baseline stability in the face of changes in temperature and flow rate. With non-absorbing solvents, they can be used for gradient elution. These advantages often make it worthwhile to make derivatives with appropriate chromophores (*see* below).

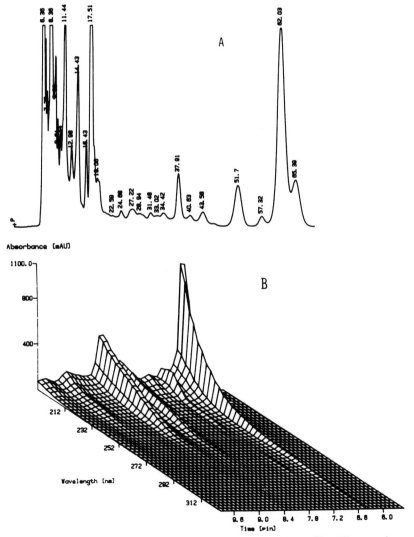

Fig. 4 (A) The 190 nm urinary carboxylic acid profile. The peak at 17·51 min is uric acid while the peak at 62·03 min is hippuric acid and 4-hydroxyphenylacetic acid; (B) three-dimensional profile of the 5·5–10 min interval of the chromatogram. The peak at 8·36 min is 2-oxoglutaric acid. (Reproduced with permission from Buchanan D. N., Thoene J. G. (1985). *J. Chromatogr*; **344**: 23.)

Fluorescence Detectors (*See* Chapter 11). The high high level of sensitivity, about 100 times greater than in UV absorption, makes fluorimetry a very popular technique in biochemical analysis, in spite of problems arising from quenching effects and background fluorescence. The use of two wavelengths, for excitation and emission, makes the analysis more specific, and aids identification. Under favourable conditions detection limits in the femtogram region may be achieved.

The detection limit for a particular compound will depend on the chemical environment of the compound (type of solvent, pH) and on the instrument configuration: design of the flow cell, choice of the excitation source, and the method of wavelength selection for both excitation and emission. Xenon and deuterium are the most commonly used light sources, and wavelength selection by filters is simpler and cheaper than by monochromators, but less selective.

As with UV absorption, monitoring at multiple wavelengths greatly improves both the qualitative and quantitative information obtainable. This can be done by a stop-flow method or by video fluorimetric monitoring of effluents. This procedure allows detailed fluorescence fingerprints of materials 'on-the-fly' in a system that uses three dimensions: retention time, excitation wavelength, and emission wavelength.[10]

The use of laser excitation in fluorimetry increases sensitivity and selectivity. It also makes it possible to design flowcells of submicrolitre dimensions for use with microcolumns. The very low detection limits which can be reached by fluorimetry, make it particularly attractive to form derivatives of compounds without native fluorescence.

Refractive Index Monitors. Differential refractometers are almost universal in their field of application, but their sensitivity is limited by the fact that, like the katharometer in gas chromatography, they are 'bulk property' detectors: they measure the change in refractive index when a small amount of sample appears in what is always a large excess of solvent. The refractive index changes with temperature, and for maximum sensitivity the temperature of the detector should be rigidly controlled. Changes in solvent composition will affect the refractive index, causing baseline drift. The refractive index detector is, therefore, not suitable for gradient elution work.

Electrochemical Detectors. The biological activity of many compounds is due to their ability to take part in electron transfer reactions. It is, therefore, not surprising that electrochemical detectors are particularly useful in biochemical analysis. Detectors based on *controlled potential amperometry* are being used increasingly in the analysis of catecholamines, analgesics, antibiotics, anti-cancer drugs, β-blockers, phenothiazines, etc. They work by measuring the current resulting from the oxidation or reduction of a fraction of the sample when the appropriate potential is applied in a flow-through cell (Fig. 5). The active volume of these cells can be made very low, between 1 and 0.1 μl. This is a great advantage in systems with very small dead volumes, e.g. microbore columns.

A simplified circuit diagram is shown in Fig. 6. The preferred material for the working electrode is glassy carbon, made by heating a resin to 1200°C in an inert atmosphere. It is a hard substance similar to graphite, but has some crosslinked bonding similar to diamond. It can be used over a wide potential range and is resistant to most solvents. The working electrode is usually Ag/AgCl. The potentials at which the eluent is oxidized or reduced limit the operating range of the detector, and at potentials more negative than about 0.2 V versus Ag/AgCl, the reduction of molecular oxygen dissolved in the eluent gives rise to a high background current. The complete removal of oxygen from the system is not easy, and the detector is generally used in the oxidative mode.

The potential suitable for the oxidation of the sample can be found by plotting a graph of the current produced in an electrochemical cell containing the

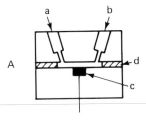

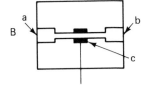

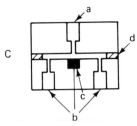

Fig. 5 Flow-through cells for amperometric detectors: A, channel, B, tubular, C, 'wall-jet'; a, entrance; b, exit, c, working electrode; d, spacer. (Reproduced with permission from Weber S. G., Purdy W. C. (1981). *Ind. Eng. Chem. Prod. Res. Dev*; **20**: 593).

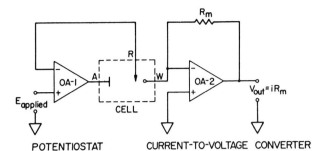

POTENTIOSTAT **CURRENT-TO-VOLTAGE CONVERTER**

Fig. 6 Fundamental operational amplifier circuit for controlled-potential electrochemistry. OA-1: first amplifier, OA-2: current-to-voltage converter, A: auxiliary electrode, R: reference electrode, W: working electrode. (Reproduced with permission from Kissinger P. T. (1983). Electrochemical detectors. In *Liquid Chromatography Detectors, Chromatographic Science Series* (Vickery T. M., ed.) **23**: 137. New York: Marcel Dekker.)

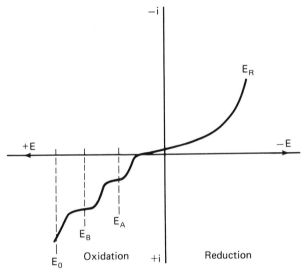

Fig. 7 Current-voltage curve for a mixture of compounds A and B: when the potential is set at E_A, a current due to the oxidation of A will flow, and compound B will not be detected. At potential E_B, both A and B will be detected. E_0 and E_R indicate the potential range of the solvent.

sample when the potential is gradually increased. For detection of an oxidizable compound, the working electrode is maintained at a selected potential in the limiting current plateau for the oxidation of the sample. The detector can be used selectively for compounds with different oxidation potentials (Fig. 7). The current resulting from the reaction will be proportional to the concentration of the sample in the detector. It will also be affected by the cell design, the flow rate of the mobile phase, and the temperature.

A dual or multiple electrode system can be used to improve selectivity, detection limits, and peak identification, and to extend the accessible potential range.

Detection of Radioactive Compounds. Sensitivity of radioactive monitoring is improved by having a large volume of sample and counting over a long period of time. This conflicts with the requirements for an HPLC detector, where volumes should be small and flow is fast. Studies of cell design, counting methods and the relation between chromatographic parameters and sensitivity, aimed at finding the best compromise between the conflicting requirements, have led to the design of on-line continuous monitoring systems and the application of such systems in pharmacokinetic and metabolism studies. These consist of either post-column reactors (*see* below), where a miscible scintillation solution is added to the column effluent, or a solid scintillator packed into the detector cell. The sensitivity of on-line systems must ultimately be limited, and a high-sensitivity radioassay of off-line measurement by automated fraction collection on filter paper impregnated with scintillator and subsequent autoradiography has recently been described.[11]

Formation of Derivatives. One of the main attractions of HPLC is the claim that it can deal with samples without derivatization. With the increasing application of reverse-phase ion-pair systems there is rarely any need to form derivatives in order to improve chromatographic performance.

Nevertheless, the formation of fluorescent or UV-absorbing derivatives is often worthwhile in order to exploit the sensitivity of the available detectors to the full. Enrichment and specificity may be added advantages. Comparison of retention data before and after derivatization and comparison with standards can be used to confirm identity. The choice of useful reactions is obviously very wide. It should be possible to make a derivative of almost any hydroxyl or amino group with an appropriate aroyl chloride to confer an adequate extinction value of suitable wavelength on the parent compound. This will make it possible to devise routine procedures using a low-cost fixed wavelength UV detector. Reactions with reagents to confer fluorescence on the compound of interest, e.g. reactions with dansyl chloride or o-phthalaldehyde, are well established in biochemical analysis, and a wide range of derivatives is used in therapeutic drug analysis.

The preparation of derivatives can be seen to have many advantages. It is, however, time-consuming; not readily automated, and, with multi-functional compounds, may give rise to multiple products or artifacts.

Post Column Reactors. The disadvantages of pre-column derivatization listed above can be overcome by adding the reagent between the column and the detector.[12] Such a system can be automated, and multiple reaction products or incomplete reactions are acceptable as long as they are reproducible, but the choice of eluents and reagents is restricted. The reagent and the eluent must not interfere with detection, the reaction must be fast, and give a high yield of stable products. (A familiar form of this method of detection is the amino acid analyser, which uses the colour reaction with ninhydrin.) The reactor and its connections with the rest of the apparatus must be designed to give the best possible compromise between the conflicting requirements for good mixing and fast analysis. Fast reactions (less than 30 s) are best carried out in a capillary coil, packed bed reaction chambers can be used for reactions taking up to 5 min, and reactions needing about 8 min can be used with gas-segmentation of the effluent. Recent developments include the use of enzymatic and photochemical reactions.

Liquid Chromatography—Mass Spectrometry. Mass spectrometry is the most conclusive method for peak identification. Collecting fractions for subsequent analysis is easier in LC than in GC, and construction of a direct interface more difficult because the excess of mobile phase over sample is greater. Most mass spectrometric analysis of LC fractions is carried out off-line. The obvious advantages of on-line operation in speed, devolution of unresolved peaks, and the examination of complex mixtures have stimulated research in the design of suitable interfaces.[13] Moving belt interfaces, where excess eluent is removed before entering the mass spectrometer inlet, are compatible with conventional column diameters and a wide range of eluents. Direct liquid introduction has been used in conjunction with microbore and microcolumns, but the most promising method appears to be the thermospray interface, where the LC effluents are sprayed directly into the ion source. It is particularly useful for non-volatile, thermally labile molecules in systems with aqueous eluents containing electrolytes, which makes it applicable to the usual reverse-phase systems.

STATIONARY PHASES

The Evolution of Modern Packings

In gas chromatography, the mobile phase does not play an important part in the separation, and interest centres on finding the appropriate stationary phase.

Liquid chromatography has greater flexibility, because both phases contribute to separation. Until recently, the choice of stationary phase was dictated by the nature of the sample: large molecules could only be separated by size-exclusion chromatography, ion exchangers were used for the separation of bases, nucleic acids and amino acids. Chromatography with a polar stationary phase, using cellulose (paper), silica gel, etc., was very successful in the separation of compounds of biochemical interest like sugars and amino acids, which had previously been very difficult to isolate. With the advent of TLC, systems based on polar adsorbents, particularly silica, were found to have a wide range of application, and HPLC was first developed on this basis. This led to the view that a situation where the stationary phase is more polar than the mobile phase is 'normal'.

Such 'normal' systems were, however, not suitable for the separation of less polar compounds, such as lipids. When it was found that solids coated with non-polar liquids like undecane or silicone oil, similar to gas chromatography column packings, could be used as stationary phases, together with more polar mobile phases, for the separation of non-polar compounds, such systems were called 'reverse phase'. The term has been retained, even though non-polar stationary phases are now used much more frequently than polar adsorbents.

A number of problems are associated with using 'mechanically' coated stationary phases in liquid chromatography: it is often difficult to maintain a constant proportion of stationary phase, even when using precolumns, changes in temperature will affect the equilibrium between stationary and mobile phase, the presence of stationary phase in the eluent may interfere with the detector, the thickness of liquid film may give poor values for the efficiency of the columns, the choice of phases is limited by the requirement that the components must be immiscible, and gradient elution is not practicable with liquid stationary phases. Chemically bonded phases are therefore preferred.

Reverse-phase packings with alkyl groups chemically bonded to silica were first developed to deal with non-polar compounds, but the use of selective secondary equilibria, such as ionization, ion-pair formation and ligand exchange makes it possible to deal with a wide variety of compounds, even proteins of mol. wt. up to 25 000, by using the same column with different mobile phases. In certain contexts the same column can even be used to concentrate the sample and then to separate the components by the appropriate choice of eluents.

The situation is now the opposite to gas chromatography: one type of stationary phase (hydrocarbon bonded to silica) is the equivalent of the inert gas mobile phase in gas chromatography, and interest centres on finding the appropriate mobile phase for the problems in hand. Mobile phases can be changed—and mixed—more readily than column packings, and there has thus been no loss in flexibility.

Bonded phases have further advantages over unmodified silica: equilibration is rapid and easily controlled: only 5–10 column volumes are required after a change in mobile phase, compared with over 100 in the case of silica. This makes them suitable for use in gradient elution and column switching systems.

Polar bonded phases, containing phenyl or nitrile functional groups, have been developed to exploit these advantages, and packings containing chiral groups can be used for direct enantiomeric separation.

Particle Size and Shape

Much of the pioneering work in HPLC was carried out using porous particles of about 40 μm diameter. These are the smallest particles which can be packed dry by a 'tap, rotate and fill' method.

The structure of the packing contributes to band broadening by providing pathways of differing resistance to the flow of molecules in the mobile phase. A complex flow pattern is produced by the differences in mobility in different regions of the packing, particularly within the pores of the particles.

Before the problems of packing very small particles were overcome, porous layer beads or pellicular supports, consisting of solid cores surrounded by a thin porous layer, were developed. They had diameters large enough to allow dry tap-fill packing, and showed increased efficiency compared with porous particles of the same size due to the reduction in path lengths for the solutes. Because of their small surface area they have the disadvantages of low sample capacity (less than 1 mg per gram of packing). Since methods for packing small particles have been developed porous layer beads are now used only for some special purposes, e.g. as guard columns or in column switching procedures.

Theoretical considerations and practical experience have shown that the fastest, most efficient separations can be obtained by using rigid, small, porous particles of uniform particle size and large surface area, typically with diameters of 5 or 10 μm and surface areas of the order of 400 m²/g.

The shape of the particles depends on their method of manufacture. Spherical particles can be packed more easily than irregular ones to give columns requiring low operating pressures and having greater physical stability, but very good results have been obtained with irregular particles. A column packed with very small particles requires a higher pressure than one of the same length packed with larger particles, but the gain in efficiency per unit column length is so great that short columns (about 30 mm) may produce very efficient separations using pressures of about $1\cdot4 \times 10^7$ Pa (2000 p.s.i.). The smaller the particle size, the greater is the need for very careful design to avoid dead volumes in the rest of the system.

Because of their large surface area, porous microparticulate packings have a high sample capacity, and can be used with a wide range of sample sizes. This makes them useful for trace analysis: relatively large volumes of dilute solutions can be applied without reducing separation efficiency. Alternatively, these columns can be used in semipreparative work to separate milligram amounts of materials from impurities.

A large number of microparticulate packings are now available. They vary in pore size and surface area, factors which will affect efficiency, resolution and sample capacity. Columns packed with particles of 3 μm diameter are now commercially available. They are capable of giving very fast, efficient separations, and are proving very useful in the analysis of biological samples.

Porous Solids

The oldest chromatographic technique is percolation through porous solids. Separation is based on adsorption of solutes by their interactions with a solid surface.

Liquid–solid chromatography is particularly useful in the separation of compounds of different chemical types and of isomers. This can be understood if the adsorption process is seen as the result of competition between the sample and the solvent for a place on a rigid adsorbent surface which contains fixed active sites.

A great deal of information about chromatographic systems with silica as the stationary phase is available in the literature of column and thin layer chromatography.

The adsorbents most commonly used in modern liquid chromatography are silica and alumina. They are available as particles of varying size, pore size, surface area and shape. The particles may be irregular or spherical or they may have a solid core surrounded by a porous layer. The relative merits of these variations have been discussed above. Silica and alumina are polar adsorbents, and compounds are eluted in order of their polarities: (fastest) alkanes > alkenes > arenes > ethers > carbonyls > alcohols and amines (most strongly retained).

Surface silanols on silica are acidic and will therefore retain basic compounds very strongly. Amines may be irreversibly adsorbed or give rise to tailing peaks. Similarly, acid samples, e.g. phenols and carboxylic acids, will be very strongly retained by (basic) alumina.

These properties can be exploited by using aqueous eluents, and adjusting separation of silica by using amines as modifiers[14] and by using alumina as an amphoteric ion exchanger.[15]

Adsorbents may act as catalysts and cause changes in the solvent or the sample. Their water content is a critical factor when using non-polar eluents, and can have spectacular effects on separation. Results will not be reproducible unless care is taken to control it. The slow rate of equilibration of adsorbents with eluent mixtures of different polarities is a serious disadvantage.

Chemically Bonded Stationary Phases

Modification of the silica by reaction with the surface hydroxyl groups (silanol, Si-OH) makes it possible to overcome the difficulties described above. Stationary phases with surfaces of any desired polarity can be made by treating silica particles with organochlorosilane or similar reagents:

$$-\underset{|}{\overset{|}{Si}}-OH + Cl-\underset{\underset{R_3}{|}}{\overset{\overset{R_1}{|}}{Si}}-R_2 \rightarrow \underset{\underset{R_3}{|}}{\overset{\overset{R_1}{|}}{Si}}-O-\underset{\underset{R_3}{|}}{\overset{\overset{R_1}{|}}{Si}}-R_2$$

By using appropriate substituents for R_1, R_2 and R_3, packings with different functionalities and physical properties can be produced. The most widely used stationary phases in analytical liquid chromatography are those substituted with alkyl groups, which can be considered as effectively non-polar. Such materials, marketed under the description 'reverse phase' packings have been found to differ considerably in retention and selectivity. These differences can be correlated with the methods and materials used in their preparation. They are due to residual silanol groups, to differences in the chain length of the bonded alkyl groups, and in the thickness and the structure of the bonded layer. Not all silanols will react with the organic modifier for steric reasons, and the pore structure of the silica will affect the extent of surface coverage because very small pores will not be accessible to the reagent. The most hydrophobic packings are produced by reaction with a dimethylarylchlorosilane

$$\underset{\underset{\underset{\underset{=Si-OH}{|}}{O}}{\overset{\overset{\overset{=Si-OH}{|}}{O}}{|}}}{-Si}-OH + Cl-\underset{\overset{|}{CH_3}}{\overset{CH_3}{\underset{|}{Si}}}-C_nH_{2n+1} \rightarrow \underset{\underset{\underset{\underset{=Si-OH}{|}}{O}}{\overset{\overset{\overset{=Si-OH}{|}}{O}}{|}}}{-Si}-O-\underset{\overset{|}{CH_3}}{\overset{CH_3}{\underset{|}{Si}}}-C_nH_{2n+1}$$

followed by a small silanizing reagent used to 'endcap' some of the remaining silanols;

$$\equiv SiOH + ClSi(CH_3)_3 \rightarrow \equiv SiOSi(CH_3)_3$$

Alternative methods employ trichloro- or alkoxysilanes, which may produce additional silanol groups and give packings with different physical properties due to polymerization of the side chains.

Residual silanol groups will increase the retention of polar compounds relative to non-polar ones. Such differences in selectivity may be exploited but they are outweighed by the disadvantages: peak tailing, particularly with basic substances, and reduction of the chemical stability of the column.

The presence of residual silanol groups in a reverse-phase column can be detected by using it as an adsorbent for small polar molecules with dry heptane as the mobile phase. Capacity factors for compounds like methanol, benzyl alcohol, or acetone should be less than 0·5, and the relative retention of nitrobenzene to benzene should be less than 2.

The most commonly used packings have alkyl chains with 18 or 8 carbons. The relationship between carbon content, chain length, and solute retention properties is complex. With a given mobile phase,

a phase with a high carbon content, e.g. C_{18}, will give greater retention and better selectivity for compounds that differ in size and structure of alkyl groups. It is more suitable than C_8 for ion pair work, because the silica matrix is better protected against attack by components of the mobile phase.

Separations on C_8 phases are fast and are therefore useful for method development. Packings with very short alkyl chains, C_4 or C_3, are particularly useful in protein separations, because they allow fast elution with a low proportion of organic solvent in the mobile phase, and are therefore less likely to cause structural changes or denaturation.

More than one type of interaction is involved in retention by these stationary phases; the primary one being hydrophobicity. In a polar eluent with a hydrogen bonding network, the non-polar areas of the solute are forced into the hydrocarbon stationary phase. The strength of this force will depend on the surface tension of the eluent and the surface area of the solute. It will be opposed by interaction of a polar functional group of the solute with the polar eluent. Solutes with polar functional groups will therefore elute faster than less polar compounds. In contrast, compounds with bulky non-polar substituents will be retained more strongly than the parent compound. It is this mechanism which relates chromatographic retention to the study of biological activities.[13] The unreacted silanol groups in the stationary phase will give rise to 'silanophilic' interactions, causing irregular retention behaviour of compounds like crown ethers and aminopeptides.[16,17] Regular retention behaviour is obtained by blocking the silanol groups with suitable amino compounds in the eluent.

Bonded phases containing aminopropyl, cyanoalkyl and phenyl, show retention behaviour similar to polar adsorbents when used with elements of low polarity, and behave like reverse phases with water–methanol systems. Bonded phases with $-NH_2$ substituents have been found particularly useful for carbohydrate separations.

Phenylsilane columns exhibit special selectivities due to the possibility of π–π interactions.

Column packings with chiral molecules bound to the solid phase, e.g. polystyrene, polyacrylamide, covalently bound chiral ligands which can complex with Cu^{2+} ions, crown ethers, or cyclodextrins can be used to carry out direct enantiomeric separations.[18] This procedure is faster than traditional methods, needs less sample, and avoids errors due to enantiomeric contamination of derivatizing agents.

Ion-exchange Packings for HPLC

The topic of ion-exchange chromatography is dealt with in Chapter 24, but it is appropriate to include here a description of packings specially developed for high performance work.

Considerations of efficiency of ion-exchange separations and their automation, e.g. the amino acid analysis by Moore and Stein, preceded and probably inspired the interest in improvements in adsorption and partition chromatography. Separations using porous resin particles are slow, and the application of pressure to compressible materials causes difficulties. The idea of speeding separations by using a particle consisting of a solid core surrounded by a thin skin or pellicle of active material originated in the ion-exchange field. Such pellicular and superficially porous ion exchangers can give fast, efficient separations but their ion-exchange capacity is generally low, between 0·01 and 0·1 milliequivalents per gram, which makes them unsuitable for the direct analysis of complex biological fluids, such as urine. Special pellicular ion-exchange packings have been developed for use in *ion-chromatography* which can be used for organic compounds, e.g. amines, amino acids, carbohydrates, as well as inorganic ions.

Packings have now been produced by bonding ion exchangers to the surface of porous microparticles. These have exchange capacities of the order of 1 milliequivalent per gram, and can give fast, efficient separations at ordinary temperatures.

Materials for Size Exclusion (*see* Chapter 25)

Packings for HPLC must be sufficiently rigid to withstand the pressures required. Particles of cross-linked styrene–divinylbenzene copolymers for use with non-aqueous solvents (gel permeation) are available in pore sizes that will fractionate a molecular weight range of about 50×10^7. The materials commonly used for size exclusion of water-soluble compounds (gel filtration), porous gels like dextrans or polyacrylamides, are not suitable for operation under appreciable pressures, but columns packed with particles of a rigid, hydrophilic, spherical, and porous gel, spherogel-TSK SW(Varian, Toyo Soda), are now available for the separation of proteins, enzymes, saccharides, etc.

Problems of adsorption with glass or silica-based packings for size exclusion have been largely overcome by surface modification with glyceryl groups (Glycophase-G/GPC, Pierce), carbohydrate (Synchropak, Syn-Chrom), diol (Lichrosorb Diol, Merck) or aliphatic ether groups (μ Bondagel, Waters Assoc.). The latter can be used with aqueous and non-aqueous solvents.

Glyceryl propyl silica and controlled pore glass with large pore sizes can be activated and coupled to functional amino groups with the formation of affinity chromatography supports.

The separation of low-molecular-weight compounds on size-exclusion packing usually involves mechanisms other than simple exclusion, but as they present a larger retention surface for smaller than for larger molecules, they can be used as pre-columns in complex separations to replace back-flushing or pre-injection clean up.

MOBILE PHASES

Possibilities and Constraints

In HPLC the mobile phase is the part of the chromatographic system which can be most easily changed or modified, and which has the greatest potential for controlling separation.

At first sight the possibilities for choosing mobile phases appear unlimited and the prospect is both promising and confusing, but the choice is limited by the constraints dictated by the nature of the process and the equipment, and helped by guidelines resulting from the studies of solute–solvent interaction. Eluents are chosen to effect separation on the basis of solubility or hydrophobicity, polarity, donor and acceptor properties, pH, and ionic strength.

The detection system imposes certain constraints on their selection: solvents which absorb in the wavelength region of interest cannot be used with UV detectors; buffers containing inorganic salts will cause interference with transport detectors, the refractive index of the mobile phase must differ significantly from that of the sample to give adequate sensitivity in RI detectors, changes in mobile phase composition will cause base line drift with RI detectors, and the mobile phase must have high electrical conductivity for use with electrochemical detectors. Post-column reactors will also influence the choice of eluents.

Strong acids and halides, and mixtures of carbon tetrachloride with solvents will corrode stainless steel, and solutions with pH above 8 and below 3 will attack bonded column packings.

Considerations of efficiency indicate that the viscosity should be as low as possible, but low viscosity is associated with low boiling points, and very volatile solvents may cause trouble due to the formation of bubbles in the system, and change in composition due to evaporation.

Water and solvents used in mobile phases must be free from impurities or additives, such as antioxidants in ethers. HPLC-grade solvents are commercially available, and mixtures should be made up fresh before use to avoid the formation of reaction products. It is obvious that hazards, e.g. reactivity, toxicity, and flammability must be kept in mind. Last and not least, the solvent must be able to dissolve the sample.

Solvent Strength

A strong solvent gives overall fast elution, and a selective one gives good separation, within a convenient analysis time. Different theoretical models are used in the discussion of strength and selectivity with polar adsorbents like silica or alumina and non-polar bonded stationary phases, but considerations of eluent strength are broadly applicable to both modes of chromatography.

In the context of chromatography, the term 'polarity' is used somewhat loosely to describe the strengths of the interactions between all the components of the system. It refers to the resultant of all the molecular forces called into play: not only dipole–dipole and induced dipole interactions, but also dispersion, hydrogen bonding and charge transfer. Snyder[19] has proposed a parameter, P', for the estimation of 'polarity' or chromatographic strength based on experimental solubility data.

With a polar stationary phase, solvent strength, the ability to move compounds along the column, will increase with polarity in the order: hydrocarbons < chlorinated hydrocarbons < ethers < nitriles < alcohols < water. The strength of the mobile phase can be varied by mixing solvents of different polarities. With adsorbents like unmodified silica, the addition of a very small amount of a strong solvent to a weak one will cause a marked increase in solvent strength. This can be understood if the adsorption process is seen as the result of competition between the sample and the solvent for active sites on the rigid adsorbent surface. The marked effect of traces of water on separation is a case in point. This model also explains the fact that adsorption systems are useful in isomer separations.

The order of eluent strength is reversed when using a hydrocarbon-bonded non-polar stationary phase: water is a weaker eluent than methanol, and hydrocarbons are so strong that they will strip any retained material from the column.

The surfaces of bonded phases are more homogeneous than those of untreated silica or alumina, and the eluent strength of mixtures varies linearly with composition.

Exploitation of Secondary Equilibria

The separation of ionizable compounds on ion exchangers is slow, peak tailing causes poor separation in adsorption systems, and they are eluted too quickly in ordinary reverse-phase systems. The control of retention through control of pH of the mobile phase and addition of ion pair reagents has extended the scope of the application of reverse-phase packings from non-polar to a wide range of ionizable compounds. Enantiomers may be separated with mobile phases containing chiral additives.

Control of Retention through pH. The distribution of weak acids or bases between a polar mobile phase and a non-polar stationary phase, and therefore retention and selectivity can be controlled by adjusting the pH of the mobile phase through the addition of suitable buffers, *ion suppression*: in the case of a weak acid, an increase in pH above its pK, will reduce retention, and for a weak base retention will increase with increasing pH, the retention of neutral compounds will not be greatly affected. The method is not suitable for strong acids or bases, because the corresponding pH values are beyond the tolerance

of the bonded phase packings, but recently resin-based packings, stable at pH 1 to 13, have been developed for use with basic compounds at pH 11, using triethylamine.

Ion Pair Chromatography. This technique, particularly in the reverse-phase mode, has many advantages pertinent to drug monitoring: it can deal with ionizable compounds, including strong acids and bases, in crude aqueous solutions, solvent strength and selectivity are easily and predictably varied by changes in counter ion structure and concentration, and pH, neutral and charged solutes can be analysed in the same chromatogram, and a single column can be used for this and ordinary reverse-phase operation.

The principles of ion pair extraction were first applied to modern liquid chromatography by Schill and his co-workers,[20] who pointed out that the distribution of a comparatively large ion containing a non-polar group between two phases can be altered by the addition of a counter ion of opposite charge also containing a large, non-polar group. The two ions will form a hydrophobic association species, an ion pair, which will tend to be forced into the non-polar stationary phase by the aqueous mobile phase, thus increasing retention. A cation (A^+) is retained by a non-polar stationary phase as an ion pair (A^+B^-) formed with a counterion (B^-).

$$A^+ + B^- \rightleftharpoons (AB)$$
$$\text{aqueous} \qquad \text{organic}$$

The distribution of the cation A^+ (as ion or part of the ion pair) between two phases, which controls its retention, will be a function of the equilibrium constant of this reaction, the extraction constant

$$E_{AB} = \frac{[AB]}{[A^+][B^-]}$$

E_{AB} will vary with the structure of the counter ion, B^-, the pH and ionic strength of the mobile phase and the proportion and kind of organic modifier in it. The equilibrium, and therefore E_{AB}, will also be affected by changes in temperature.

A more sophisticated model involving the formation of a dynamic ion-exchange medium in the hydrophobic stationary phase has been shown to account for a number of phenomena observed in the process, but the simple concept of the formation of an ion pair and its partitioning between the phases is helpful in choosing appropriate conditions for analysis. Commonly used counter ions for the separation of acidic compounds are quaternary amines which differ in the size of their substituents (tetramethyl or tetrabutyl ammonium ions), and alkyl sulphates or sulphonates for the separation of bases. As a general rule, retention of ionizable compounds will be increased by increasing the size and (up to a limit) the concentration of the appropriate counter ion. For most compounds it will be increased by decreasing the proportion of organic modifier in the mobile phase, decreasing the temperature and by using a stationary phase with a higher degree of coverage. The effect of pH will depend on the nature of the solute. An increase in pH will increase the retention of anions and decrease that of cations, and different compounds will be affected differently. It can be seen that an understanding of this technique makes it possible to devise separation methods for a wide variety of compounds.

Ion pair chromatography can also be carried out using unmodified (polar) porous silica packings, which makes it possible to use UV-absorbing or fluorescing counter ions for detection of non-absorbing sample compounds, but reverse-phase systems are usually preferred because of their other advantages.

Chiral Additives. Demand for optically pure pharmaceuticals and the importance of enantiomeric analysis in protein research has stimulated investigations into enantio[18] separations. These can be carried out using chiral stationary phases but the preferred method appears to be based on the addition of optically active mobile phase additives, such as complexes of Cu^{2+} with N,N-dialkyl-α-amino acids.

EVALUATION OF PERFORMANCE

Definitions

The many factors contributing to separation have been discussed in the preceding sections. It is necessary to have well-defined criteria for the comparison of the performance of chromatographic systems and procedures, so as to be able to choose the best conditions for any given separation problem.

The objective is to relate the achievement of separation as displayed by the chromatogram to the many parameters which can be varied to give appropriate working conditions.

The chromatogram is a plot of the separated solute concentrations against time, as 'seen' by the detector when the solutes leave the column (Fig. 8). Column performance can be assessed by using the following definitions and relationships derived from measurements of retention times, t_R, and peak widths, w, i.e. measurements carried out on the chromatogram (i-vii) and others which include column geometry and flow rate.

i. adjusted retention time
$$t_R{'} = t_R - t_0$$

ii. capacity factor or distribution ratio
$$k' = \frac{t_R - t_0}{t_0} = \frac{t'_R}{t_0}$$

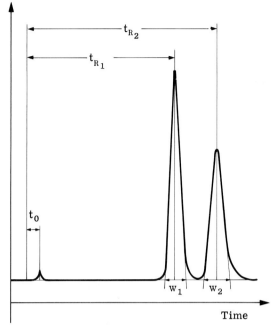

Detector Response

Fig. 8 Chromatogram t_{R1}, t_{R2}: retention times of samples. t_0: retention time of non-retarded peak. w_1, w_2: peak widths, measured on the base line between the tangents to the peaks at the points of inflection.

iii. separation factor for compounds 1 and 2
$$\alpha = \frac{t_{R2} - t_0}{t_{R1} - t_0} = \frac{k_2{'}}{k_1{'}}$$

iv. efficiency or no. of theoretical plates
$$N = \frac{16 t_R^2}{w^2}$$

v. resolution
$$R_s = \frac{t_{R2} - t_{R1}}{\frac{1}{2}(w_1 + w_2)}$$

vi. peak capacity
$$\phi = f(\sqrt{N}, \alpha)$$

vii. height of the (equivalent) theoretical plate
$$H = \frac{L}{N}$$
(L = column length)

viii. retention volume
$$V_R = T_R \times F_c$$
(F_c = volume flow rate of mobile phase)

The Relations between Definitions and Performance

i. The *adjusted retention time*, $t'_R = t_R - t_0$, the difference between the retention time of a sample and time taken by a non-retarded substance, is a measure of the retardation experienced by the sample. This retardation is the result of the interactions between the sample and the two phases, the process which causes chromatographic separation. It is therefore a more suitable value for assessing column performance than the total retention time.

ii. The *capacity factor* or *distribution ratio*, k', is another function based on retention times, a measure of the capacity of the column to retain a given sample. It is used in preference to retention time because it can more easily be related to both efficiency and resolution, and is independent of flow rate and column length. The first priority in choosing a system is to obtain an appropriate value for k'. A very large value for k' is another expression for a very long retention time, and a very small value for k' implies that the samples are hardly retarded at all and emerge from the column close to each other and to non-retarded materials. Both these situations are clearly undesirable if separation is to take place in a reasonable time. In practice, the time, t_0, taken by a non-retarded peak in a typical column is of the order of 1 minute, and values of k' between 1 and 10 are generally acceptable. It can be shown that k' values between 2 and 5 are preferable from the point of view of obtaining good resolution.

It can be shown that k' is equal to the distribution ratio, i.e. to the ratio

$$\frac{\text{(amount of sample in stationary phase)}}{\text{(amount of sample in mobile phase)}}$$

The ratio is the product of the distribution constant K, and the volume ratio of the two phases:

$$K = \frac{Cs}{Cm}, \quad k' = \frac{CsVs}{CmVm}$$

where Cs = conc. of sample in stationary phase.
Cm = conc. of sample in mobile phase.
Vs = Vol. of active stationary phase.
Vm = Vol. of mobile phase.

The geometry of the column packing will therefore have an effect on k': packings with relatively low volumes of stationary phase, e.g. porous layer beads will have low values of k' (short retention time) compared with those for totally porous beads, and bonded phases with polymeric layers or long carbon chains will give higher values of k' than those with small alkyl groups.

In adsorption chromatography, surface area is analogous to stationary phase volume, and packings with large surface areas will have high values of k'.

iii. The extent of separation of any two compounds can be expressed as the ratio of the two adjusted retention times, the *separation factor*

$$\alpha = \frac{t_{R2} - t_0}{t_{R1} - t_0} = \frac{k_2'}{k_1'}$$

For a given column, the volume ratio Vs/Vm is constant, and

$$\frac{k_2'}{k_1'} = \frac{K_2}{K_1}$$

The separation factor is thus equal to the ratio of the distribution constants (or partition coefficients) of the components of the sample mixtures between the two phases. The only way to change these is to change the chemical nature of the phase system or the temperature. To obtain differences in the ratio k_2'/k_1', it is necessary to choose solvents which differ in selectivity rather than strength.

iv. The *efficiency*, N, of a column with respect to a given sample is the function of both the retention time and the peak width. The narrower the peak after a given retention time the greater the efficiency. This function is referred to as the number of theoretical plates, N, a name derived from the plate model of chromatography proposed by Martin. This model gives a vivid and easily accessible picture of chromatographic separation, but it does not enable us to relate many of the experimental conditions with performance. The term 'theoretical plate' is, however, firmly established in the literature and the efficiency is defined as $N = 16(t_R)^2/w^2$.

v. The ultimate objective of any chromatographic method, the *resolution*, R_s, between the two compounds, depends not only on the distance between the peak maxima, $t_{R2} - t_{R1}$, but also on the narrowness of the peaks, i.e. the average of the inverse of the peak widths. It is defined as

$$R_s = \frac{t_{R2} - t_{R1}}{\frac{1}{2}(w_1 + w_2)}$$

vi. There must clearly be a limit to the number of peaks which can be separated in a chromatogram. This limit is expressed as the *peak capacity*, ϕ, the maximum number of components that can be separated in a single operation. This will depend on a small band width, a function of N, and on the separation factor α, and can be increased by any change which will increase N and/or α. In exclusion chromatography, the fraction capacity is limited by the total volume of solvent in the column and, the only ways of increasing it are increasing the column length or recycling. In other forms of chromatography, the ultimate limitations will be the time and money which can reasonably be spent on a separation.

vii. The ratio of the column length, L, over the efficiency, N, is defined as H, the *height equivalent of a theoretical plate*. This term like N, is derived from the plate theory. It can also be considered as the resultant of the factors which contribute to band broadening.

These factors also depend on the flow rate, or, more precisely, on the linear velocity, u^*, of the

---

* Linear velocity,
$$u = \frac{\text{Flow rate} \times \text{column volume}}{\text{Area of cross section} \times \text{interstitial volume}} \approx L/t_0$$

mobile phase. It has been found empirically that the relationship between plate height and linear velocity is of the form $H = Du^n$.

D and n are constants for a given column and solvent. The value of n, usually about 0·4, can be obtained from the plot of H against log u, and D can thus be found for a given column by determining the efficiency at different flow rates. D is a measure of overall efficiency. It can be used to compare different column packings.

viii. The volume needed to elute a given compound at constant flow rate, Fc, *the retention volume*, V_R, is characteristic for the compound and independent of the flow rate: when the flow rate is increased in a given system, the retention time will be correspondingly reduced. Corresponding values are V_R', the adjusted retention volume, and V_0, the volume required to elute a non-retarded compound. It can be seen that V_0 is the volume of mobile phase in the column, or, except in the case of exclusion chromatography, the interstitial volume.

ix. The *minimum weight* of sample which can be detected, the *detection limit*. D^*, depends not only on the sensitivity of the detector but also on the efficiency of the total system. For reliable detection, the signal to noise ratio should be at least 5 : 1. The expression[21]

$$D^* = \frac{5\sqrt{(2\pi)}V_R G}{(\sqrt{N})S}$$

where G = noise level on the base line in mV; and S = detector response in mV for unit change in solute concentration, relates this requirement to the retention volume, the column efficiency, the absolute sensitivity of the detector and the noise.

The minimum detectable concentration will depend on D^* and on the maximum volume of sample which can be injected without causing peak broadening. This volume may be as high as 100μl or even greater, and this may compensate low detector sensitivity.

SEPARATION STRATEGY

When developing a spectroscopic method of analysis, the choice of operating parameters is usually confined to the selection of a suitable solvent from a limited range and an appropriate sample concentration. The procedure will be identical for many different types of sample, results are recorded automatically and the intellectual problems are deferred to their interpretation.

In contrast, when devising a chromatographic procedure, many parameters have to be considered, and choices have to be made which are based on an understanding of the separation process, the parts played by all the components of the system, the chemical nature of the sample and of the components of the system. These problems have to be solved *before* the

analysis is carried out. Once a good chromatogram has been obtained, interpretation is easy. The advantages of this type of analysis in terms of speed, selectivity, specificity, and sensitivity, may have to be paid for by a considerable investment in time spent in developing the best possible separation procedure.

The chromatographer wants to obtain narrow peaks well separated from each other which can only be achieved if conditions are chosen to optimize the efficiency and selectivity.

The attainment of narrow peaks—efficiency—is achieved by reducing all the factors which contribute to band broadening. These factors are largely due to the engineering aspects, i.e. geometry, and the mechanics of the system, and are commonly referred to as kinetic factors.

The separation between the centres of chromatographic zones, the selectivity of the system, is a function of the relative strengths of the forces acting between the sample, the stationary phase, and the mobile phase, i.e. of the equilibrium distribution of the sample between the two phases, the 'rate processes' or the thermodynamic properties of the system. They depend on the chemical nature of the phase system and on the temperature.

The Choice of an HPLC Mode

The choice of a mode of separation is dictated by the properties of the compounds of interest and of the matrix in which they are present. It may be advisable to reconsider the mode traditionally used in a particular chromatographic method so as to be able to take advantage of the new techniques.

The new HPLC methods are so flexible that many separation problems can be solved in more than one way, and the demarcation lines between different modes are increasingly difficult to define.

Reverse-phase packings with aqueous stationary phases containing varying amounts of methanol, acetonitrile or tetrahydrofuran are by far the most commonly used systems at present. The addition of buffers and ion-pairing reagents has extended their range of application to ionic compounds.

Reverse-phase systems can be used to separate peptides and proteins; these separations involve complex distribution equilibria, specific solvation equilibria, solute–solute interactions and susceptibility of the solutes to specific changes in pH, and are affected by the structure of the silica matrix. The advantages of reverse-phase systems are that one column can be used for many different types of separation, and that aqueous samples can be injected without disturbing the column, and many interfering substances, which are often highly polar compounds, are eluted faster than drugs and their metabolites and do not accumulate on the column. These factors constitute a great advantage in clinical analysis, where many compounds of interest are not easily extracted into organic solvents. Clean-up procedures can be simplified, may be more easily automated, or sometimes even eliminated.

Compounds of low polarity can also be separated on hydrocarbon-bonded stationary phases, but more usually on polar-bonded phases or unmodified silica, with non-aqueous mobile phases. Such volatile organic solvents are more easily removed at the end of the analytical procedure, and this is an advantage in preparative work, or in conjunction with certain methods of detection, i.e. MS, FTIR or NMR.

Polar stationary phases can be used in both the normal and reverse-phase mode, this makes it possible to deal with multicomponent mixtures with a single stationary phase and a limited number of mobile phase solvents.[22]

The Resolution Equation

It is possible to derive equations connecting the resolution, R_s, the separation factor, α, the efficiency, N, and the capacity ratio or distribution factor, k'. An approximate form of such an equation can be used when discussing the separation of a pair of poorly separated compounds, when α is close to unity, and the capacity ratios are similar ($k'_1 \approx k_2'$).

$$R_s = \tfrac{1}{4}(\alpha - 1)\sqrt{N}\left(\frac{k'}{1 + k'}\right)$$

This equation makes it possible to improve resolution by considering the effects of k', N, and α separately.

Control of k' and its Effect on Resolution

The difficulties likely to arise in the separation of mixtures containing a limited number of components are of three kinds:

1. Elution is too fast, i.e. k' is too small.
2. Elution is too slow, i.e. k' is too large.
3. The overall elution time is acceptable, but resolution is not adequate.

1. and 2. can usually be remedied by altering the strength of the mobile phase: k' will be increased by increasing the water content in a reverse-phase system; with a polar stationary phase it usually means increasing the proportion of hydrocarbon in the eluent. Conversely, elution in a reverse-phase system will be speeded up by an increase in the proportion of organic modifier, and in a normal system by increasing the proportion of the more polar constituent of the mobile phase.

The stationary phase will also affect k'. Increase in particle surface area and the number of carbons in each silyl chain of a bonded phase will increase k'. It is not only evident from the term $k'/(1 + k')$ in the equation, but also from common sense, that increasing k' will only improve resolution when k' is small (less than about 5).

In the case of (3), resolution can only be improved by increasing N, the efficiency or α, the selectivity.

Attainment of High Efficiency

The equation shows that resolution can be increased by increasing N. This can be done by increasing the length of the column, L, and, as in the case of k', by using particles with smaller diameter and greater surface area. It can be seen that column length has to be increased fourfold to double the resolution. Increasing column length will result in longer retention times and/or the requirement for higher pressures.

The effect of column dimensions on efficiency has been discussed in the section dealing with columns. Commercial columns packed with $5\,\mu m$ particles should be capable of giving 60 000–100 000 plates per metre, and $3\,\mu m$ packings up to 150 000 plates per metre. In exclusion chromatography and in some cases of other modes, N may be increased by recycling.

The smaller the column and the particle diameter, the more important it is that the column should be well packed and that the extra-column dead volume in the system, i.e. the injector, pipework, and detector should be as low as possible. The manufacturers are usually responsible for these aspects of HPLC. They often claim specific values of N for their products, but it should be kept in mind that the value of N can be calculated in different ways and that it will depend on the nature of the sample, the viscosity of the mobile phase, and the temperature.

Selectivity

It can be seen from the resolution equation that quite a small change in α will have a considerable effect on resolution: a change in α from 1·1 to 1·2 will almost double the resolution. Changing α implies changing one or both of the two phases or the temperature.

Qualitative consideration of the relative importance of the various intermolecular interactions between both phases and the sample (polar and ionic effects, solvophobicity, and the use of additives to exploit secondary equilibria) may make it possible to change the phase system so as to improve selectivity for a given mixture of compounds while keeping k' within an acceptable range.

Mobile phase composition is the most accessible factor in this context. Snyder[19] has classified the solvent properties of common liquids with reference to their behaviour as proton donors, proton acceptors, and their ability to take part in dipole interactions. Because of the constraints discussed earlier, the choice is usually limited to water with methanol, acetonitrile, and tetrahydrofuran as modifiers in reverse-phase systems, and to n-hexane as carrier with methyl t-butyl ether, chloroform, and methylene chloride as modifiers. An optimization triangle

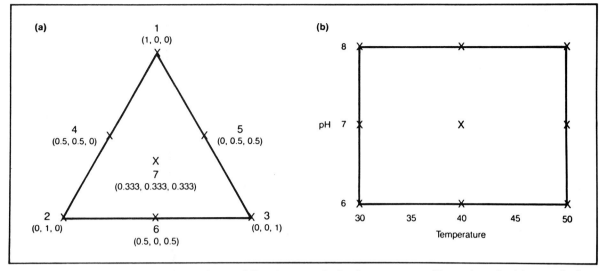

Fig. 9 Mixture design experiments for mobile phase optimization strategy. (Reproduced with permission from Glajch J. L., Kirkland J. J. (1983). *Anal. Chem*; **55**: 319A.)

approach (Fig. 9) can be used to find the optimum mobile phase composition of a carrier and three modifiers. The apexes of the triangle correspond to mixtures of the carrier with each of the modifiers, chosen to give equal eluent strengths (ranges of k'). These three solutions as well as four more made by combining them in the ratios shown in Fig. 9 are then used to carry out a total of seven chromatographic runs. It should then be possible to improve the solvent composition for the given separation.

In the case of many of the factors listed above the effect of one depends on the value of others, e.g. the pH and the concentration of the counter ion in ion pair chromatography, and it is not possible to find the best possible conditions by studying one factor at a time. For complex mixtures of unknown composition the physicochemical data are not available for consideration.

Statistical methods for finding the optimum mobile phase composition from a limited number of experiments have been developed[23] and, in some cases, incorporated in microprocessor controlled equipment.

Gradient Elution

No one set of conditions is likely to meet the requirements for the fast separation of all the components of a complex mixture, and some form of gradient or multistep procedure has to be devised. Gradient elution makes it possible to deal with mixtures of compounds with a wide range of values of k'. A weak solvent is used to elute the fast components of the mixture. The composition of the mobile phase is then changed continuously, so that the more strongly retained compounds are eluted with appropriate values of k'. This procedure is also useful for finding a suitable mobile phase composition for isocratic separation.

Gradient elution presents obvious advantages, but it must be kept in mind that varying conditions are not as easily reproducible as constant ones, and that, as in temperature programming in gas chromatography, the time required for the system to return to its original conditions and be ready for another sample, is often longer than the analysis time and must be included in the time required for an analysis.

Column Switching

The peak capacity of a number of sequential steps is equal to the product of the peak capacities of the individual steps, as long as the processes underlying separation are different. Methods employing different modes of chromatography in sequence: ion exchange, molecular exclusion, adsorption and partition using different systems (e.g. two-dimensional thin layer chromatography) have traditionally been used in trace analysis, and similar reasoning can be applied to using different modes in sequence in column chromatography. Sequential analysis procedures employing molecular exclusion as a preliminary step, ion pair partition following adsorption, trace enrichment etc. by means of column switching and backflushing techniques can be used to replace preliminary separation and cleanup steps.

A system for the automated analysis of antiepileptic drugs is shown in Fig. 10. The sample is transferred automatically from the autosampler(S) to the sample loop (L) by the peristaltic pump (PP) with excess going to waste (W). Simultaneously the extraction column (EC) is equilibrated with flushing solvent. The loading valve (V_1) is then rotated to wash the sample on to the reverse-phase extraction column, where the analytes are retained while hydrophilic substances are washed through to waste (W). The injection valve is next reversed and the sample components are back-flushed on to the analytical column

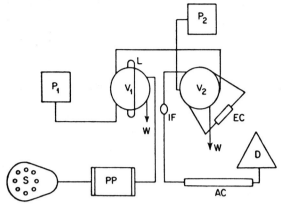

Fig. 10 Configuration of the fully automated HPLC system with on-line, solid-phase sample cleanup. S, autosampler; PP, peristaltic pump; L, sample loop; V_1, and V_2, six-port switching valves; W, waste; P_2, mobile-phase pump; P_1, wash pump; EC, extraction column; AC, analytical column; IF, in-line filter; and D, detector. (Reproduced with permission from Nazareth A. *et al.* (1984). *J. Chromatogr*; **309**: 357.)

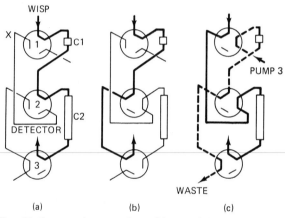

Fig. 11 Connections and positions of the three high-pressure valves used for column-switching HPLC of oxidized pterins. Status (a), 0–2 min injection of sample with columns C1 and C2 in series. Status (b), 2–12 min gradient elution of slow-moving compounds from C1 into detector. Status (c), 12–32 min elution of faster moving compounds from C2 into detector, with simultaneous cleaning of C1. (Reproduced with permission from Niederweiser *et al.*[24])

for separation and analysis. Using this system, it was possible to carry out the continuous analysis of primidone for over 2000 serum samples at the rate of twelve samples per hour.

A similar system has been used to deal with a mixture of compounds with a wide range of k',[24] where the effluent from the first column goes through the analytical column for analysis of fast-eluting compounds, while the slower ones are retained on the column (Fig. 11). After an appropriate interval the flow pattern is changed so that the more strongly retained compounds go from the first column through a by-pass to the detector. The resulting chromatogram will present a group of strongly retained com-

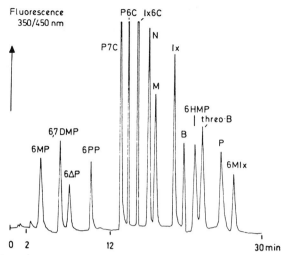

Fig. 12 HPLC of a mixture of oxidized pterins using the column-switching programme. Between 2 and 12 min the slow-moving compounds were eluted first from the short column C1. The amounts injected varied in this mixture from 5 to 20 ng. (Reproduced with permission from Niederweiser *et al.*[24])

pounds *before* the compounds which are more easily eluted. An example of this is shown in Fig. 12.

OUTLOOK

There has been a spectacular increase in the use of HPLC in biochemical analysis since the first edition of this book was published. The wide range of applications includes the monitoring of levels of drugs and their metabolites, analytical toxicology, analysis of peptides and proteins, catecholamines, antibiotics, and the investigation of structure–activity relationships.

Separation technology is still advancing very rapidly, particularly in the development of detection systems, the use of additives to the mobile phase for specific selectivity, optimization of conditions, data handling, and the combination of different HPLC modes with each other and with other analytical procedures, e.g. immunoassay[25] and automation of all these features.

Very versatile forms of apparatus are now available, and are used extensively both in research and routine analysis. The design of dedicated equipment for a particular type of analysis, e.g. Waters Catecholamine Analysis system, should be particularly useful in routine work. It seems likely that these developments will lead to a further expansion of the use of HPLC in clinical laboratories.

REFERENCES

1. Martin A. J. P., Synge R. L. M. (1941). A new form of chromatogram employing two liquid phases. *Biochem. J*; **35**: 1358.
2. Done J. N., Kennedy G. J., Knox J. H. (1972). The revolution in liquid chromatography. *Nature*; **237**: 77.

3. Kaliszan R. (1984). High performance liquid chromatography as a source of structural information for medicinal chemistry. *J. Chromatogr. Sci*; **22**: 362.

4. Katz E., Ogan K. L., Scott R. P. W. (1984). Liquid chromatography column design. *J. Chromatogr*; **289**: 65.

5. Simpson R. C., Brown P. R., Schwartz M. K. (1985). Evaluation of HPLC column performance for clinical studies. *J. Chromatogr. Sci*; **23**: 89.

6. Borman S. A. (1984). Microcolumn liquid chromatography. *Anal. Chem*; **9**: 1031A.

7. Scott R. P. W. (1985). An introduction to small-bore columns. *J. Chromatogr. Sci*; **23**: 233 (and further papers in this issue).

8. Jinno K., Phillips J. B., Carney D. P. (1985). Temperature controlled high-speed liquid chromatography. *Anal. Chem*; **57**: 574.

9. Rabel F. M. (1980). The use and maintenance of microparticulate HPLC columns. *J. Chromatogr. Sci*; **18**: 394.

10. Hershberger L. W., Callis J. B., Christian G. D. (1981). Liquid chromatography with real-time video fluorometric monitoring of effluents. *Anal. Chem*; **53**: 971.

11. Karmen A., Malikin G., Lam S. (1984). High-sensitivity radioassay in chromatographic effluents. *J. Chromatogr*; **302**: 31.

12. Frei R. W., Jansen, H., Brinkman U. A. Th. (1985). Postcolumn reaction detectors for HPLC. *Anal. Chem*; **57**: 1529A.

13. Karger B. L., Vouros P. (1985). A chromatographic perspective of high performance-liquid chromatography-mass spectrometry. *J. Chromatogr*; **323**: 13.

14. Bidlingmeyer B. A., Del Rios J. K., Korpi J. (1982). Separation of organic amine compounds on silica gel with reverse-phase eluents. *Anal. Chem*; **54**: 442.

15. Billiet H., Laurent C., de Galan L. (1985). A reappreciation of alumina in high-performance liquid chromatography. *Trends Anal. Chem*; **4**: 100.

16. Nahum A., Horvath C. (1981). Surface silanols in silica-bonded hydrocarbonaceous phases. *J. Chromatogr*; **203**: 53.

17. Bij K. E., Horvath C., Melander W. R., Nahum A. (1981). Irregular retention behaviour and effect of silanol masking. *J. Chromatogr*; **203**; 65.

18. Allenmark S. G. (1985). Analytical applications of direct chromatographic enantio separations. *Trends Anal. Chem*; **4**: 106.

19. Snyder L. R. (1978). Classification of the solvent properties of common liquids. *J. Chromatogr. Sci*; **16**: 223.

20. Eksborg S., Lagerstrom P., Modin R., Schill G. (1973). Ion pair chromatography of organic compounds. *J. Chromatogr*; **83**: 99.

21. Karger B. L., Martin M., Guiochan G. (1974). The role of column parameters and injection volumes on detection limits in liquid chromatography. *Anal. Chem*; **46**: 640.

22. De Smet M., Hoogewijs G., Puttemans M., Massart D. L. (1984). Separation strategy of multicomponent mixtures by liquid chromatography with a limited number of mobile phase solvents. *Anal. Chem*; **56**: 2662.

23. Glajch J. L., Kirkland J. J. (1983). Optimization of selectivity in liquid chromatography. *Anal. Chem*; **55**: 319A.

24. Niederwieser A., Staudenmann W., Wetzel E. (1984). High-performance liquid chromatography with column switching for the analysis of biogenic amine materials and pterins. *J. Chromatogr*; **290**: 237.

25. Wehmeyer K. R., Halsall H. B., Heinemann W. R. (1985). Heterogeneous enzyme immunoassay with electrochemical detection. *Clin. Chem*; **31**: 1546.

FURTHER READING

Books

Brown P. R., Krstulovic A. M. (1982). *Reverse-Phase High Performance Liquid Chromatography Theory, Practice, and Biomedical Application*. New York: Wiley.

Frei R. W., Lawrence J. F. (1981, 1982). *Chemical Derivatisation in Analytical Chemistry*, Vols 1 and 2. New York and London: Plenum.

Hancock W. S., Sparrow J. T. (1984). *HPLC Analysis of Biological Compounds*, Chromatographic Science Series 26. New York: Marcel Dekker.

Kucera P. (1984). *Microcolumn HPLC*. Amsterdam: Elsevier.

Poole C. F., Schuette S. A. (1984). *Contemporary Practice of Chromatography*. Amsterdam: Elsevier.

Snyder L. R., Kirkland J. J. (1979). *Introduction to Modern Liquid Chromatography*, 2nd edn. New York: Wiley-Interscience.

Vickrey T. M. (1983). *Liquid Chromatography Detectors*. Chromatographic Science Series 23. New York: Marcel Dekker.

Wong S. H. (1985). *Therapeutic Drug Monitoring and Toxicology by Liquid Chromatography*. New York: Marcel Dekker.

Reviews

Deming S. N., Bower J. G., Bower K. D. (1984). Multifactor Optimisation of HPLC Conditions. In *Advances in Chromatography*, vol. 24, Ch. 2. New York: Marcel Dekker.

Deyl Z., DeSilva J. A. F. (eds) (1985). Drug Level Monitoring. *J. Chromatogr*; **340**: (special volume).

Krstulovic A. M., Colin H., Guiochon G. A. (1984). Electrochemical Detectors for LC. In *Advances in Chromatography*, vol. 24. New York: Marcel Dekker.

Lingeman H., Underberg W. J. M., Takadate A., Hulshoff A. (1985). Fluorescence Detection in HPLC. *J. Liq. Chromatogr*; **8**: 789.

24. Ion-exchange Chromatography and Gel Filtration

A. M. Stokes

ION EXCHANGE CHROMATOGRAPHY
INTRODUCTION

The components of a mixture are distinguished from each other in ion-exchange chromatography on the basis of the net charge on each molecule which is available for interaction with the ion-exchanger under the conditions imposed. Molecular size and the distribution of charges are also important factors. Separation in ion-exchange chromatography is similar to that obtained in other separation methods which depend on charge properties, such as electrophoresis and isoelectric focusing. This similarity is illustrated in Fig. 1, showing the isoenzymes of lactate

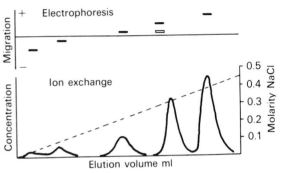

Fig. 1 Elution diagram of lactate dehydrogenase isoenzymes on DEAE-Sephadex A-50. (From Wachsmuth E. D. and Pfleiderer G., *Biochem. Z.,* **336** (1963) 545–556.)

dehydrogenase from human brain, separated by ion-exchange chromatography and also by high voltage electrophoresis.

The five isoenzymes were eluted using a continuous ionic strength gradient in an order corresponding with increasing migration towards the anode in electrophoresis, i.e. increasing net negative charge.

Frequently there are significant variations in the behaviour of substances in ion-exchange chromatography and electrophoresis, because, as the two methods of separation are generally carried out under different ionic conditions, the charge of the substance is different.

Variables other than net charge may also be involved (e.g. the diffusion coefficient and frictional interaction with the gel in the case of gel electrophoresis). Secondary forces such as hydrophobic interactions, which depend on the nature of the ion-exchanger matrix, may also be involved. Because of these variations in the behaviour of substances in ion-exchange chromatography and electrophoresis the two techniques are to some extent complementary. Thus electrophoresis may be used to evaluate the heterogeneity of fractions obtained by ion-exchange chromatography, and ion-exchange chromatography may be used in the further fractionation of components initially separated by electrophoresis.

Ion Exchange Equilibria

An ion-exchanger consists of an insoluble matrix containing chemically bound charged groups and exchangeable counter ions. A matrix which carries positive groups will contain exchangeable negative counter ions and is therefore termed an *anion* exchanger. Similarly, a matrix which carries negative groups will exchange positive counter ions and is therefore a *cation* exchanger.

When a cation exchanger in the hydrogen form (i.e. H^+ counter ions) is immersed in sodium chloride, the hydrogen ions are replaced by sodium and sodium chloride is converted into hydrochloric acid.

This type of small electrolyte ion-exchanger reaction may be described either as an *adsorption system* (obeying the Langmuir isotherm or Freundlich isotherm), or as a reaction obeying the law of *mass action*, or as a *Donnan equilibrium* between the inside of the exchanger particle and the outside solution. Each of these treatments demonstrates that the amount of an ion within an exchanger particle will be proportional to the concentration of that ion in solution. However, the Donnan theory alone provides an adequate explanation of the volume change observed when one species of counter ion is replaced by another. This phenomenon is not directly related to the dependence of volume on ionic strength and pH which is observed particularly with gel-type ion exchangers.

Exchange Kinetics

Ion-exchange kinetics consist of two basic components: (1) diffusion of the irrigating ion A in free solution, within the ion-exchanger particle and through the phase boundary; (2) chemical exchange between A and BX (B being the counter ion on the exchanger X). For small electrolytes at least, chemical exchange is effectively instantaneous. Attainment of the equilibrium position in such an ion-exchange reaction is therefore limited by diffusion and hence concentration. This may not necessarily be the case with a macromolecular poly-electrolyte.

However, in any ion-exchange experiment involving irrigation, the extent to which the system can approach equilibrium is determined by the rate of irrigation, by the particle size of the ion exchanger and by the ionic strength of the irrigating solution.

If flow rate and particle size are such as to establish a perfect equilibrium an elution curve as shown in Fig. 2a is obtained.

However, this is an ideal condition which is rarely approached in practice. Because practically useful flow rates are usually too high and particle sizes are usually too large, non-equilibrium curves such as that shown in Fig. 2b are generally obtained.* Indeed the

---

* Vertical and eddy diffusion have the same effect and thus tend to produce a band with the characteristic concentration curve, similar to a normal distribution curve. These are general pheno-

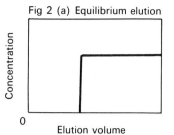

Fig 2 (a) Equilibrium elution

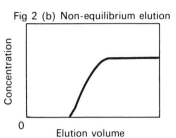

Fig 2 (b) Non-equilibrium elution

Fig. 2 (a) Equilibrium elution; (b) non-equilibrium elution.

adverse effect on resolution of increasing flow-rate in ion-exchange chromatography is due to the tendency to non-equilibrium elution under high-flow conditions.

Theories of Elution

Various theories of chromatography and chromatographic adsorption have been developed and applied to ion-exchange chromatography. These theories permit the calculation, for simple, small electrolyte ion-exchange processes, of adsorption isotherms, equilibrium constants and the number of theoretical plates. In some cases it is also possible to calculate the degree of contamination of one substance by another, the minimum length of column for a given separation and even the optimum eluant composition. This quantitative theoretical approach has, however, contributed little to practical ion-exchange chromatography. The separation of macromolecular poly-electrolytes, such as proteins and nucleic acids, in ion-exchange chromatography requires the use of conditions for which there is, as yet, no satisfactory quantitative theoretical treatment. An empirical approach to the analytical application of ion-exchange chromatography is therefore generally adopted and column dimensions, etc. are judged by trial, error and intuition.

ION-EXCHANGE MEDIA

The first ion-exchangers were silicates, either natural products such as montmorillonite clay or Fuller's earth, or synthetic alumino-silicates prepared from

---

mena in chromatography however, and will not be considered further here. An introduction to these concepts is given in Chapter 21.

aluminium compounds and sodium silicate. The inherent limitations of these materials (e.g. a tendency to dissolve at low pH) led to the commercial development of synthetic ion-exchange *resins*. Various ion-exchangers derived from *cellulose* and synthetic *gel* matrixes have been developed more recently. Ion-exchangers prepared from these matrixes (resins, celluloses and gels) are now by far the most widely used media in both analytical and preparative ion-exchange chromatography.

The type of charged group which is covalently attached to the insoluble matrix determines whether the resulting exchanger is a strong or weak, anion or cation exchanger. Phenolic hydroxyl, carboxyl and sulphonic groups are commonly used to form cation exchangers and quaternary ammonium and aliphatic or aromatic amino groups to form anion exchangers. Sulphonic and quaternary amino groups result in strongly acidic and strongly basic, cation and anion exchangers respectively. The other groups result in weak ion exchangers.

It is the physicochemical nature of the matrix however, which largely determines the type of separation for which the resulting ion-exchanger is most useful.

Ion-exchange Resins

Ion-exchange resins are essentially crosslinked polymer networks originally prepared by polycondensation reactions such as the condensation of phenol, phenol-sulphonic acid and formaldehyde using sodium hydroxide as catalyst. Vinyl type polymerization reactions are now widely used and permit greater control of both the degree of crosslinkage and the degree and type of ionic substitution.

The hydrophobic matrix, high degree of substitution and low degree of permeability to macromolecules are factors which severely limit the value of ion-exchange resins as far as biopolymer fractionation is concerned. Resin ion-exchangers are widely used, however, in the fractionation of sugars, nucleotides, amino acids etc., where their relatively rapid exchange kinetics and secondary adsorption effects occasionally permit extremely high resolution. This is illustrated in Fig. 3 which shows the fractionation of a mixture of amino acids on a sulphonated polystyrene cation exchanger.

This method serves to separate all the amino acids commonly found in proteins, because it depends not only on ion-exchange properties, but also on the adsorption of the amino acids to the resin material. The column material is sufficiently selective in its adsorption properties so that all the neutral amino acids, which cannot be separated purely on the basis of ion-exchange, are eluted from the column separately.

It is evident from theoretical considerations that several important features must be known before a particular resin can be selected for a particular analytical purpose. This information is almost invariably

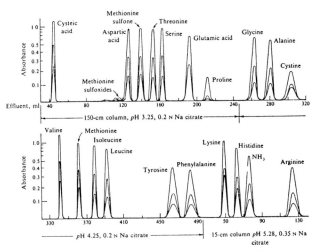

Fig. 3 Automatically recorded chromatographic analysis of a synthetic mixture of amino acids on a sulphonated polystyrene resin. (From Spackman D. H., Stein W. H., Moore S. (1958). *Anal. Chem*; **30**: 1190.)

available in pamphlets produced by the manufacturers of the resins.

Cellulose Ion-exchangers

A wide variety of ion-exchangers derived from cellulose are now commercially available. Table 1 summarizes some of these and the substituent groups that give them their ionic properties. According to literature from the manufacturers of cellulose ion-exchangers the matrix may be cotton cellulose (Whatman), wood cellulose (Serva) or both (Selectacel and Cellex). The current literature of the manufacturers should be consulted for detailed descriptions of the several grades of each type offered by each.

Most of the ion-exchange celluloses retain some degree of 'native structure' and this precludes their classification as resins, which are amorphous. Indeed one of the advantages of cellulose ion-exchangers in the fractionation of biopolymers such as proteins is the retention of an open microstructure which permits relatively easy access to the charged sites. As well as presenting a low charge density (*see below*) the cellulose adsorbents offer a supporting matrix which is hydrophilic. This minimizes the hydrophobic interactions that apparently complicate the fractionation of proteins on resin type ion-exchangers. In addition the relative freedom of movement of the charged polysaccharide chains results in a minimal particle–solution interface and permits flexibility in the accommodation of oppositely charged sites on the adsorbed macromolecule.

The degree of substitution of charged groups in cellulose ion-exchangers is generally extremely low—perhaps only 1–2% of the chemically possible level of substitution. From the point of view of capacity and working ionic-strength, which influence exchange kinetics, a considerably higher degree of substitution is desirable, but incorporation of charged

TABLE 1

CELLULOSIC ION EXCHANGERS

Anion exchangers	*Ionizable group*		meq/g*
AE-cellulose	Aminoethyl	$-O-CH_2-CH_2-NH_2$	0·3–1·0
DEAE-cellulose	Diethylaminoethyl	$-O-CH_2-CH_2-N(C_2H_5)_2$	0·1–1·1
TEAE-cellulose	Triethylaminoethyl	$-O-CH_2-CH_2-N^+(C_2H_5)_3$	0·5–1·0
GE-cellulose	Guanidoethyl	$-O-CH_2-CH_2-NH-\overset{\overset{NH}{\|\|}}{C}-NH_2$	0·2–0·5
PAB-cellulose	*p*-Aminobenzyl	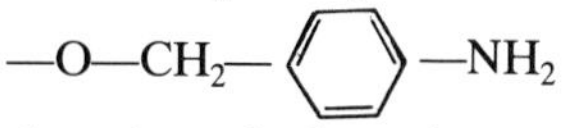 $-O-CH_2-\langle\bigcirc\rangle-NH_2$	0·2–0·5
ECTEOLA-cellulose	Triethanolamine coupled to cellulose through glyceryl and polyglyceryl chains. Mixed groups		0·1–0·5
BD-cellulose	Benzoylated DEAE-cellulose		0·8
BND-cellulose	Benzoylated-naphthoylated DEAE-cellulose		0·8
PEI-cellulose	Polyethyleneimine adsorbed to cellulose or weakly phosphorylated cellulose		

Cation exchangers	*Ionizable group*		meq/g*
CM-cellulose	Carboxymethyl-	$-O-CH_2-COOH$	0·5–1·0
P-cellulose	Phosphate	$-O-\overset{\overset{O}{\|\|}}{\underset{\underset{OH}{\|}}{P}}-OH$	0·7–7·4
SE-cellulose	sulphoethyl	$-O-CH_2-CH_2-\overset{\overset{O}{\|\|}}{\underset{\underset{O}{\|\|}}{S}}-OH$	0·2–0·3

* Acid–base capacity as indicated by manufacturer.

groups significantly above 1 mmol/g causes profound changes in the physical properties of the matrix. Interchain hydrogen bonds make cellulose insoluble in water and the substitution of any group tends to disrupt this hydrogen bonding.

Ultimately increasing substitution of the cellulose matrix leads to solubility in water, but other physical properties, which render the matrix unsuitable for use in ion-exchange columns, are encountered even at quite low levels of substitution. In cases where a higher capacity and working ionic strength are important, the disruption caused by an increased degree of substitution can be minimized if covalent crosslinkages are introduced into the cellulose matrix.

When native cellulose is substituted in such a way that the physical structure of the matrix is not significantly changed then a 'fibrous' form product is obtained. Fibrous form cellulose ion-exchangers are available in a number of particle sizes ranging from coarse, cotton-like flocs to very fine powders. Some adsorbents are available in the form of paper sheets prepared from floc mixed with native cellulose fibre to provide mechanical strength.

Some ion-exchange celluloses, e.g. DEAE-cellulose and CM-cellulose, are also available in a very finely divided 'microgranular' or 'microcrystalline'

form in which the substituted celluloses (enriched with respect to microcrystalline regions) have been chemically crosslinked. Such materials should only be used when resolution is of much greater importance than flow rate. In addition these particles must be handled with great care since they are more easily damaged by mechanical agitation than fibrous forms and this may limit their repeated re-use.

Partly because of the variability inherent in cellulose there has been an undesirable variability in the capacity, affinity and general performance of most cellulose ion-exchangers. Most of the objectionable variation had been concerned with DEAE-cellulose, because it is the most extensively used ion-exchanger and because of the occurrence of a side reaction which is difficult to control during its preparation. Present products are, however, more acceptable because of standardization and improvements introduced by manufacturers. It is nevertheless important that the user of these adsorbents be aware of past difficulties since they may still be encountered.

Ion-exchange Gels

Ion-exchange gels derived from crosslinked dextran (Sephadex) or polyacrylamide (Bio-Gel) are available with charged groups similar to those in the cellu-

TABLE 2

SEPHADEX ION-EXCHANGE GELS

Types		Description	Functional groups	Counter ion
DEAE-Sephadex	A–25 A–50	Weakly basic anion exchanger.	Diethylaminoethyl	Chloride
QAE-Sephadex	A–25 A–50	Strongly basic anion exchanger.	Diethyl-(2-hydroxy propyl)aminoethyl	Chloride
CM-Sephadex	C–25 C–50	Weakly acidic cation exchanger.	Carboxymethyl	Sodium
SP-Sephadex	C–25 C–50	Strongly acidic cation exchanger.	Sulphopropyl	Sodium

The letters A and C are added as suffixes to denote either anion or cation exchanger. They are used in conjunction with the number –25 and –50 to designate degree of porosity.

DEAE	$—C_2H_4N^+(C_2H_5)_2H$	
QAE*	$—C_2H_4N^+(C_2H_5)_2CH_2CH(OH)CH_3$	*(QAE = quaternary aminoethyl)
CM	$—CH_2COO—$	
SP	$—C_3H_6SO_3^-$	

lose ion-exchangers. A variety of Sephadex ion-exchange gels are listed in Table 2.

Like the cellulose ion-exchangers those derived from Sephadex gels present a neutral, hydrophilic matrix and exhibit minimal non-ionic adsorption. In contrast to cellulose-based materials, however, the covalent cross-links of Sephadex prevent solubilization and thus permit a degree of substitution of charged groups several times that of cellulose ion-exchangers. This is an advantage since it leads to an increased affinity for poly-electrolytes, making adsorption of biopolymers possible at significantly higher ionic strength. The use of a higher working ionic strength is in itself an advantage since it leads to minimal protein–protein interaction, greater potential resolution via an effect on exchange kinetics, and minimizes the bed-volume changes characteristic of gel-type ion-exchangers.

Sephadex ion-exchangers are prepared from Sephadex G-25 and Sephadex G-50 and the swelling properties of the ion-exchange gels are related to those of the parent Sephadex types. Thus the ion-exchangers swell in aqueous solvents and the degree of swelling is dependent on the degree of crosslinking. The capacity of an ion-exchanger is an important parameter since it is a quantitative measure of its ability to take up exchangeable counter ions (Table 3).

The *total capacity* is directly determined by the degree of substitution whereas the *available capacity* is the actual capacity obtainable under specified experimental conditions. The available capacity varies with the accessibility of the charged groups, i.e. the porosity of the exchanger and the size of the molecule. Ion-exchangers prepared from Sephadex G-50 are more porous than those prepared from Sephadex G-25 and thus, for molecules which are able to penetrate the −50 types more than the −25 types, the −50 type ion-exchangers have a higher available

TABLE 3

CAPACITIES OF SEPHADEX ION-EXCHANGERS

Ion exchanger		Total capacity (meq/g)	Haemoglobin capacity* (g/g)
DEAE-Sephadex	A–25 A–50	3.5 ± 0.5	0·5 5
QAE-Sephadex	A–25 A–50	3.0 ± 0.4	0·3 6
CM-Sephadex	C–25 C–50	4.5 ± 0.5	0·4 9
SP-Sephadex	C–25 C–50	2.3 ± 0.3	0·2 7

* The haemoglobin capacity is the amount of haemoglobin (MW 69 000) reversibly bound by one gram (dry weight) of ion exchanger. This value was measured for DEAE- and QAE-Sephadex in tris-HCl buffer pH 8·0, I = 0·01 and for CM- and SP-Sephadex in acetate buffer pH 5·0, I = 0·01.

TABLE 4

CHOICE OF ION-EXCHANGE GEL

Molecular weight of protein		Preferred exchanger	
Low MW	30 000	A–25,	C–25
Medium MW	30 000–200 000	A–50,	C–50
High MW	200 000	A–25,	C–25

capacity. The haemoglobin capacities given in Table 3 are therefore only a guide to the protein capacity, and Table 4 gives an approximate guide to the choice of Sephadex ion-exchanger based on molecular weight.

It has been suggested that separations on Sephadex ion-exchangers depend on both ionic interactions and differences in molecular size. Although steric factors are always involved, they only affect the separation of charged solutes by determining the available capacity for such substances. Only uncharged solutes will be fractionated according to size as in gel filtration, and then it should be noted that the fractionation range of the ion-exchanger will not correspond to the parent Sephadex type.

Unlike the parent Sephadex types, the degree of swelling of the Sephadex ion-exchangers varies with the ionic composition of the swelling medium. At low ionic strengths, repulsion between the fixed charged groups is maximum. This ionic repulsion and the consequent degree of swelling decrease with increasing ionic strength. At ionic strengths of 0·1 and above such bed volume changes are minimal, however. Because of the high degree of substitution of Sephadex ion-exchangers, it is usually possible to employ a starting ionic strength of 0·1 or greater and thus avoid excessive bed volume changes during operation. A pH-dependent swelling may also be encountered with gel type ion-exchangers. Repulsion between charged groups is maximal at pH values where the ion-exchanger is fully charged and decreases, causing a decrease in bed volume, as the charged groups become neutralized. The 'strong' ion-exchange gels QAE-Sephadex and SP-Sephadex are, however, fully charged over a very wide pH range and thus have swelling properties independent of pH.

For this reason they are frequently selected when a pH gradient is to be employed for an ion-exchange fractionation.

Since the Sephadex ion-exchangers are derived from neutral, synthetic types they are all in bead form and thus have good mechanical chromatographic properties. In addition the variability inherent in ion-exchange media derived from natural products is not encountered with the Sephadex ion-exchange gels.

PREPARATION OF ION-EXCHANGE MEDIA

The preparation of an ion-exchanger for use essentially consists of: (1) removal of contaminants, whether they are side products from the manufacturing process or contaminants from previous use, (2) removal of 'fines' and degassing, and (3) equilibrium of the ion-exchanger with 'starting' buffer.

Washing

Ion-exchange resins, especially cation exchangers, generally contain significant quantities of iron and heavy metals. Washing with 6–8 M HCl until the washings are free of metal ions, followed by washing to neutrality with distilled water is a procedure commonly used for removing these contaminants.

All types and grades of cellulose ion-exchangers should be thoroughly washed before use. Detailed washing or 'precycling' procedures are often recommended by the manufacturer and it is advisable to follow these recommendations closely. Such washing procedures usually entail alternate exposure to 0·5 M NaOH and 0·5 M HCl for varying periods of time and in an order which varies to some extent with the nature of the ion-exchanger. In addition to the

possibility of contamination by side products of the manufacturing process cellulose ion-exchangers usually contain oxidative degradation products.

These impurities will generally be seen as a yellow colour in the supernatant during washing with alkali. If the original material or washings are strongly coloured it may be advisable to filter the suspension on a coarse glass sinter and continue washing with alkali until no more colour is removed. Finely divided cellulose ion-exchangers, particularly DEAE-cellulose powder, are extremely difficult to filter in strong alkali, however, and centrifugation may then be used instead. Even after the type of washing procedure described above, cellulose ion-exchangers are likely to contain sufficient metal ions to interfere with experiments involving trace metals. In such cases washing with a suitable chelating agent may also be necessary.

Sephadex ion-exchange gels do not require precycling. Contaminants from previous experiments can generally be removed by washing with a solution with an ionic strength of about 2, if they are bound by ionic forces. Contaminants such as lipids and precipitated protein can be removed by washing with aqueous alcohol or non-ionic detergents.

Removal of 'Fines'

Undue mechanical agitation of any ion-exchanger should be avoided as this will lead to the generation of very small fragments or 'fines', which in any significant quantity will markedly reduce the flow-rate obtainable when the material is packed in a column. All ion-exchange resins, even analytical grade resins of a given mesh size should therefore be stirred with water and allowed to settle and the 'fines' removed by decanting.

A similar procedure is usually necessary with cellulose ion-exchangers but in this case it is impossible to be precise about how long a suspension should be allowed to stand before decanting since the distinction between the usuable fraction and the fines may be difficult to establish. Generally the time required for each sedimentation can be regarded as being of the order of 1 hour. Detailed recommendations for each type and grade of cellulose ion-exchanger are often made by the manufacturer.

Decantation of fines is normally unnecessary with Sephadex ion-exchange gels.

Degassing

It is advisable to remove occluded air or carbon dioxide from most ion-exchangers and buffers by means of a gentle vacuum.

Equilibration

Conversion of a cation-exchange resin to the hydrogen form is readily carried out by washing with HCl (which is a necessary pre-treatment anyway) and washing to neutrality with distilled water. The sodium form of a strong cation exchanger can be prepared by reacting the hydrogen form with NaCl, which will liberate HCl, or with NaOH.

With carboxylic resins hydrolysis occurs as with weak acids, and if the sodium form is required the reaction must be carried out with the necessary amount of NaOH. If such a column is then washed with water some of the Na^+ is lost due to hydrolysis and the washings will react alkaline even without excess NaOH.

Strongly basic anion exchange resins are converted into the OH^- form only with an excess of NaOH (in the absence of carbonate which, being divalent, absorbs more strongly than OH^-). Weak anion exchange resins can be converted into the free amino form by washing with NaOH or even ammonia. Final equilibration so that the ionic strength and pH of the effluent match those of the irrigant can be carried out in the column.

Equilibration of acid-and-base treated cellulose ion-exchanger can often be accomplished simply by washing the exchanger with several volumes of starting buffer. However, the volume of buffer required for this procedure becomes excessive on a normal laboratory scale when such adsorbents as DEAE-cellulose are to be adjusted over a considerable pH interval by interaction with a dilute starting buffer. In such a case the suspension of adsorbent in starting buffer can be titrated back to the desired pH with small volumes of relatively concentrated solutions of the acidic or basic components of the buffer. Equilibration of most of the cellulose ion-exchangers is reasonably rapid and the pH can be measured in a minute or two, but care should be taken to ensure effective stirring during the procedure.

Some types (e.g. ECTEOLA-cellulose) require more time for equilibration and the pH reading may drift for a few minutes. When the suspension has been adjusted to within 0·1 pH unit of the desired value, it is filtered and/or packed into a column and washed with starting buffer to complete equilibration with respect to both conductivity and pH.

Sephadex ion-exchange gels are supplied with Cl^- (DEAE- and QAE-Sephadex) and Na^+ (CM- and SP-Sephadex) counter ions respectively. The equilibration procedure depends on whether or not the counter ions are to be changed. If not, the required amount of ion-exchanger is stirred into an excess of starting buffer which must contain the appropriate counter ion. The supernatant should be replaced with fresh buffer several times during the swelling period, which takes 1–2 days at room temperature or 2 hours on a boiling-water bath. Alternatively the ion-exchanger can be washed extensively on a filter after the initial swelling. If the counter ion is to be changed the exchanger should be swollen in an excess of 0·5–1·0 M solution of the salt of the new counter ion. The fully swollen exchanger is then washed extensively with starting buffer. In both cases final equilibration with respect to pH and conductivity can be performed in the column.

Storage

In prolonged experiments and during storage in the wet state an antimicrobial agent should be added to the ion exchanger.

In some cases removal of buffer substrates and phosphates may be sufficient to prevent growth. When an antimicrobial agent is necessary it should be chosen so that it is not bound by the ion-exchanger. Phenyl mercuric salts (0·001% in weakly alkaline solution) and Hibitane (chlorhexidine, 0·002%) are suitable for anion exchangers. Sodium azide (0·02%) and merthiolate (0·005% in weakly acidic solution) are suitable for cation exchangers.

CHOICE OF OPERATING CONDITIONS

General Considerations

More often than not there is very little information available about the physical properties of the components of a mixture extracted from a biological source. Since the selection of a logical fractionation procedure must be based on such properties the choice of operating conditions for an ion-exchange experiment must be largely empirical. It is however advisable to acquire some information about the stability of the molecules of interest and the effect of pH, ionic strength and buffer composition on the solubility and 'activity'. In many cases one or more of the following precautions may be necessary; (1) rapid separation from proteolytic activities, (2) addition or removal (by chelation) of metal ions, (3) addition of sulphydryl compounds or antioxidants and (4) replacement of buffer ions that are likely to be used in the fractionation. Furthermore, it is not uncommon for biopolymers to become less stable as their purity increases and additional evaluation of operating conditions from the point of view of stability may then be necessary.

Choice of Adsorbent

Basically molecules which carry a net negative charge are chromatographed on anion-exchangers and molecules which carry a net positive charge are chromatographed on cation-exchangers. If ion-exchange fractionation has been preceded by electrophoresis valuable information concerning the distribution of charged species within a mixture may be available. For the preliminary fractionation, molecules that migrate towards the anode at neutral pH or above should be adsorbed on an anion exchanger at the same pH and those that migrate towards the cathode, or very slowly towards the anode, under such conditions should be adsorbed on a cation exchanger.

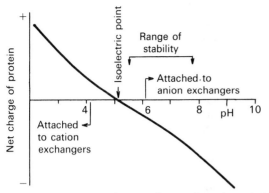

Fig. 4 The net charge of a protein as a function of pH.

An example of the way in which the net charge on a protein varies with pH is shown in Fig. 4. An arbitrary pH range of stability is shown and in this case restricts the choice of adsorbent to an anion exchanger. This example is not unusual since many proteins have a greater range of stability above their isoelectric points than below. For this reason anion exchangers (particularly DEAE-cellulose and DEAE-Sephadex) are by far the most widely used type of adsorbent for ion-exchange work.

The net charge on a molecule is not, however, the only critical factor. Affinity for a particular adsorbent can be determined by the most effective pattern of charges that can be presented by a molecule for interaction with the charges on the absorbent. For example, human carboxyhaemoglobin (isoelectric point 6·5) is tightly adsorbed to CM-cellulose at pH 7·0 in 0·01 M sodium phosphate, even though its net charge is negative. Some region of the surface of the molecule is presumably sufficiently positively charged to interact effectively with the negatively charged absorbent.

Definite information concerning the choice of ion-exchanger can be obtained from simple experiments on both anion and cation exchangers at the appropriate pH (about pH 8 for the anion exchanger test and pH 5 for the cation exchanger test). Measurements of absorbance at 280 nm may be sufficient to indicate uptake of protein by an ion-exchanger. If several proteins are present, determination of enzyme activities etc. may be necessary to provide specific information about the behaviour of the components of interest.

Choice of Buffer

The stability and solubility of the material to be fractionated often determines the operating pH for ion-exchange. This in itself restricts the choice of buffer species if good buffering action is to be provided. The exact pH and ionic strength are normally chosen so that the substances of interest are adsorbed but not too tightly. For cellulose ion-exchangers, a starting ionic strength of 0·001 to 0·01 M is not uncommon whereas an ionic strength of about 0·1 M is frequently used with Sephadex ion-exchangers.

It is often claimed that the use of a buffer system in which the buffering ion carries the same charge as the absorbent is an advantage (e.g. alkyl amines with DEAE-Sephadex, acetate with CM-Sephadex). Such practice would undoubtedly reduce the incidence of false pH and ionic strength fronts but would also eliminate many of the systems which have provided effective fractionation. Providing that adequate measures are taken to ensure equilibration and hence reproducibility the only real criterion for the evaluation of an ion-exchange system is its success and efficiency in performing the required separation.

COLUMN CHROMATOGRAPHY AND BATCH OPERATION

Bed Volume

The volume of adsorbent required for the fractionation of an adsorbed mixture depends on the available capacity of the adsorbent for the sample substances. Generally no more than 10–20% of the available capacity should be used and the choice of bed volume and sample size (amount) are interdependent. The available capacity can readily be determined by adding a quantity of adsorbent to an excess of the sample and measuring the uptake of material.

Overloading is one of the most common causes of unsatisfactory separation in ion-exchange chromatography and yet may be readily avoided.

Column Geometry

When the affinities of the substances to be fractionated are sufficiently different, adequate resolution may be obtained under conditions far removed from equilibrium elution, as when steep ionic strength gradients are employed. In this case column geometry is unimportant as far as resolution is concerned and the use of short, broad columns is advantageous practically. When the affinities of the substances for the adsorbent are closely similar, and an attempt is made to approach equilibrium elution, longer beds may be required. In a preliminary fractionation the choice of more conventional column geometry is advisable to prevent loss of resolution. Normally the conditions are such that the sample substances are adsorbed in the upper 1–2 cm of the ion-exchanger bed and a bed height of 20 cm is often sufficient. Column diameter can then be calculated on the basis of bed height and volume.

Packing the Column

Providing the column is mounted vertically and precautions are taken to ensure that air is not trapped under the bed support, few problems should arise in packing an ion-exchange column. The consistency of the suspension should be thick but not so thick that air bubbles are trapped by the ion-exchanger when it is poured. Packing from a thin suspension introduces problems of convection currents arising during sedimentation. Irregularities in ion-exchange gel beds can normally be seen in light transmitted from a lamp held behind the column.

Batch Operation

Batch ion-exchange procedures and stepwise column elution are essentially similar preparative rather than analytical fractionation methods. Either the substance of interest or the contaminants may be adsorbed by stirring the adsorbent (previously equilibrated) with the sample solution until the mixture has reached equilibrium which generally takes about 1 h. The slurry is then collected by filtering or centrifuging and washed with the appropriate buffer solutions.

Although batch procedures are less efficient than column techniques, they have certain practical advantages, particularly in pilot and production scale processes. Thus batch separation is a very rapid procedure requiring a minimum of specialized equipment and in which bed volume changes present no technical difficulties.

THE SAMPLE

Sample Size

The amount of sample that can be fractionated is dependent on the available capacity of the column. Either the column size or the amount of sample must be decided first. If the fractionation is to be performed under starting conditions the sample volume is important and must be determined in conjunction with the amount of sample. When gradient elution is employed, starting conditions are normally such that the substances of interest are adsorbed at the top of the bed. In this case the actual sample volume is of very little importance. For example, if a mixture of haemoglobins is to be fractionated on SP-Sephadex C-50 at least 0·7 g haemoglobin can be fractionated per g (dry weight) ion exchanger (0·7 g is 10% of the haemoglobin capacity of the ion exchanger). Whether the 0·7 g haemoglobin is applied in 2 ml or 50 ml is unimportant since all the protein will be bound at the top of the bed. In practice, this means that large volumes of dilute solutions (such as pooled fractions from a preceding gel filtration step) can be applied to the ion exchanger without a separate concentration step.

Sample Composition

The ionic composition (pH and ionic strength) of the sample should be the same as that of the starting buffer. If it is not it should be changed by gel filtration on Sephadex G-25, dialysis or possibly by simple dilution and pH adjustment. The latter procedure should not be used when resolution in the early part of the fractionation is important, and peaks eluted in the early part of a subsequent gradient must be evaluated with appropriate reservation.

Sample Application

When the adsorbent does not completely fill the column space the sample may be applied with a pipette or syringe to the drained surface of the bed. Alternatively, provided the sample is denser than the eluting buffer or is made denser by the addition of, for example, glucose, it may be layered carefully below excess eluant on top of the ion-exchanger. In either case even loading is the prime requirement and this is more likely to be achieved if the column outlet is first closed.

When the ion-exchanger bed completely fills the column space and is in contact with a fixed porous disc at the top and bottom the sample may be added directly through the feed tubing and this is often the most convenient arrangement.

ELUTION

Unadsorbed Components

Sample application should be followed with small initial washes with starting buffer and then by irrigation with a substantial volume of starting buffer. This volume should be sufficient to elute both unadsorbed and lightly adsorbed components and provides an opportunity to determine whether any of these substances migrate in adsorption equilibrium with the adsorbent under starting conditions. It also eliminates or diminishes any spurious pH or ionic strength fronts that might have arisen as a result of incomplete equilibration of the sample or changes accompanying the adsorption process. When the system is well characterized it may be possible to reduce the volume of starting buffer employed at this stage but preliminary experiments should be conducted as described above.

Gradient Elution

The range of adsorption affinities encountered in a mixture of biopolymers is almost invariably too great to permit differential elution of all components with a single eluant. Stepwise or continuous increases in ionic strength or changes in pH must therefore be used. Continuous pH gradients alone are rather difficult to produce since simultaneous changes in ionic strength, although small, normally occur. Linear pH gradients are not obtained by mixing buffers of different pH in linear volume ratio since the buffering capacities of the systems produced are pH dependent.

Stepwise pH gradients are rather easier to produce and may therefore be preferred. Continuous ionic strength gradients can be prepared by mixing two or more buffers of different ionic strength. If the volume ratio is changed linearly, the ionic strength is changed linearly. Convex gradients can readily be generated by means of a constant-volume mixing vessel. A two-chamber device (similar to those used for the generation of linear gradients) will produce concave gradients if the cross-sectional area of the mixing vessel is greater than that of the reservoir. When the object of a fractionation is to separate all the components of a complex mixture a 'shaped' or compound gradient may be required, whose shape must be determined by a succession of trials. A number of devices for the generation of compound gradients are now commercially available. The total volume of eluant in gradient elution should generally be 5–10 times the bed volume of the ion-exchanger.

Stepwise Elution

Stepwise ionic-strength elution is technically simpler than continuous gradient elution but it has disadvantages. Substances released from an adsorbent by a change of pH or ionic strength are eluted with sharp fronts. The appearance of false or spurious peaks may occur if a buffer change is introduced too early.

Flow-rate

Resolution in ion-exchange chromatography is critically dependent on flow-rate. For practical purposes the optimal linear flow-rate on, for example, Sephadex ion exchangers is 5–8 cm/h. A pronounced decrease in resolution may result if this flow-rate is significantly exceeded. This is illustrated in Fig. 5.

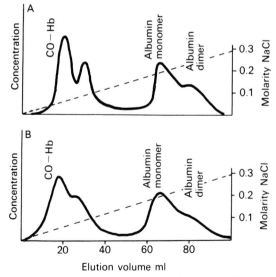

Fig. 5 Separation of haemoglobin and albumin on DEAE-Sephadex A-50. The sample consisted of a mixture of O_2-haemoglobin CO-haemoglobin, albumin monomer and albumin dimer. The two examples differed only in flow rate. In A flow rate was 8 cm/h and in B 20 cm/h.

The linear flow-rate (cm/h) is the same as flow in ml per cm^2 cross-sectional area per hour and is governed by: (1) particle size, (2) column geometry, (3) the pressure drop over the bed and (4) the eluant viscosity and other factors.

Variations in flow-rate due to absorbent volume changes can be eliminated by using a pump instead of gravity feed.

GEL FILTRATION
INTRODUCTION

Gel filtration is a chromatographic method in which materials are separated primarily on the basis of differences in molecular size and shape. Depending on which particular aspects of the method are being stressed a variety of names are used. Thus molecular-sieve chromatography, restricted-diffusion chromatography, exclusion chromatography, gel-permeation chromatography and gel chromatography are all commonly used terms. For historical reasons gel filtration continues to be the most widely used name despite the fact that the designation filtration is somewhat misleading.

Gel filtration gained remarkably rapid recognition as a standard procedure following its introduction in 1959. This is largely because the characteristic properties of the technique are just those required of a successful method for the fractionation of biopolymer mixtures. Thus gel filtration is technically simple to perform and is relatively insensitive to the composition of the eluant and to temperature. Conditions may generally be employed therefore, under which even the most labile components of a sample are not destroyed. In addition, variation of the gel matrix permits fractionation within very wide limits of molecular size. The most dense micro-reticular gels are capable of fractionating substances with molecular weights of up to 1000. At the other end of the scale, gels capable of fractionating particles and molecules with molecular weights of up to 40×10^6 are available.

The introduction of gel filtration also provided a new solution to some classical biochemical problems. Perhaps the best-known examples are the desalting of solutions of proteins and other high-molecular-weight substances, and the determination of molecular weights of macromolecules, particularly proteins.

Mechanism of Gel Filtration

For most groups of substances in gel filtration a very close correlation is found between molecular weight and elution behaviour, large molecules emerging first from the bed while smaller molecules are retarded. For practical purposes the elution volume is usually determined entirely by the molecular weight and this can be adequately explained by the simple steric model of gel filtration. According to this model the partition coefficient of a solute between the gel phase and the liquid phase is governed exclusively by steric effects. Steric restrictions to the mobility of solutes within the stationary phase may be considered to arise in various ways. In the case of crosslinked gels the gel-matrix occupies a great deal of space in the vicinity of the crosslinks and large molecules are unable to penetrate these regions. Alternatively the gel particles may be considered as rather solid spheres with conically shaped pores. Another approach considers the gel to be a matrix of randomly distributed straight rods of infinite length.

However they arise, such steric restrictions may be taken to divide the stationary phase into permitted and forbidden regions. The larger the molecular dimensions of a solute, the greater the proportion of the gel constituting the forbidden region. The solute is assumed to be evenly distributed between the interstitial liquid and the permitted region of the stationary phase. This model leads to the definition of a constant (K) for gel filtration as the fraction of the stationary phase volume accessible to a given molecular species.

The steric approach does not take account of other factors which can influence the distribution of a solute between the stationary and mobile phases. Particularly for gels of low water regain, which have a high content of gel matrix, the steric approach is unsatisfactory, because the effects on these gels of differences in the affinity of a solute for the solvent and the gel matrix are often just as great as the steric effects. There are considerable advantages in treating gel filtration as a kind of partition chromatography. A unified treatment becomes possible both for substances that behave as one would expect from steric considerations and for those with behaviour differing from that. In addition if K-values are not regarded as fractions of space in the gel but as partition coefficients, K-values of greater than 1 are no longer an anomaly. Since the partition isotherms are linear both for substances with high and for those with low K-values, such a treatment is also theoretically justified.

Definitions and Parameters

The flow rate through a chromatographic bed is usually measured in ml/min or ml/h. The linear flow rate or flow rate per unit cross-sectional area is a useful parameter which permits a direct comparison of experiments performed on columns of different diameter. Linear flow rate has units $ml/h/cm^2$ or cm/h. The linear rate of migration of a substance that is completely excluded is obtained by dividing the linear flow rate by the fraction of the bed volume that is occupied by the interstitial space.

V_t— *total bed volume.* For practical reasons in accurate work this parameter should be determined directly rather than calculated from column dimensions.

V_0—the *void volume.* This is the volume of liquid in the interstitial space between the gel beads. It can be determined by measuring the elution volume of a substance that is not retarded by the bed material (i.e. that is completely excluded). High molecular weight proteins or a material especially intended for this purpose, Blue dextran 2000 (mol wt 2×10^6, Pharmacia) may be used for V_0 determinations.

V_x—the *volume of the gel phase.* This is obtained as the difference between the total bed volume and the void volume

$$V_x = V_t - V_0.$$

V_i— the *inner volume.* This is the partial volume of liquid in the gel phase and can be estimated by subtracting the partial volume of the gel matrix from the volume of the gel phase.

$$V_i = V_x - M_g V_g$$

where M_g is the weight and the V_g the partial specific volume of the gel matrix. This parameter may also be obtained as

$$V_i = M_g W_r$$

where W_r is the water regain of the gel. Since accurate determinations of W_r are difficult to perform this equation is of limited value.

V_i— the *inner volume.* This is the partial volume of most important variable and is determined directly from the raw data obtained from an experiment (a plot of some variable related to solute concentration versus effluent volume). For small sample volumes that can be neglected in comparison with V_e, the volume of liquid that has passed through the column between sample application and the elution of the maximum concentration of substance is the elution volume, if the elution curve is symmetrical. If the sample volume is so large that the elution curve reaches a plateau region, the elution volume is that volume eluted from the onset of sample application to the inflection point, or half height, of the elution curve (*see* Fig. 9). For samples of intermediate size, not forming plateau regions in their elution curves, the elution volume should be measured from the point where half the sample volume has been applied until the maximum of the elution curve is reached.

The elution volume can be used to characterize a substance but is of limited significance as it depends on the geometry and packing characteristics of the chromatographic bed. The theory of partition chromatography provides a correlation between elution behaviour and the partition coefficient (K) of a solute between the stationary and mobile phases.

$$V_e = V_0 + KV_s,$$

where V_s is the volume of the stationary phase. The partition coefficient derived from this equation is the most useful parameter for characterizing the behaviour of a given solute.

In gel filtration, two different partition coefficients are used depending on the definition of the stationary phase. If the entire gel phase is assumed to be the stationary phase the partition coefficient (K_{av}) is given by:

$$K_{av} = \frac{V_e - V_0}{V_x}$$

If, on the other hand, only the liquid imbibed in the gel is assumed to be the stationary phase the partition coefficient (K_d) is given by:

$$K_d = \frac{V_e - V_0}{V_i}$$

K_{av} and K_d are useful theoretically for the characterization of a substance. From a practical standpoint K_{av} is often preferable as the determination of V_i involves measurements with considerable uncertainties. However, for historical reasons, K_d has been much used and is found in many of the early papers on gel filtration.

Graphical Representation

Several graphical representations for the relationship between molecular size and gel filtration behaviour have been proposed. For practical purposes the most useful presentation is one in which a parameter linearly related to the elution volume, such as K_{av}, is plotted as a function of molecular weight on a logarithmic scale (Fig. 6).

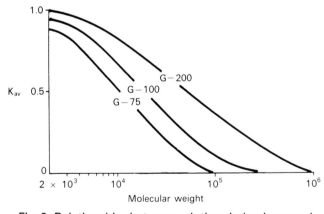

Fig. 6 Relationship between elution behaviour and molecular weight (on a logarithmic scale) for globular proteins on Sephadex G-75, G-100 and G-200.

The advantages of this method of presentation are that the errors are relatively constant along both axes and a clear picture is given of the working ranges of the various gels. The central part of the curve has a negative slope and a variation in molecular weight here corresponds to a variation in elution volume. The slope of the curve is a very important characteristic for a given gel. A gel that has a very steep curve within the working range will be very effective for the fractionation of substances within that range. However, the fractionation range will be much narrower for this type of gel. A reasonable compromise between steepness and fractionation range is obviously desirable.

GEL FILTRATION MEDIA

Gel Classification

The types of gel which are important in gel filtration are xerogels, aerogels and xerogel–aerogel hybrids. Xerogels, which are gels in the classical sense, shrink on drying to a compact material, containing only the gel matrix. Aerogels, strictly speaking, are not gels at all and on drying do not shrink. Instead the surrounding air penetrates into the gel.

Xerogels were the first gels to be used in gel filtration. A xerogel typically consists of a solution of linear macromolecules whose movement, relative to one another, is restricted either by crosslinking or by physical interaction. Such a gel is partly solvent and partly a three-dimensional space network of solvated polymer chains. Although xerogels generally appear to be soft-solids, diffusion of various solutes may occur within the gel, just as in the case of a normal liquid. Aqueous gels based on crosslinked dextran and crosslinked polyacrylamide are typical examples. Gelation is necessarily a process of restricted dissolution and a given polymer matrix will form gels in the range of solvents in which the individual polymer chains are soluble.

Aerogels typically consist of a rigid preformed matrix containing pores into which a solvent has been introduced (e.g. porous glass). Aerogel formation does not depend on restricted dissolution of the matrix which will, therefore, form aerogels in any solvent.

Xerogel–Aerogel hybrids have features common to both xerogels and aerogels. The polymer matrix from which they are formed is frequently a semi-rigid structure which undergoes minimal dissolution on constituting the gel. Agarose gels and crosslinked polystyrene, produced by a macroreticular polymerization technique, are typical examples.

From the point of view of chromatographic properties the distinction between macroreticular and microreticular gels is important. Macroreticular gels have properties which indicate that the microstructure is strongly heterogeneous, with regions where the matrix material is aggregated and regions where there is very little gel matrix present. This type of structure, with large spaces within the gel virtually free from gel matrix gives rise to gel filtration media with very high exclusion limits. In contrast, microreticular gels have properties that indicate that the gel matrix is relatively evenly distributed. They fractionate in lower-molecular-weight ranges than macrore-

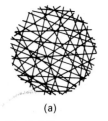 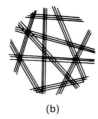

(a)   (b)

Fig. 7 Microstructure of a typical micro-reticular xerogel (a) and of agarose (b), macroreticular xerogel–aerogel hybrid.

ticular gels and are usually softer. The macroreticular gels are usually aerogels or xerogel–aerogel hybrids, while the microreticular gels usually seem to be xerogels. Examples of the microstructure of each type are shown in Fig. 7.

Commercial Gel Filtration Media

Relatively few of the large number of gels that exist or could be synthesized, are suitable for gel filtration. The following practical requirements are met by most of the commercially available gel-filtration media.

The matrix of the gel must be inert, in order to minimize chemical interaction between the bed material and the solutes; such interaction might lead to irreversible binding of solutes to the bed material or to chemical alteration of labile substances. Weak reversible interactions between a solute and the matrix give rise to larger elution volumes than would be expected from a knowledge of molecular size and steric model of gel filtration. Such weak interactions (e.g. those between aromatic substances and dextran or polyacrylamide gels in aqueous solution) may occasionally improve the separation of substances which are difficult to fractionate purely on the basis of size.

The gels should be chemically stable to permit re-use over a period of months or years. A reasonable range of pH and temperature stability is desirable to permit free choice of working conditions. In addition, leaching of material from the bed should be as low as possible to minimize contamination of fractionated substances with leached materials.

A low content of ionic groups is required to avoid ion-exchange effects. It is impossible to avoid charged groups completely but a working ionic strength of 0·02 or higher is generally sufficient to avoid ion-exchange or ion-exclusion effects.

The particle size distribution should be carefully controlled. Large particle sizes give rise to zone broadening and loss of resolution, but resistance to flow is greater with small particle sizes. Consequently it is necessary to reach some compromise between zone resolution and required flow characteristics.

Crosslinked Polyacrylamide—Bio-Gel P. Bio-Gel P
is a bead-formed, crosslinked polyacrylamide prepared by suspension polymerization of acrylamide

and N,N-methylene-bis-acrylamide in aqueous solution. The matrix is inert and intensely hydrophilic, readily forming xerogels in water but not in organic solvents.

The polyacrylamide matrix is chemically stable under normal operating conditions but at extremes of pH the primary amide residues undergo hydrolysis to carboxylic acid groups. Such extremes of pH however are not normally encountered in gel filtration. Since polyacrylamide copolymers are synthetic they are very resistant to attack by microorganisms.

Crosslinked Dextran—Sephadex. Sephadex, crosslinked dextran gels were the first gels to have their chromatographic behaviour systematically investigated and exploited. Dextran is a linear glucose polymer in which the glucose units are joined by α-1,6-glucosidic linkages. The dextran used for the manufacture of Sephadex has rather infrequent branches joined to the main chain by 1,3-glucosidic linkages. Sephadex is prepared in bead form by carrying out a crosslinking reaction with epichlorhydrin in an aqueous mixture dispersed as droplets in a cold organic solvent. Crosslinked dextran is much less sensitive to extremes of pH than crosslinked polyacrylamide but is degraded by strong mineral acids due to hydrolysis of the glucosidic linkages. The matrix is to some extent susceptible to attack by oxidizing agents and microorganisms.

Sephadex is the most popular chromedium for aqueous gel filtration. It does not swell substantially, and is thus not useful, in the common organic solvents. However, it will form xerogels in formamide, dimethylformamide and dimethyl sulphoxide, although the solvent regain in these solvents is not equivalent to the water regain. Sephadex LH-20 is the hydroxypropyl ether of Sephadex G-25. The letters L and H signify that the matrix is compatible with both lipophilic and hydrophilic solvents. Maximum swelling takes place in dimethylsulphoxide and pyridine followed by dimethyl formamide, water and methanol. The matrix is less expanded in chloroform and still less in tetrahydrofuran. The derived xerogels are all suitable for gel filtration, however. The exclusion limit for Sephadex LH-20 is generally quoted as about 5000. This limit varies considerably from solvent to solvent depending on the degree of swelling and is therefore very approximate.

Agarose Gels—Sepharose, Bio-Gel A, Sagavac and Gelarose. Agarose is a seaweed polysaccharide consisting of alternating 1,3-linked β-D-galactose and 1,4-linked 3,6-anhydro-α-L-galactose residues. Agarose is soluble in hot water, and on cooling, gelation occurs. Gelation of agarose in bead form is induced by dispersing a hot, aqueous solution of the polysaccharide as droplets in a cold polar organic solvent (Sepharose, Bio-Gel A, and Gelarose). Sagavac is supplied in the form of crushed particles.

Gelation of agarose involves hydrogen bonding

between the individual polysaccharide chains which leads to linear agglomeration and the formation of microscopic strands. This results in a matrix of considerable mechanical stability but large pore size. The effective pore size of a xerogel–aerogel hybrid such as agarose depends less on the nature of the solvent than in the case of a xerogel. Consequently agarose gels do not shrink drastically on equilibration with polar organic solvents such as acetone, ethanol and methanol. Agarose gels do however, 'melt' on heating which can be a disadvantage.

Crosslinked Agarose Gels—Sepharose CL. Sepharose CL is prepared from Sepharose by reaction with 2,3-dibromo-propanol under strongly alkaline conditions. This produces a crosslinked agarose gel with substantially the same porosity as the parent gel, but with greatly increased thermal and chemical stability. The material may be used at temperatures of up to 100°C, in strongly denaturing media in the range pH 3–14 and most organic solvents. The exclusion limits for proteins and dextrans in aqueous solution are the same as for the parent Sepharose gels.

Fractionation Ranges of Commercial Gels

The fractionation ranges and some properties of the most widely used commercial gel filtration media are summarized in Table 5.

EXPERIMENTAL TECHNIQUE

The Gel

For methodological purposes it is useful to distinguish two types of gel filtration separation; group separation and fractionation.

In *group separation*, substances are separated into a few large groups. Frequently there will be just two groups, those substances of larger molecular weight which are excluded from the gel and eluted in the void volume (V_0), and low-molecular-weight substances which permeate the gel phase virtually completely and are eluted at a volume close to the total bed volume (V_t). This type of separation is often referred to as desalting, even when no salts are involved, since one of the most common applications is the removal of salts from protein solutions. Gels suitable for this purpose are Sephadex G-25 and G-50 and Bio-Gel P-6 and P-10. For desalting peptides and other materials in the molecular weight range 1000–5000 Sephadex G-10 and G-15 and Bio-Gel P-2 and P-4 are suitable. Since the separation of compounds of high and low molecular weight is very good, large sample volumes may be used, often up to 30% of the total bed volume (V_t).

In group separation, the high-molecular-weight substances fall on the horizontal part of the fractionation curve (*see* Fig. 6) at $K_{av} = 0$. Low-molecular-weight substances fall on the horizontal part of the curve close to $K_{av} = 1$. Ideally no substance should fall on the inclined part of the curve.

In *fractionation*, the substances to be separated are more closely similar and a gel should be chosen so that the substances fall within the fractionation range of the gel, i.e. on the inclined part of the fractionation curve. Generally the component(s) of interest should fall fairly close to the exclusion limit of the gel since the peaks are sharper and the resolution greater in this situation.

Sephadex and Bio-Gel are supplied as dry powders and before use must be swollen in the eluant solution. The most convenient method is to warm a slurry of the gel in a boiling-water bath to a temperature close to 100°C, when the swelling will be complete in a couple of hours rather than days (for loosely cross-linked gels). Additional advantages of this method are probable sterilization and de-aeration of the slurry which makes a separate de-gassing operation unnecessary. If the eluant solution is unstable to heating, the gel should be swollen in hot distilled water and, after cooling, washed repeatedly with de-aerated eluant.

Agarose gels are supplied swollen and only require equilibration with solvent before use. 'Fines' should be removed from all gels at this point in the procedure if necessary. After gentle stirring the gel is allowed to sediment and the 'fines' and supernatant removed by decanting or under vacuum. It may be necessary to repeat this procedure.

Prevention of Microbial Growth. Microbial growth rarely occurs in running columns but steps should always be taken to prevent infection of packed columns and gel suspensions during storage. Sodium azide (NaN_3) 0·02% is very widely used. It does not interact noticeably with proteins or carbohydrates or affect their chromatographic behaviour. Sodium azide does however interfere with fluorescent labelling of proteins, the anthrone reaction, and inhibits certain enzymes. Chloretone (trichlorobutanol) 0·05% and merthiolate (ethyl mercuric thiosalicylate) 0·005% are most effective in weakly acidic solutions. Hibitane (chlorhexidine), 0·002% is an extremely effective antimicrobial agent which is compatible with most substances.

The Column

A variety of chromatographic columns are now commercially available, most of which possess the following required features. (1) Precision bore tubing and a dead space volume at the outlet which is less than 0·1% of the column volume. This minimizes dilution and prevents remixing. (2) A suitable bed support (e.g. nylon fabric) which does not clog during use. (3) Flow adaptors (i.e. an adjustable end piece) to permit upward flow experiments and automatic or semi-automatic sample application.

TABLE 5
COMMERCIAL GEL FILTRATION MEDIA

Trade name and manufacturer	Nature	Operating solvents	Fractionation range or exclusion limit	
Bio-Rad Labs				
Bio-Gel P2	Cross-linked	Aqueous	200–	2 500
Bio-Gel P4	Polyacrylamide		500–	4 000
Bio-Gel P6			1 000–	5 000
Bio-Gel P10			5 000–	17 000
Bio-Gel P30			20 000–	50 000
Bio-Gel P60			30 000–	70 000
Bio-Gel P100			40 000–	100 000
Bio-Gel P150			50 000–	150 000
Bio-Gel P200			80 000–	300 000
Bio-Gel P300			100 000–	400 000
			(refers to peptides and proteins)	
Pharmacia Fine Chemicals, AB				
Sephadex G–10	Cross-linked	Aqueous	–	700
Sephadex G–15	dextran	(DMF)	–	1 000
Sephadex G–25	(xerogel)	(DMSO)	1 000–	5 000
Sephadex G–50			1 500–	30 000
Sephadex G–75			3 000–	70 000
Sephadex G–100			4 000–	150 000
Sephadex G–150			5 000–	400 000
Sephadex G–200			5 000–	800 000
			(refers to peptides and proteins)	
Sephadex LH–20	Hydroxypropyl ether of Sephadex G–25 (xerogel)	Polar-organic	up to 5 000 (Solvent dependent)	
Bio-Rad Labs.				
Bio-Gel A–0·5	Agarose gel	Aqueous	10 000–	500 000
Bio-Gel A–1·5			10 000–	1 500 000
Bio-Gel A–5	(xerogel–aerogel		10 000–	5 000 000
Bio-Gel A–15	hybrid)		40 000–	15 000 000
Bio-Gel A–50			100 000–	50 000 000
Bio-Gel A–150			1 000 000–	150 000 000
			(refers to dextrans in water)	
Pharmacia Fine Chemicals AB				
Sepharose 6B	Agarose gel	Aqueous	4 000 000	
Sepharose 4B	(xerogel–aerogel		20 000 000	
Sepharose 2B	hybrid)		40 000 000	
			(refers to proteins)	
Sepharose Cl–6b	Cross-linked	Aqueous or	4 000 000	
–4b	Agarose gel	Organic	20 000 000	
–2b	(xerogel–aerogel hybrid)		40 000 000	
			(refers to proteins)	

Column Dimensions. The length of a column determines the resolution that can be obtained. The resolution of small samples will generally be improved approximately in relation to the square root of the length of the bed. Long columns however, imply greater dilution and longer running times. The appropriate column length for a given application is usually found by systematic trial and error. As a general guide a bed length of 20–30 cm is usually sufficient for group separation experiments. Bed lengths of about 100 cm are used in many fractionation experiments but may occasionally be as long as 200 or 300 cm. Such long columns are however rather difficult to handle and if a very long bed length is required it may be more convenient to connect a number of columns in series or use a recycling system.

A column diameter of about 1 cm is usual for analytical gel filtration. Narrower columns are used but wall effects begin to affect resolution at very small diameters. Very narrow columns are useful only when the amount of sample available is very limited.

In preparative applications the column diameter

is chosen to give the column sufficient capacity. Increasing the column diameter does not impair resolution even at very large diameters, although columns with diameters of 5 cm or more should preferably be equipped with flow adaptors to permit an even application of sample over the whole bed surface. Columns for gel filtration are commercially available in a range of diameter from about 1–180 cm.

Packing the Column. Most gels are best packed from a moderately thick suspension in which convection currents will be minimized. In general a volume of supernatant of 30–50% of the volume of settled gel will give a suspension of suitable thickness when stirred. The suspension should not be so thick that air bubbles are retained.

The column should be filled in one continuous operation either by pouring down a glass rod or down the inclined wall of the column. If necessary an extension tube should be used to avoid packing the column in sections since this procedure is likely to give rise to uneven beds.

After the slurry has been poured, flow through the column may be started. The flow rate at this stage should not too high and in all circumstances should be lower than the flow rate to be used during normal operation of the column. Flow rates and operating pressures are of great importance in gel filtration and the manufacturers' literature should always be consulted for information concerning limiting values of these parameters for each individual gel. Examples of the operating pressures resulting in maximum flow rates for some of the Sephadex gels are as follows: Sephadex G-200: 10% of bed height; Sephadex G-150: 15% of bed height; Sephadex G-100: 30% of bed height and Sephadex G-75: 100% of bed height (these values refer to columns with diameters up to 5 cm and lengths of up to 100 cm).

The Sample

Sample Composition. One of the principal advantages of gel filtration is the relative insensitivity of the method to sample composition. The concentration of sample that can be used is limited however, by the effect of viscosity on resolution and by solubility. A high sample viscosity causes instability of the sample zone and an irregular flow pattern. This leads to very broad and skew zones. The critical variable is the viscosity of the sample relative to the eluant; this is illustrated in Fig. 8.

Sample Size. For analytical purposes the starting zone should be as narrow as possible. A sample volume of 2–5% of the total bed volume is generally satisfactory. Using a sample volume of less than 1–2% of the bed volume does not improve the separation result.

On a preparative scale, where the objective is to

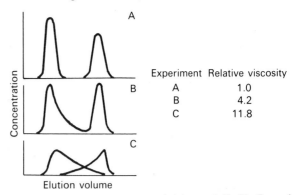

Experiment	Relative viscosity
A	1.0
B	4.2
C	11.8

Fig. 8 Separation of haemoglobin and NaCl. Experimental conditions were identical except that the viscosities were increased by adding increasing amounts of dextran. A progressive deterioration of the separation is apparent.

obtain the maximum yield with a given degree of separation, the sample should obviously be made as large as possible.

The volume which separates the elution front of one substance from that of another, i.e. the difference between their elution volumes, is called the separation volume.

$$V_{sep} = V'_e - V''_e = V_s (K' - K'')$$

Theoretically the sample size could be as large as the separation volume. Microturbulence, non-equilibrium, elution and longitudinal diffusion give rise to zone broadening however, and the sample size must therefore be smaller than the separation volume. This is illustrated in Fig. 9.

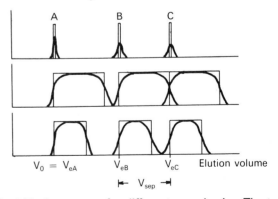

Fig. 9 Elution curves for different sample size. The top diagram corresponds to the application of a small sample. The centre diagram corresponds to the maximum sample size giving complete separation if no zone broadening were to take place. The bottom diagram corresponds to the maximum sample volume to be applied to obtain complete separation under experimental conditions. The rectangular areas correspond to the elution profiles that would be obtained if no zone broadening were to take place.

Sample Application. The simplest method of sample application is careful layering of the sample onto the drained bed surface followed by washing with a small amount of eluant. This method is perfectly satisfactory but demands technical skill.

A sharp zone can also be obtained by layering the sample on top of the gel bed, underneath the eluant. The sample must be denser than the eluant; if necessary this can be achieved by the addition of a small amount of glucose or another suitable inert material. No rinsing is required after sample application by this method since the sample is quantitatively transported into the gel bed by the eluant.

Perhaps the most convenient method of sample application is with a flow adaptor; this is the only method possible in upward-flow elution. Samples may be applied either directly through the adaptor capillary tubing or by a semi-automatic procedure if this tubing is connected to a three-way valve.

Elution

In most cases solute molecules and the gel matrix have a higher affinity for water than for each other. For practical purposes the gel matrix is shielded by a hydration layer and this is probably the reason why gels that are chemically very different have chromatographic properties which are so similar (e.g. Sephadex and Bio-Gel P). This would also explain why differences in the chemical nature of the solutes make so little difference to their chromatographic characteristics permitting elution of a gel filtration column with a single irrigant, i.e. without the necessity for gradient elution.

Completely uncharged substances can be eluted with distilled water. Substances bearing charged groups should be chromatographed at an ionic strength of 0·02 or greater since most gel filtration media contain a small number of charged groups. The separation volume in group separation is generally so large that charged substances can also be eluted with distilled water. A complete removal of salt may not be possible but the amount of ions excluded, and therefore eluted in the high-molecular-weight fraction, is so small that it can usually be neglected.

The flow of liquid in gel filtration can be produced either by hydrostatic pressure or by a pump. When the flow is maintained by gravity feed a constant pressure flask (Mariotte flask) should be used as a reservoir. In the case of a Mariotte flask the operating pressure corresponds to the vertical distance between the lower end of the flask air inlet tube and the free end of the column outlet tubing.

When a pump is used (e.g. where the constancy of flow obtained with gravity feed is unsatisfactory) it should be a precision metering pump. For laboratory scale work peristaltic pumps are usually satisfactory. In this case the flow rate should not exceed approximately 70% of the flow rate obtainable under gravity feed.

High flow rates and coarse bed material (large particle size) invariably give rise to zone broadening,

especially in small columns with small samples. For analytical purposes the smallest suitable particle size and minimum convenient flow rate should be used. The effects of flow rate and particle size are shown in Figs 10 and 11 respectively. For preparative purposes the convenience of rapid separation often outweighs the consequent loss of resolution.

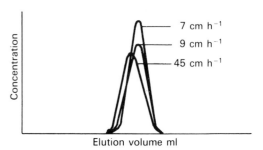

Fig. 10 Elution profiles of glucose on Sephadex G-25 at different flow rates. A slight displacement of the peak is observed, indicating that a complete diffusion equilibrium has not been attained.

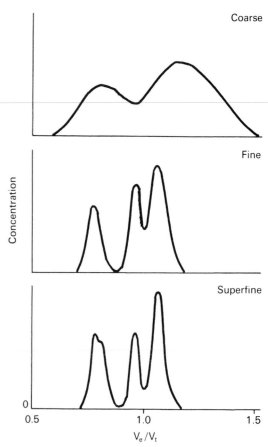

Fig. 11 Gel filtration of cytidylic acid, cytidine and cytosine on Sephadex G-25 of different grades. On the coarse grade only cytosine and cytidylic acid were chromatographed.

FURTHER READING

Determann H. (1968). *Gel Chromatography*. New York: Springer Verlag.

Fischer L. (1969). An introduction to gel chromatography. In *Laboratory Techniques in Biochemistry and Molecular Biology*, Vol. 1, pp. 157–396. (Work T. S., Work E., eds). Amsterdam and London: North Holland Publishing Co.

Giddings J. C. (1965). *Dynamics of Chromatography. Part I, Principles and Theory*. New York: Dekker.

Lederer E., Lederer M. (1962). Ion exchange chromatography. In *Comprehensive Biochemistry*, Vol. 4, pp. 107–150. (Florkin M., Stotz E. H., eds). Amsterdam, London and New York: Elsevier.

Osborn G. H. (1961). *Synthetic Ion Exchangers*, 2nd edn, London: Chapman and Hall.

Peterson E. A. (1970). Cellulose ion exchangers. In *Laboratory Techniques in Biochemistry and Molecular Biology*, Vol. 2, pp. 223–400. (Work T. S., Work E., eds). Amsterdam and London: North Holland Publishing Co.

25. Affinity Chromatography
Yannis D. Clonis and C. R. Lowe

INTRODUCTION

Progress in biotechnology may be largely attributed to the development of modern purification and analytical techniques. The isolation of individual substances, such as enzymes from complex biological mixtures has been performed traditionally by conventional techniques whose resolving power relies upon differences in the overall physicochemical properties of the molecules to be isolated. However, the tertiary structure of enzymes not only dictates their physicochemical properties but also endows them with biological specificity. The technique of affinity chromatography resolves and purifies enzymes and other proteins by exploiting this biological specificity as expressed in binding substrates, coenzymes, allosteric effectors, metal cations and other ligands specifically and reversibly. The technique is realized by chemically immobilizing the ligand often via a spacer molecule to a water-insoluble hydrophilic polymeric matrix and packing it into a chromatographic column (Fig. 1). In principle, only enzymes or proteins which

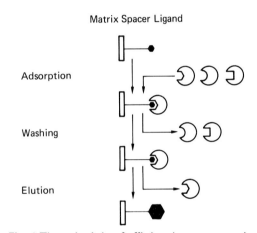

Fig. 1 The principle of affinity chromatography.

display appreciable affinity for the immobilized ligand will be retained on such a column, whilst other biological molecules displaying little or no affinity will pass through unretarded. The specifically adsorbed protein can then subsequently be released by altering the mobile (liquid) phase to favour dissociation of the bound complex. In principle, the technique can be applied in all cases where a ligand specifically and reversibly interacts with a complementary biomolecule. Thus, affinity chromatography has been applied to resolve and purify proteins, glycoproteins, enzymes, antibodies, peptide hormones, polynucleotides, nucleic acids, glycolipids, polysaccharides, receptors, viruses, subcellular particles and whole cells.

The potentially facile, rapid and almost quantitative isolation of the desired biomolecule from the bulk of contaminants depends largely on how closely the chosen experimental conditions allow the ligand–

TABLE 1

EXAMPLES OF THE USE OF GROUP-SPECIFIC LIGANDS IN AFFINITY CHROMATOGRAPHY

Immobilized ligand	*Biomolecule specificity*
Amino acids and their analogues Arginine, aspartate, histidine, lysine, phenylalanine, tryptophan	Amino acid-binding enzymes (e.g. certain synthetases and transferases), some plasma proteases and factors (e.g. plasminogen, plasminogen activator, prekallikrein, prothrombin, maturation promoting factor), bromelain, carboxypeptidase, chymotrypsin
Boronic acid analogues e.g. *p*-aminophenylboronic acid	Glycoproteins, nucleic acid components, sugars and other polyols. General support for polyolic ligands in affinity chromatography
Calmodulin	Calmodulin-binding enzymes (e.g. several protein kinases, ATPases, phosphodiesterases, neurotransmission-system proteins and spectrins)
Coenzymes and their analogues Biotin, cobalamin, flavin, folates, porphyrins, lipoic acid, pyridoxal coenzymes	Complementary enzymes and proteins, (e.g. avidin, ribonucleotide reductase, flavokinase, dihydrofolate reductase, haemopexin, lipoamide dehydrogenase, glutamic-oxalo-acetic apotransaminase)
Heparin	Coagulation proteins, lipoproteins, lipases, nucleic acid-binding enzymes (e.g. restriction endonucleases)
Lectins e.g. Castor bean, concanavalin A, *H. pomatia*, horseshoe crab, *L. culinaris*, peanut, pea, soyabean, wheat germ	Glycoproteins, glycolipids, polysaccharides, subcellular particles and cells
Nucleic acids, oligo- and poly-nucleotides DNA, oligo- and poly-dA, dC, dG, dI, dT, A, C, G, I, T	DNA and RNA-binding proteins, DNA, RNA, complementary nucleotide sequences
Nucleotides and nucleotide coenzymes Mono-, di-, tri-phosphoanalogues of adenosine, cytidine, guanosine, inosine, thymidine, uridine. Coenzyme A, nicotinamide adenine- and nicotinamide adenine phosphate-nucleotide (NAD^+ and $NADP^+$)	Nucleotide-binding enzymes (e.g. dehydrogenases, kinases, synthetases, transferases, DNases and RNases)
Organomercurials e.g. aminophenylmercuric acetate, chloromercuric acetate, chloromercuribenzoate	Binding by covalent mercaptide bond to biomolecules with free sulphydryl functions (e.g. cathepsin, deaminase, DNA polymerase, papain, platelet factor)
Protease-binding ligands Aminobenzamidine, trypsin inhibitor	Various proteases (e.g. chymotrypsin, endopeptidase, enterokinase, human complement factor, thrombin, urokinase)
Protein A	IgG, IgG subclasses and fragments
Triazine dyes Cibacron blue F3G-A and 3G-A, Procion range (e.g. yellow MX-8G, brown MX-5BR, orange MX-G, red H-3B, red H-E3B, red H-8BN, blue H-B, blue MX-3G, blue MX-4GD, green H-4G, green H-E4BD	Nucleotide- and nucleic acid-binding enzymes, albumin, coagulation factors, interferons

chlorohydrin, bis-oxiranes 1,1'-carbonyldiimidazole, 1,3,5-trichloro-*s*-triazine, tosyl chloride and tresyl chloride are popular choices.

The importance of the immobilized ligand concentration (μmol ligand/g moist gel) on the successful application of the affinity adsorbent necessitates an accurate method for determining the bound ligand. Depending on the resistance of the gel to chemical hydrolysis and the stability of the ligand under the conditions employed, one may usually choose either to hydrolyse the gel completely in acid or alkali at elevated temperatures and subsequently measure the absorbance of the neutralized solution at the $\lambda_{max.}$ of the ligand or to suspend the gel intact in glycerol (50%(v/v)) or DMSO (usually for silica-based matrices) and read the absorbance against unmodified gel treated in the same way. In both procedures, the extinction coefficient of the immobilized ligand must be known. Alternatively, ligand concentration may be measured radioactively or fluorophotometrically.

ADSORPTION OF THE COMPLEMENTARY MACROMOLECULE

Optimal conditions for adsorption of the complementary protein to the immobilized ligand are governed partly by its interaction with the ligand. The buffer used to equilibrate the column, its ionic strength, pH and temperature should reflect both the stability range of the macromolecule and the optimal conditions for the enzyme–ligand interaction. The sample to be applied should be dialysed against the equilibrating buffer prior to its application to the column and following the passage of several column volumes of buffer through the gel bed to remove non-adsorbed proteins, the desired protein can be eluted by a change in the irrigant solution. However, there are several parameters which influence the adsorption of macromolecules to affinity matrices.

Column Geometry

The interaction between a complementary protein and an immobilized ligand can be profoundly influenced not only by the concentration of the ligand but also by the total amount of ligand contained within the gel bed and its geometrical disposition. Particularly, for interacting systems of low affinity the length of gel bed through which the enzyme percolates may be a critical parameter for reproducible purifications. Optimum column dimensions will depend on the enzyme under examination, the adsorbent and the conditions of elution. Nevertheless, in many cases, 'short' and 'wide' beds are used.

Dynamic Factors

In some cases the adsorption equilibrium between the specific ligand and the complementary protein is reached at a very slow rate. This is because it is essential for the active site of the protein to be in close alignment with the specific ligand for adsorption to occur. Also the restriction of static films around the solid support means that diffusion is an important factor in the overall kinetics of the reaction. For these reasons it is desirable to use the lowest practicable flow rate, particularly when columns are being loaded with large amounts of protein. Thus the appearance of traces of enzyme in the void volume, when samples containing high concentrations of enzyme are applied at high flow rates, can often be prevented by using lower flow rates or by applying more dilute enzyme samples. Alternatively, the complementary macromolecule may be applied and left in contact with the column material for some time prior to elution. This treatment may improve the subsequent resolution achieved on elution.

Protein Concentration

Under quasi-equilibrium conditions, the applied sample becomes more concentrated until a sufficiently strong interaction with the ligand arrests the downward migration of the enzyme through the column. The adsorbed enzyme thus appears as a narrow zone at the top of the column and while for interacting systems of moderate affinity this process is critically dependent on ligand concentration, it is virtually independent of the initial concentration of the free macromolecule. Furthermore, experience has shown that generally the adsorption of a complementary macromolecule is independent of the presence or absence of inert proteins. The chromatographic behaviour of a purified protein often parallels the behaviour of the same protein in a crude tissue extract.

Biospecific Effects

Incorporation of a counter ligand that enhances the binding of the enzyme to the immobilized ligand, provides a means of increasing the selectivity of the adsorption process. Thus, bovine carboxypeptidase B(EC 3.4.12.3) is strongly bound to agarose–phenylalanine only in the presence of a lysine analogue at low concentration. Similarly, yeast hexokinase binds to agarose–Procion green H-4G only in the presence of Mg^{2+} ions. In both examples, removal of the free counter ligand elutes the enzyme from the adsorbent. Many more similar examples may be found in the literature.

ELUTION OF THE ADSORBED MACROMOLECULE

The elution conditions chosen, whether performed isocratically, pulse-wise or by forming a gradient, should be tolerable by the affinity adsorbent and effective in desorbing the biomolecule, undenatured and in good yield. Elution methods can be divided into non-specific and biospecific methods. The former involve: (1) changing the ionic strength; usually by increasing the buffer's molarity or including salt, (2) altering the polarity of the irrigating buffer by employing, for example, ethylene glycol or organic solvents, (3) introducing chaotropic agents such as urea or thiocyanate, or varying (4) the pH or (5) the temperature.

Non-specific elution methods, although economical, result in co-elution of proteins non-specifically bound to the adsorbent and thus compromise the purity of the final product. Such methods are better suited to high affinity systems, whereas, for group-specific affinity adsorbents, which inherently exhibit decreased adsorption selectivity, biospecific elution methods are recommended.

These are realized by introducing free ligand(s) which either compete with the immobilized ligand for the same site in binding the complementary enzyme or forming with the adsorbed enzyme such a complex that weakens the immobilized ligand–enzyme interaction. The free ligand or mixture of ligands should preferably be different and exhibit higher affinity than the immobilized ligand; 'double specificity' is thus employed during the adsorption–desorption processes. For example, the high affinity of lactate dehydrogenase for NADH and immobilized AMP was successfully exploited in the resolution of the five isoenzymes from an agarose-immobilized N^6-(6-aminohexyl)-AMP adsorbent by an NADH gradient. Alternatively, lactate dehydrogenase was recovered from the same affinity adsorbent by a mixture of NAD^+ and pyruvate whilst NAD^+ alone proved ineffective. Likewise, adenylosuccinate synthetase was quantitatively eluted from agarose–Procion blue H–B only in the presence of all three substrates, IMP, GTP and L-aspartate. However, if the adsorption process was promoted by a free counter ligand such as a metal ion, then by omitting that ligand or by using chelating agents (EDTA), elution of the enzyme can be effected. This method is called 'negative elution' and has proved particularly effective in some cases. For example, RNA ligase adsorbed on ADP–agarose in the presence of Mg^{2+} ions was then eluted in pure form by simply omitting the metal cation. Similarly, thymidylate synthetase adsorbed on immobilized tetrahydromethotrexate in the presence of dUMP was subsequently eluted by omitting dUMP from the irrigating buffer.

Biospecific elution is not always the most efficient method. Consecutive affinity chromatography using combinations of non-specific and biospecific elution techniques has proved advantageous.

APPLICATIONS OF AFFINITY CHROMATOGRAPHY

Protein Isolation and Purification

In principle, the technique can be employed whenever a specific reversible interaction occurs between any two biomolecules. Consequently, the literature abounds with a plethora of examples where this technique has been applied (Table 1). Among the numerous examples of enzyme purification, the isolation of transcobalamin II from human plasma with a 2×10^6-fold purification is most impressive.

The technique has also found application in the purification of enzymes used in diagnostic kits for clinical analysis. Thus, for example: cholesterol esterase can be purified on palmitoyl–cellulose after elution with Triton X-100; cholesterol oxidase on succinylcholesterol–ethylenediamine–agarose after elution with 0.5% sodium deoxycholate at pH 8.1; lactate dehydrogenase on two consecutive columns of Matrex Gel Green-A and Cibacron blue F3G-A–agarose after elution with NADH and KCl respectively; malate dehydrogenase on Procion red H-E3B–agarose after elution with a mixture of the substrates NAD^+ and L-malate; alkaline phosphatase on Cibacron blue F3G-A–agarose after desorption with inorganic phosphate or α-naphthyl phosphate; glycerokinase on Procion blue MX-3G–agarose after elution with ATP; and urease on hydroxyurea–agarose after elution with 0.2M phosphate buffer at pH 4.6 containing 1mM β-mercaptoethanol. Similarly, affinity chromatography has been successfully applied in the purification of medically important enzymes; for example, the human urine thrombolytic enzyme urokinase was purified on β-naphthamidine–agarose or p-aminobenzamidine–agarose after elution in acidic conditions, whereas, human placenta β-glucuronidase was purified on the immuno-adsorbent anti-β-glucuronidase antibody–agarose after desorption with 6M urea.

The selection and immobilization of a suitable ligand sometimes requires considerable expertise and the resulting adsorbents are sometimes costly, with moderate capacity for large-scale use and liable to microbial degradation. Furthermore, when plasma fractions are processed to produce therapeutic proteins the dual risks of viral contamination and of contamination with adsorbent exudates has delayed the widespread use of this technique so far. Nevertheless, affinity chromatography now finds successful application in the large-scale recovery of albumin from Cohn Fraction IV on Cibacron blue F3G-A–agarose (16l column), plasma antithrombin III and plasminogen from Cohn Fraction I on heparin–agarose and lysine–agarose, respectively, and coagulation Factor VIII on mouse monoclonal anti-IgG antibodies immobilized to agarose (1.5l column). Furthermore, the technique is becoming increasingly important in the purification of tissue culture and genetically engineered proteins where crude products are often very diluted. Thus, human leucocyte interferons (HuINF α) were purified on polyclonal anti-interferon antibody immunoadsorbents and, almost a decade later, on monoclonal immunoadsorbents developed with the aid of hybridoma technology. The latter remains the favoured means of purifying interferon in a single step (200 ml column, 500-fold purification). Similarly, fibroblast interferon (HuINF β) produced both by cell culture and recombinant-DNA bacteria was purified by a combination of concanavalin A–agarose and zinc-chelate–agarose.

Isolation and Resolution of Supramolecular Structures

Affinity chromatography is also proving effective in the resolution of viruses, phages, organelles, and whole cells. For example, agarose-immobilized D-mannose-specific lectin from *Vicia ervilia* was employed to purify influenza virus whereas other lectins were effective for bovine diarrhoea viruses. Furthermore, the problem presented by hepatitis-B virus for blood protein fractionation was successfully eliminated by adsorption of the virus on octanoic acid hydrazide–agarose (3l column) or by combining Concanavalin A–agarose and ω-aminononyl–agarose columns (3.5l columns). Likewise, functionally distinct cells may be resolved on immobilized ligands that recognize certain receptor sites present on the cell surface. Thus, human peripheral blood lymphocytes were resolved into two distinct populations on immobilized human immunoglobulin, whereas, rat and mice thymus-dependent (T) and thymus-independent (B) lymphocytes were resolved on Magnogel-immobilized anti-immunoglobulin antibody; that is because B cells exhibit higher amounts of surface immunoglobulins than the T cells.

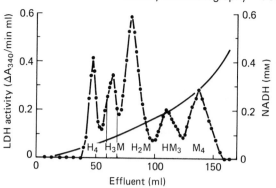

Fig. 2 The resolution of the five isoenzymes of lactate dehydrogenase by affinity chromatography on an immobilized-AMP adsorbent. Protein (0.2 mg) in 0.2 ml 0.1 M sodium phosphate buffer (pH 7.0), 1 mM 2-mercaptoethanol and 1 M NaCl was applied to an N^6-(6-aminohexyl)-AMP–agarose column (6 mm × 140 mm, containing 2.5 g wet gel) equilibrated with 0.1 M sodium phosphate buffer (10 ml) and the isoenzymes eluted with a concave gradient of NADH (0–0.5 mM) in the same buffer containing 1 mM 2-mercaptoethanol. Fractions (1 ml) were collected at 3.4 ml/h. Reproduced with permission from Brodelius and Mosbach (1973). *FEBS Lett*; **35**: 223.

Analytical Applications

The isoenzyme complement of each cell is genetically determined and the level of the isoenzymes of a particular enzyme in the various organs or tissues may reflect the pathological status of a patient. Although traditionally, isoenzyme detection is performed electrophoretically, such analysis may now be performed by affinity chromatography as shown, for example, in Fig. 2 for the five isoenzymes of lactate dehydrogenase. The same adsorbent, N^6-(6-aminohexyl)-AMP–agarose may also be used to resolve the isoenzymes of alcohol dehydrogenase by elution with a mixture of NAD^+ and cholic acid as well as to resolve cytoplasmic and mitochondrial malate dehydrogenase with a NADH gradient. Immunoassay techniques have been widely used in clinical analysis primarily because of their high sensitivity; however, affinity chromatographic methods are faster and the columns reusable and may thus prove to be competitive in many instances. For example, a commercial kit based on affinity chromatography is now available for the detection of total glycosylated haemoglobins (HbA_1) in blood. Only the glycosylated biomolecule is specifically adsorbed on immobilized phenylboronic acid and then eluted in the presence of sorbitol. The method is a more reliable indicator of diabetic control than blood or urine glucose levels. Finally, rapid analysis of thromboxanes, potent vasoconstrictor and platelet agonists, is now possible by selective extraction on silica-immobilized phenylboronic acid from small volumes of urine.

Medical and Therapeutic Applications

An attractive application of affinity chromatography is the removal of pyrogens such as the lipopolysaccharide endotoxins released from the cell wall of gram-negative bacteria upon cytolysis. Thus, for the safe parenteral administration of medicaments produced from natural sources endotoxin elimination is essential. This may be achieved by passing endotoxin-containing products through a polymixin-B–agarose or aminohexyl–histamine–agarose column which both specifically adsorb endotoxins. Recently, affinity chromatography has found an interesting application as a therapeutic tool in the purification of allergens for immunotherapy of patients with several allergies. Accordingly, after adsorption of the patient's IgE on an anti-IgE antibody gel, a mixture of different allergens is passed through the column. Allergens that adsorb onto the IgE and are subsequently eluted along with IgE are those responsible for the patient's allergy and, thus, could be used for immunotherapy. The affinity technique has also been exploited in the separation of mature T-lymphocytes from peripheral blood on a soybean-lectin–agarose. This application is important because the removal of these cells from bone marrow prevents graft-*vs*-host disease in transplantation. Progress in the design and applications of extracorporeal blood detoxification units is mainly due to the development of affinity chromatographic adsorbents. Appropriate ligands (e.g. UDP-glucuronyl transferase, NADP-cytochrome-C-reductase, cytochrome-P_{450}, albumin, Protein A, LDL-antibodies and heparin) specific for the toxin to be removed were immobilized on agarose beads and patients's whole blood or plasma then passed through the affinity adsorbent, resulting in selective adsorption and elimination of toxins such as, for example, phenols, benzphetamine, hexobarbital, unconjugated bilirubin, chenodeoxycholic acid, IgG and LDL-cholesterol. Likewise, passage of plasma, obtained from a patient suffering from systemic lupus erythematosus, through a poly(vinyl alcohol)-immobilized phenylalanine column resulted in the removal of pathogenic substrates and consequently in a marked improvement in the patient's condition.

EPILOGUE

The specificity and reversibility of ligand–macromolecule interactions has been exploited in affinity chromatography for the resolution and purification of numerous biomolecules. Recently the affinity concept has also been extended in other biotechnological fractionation processes which seek to circumvent some problems associated with scaling-up and speed of resolution. Particular attention is now being paid to techniques such as high-performance liquid affinity chromatography, affinity partition, ultrafiltration affinity purification, and affinity precipitation.

FURTHER READING

Review articles

Clonis Y. D. (1982). General ligand affinity chromatography. *Chim. Chron.* N S; **11**: 87.

Clonis Y. D. (1987). Large-scale affinity chromatography. *Biotechnology;* **5** (in press).

Clonis Y. D. (1987). High performance affinity chromatography. In *HPLC of Macromolecules—A Practical Approach* (Oliver R. W. A., ed.) Chap. 6. Oxford: IRL Press.

Lowe C. R. (1981). Immobilised coenzymes In *Topics in Enyzme and Fermentation Biotechnology* (Wiseman A., ed.) Vol. 5, pp. 13–146. Chichester: Ellis Horwood.

Lowe C. R. (1984). Application of reactive dyes in biotechnology. In *Topics in Enzyme and Fermentation Biotechnology* (Wiseman A., ed.) Vol. 9, pp. 78–161. Chichester: Ellis Horwood.

Lowe C. R. (1984). New developments in downstream processing. *J. Biotechnol*; **1**: 3.

Lowe C. R., Clonis Y. D. (1985). Affinity chromatography. In *Bioactive Polymeric Systems* (Gebelein C. G., Carraher C. E., eds) pp. 203–22. New York: Plenum Press.

Books

Clonis Y. D., Atkinson, A., Bruton C. J., Lowe C. R. (eds) (1987). *Triazine Dyes in Protein and Enzyme Technology*. Basingstoke: Macmillan.

Dean P. D. G., Johnston W. S., Middle F. A. (eds) (1985). *Affinity Chromatography—A Practical Approach*. Oxford: IRL Press.

Jakoby W. B. (ed.) (1984). *Enzyme Purification and Related Techniques. Methods in Enzymology*. Vol. 104. London: Academic Press.

Lowe C. R., Dean P. D. G. (1974). *Affinity Chromatography*. Chichester: Wiley.

Scouten W. H. (1981). *Affinity Chromatography-Bioselective Adsorption on Inert Matrices*. Chemical Analysis Monograph Series. Vol. 59. New York: Wiley.

Turkova J. (1978). *Affinity Chromatography*. Journal of Chromatography Library. Vol. 12. Amsterdam: Elsevier.

26. Electrophoresis
A. W. Walker

INTRODUCTION

Electrophoresis is the migration of particles under the influence of a direct electric current. To apply the technique, two simple requirements must be met. First, the particles which it is wished to study must be charged or be capable of accepting a charge. Many compounds of biological interest, e.g. proteins and amino acids, meet this requirement. Secondly, the medium in which the electrophoresis is performed must be capable of carrying an electric current.

Historical

Although the widespread application of electrophoresis in science and in medicine followed the publication in 1937 of the work of Tiselius, the phenomenon had been demonstrated many years before. It has been reported that in 1809, Reuss had found that fine sand particles would migrate under the influence of an electrical current. The first conscious exploitation of the technique, however, came with the work of Picton and Linder reported in 1892. Using a simple apparatus consisting of a glass tube with a platinum electrode at each end, they reported 'a remarkable property we have observed in some solutions; this consists in the repulsion of the dissolved substances as a whole from one pole to another when we immerse in the liquid electrodes connected with a Galvanic battery'. The use of the technique enabled these workers to conclude that there was no hard and fast dividing line between colloidal and crystalloid solution.

Electrophoretic studies made by Hardy at the turn of the century helped to establish the amphoteric nature of proteins and the concept of the isoelectric point, but it was not until 1937 that Tiselius applied the technique to clinical purposes with his analysis of serum proteins and their variation in disease. Tiselius had developed a refined apparatus for the conduct of the procedure, and by the use of this and closely related instruments, the best conditions for the separation of serum proteins were thoroughly investigated, particularly by Longsworth and his co-workers.

As a result of the seminal influence of the work of Tiselius, it has been frequently imagined that the technique of free electrophoresis antedates that of zone electrophoresis, i.e. electrophoresis conducted in some stabilizing medium. In fact, the latter technique is of roughly equal ancestry as Lodge in 1886 had used a gelatin–acetic acid jelly as a stabilizing medium in a study of ionic migration and the determination of absolute ionic velocity. The use of agar as a supporting medium was employed by Kendall in an extensive series of studies on the separation of isotopes in the twenty years from 1919 and in 1934 Susan Veil employed the technique of autoradiography as a means of detecting separated isotopes. The application of these zone electrophoretic techniques did not, however, become widespread.

The Tiselius approach, although precise and quantitative, had the disadvantage of requiring complex apparatus. After 1945, several simplified versions of the Tiselius apparatus appeared, for example that of Antweiler. These versions eliminated some of the laborious parts of the Tiselius technique but were less satisfactory in other ways and were not widely adopted.

König in 1939–40 published several papers describing electrophoresis on paper, but it was the publication in 1946 of the work of Consden, Gordon and Martin using silica jelly as an anti-convection medium for the separation of amino acids and peptides from wool hydrolysates, which brought the potential of zone electrophoresis to wide attention. Their paper discussed fully the theory of electrophoretic separation and emphasized the possibility of separating substances with only small differences in electrophoretic mobility.

The use of electrophoresis in clinical biochemistry became widespread in the fifties with the adoption of paper electrophoretic techniques for the study of serum proteins. Subsequently cellulose acetate membrane was substituted for paper and although this offered a number of advantages it did not give appreciably greater resolving power. The technique of agar immunoelectrophoresis, in which precipitating antibodies are introduced into the medium for the location and characterization of the separated protein components, allows the detection of perhaps 30–40 proteins in serum as opposed to the five components discriminated by paper, cellulose acetate or simple agar electrophoresis. A similar high resolution was offered by starch and polyacrylamide gel electrophoresis, introduced in about 1955 and 1959 respectively.

A further advance was the introduction of isoelectric focusing in the early 1960s and a combination of this technique with high resolution polyacrylamide gel electrophoresis in two-dimensional separations opened the possibility of resolving mixtures containing thousands of components.

These high resolution techniques, although a powerful tool to improve our understanding of the complex alterations in protein metabolism that occur in disease have yet to establish a role in clinical diagnosis and monitoring. However, high resolution electrophoresis is currently used to separate DNA fragments during DNA hybridization techniques[1] which are likely in future to play a large part in the clinical laboratory for the diagnosis of infectious, inherited, and neoplastic disease.

GENERAL THEORETICAL CONSIDERATIONS

This section outlines the basic theoretical background of all forms of electrophoresis. Further theoretical discussion of any factor which is particularly important in an individual electrophoretic technique will be found under the description of that technique.

The term 'particle' is used throughout this chapter to embrace ions and molecules in addition to objects of microscopic size.

For electrophoretic separation to be possible the particle must either be charged or be capable of accepting a charge. Neutral molecules may, however, be induced to move in an electric field by the formation of complexes between the molecule and a charged ion, a well-known example being the complexing of carbohydrates with borate ions. With organic molecules the number of charges present is closely related to the degree of ionization of the chemical groups of which the molecule is composed; this in turn reflects the chemical environment surrounding the molecule. A minimum requirement of this environment is that it must be capable of conducting an electric current. Hence it is not possible to discuss the behaviour of a molecule in an electric field without consideration of the nature of the surrounding electrolyte.

The Charge on the Particle

The behaviour of a particle in an electric field depends mainly on the sign of the charge on the particle. Negatively charged particles will, in the absence of countervailing forces, migrate to the positively charged anode and vice versa, i.e. the direction of migration is dictated by the sign of the charge.

The rate of migration in an electric field is dictated by the number of charges on the particles. In general, charged particles do not accelerate continuously in an electric field. Thus the driving force exerted by the applied potential on the charged particle is at some point balanced by retarding forces brought into play by the movement of the particle. These latter forces will be discussed below.

Charged groups may be pre-existing or induced by the presence of the electrolyte. Mobility will be related to the degree of dissociation of the potentially ionizable groups on the particle, which in turn is governed by the pK of the groups and the pH of the electrolyte solution. The latter will determine whether a particular group is charged, e.g. for an acid group.

$$\underset{\substack{\text{Neutral} \\ \text{molecule}}}{HA} + H_2O \rightleftharpoons \underset{\text{Ions}}{H_3O^+ + A^-}$$

Charged groups of opposite sign may exist on the same molecule. Hardy in 1899 noted that 'proteid particles therefore have this interesting property that their electrical characters are conferred upon them by the nature of the reaction, acid or alkaline of the fluid. If the latter is alkaline the particles will become electro negative and vice versa', i.e. proteins and the amino acids of which they are composed are amphoteric, acting either as proton donors (acids) or as proton acceptors (bases).

This can be represented as follows:

$$\underset{\text{(cation)}}{protein^+} \rightleftharpoons H^+ + \underset{\text{(zwitterion)}}{{}^+protein^-} \rightleftharpoons 2H^+ + \underset{\text{(anion)}}{protein^-}$$

$$\text{increasing pH}$$

The pH of net neutrality, i.e. when there is an equal number of positive and negative charges, is known as the isoelectric point. The rate of migration will depend on the degree of ionization of the charged groups at the pH of the surrounding electrolyte solution.

The choice of pH for the electrolyte is not, however, determined only by a wish to maximize the electrophoretic mobility. In clinical biochemistry the aim will be to achieve the maximum separation of components in a mixture. In practice, for the separation of a biological mixture, this is something which has to be explored experimentally. The theoretical basis of a choice of pH to produce the maximum difference in mobility between two components under idealized conditions has been discussed by Consden.

The Driving Force

Movement of the charged particle is brought about by the action of the electrical force. The driving force (DF) exerted on the particle is equal to the product of the field strength X and net charge on the particle Q. The field strength is the applied electrical potential (V, expressed in volts) divided by the distance between the electrodes (d, expressed in centimetres), i.e. $DF = XQ = V/d \times Q$. Other factors being constant, the migration velocity is, therefore, dependent on the field strength, which can be increased either by increasing the applied potential or by decreasing the distance between the electrodes. As there are inevitably losses and discontinuities in electrophoretic assemblies, due to connecting wicks, etc., it is important to remember that in practice the applied potential V has to be measured between the ends of the filter paper, gel slab, etc., and is not equal to the voltage registered on the power pack.

The passage of an electrical current inevitably generates heat;

$$\text{Heat produced} = kI^2Rt = kVIt$$

where k = a constant (dependent on the units used),
$\quad I$ = the current,
$\quad R$ = resistance,
$\quad t$ = the time in seconds,
$\quad V$ = the voltage.

The higher the voltage the greater the current carried and the quantity of heat produced. As the driving force is proportional to the applied voltage (and through Ohm's law to the current) the heat produced is proportional to the square of the current. Increasing the migration velocity by increasing the applied potential necessitates a faster dissipation of the heat produced.

The concentration of electrolyte used, best considered in terms of its ionic strength (see below), also influences the amount of heat generated. The more dilute the electrolyte, the lower its actual conductivity and the lower, therefore, the current carried, i.e. use of a more dilute electrolyte will minimize heating effects or allow the use of higher potential gradients. However, the electrolyte has to perform other functions such as maintaining the pH and solubilizing the components being separated. The use of ampholytes (see below) at their isoelectric points provides one method whereby adequate conductivity can be obtained in the presence of low ionic strength, allowing higher voltage gradients at lower current flow.

Increase in temperature has a number of effects. Electrophoretic mobility is increased, the pH of the buffer solution decreases, and the current increases, if the voltage is kept constant. However, in certain electrophoretic systems there may be other effects. The increased heat may cause an increased evaporation of solvent from a paper or a cellulose acetate strip. This results, of course, in an increased concentration of electrolyte which decreases the mobility of the particles (see below), and may also result in the syphoning of electrolyte into the support from the buffer reservoir. This problem will be discussed more fully under the section on paper electrophoresis.

Evaporation may be reduced by enclosing the electrophoretic strip in an atmosphere fully saturated with water, but with higher voltages, most electrophoretic systems require to be cooled.

The Retarding Force

The force (RF), referred to above, which retards the movement of particles in an electric field is proportional both to the molecular size and to the viscosity of the medium. It can be represented by Stokes Law:

$$RF = 6\pi r\eta v$$

where r = radius of migrating particle,
$\quad \eta$ = coefficient of viscosity of the solution,
$\quad v$ = velocity of migration.

The velocity becomes constant when the retarding force equals the driving force (DF) produced by the applied potential and the charge on the ion.

i.e. when $\qquad XQ = 6\pi r\eta v.$

The migration velocity is then

$$v = \frac{XQ}{6\pi r\eta}$$

i.e. the rate of migration is directly proportional to the field strength and to the net charge on the particle, and inversely proportional to the size of the particle and the viscosity of the solution.

In starch and polyacrylamide gel electrophoresis, molecular sieving plays a significant role. These media form a barrier to movement of particles as the pores in the gel approach the size of the particles. High-molecular-weight particles are retarded relative to smaller particles. This effect is of course the reverse of that found in Sephadex gel diffusion where smaller particles are retarded by their penetration into the matrix of dextran beads and the consequent extension of their distance of movement.

Enhanced separation between the components of mixtures may also be achieved by chemical and immunological modification of the migrating particle, a well-known example being the complexing of carbohydrates with borate ions. The isoenzymes of alkaline phosphatase have also been studied electrophoretically after modification of their protein structure by acetylation, treatment with neuraminidase, and reaction with antiserum directed against one component of the mixture. These modifications either alter the number of charged groups on the molecule or drastically alter the molecular size, a change which can be exploited in those electrophoretic techniques where molecular sieving plays a prominent part. Indeed, in these media it may be useful to abolish significant differences in charge between the particles being separated. This may be achieved by surrounding the protein or polypeptide with detergent ions, such as those of sodium dodecyl sulphate (SDS), allowing separation to take place purely on the basis of molecular weight.

The Nature of the Electrolyte

In addition to charged particles electrophoresis requires a medium capable of carrying an electric current—the electrolyte. The influence of the electrolyte in inducing charge on the particles has been discussed above. However, the electrolyte may also have to serve other purposes and may produce some less desirable side effects. The electrolyte may be required to dissolve the material being investigated and to act as a buffer to resist chemical change brought about during the electrophoresis by electrode breakdown products or local variation in the concentration of particular molecules.

A charged particle attracts particles of opposite charge around it setting up a double layer. The effect is described by the Helmholz Gouy double layer theory and increases as the concentration of the electrolyte increases. For example, negative charges on the surface of the particle create around the particle a layer of immobile positive ions which cause a resisting force (Fig. 1).

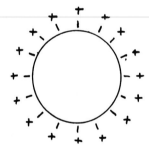

Fig. 1 Illustration of a negatively charged particle surrounded by a layer of immobile positive ions which cause a resistance to electrophoretic migration.

Electrophoretic mobility is inversely related to the square root of the ionic strength, μ, which is a function of the charge and concentration of the ions present.

$$\mu = \tfrac{1}{2}\Sigma C_i Z_i^2$$

where C_i = concentration of ion i,
Z_i = valence of ion i.

But, in addition to decreasing mobility, an increase in ionic strength also tends to sharpen the zones of separated components of a mixture. Increased ionic strength reduces the diffusion which would otherwise

result from charged particles binding ions of opposite charge. Again it must be stressed that optimum separation rather than maximum mobility is what is usually required of electrophoresis. A reduction in the concentration of electrolyte will increase mobility and decrease heat generated, but will also reduce buffering power and increase diffusion. Molecular association or precipitation of the components being separated may also occur, and adsorption on to the stabilizing medium may increase.

Diffusion

Diffusion, which is the movement of particles from a region of high to one of low concentration, is often the limiting factor in the degree of resolution that can be obtained by electrophoresis. The extent of diffusion can be specified for idealized particles by the Sutherland–Einstein equation.

$$D = \frac{RT}{6\pi\eta r N}$$

where D = diffusion coefficient,
R = universal gas constant,
T = absolute temperature,
η = coefficient of viscosity,
r = the radius of the diffusing particle
and N = Avogadro's number;

i.e. diffusion is directly proportional to temperature, and inversely proportional to particle size and solution viscosity.

However, dispersion of particles during electrophoresis is not governed simply by the above diffusion theory. Increase in temperature may not be evenly spread throughout a system, but may be localized, giving rise to convection currents which may cause substantial dispersion of particles. This is, of course, a severe limitation in free electrophoretic systems and is the reason for the use of stabilizing media—frequently referred to as anticonvection media.

The use of such media reduces the dispersion of particles in a variety of ways. The particle may be adsorbed onto the surface of the medium or partially immobilized by the 'pores' of the medium which may approximate in size to the diameter of the particle. These pores can be thought of as simple obstructions to the free movement of the particle or as forming tortuous capillary pathways of non-uniform diameter, which provide a greatly increased migration distance. Whatever the mechanism the effect is that, on media such as polyacrylamide and starch, the effect of particle size on electrophoretic mobility is of great importance.

Adsorption

Adsorption of the particles onto the stabilizing medium is a frequent occurrence. Although, like the 'sieving' effect mentioned above, this decreases the electrophoretic mobility, it can also be exploited to enhance the separation of the components of a mixture. Adsorption can be detected by running the electrophoresis for a period, followed by reversal of the direction of the current. The presence of trailing edges will show that adsorption of the particles onto the stabilizing medium has occurred.

Electro-endosmosis

Charged groups may also exist on the surfaces of glass or on stabilizing media. As these are fixed, an opposite charge is induced in the electrolyte in the vicinity of the fixed charge, and the particle carrying the induced charge moves towards the opposite electrode. The phenomenon is known as electro-endosmosis. In electrophoresis under alkaline pH conditions, these fixed charges are negative, and result in a flow of electrolyte to the cathode, i.e. in opposition to the movement of the negatively charged particles towards the anode. Uncharged or weakly charged particles will be carried along by this flow. The phenomenon is particularly prominent with support media such as agar or paper. The effect increases with increasing pH which increases the degree of ionization of the potentially charged carboxyl groups present on the surface of the paper or agar.

The charges on the surface of glass are not of significance unless the electrophoresis is being conducted in tubes of narrow bore or between closely placed glass plates. The presence of electro-endosmosis can be detected by studying the behaviour of substances, such as the widely used blue dextran, which are effectively uncharged under the particular conditions used.

Electro-endosmosis will reduce the electrophoretic mobility but as with the other factors mentioned above this can be exploited to aid separation. The excellent results achieved in the separation of the main immunoglobulin classes, and their detection by specific antiserum on agar gel electrophoresis, is largely due to the beneficial effects of substantial endosmosis on the separation of these lightly charged components from other, more highly charged, serum proteins.

Zone-sharpening Techniques—Discontinuous Electrophoresis

The aim of electrophoresis is to obtain the maximum separation between the components of a mixture and this is aided if the separated components are concentrated in zones as narrow as possible at the end of an electrophoretic run. Careful attention to all the electrophoretic conditions are necessary to achieve this end, but in particular special buffer systems may aid 'zone-sharpening' of components in a variety of electrophoretic media. Generally, such systems make use of discontinuities of conductivity or of pH, some-

times in association with gel concentration discontinuities in the case of polyacrylamide gel electrophoresis. These zone sharpening techniques may be categorized as follows:

1. Where the sample is applied in dilute solution;
2. Where discontinuous buffer systems are used;
3. Where discontinuities of buffer pH and gel concentration are employed.

When the sample is applied in dilute solution, the conductivity within that solution is very much less than that of the preceding or following buffer zones. This sets up a voltage discontinuity which causes zone sharpening because the rear of the sample zone will be accelerated relative to the front of the sample zone. This technique is very simple to employ, particularly in gel electrophoretic systems.

The discontinuous buffer system devised by Poulik was initially used for starch gel electrophoresis, though similar buffer systems may give equally good results on polyacrylamide gel. The gel buffer contains citrate ions which have higher mobility than the borate ions in the electrode compartment. On electrophoresis a sharp boundary exists between the two ions and this remains sharp and stable according to the Kohlrausch regulating function. A leading (higher mobility) ion migrating in front of a trailing (lower mobility) ion 'regulates' the mobility of the latter which is accelerated to the mobility of the faster ion by the increased voltage gradient at the boundary between the ionic species. Such discontinuities can be observed either as a Schlieren front or, in the Poulik system on starch gel, as a brown line. When the discontinuity overtakes the protein components a zone-sharpening effect is obtained.

The application of a sample in dilute solution and the use of discontinuous buffer systems have been combined in the technique of Allen using polyacrylamide gel. In this method the electrophoretic conditions are arranged so that the boundary between the solutions of the two ions does not overtake the sample until the latter has entered the small pore separation gel.

The use of discontinuities of voltage and pH combined with layers of polyacrylamide gel of different concentration has been exploited in the Ornstein and Davis technique of polyacrylamide gel electrophoresis. This technique is often referred to as 'disc' electrophoresis by virtue of the above discontinuities. The system is based on a complex arrangement of gel layers with different buffer systems and pH. The pH conditions within the system are arranged so that the sample is initially sandwiched between 'leading' and 'trailing' buffer ions. On entry of the sample into a small pore separation gel the conditions of pH change abruptly and the degree of dissociation and mobility of the trailing ion increases. The zone then overtakes the components and exerts a sharpening effect.

For a full discussion of the theoretical basis of the

technique see Whipple[2] (especially the chapter by Ornstein) and Maurer.[3]

SEPARATION METHODS

Electrophoresis in Free Solution

The discussion of this technique will be brief, as although still useful to physical chemists and in cell research it is of largely historical interest to clinical chemists.

The apparatus to be described is Longsworth's modification of the 'Tiselius' apparatus (Fig. 2). This

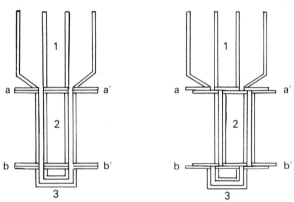

Fig. 2 Schematic representation of the Tiselius apparatus as modified by Longsworth. See text for description of apparatus and method.

consists basically of a U-shaped glass tube divided into three sections (1, 2, 3). Section 2 may be isolated from the other sections by being moved out of alignment. Precision ground glass plates greased with a little Vaseline are at a—a' and b—b' and these join section 2 to the other two sections. This sectional construction allows the introduction of protein solutions or buffer at different levels of the U-tube without significant mixing with other components.

The stages in the electrophoretic separation are illustrated diagrammatically in Fig. 3.

Initial boundaries between the buffer and protein mixture are established at a' and b. Application of the potential causes the boundary on one side to rise and on the other to fall. If electrophoresis of proteins is being conducted at a pH greater than 7, the components are negatively charged and the boundary will rise towards the anode and fall towards the cathode.

The initial single boundary at a' and b is replaced by a series of boundaries. In the idealized case the first ascending boundary is between the buffer and component A, the second between A and component B and the third between B and component C.

It should be noted that protein 'separation' is achieved only in the upper portions of the two arms of the U tubes, containing isolated fractions of the fastest and slowest moving protein respectively. However, variations in the refractive index caused by the different concentrations of protein at the boun-

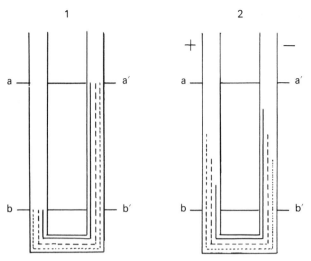

Fig. 3 Electrophoretic separation of a three component mixture in the Tiselius apparatus. (1) The initial situation; (2) the situation at the end of the run.

daries between the components can, with various optical methods, be observed as 'schlieren' or shadows. The schlieren can be represented in the form of bands at each boundary, or by means of the schlieren scanning device introduced by Longsworth, the boundaries can be represented as a series of peaks giving the now-familiar serum electrophoretic pattern. The area under the peak is proportional to the concentration of the particular protein, although identical amounts of different proteins may produce different changes in the refractive index.

It must be emphasized that the Tiselius apparatus incorporated several important improvements of earlier free electrophoresis devices. A glass tube of narrow rectangular section allowed excellent temperature control if the apparatus was immersed in a cooling bath at 4 °C. Disturbance to the boundaries by diffusion and convection currents was thus minimized, and increased potential gradients could be applied. The sliding section allowed the introduction of sample and buffer with the minimum of mixing, and also allowed the isolation and removal of separated components. Finally, the schlieren optical system allowed detection, and with some qualification the quantitation of the invisible components. The method was very suitable for physicochemical measurements, such as determination of isoelectric point, as minimum resistance was offered to the free migration of particles. However, the incomplete separation of the components and the expensive nature of the apparatus were distinct disadvantages.

Although a variety of simplified apparatus became available commercially in the late 1940s and 1950s, and were used in a number of clinical biochemistry laboratories, it is fair to say that the technique was always extremely laborious, and only a limited number of serum specimens could be examined in the course of a day. As a result of these drawbacks, the technique did not achieve widespread use in clinical biochemistry.

However, the separation of serum proteins into albumin, alpha 1, alpha 2, beta and gammaglobulin was achieved, and the variation of these groups of proteins in disease thoroughly documented. With the exception of the albumin fraction all the fractions identified were in fact mixtures of protein molecules. Further progress in resolution of these mixtures could be achieved only by the use of higher potential gradients or by the introduction of some further discriminating principle. Neither was possible with the free electrophoresis system.

Electrophoresis in Stabilizing Media

The disadvantages of free electrophoresis, expense, laboriousness, and inability to employ high potential gradients, were overcome by the introduction of electrophoresis on support media—often referred to as stabilizing or anticonvection media. A wide range of materials has been employed. The list includes gelatin, agar, paper, silica gel, glass beads and glass powder, kieselguhr, cellulose acetate, starch in block and gel form, and polyacrylamide. Only the most widely used media will be discussed. These are paper, cellulose acetate, agarose, starch gel, and polyacrylamide gel.

Paper Electrophoresis. An advantage of paper electrophoresis compared with free electrophoresis, is that small volumes (10 µl or less) of serum and other samples can be studied. Unlike electrophoresis in free solution, zones of protein may be completely separated by the technique. Although the popularity of paper electrophoresis has greatly declined with the advent of cellulose acetate it still has advantages for certain applications.

A wide variety of paper types has been employed for electrophoretic separation. Resolving power is greatest when the electrophoresis is conducted in the predominant fibre direction. The paper may be suspended in an atmosphere saturated with water vapour (the so-called open strip method), enclosed between glass plates, or immersed in a non-conducting fluid. Contact between the paper strip and the electrode vessels may be made directly or through a filter paper or sponge wick.

With all open strip methods it is important that the air space in the electrophoresis tank is kept to a minimum and that the atmosphere is saturated with water vapour as far as possible before the electrophoresis is commenced. Additional filter paper pads soaked in buffer and placed in the electrophoresis tank may help to achieve this end. The lid of the tank should either be sloped or covered with a sponge material to prevent condensed vapour dropping on to the paper.

With enclosed strip methods the paper strip is held between plates which must serve both as conductors

of heat and electrical insulators. In general, two components will have to be employed to achieve this end, as glass, for example, is a good electrical insulator but a poor heat conductor, and metal plates are good heat conductors but bad electrical insulators. Hence it is common to find the strip held between glass plates which in turn are sandwiched between two metal cooling tanks but separated from them by thin polythene sheets which act as insulators.

In order to control the moisture content of the paper strip, pressure is often applied to the sandwich in some way. It is important that the pressure is applied evenly. A common method adopted is to compress an inflatable rubber bag between the top surface of the sandwich and an adjustable pressure plate. The moisture content of the paper may be varied by adjusting the applied pressure by movement of the pressure plate.

When voltage gradients in excess of about 20 volts per centimetre are applied, the technique is termed '*high-voltage electrophoresis*'. Power packs supplying voltages of between 1000 and 10 000 volts and 100–500 milliamps are required for this technique. In comparison with low-voltage electrophoresis a relatively dry paper is used.

The main problem with high-voltage electrophoresis is the difficulty of ensuring adequate heat dissipation. Frequently this is achieved by using the cooling technique outlined above, i.e. placing the paper in intimate contact with a cooled plate or plates. An alternative is to immerse the paper in a non-polar organic solvent, which itself may be subjected to cooling. Such organic solvents must not be miscible with or denser than water, or conducting, and should not act as solvents for any of the buffer constituents employed. It is also desirable that they be relatively volatile.

Another major problem is to ensure adequate operator safety. High voltages used in the presence of conducting fluid pose a particular threat. It is essential that safety features be built into the apparatus.

Most commercially available and many 'home made' examples have devices whereby the current is switched off automatically if any attempt is made to open the apparatus when in use, or if the coolant pressure drops. The use of organic solvents as coolant poses an additional fire hazard, although the relative simplicity of the apparatus is an advantage.

High-voltage electrophoresis has proved to be most useful in the separation of compounds of relatively small molecular weight such as monosaccharides, oligosaccharides, amino acids and oligopeptides. Protein separation is not generally possible because of denaturation of the proteins by a combination of the relatively dry paper and local heating effects. The apparatus is relatively costly, but can yield an excellent solution to many separation problems.

Better separation of the components of a mixture

may be achieved by following an initial low- or high-voltage electrophoretic run in one direction by a second run, using different conditions in a direction at 90° to the first—*two-dimensional electrophoresis*. Alternatively, electrophoresis may be followed by *chromatography*. The latter approach is frequently useful as the principles by which separation is achieved in the two techniques are different.

Either two-dimensional electrophoresis, or the combination of electrophoresis with chromatography in a second dimension, can be carried out on one piece of paper or by attaching either the whole or a portion of the original electrophoretic paper to a second paper. In order to give a thin starting zone the strip transferred should be as narrow as possible. The term 'finger printing' is often used with respect to the analysis of hydrolysates of macromolecules by this technique.

In general, an advantage that paper electrophoresis enjoys over paper chromatography is speed of separation. In clinical work another important advantage is that separation of carbohydrates, amino acids or indoles from urine, either by electrophoresis alone or by electrophoresis followed by chromatography in a second dimension, obviates the need for the tedious desalting generally necessary where chromatography alone is used. During electrophoresis salts rapidly move off the paper leaving a de-salted sample.

Cellulose Acetate Electrophoresis. The technique of cellulose acetate electrophoresis was introduced by Kohn in 1957. The material had previously been employed as a filter membrane, and hence the technique is sometimes referred to as membrane filter electrophoresis.

The cellulose of the strip has some or all of its free hydroxyl groups acetylated. Although this detailed specifications, and the choice of a particular product must be made empirically.

Cellulose acetate membrane enjoys distinct advantages over paper. The material is in the form of a fine film, allowing the separation of very small amounts of material. This advantage combined with minimal adsorption of protein generally results in sharper zones. The material is easily cleared or dissolved which is an advantage if the separated components are to be quantitated. However, as mentioned above all cellulose acetate membranes do not respond to the same treatment. The material is more costly than paper, although this additional expense may be more than balanced by the ability of the material to handle a much larger number of samples for a given area. The time required for separation is also greatly reduced.

Almost invariably cellulose acetate electrophoresis is carried out with the membrane in the *horizontal position*. The general arrangement is, therefore, very similar to that used with paper. Certain precautions specific to cellulose acetate have to be adopted. The strips must be moistened by holding the strip in a gentle curve and floating it without immersion on the surface of the buffer solution. The buffer then permeates the strip from below and air is not trapped in the interstices of the membrane. When permeation is complete the strip may be fully immersed in the buffer. If inadvertently the strip is plunged under the surface of the buffer it is best to discard the strip, as the entrapped air (shown by white patches in the strip) may not disappear for several hours, if at all.

Before use the strip must be lightly blotted and placed in the electrophoresis tank. Compared with paper, cellulose acetate has the advantage that, in the horizontal position, it is much easier to stretch between two supports. A common arrangement is illustrated in Fig. 4. The cellulose acetate membrane

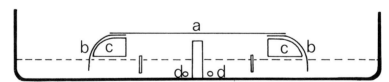

Fig. 4 Cellulose acetate electrophoresis. (a) Cellulose acetate membrane; (b) filter paper wicks; (c) support shoulders; (d) electrodes.

should give a very consistent and uniform structure, laboratory workers are very familiar with differences between one batch of membrane and another and also between the products supplied by different manufacturers. These latter differences are often marked, both with respect to the physical properties of the material, its resolving power and the different procedures necessary for clearing the strip prior to densitometric evaluation. Presumably these differences result largely from variations in pore size of the strip and in the degree of derivatization of the hydroxyl groups. Manufacturers of cellulose acetate membrane for electrophoretic purposes do not issue adheres satisfactorily to the filter paper covering the support shoulders and no further support is necessary. However, some arrangements involve the membrane supported on a glass plate.

Because of the thinness of the strip great care has to be taken to minimize evaporation during the electrophoretic run. In the apparatus designed by Kohn the cellulose acetate strip is suspended over the surface of the buffer for the greater part of its length. A well-sealed lid is applied and the air space above the strip is minimal. The lid may also with advantage have a soaked sponge attached.

The sample may be applied with a glass capillary

or micro pipette, but the applicator designed by Kohn and marketed by Shandon is very much more convenient, allowing reproducible amounts of serum to be applied with great rapidity and the minimal amount of skill. Similar multi-sample applicators provide a very economical method for the simultaneous electrophoresis of a large number of serum samples. A variety of other applicators are available, many based on a system of parallel wires. These tend to be rather more fragile than the Kohn applicator, but if properly adjusted give excellent results.

In general, buffers similar to those used in paper electrophoresis are effective.

Gel Electrophoresis. The stabilizing media described above are all available in 'ready to use' form. Paper and cellulose acetate strips merely require to be soaked in the relevant buffer, and inserted into the electrophoresis apparatus. They are then ready for sample application. The group of materials to be discussed below are used in the form of *gels*, and require additional preparative steps. In return for this extra effort, however, they offer a number of advantages.

Agar and agarose gels are relatively transparent and do not significantly retard the diffusion of antigen and antibody. They are therefore ideal for the application of immunoprecipitation detection reactions. Electrophoretic separation in such gels takes place essentially on the basis of electrical charge, although a useful molecular sieving effect occurs with very large particles.

The other two gel media to be discussed, starch and polyacrylamide, allow separation to be effected by a combination of electrical charge differences and molecular sieving. They, therefore, offer a quality of resolution unobtainable with any preprepared medium.

A gel consists of a matrix of hydrophilic material holding a substantial water content. As such it must be distinguished from a slurry, which is simply a dispersion of small particles in a liquid. Under certain conditions slurrys of certain materials can be induced to form true gels. The transformation can be effected in the case of agar, gelatine, and low concentrations of starch by solution in water with heat, followed by cooling. Such gels are known as thermal gels. Gels may also be formed by a chemically catalysed process, a typical example being the formation of polyacrylamide gel from acrylamide and bisacrylamide. A thick slurry of some materials such as starch will form a gel on standing. Such gels are known as thixotropic gels. A thixotropic starch gel differs in nature from a thermal starch gel.

With the exception of polyacrylamide gel, the detailed structures of the gels used in electrophoresis are not known. They are presumed to consist of a mesh, the density of which may limit the movement of particles through the gel. For the sake of convenience the interstitial space will be referred to as the 'pore size'. The pore size is unlikely to be uniform throughout, though gels of a particular concentration can be assumed to have an average effective pore size. The 'pore' size is inversely proportional to the concentration of the gel, although the relationship may not be a simple one as for example in the case of polyacrylamide.

Agarose gel electrophoresis.[4] Agarose is a term applied to a variety of preparations derived from agar, a galactan polysaccharide obtained from red algae, and distinguished from it by a reduced content of sulphate and carboxyl groups. The charged groups in the native agar cause a considerable electro-endosmosis when the material is used as a support medium for electrophoresis. For many years immunoelectrophoresis in agar gel was widely used for the identification of clinical abnormalities of immunoglobulin synthesis where the electro-endosmosis was an advantage in increasing separation in the beta and gamma globulin regions. However, the technique of immunofixation (*see* p. 419), usually carried out on cellulose acetate, has largely replaced immunoelectrophoresis for clinical purposes, and as a result the use of agar has declined.

Although often described as a purified material it must be stressed that the term agarose describes a range of products derived from native agars of ill-defined and possibly varying composition, and the products of one manufacturer may differ considerably from those of another. Manufacturers tend to offer a range of products varying in the degree of electro-endosmosis they produce but it is rash to assume that this is the only difference between the preparations. Different binding properties for the substances being separated may be exhibited, and therefore an individual brand may show an advantage for a particular separative purpose.

Despite the extensive use of acrylamide as a support medium, agarose has remained in wide use. One reason is simplicity of preparation. Solid agarose in the proportion of $0·2–1·5\,g/100$ ml buffer, is dissolved by heat and poured onto a suitable support such as glass or hydrophilic polyester sheet (for example Gel Bond, FMC) when the gel forms on cooling. The material, unlike acrylamide monomer, is non-toxic and gelation does not require catalysts of variable effect which may interfere with subsequent separation. The gelation, unlike polyacrylamide, does not require the exclusion of air, and therefore gels can be cast in open trays. However, the nature of the gel may alter with time and storage must be in a humidified atmosphere.

Agarose gel has a larger pore size and much superior mechanical properties than low concentration polyacrylamide gel and is usually the medium of choice for the electrophoretic separation of large molecular weight (greater than 2M daltons) proteins, nucleic acids and virus particles. However, the absence of molecular sieving for all the largest particles also makes the medium a good support for isoelectric focusing (*see* below), although agarose of minimal electro-endosmotic properties must be used.

Agarose preparations with enhanced molecular sieving properties for low molecular weight particles have been produced by incorporation of additional hydroxyethyl groups. These materials are, however, mechanically unstable and also possess a low melting point requiring rigorous control of temperature during the electrophoretic run.

Electrophoresis using agarose does not require specialized apparatus. Most equipment devised for cellulose acetate or paper electrophoresis can be adapted for agarose work with the minimum of effort. The gel is laid in a horizontal position and contact made with the electrode compartments by filter paper, two layers of Whatman 3 MM being sufficient. In general the paper wicks will adhere satisfactorily to the top surface of the agarose if 0·5–1 cm overlap is allowed. Sample holes or slots can be cut in the agarose and the sample inserted either directly by micropipette or absorbed onto a piece of filter paper or cellulose acetate. Generally voltages of the order of 15 volts/cm may be applied. It may be desirable to place the gel on a simple cooling box in the tank through which tap water is circulated. Alternatively, the temperature may be controlled by inserting the tank in the refrigerator and by pre-cooling the buffer.

Suitable buffers for agar gel electrophoresis are listed by Smith,[5] and for agar gel immunoelectrophoresis in Crowle.[6]

Starch gel electrophoresis. Using the media discussed above, separation, for all but the largest particles, is achieved by virtue of the difference in charge between the particles, modified by endosmosis and by adsorption.

The structure of starch and polyacrylamide gels, however, is such that molecular sieving plays a significant role. Particles larger than the 'pores' of the gel are obstructed in their movement whereas smaller particles migrate essentially as in free solution.

This concept is, of course, an oversimplification. The gel 'pore' is not of regular shape and does not possess a rigid dimension. Particles larger than the pore may, therefore, be forced through by distortion of the walls of the pore under the force created by the potential on the charged particle.

It must not be assumed with either technique that molecules of different molecular weight will inevitably be separated. A large molecule whose passage through the gel is obstructed by the pore size may migrate at the same speed or faster than particles of smaller molecular weight which are less highly charged. Whether charge or molecular weight effects predominate in the separation will depend on the composition of the gel. The more concentrated the gel the greater the influence of molecular sieving.

Potato starch forms a gel if heated to greater than 65 °C and then cooled. However, it has been found that partially hydrolysed starch gives the best results

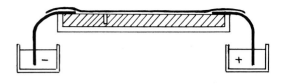

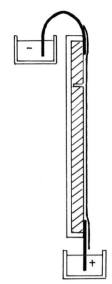

Fig. 5 Starch gel electrophoresis. Gel may be run in either the horizontal or vertical position. The gel (hatched area) sits in a perspex tray covered by a thin plastic sheet. Contact with the electrode compartments is made by multi-layer filter paper or sponge wicks.

for electrophoresis. The original authorities on the technique gave details of how to prepare potato starch for electrophoresis, but satisfactory preparations can be obtained from several suppliers.

As the technique is essentially obsolete following the introduction of polyacrylamide gel electrophoresis it will not be described in detail. Readers wishing further information should consult the first edition of this volume or for more details, Gordon.[5] Suffice it to say that the preparation of a satisfactory starch gel requires skill and good results are obtained only with experience. Setting requires some two hours and sample slots may be cut in the gel after setting or incorporated into the gel by means of a slot former.

The gel block can be run in either the horizontal or the vertical position, the basic arrangements in the two cases being shown in Fig. 5. It is generally accepted that superior resolution is achieved if the gel is run in the vertical position. As with agar gel it may be advantageous to use water cooling to permit higher voltage gradients to be applied. Heat dissipation is, of course, aided by the use of a thin gel.

Suitable buffers for use in starch gel electrophoresis are listed by Gordon.[7]

Although good results can be achieved with starch

gel techniques, it is difficult to obtain uniformity between the production of one gel (or batch of gels) and another. Regrettably, even with gels of the same starch concentration, such variations produce gels of differing separative properties.

Polyacrylamide gel. Polyacrylamide gel is formed by the polymerization of the two monomers, acrylamide and methylene-bis-acrylamide. The structures of these compounds and of the gel formed are shown in Fig. 6. The gel consists of strands of polyacrylamide

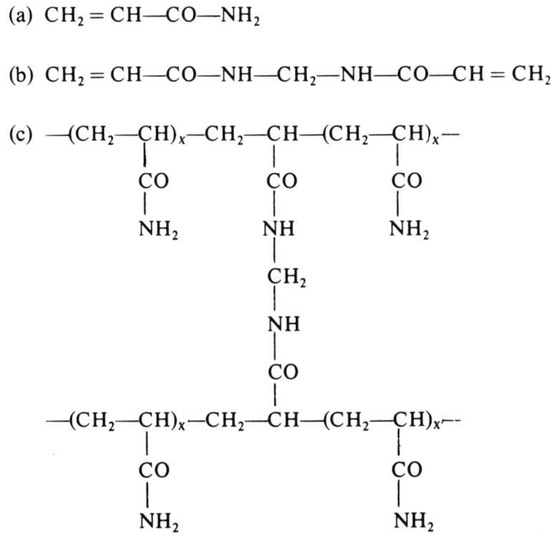

(a) $CH_2 = CH—CO—NH_2$

(b) $CH_2 = CH—CO—NH—CH_2—NH—CO—CH = CH_2$

(c)
$$—(CH_2—CH)_x—CH_2—CH—(CH_2—CH)_x—$$
with CO, NH_2, CO, NH, CO, NH_2 side groups, CH_2, NH, CO crosslink, and
$$—(CH_2—CH)_x—CH_2—CH—(CH_2—CH)_x—$$
with CO, NH_2, CO, NH_2 side groups

Fig. 6 The structure of (a) acrylamide, (b) methylene-bis-acrylamide and (c) polyacrylamide gel.

linked together at intervals by the crosslinking agent methylene-bis-acrylamide.

As with starch gels, the resultant 'mesh' impedes the passage of particles. Polyacrylamide has, however, many advantages compared with starch:

1. Its composition is relatively well defined and its ability to form gels over a wide range of acrylamide and bis-acrylamide concentration allows the preparation of gels of widely differing 'pore size' and physical properties;
2. Further variation in physical properties such as mechanical stability, elasticity and adhesion to various support materials can be obtained by substitution of alternative crosslinking agents such as N,N'-diallytardiamide (DATD) or the agarose derivative AcrylAide (Marine Colloids, FMC);
3. The transparent nature of the gel and, in most applications, the absence of significant background staining renders visual or densitometric evaluation easy;
4. The gel forms an ideal matrix for enzyme detection allowing relatively easy access of substrate and staining solution while impeding the diffusion of the separated protein components or of particulate stain;
5. The gels are relatively easy to adapt for preparative electrophoresis and, although elution of

protein components may be slow, the gel may be macerated to allow extraction;
6. The gels are tough and easily handled even in thicknesses of 1–2 mm.

Polyacrylamide gel electrophoresis is unambiguously the medium of choice where high resolution electrophoresis on the basis of charge and molecular size is required. Its qualities as a molecular sieving medium however, initially rendered the application of immunological detection methods difficult, as diffusion of antigen and antibody only occurred at a very slow rate. This difficulty was only overcome by the development of nitrocellulose electroblotting techniques (*see* section on Immunological identification below).

Polyacrylamide gel as an electrophoretic medium was introduced in 1959 (*see* Whipple[2]). Raymond used a continuous buffer system, and an acrylamide gel of one concentration in the form of a rectangular slab, whereas Ornstein and Davis employed discontinuous buffer, pH and gel systems, established in cylindrical glass tubes. By virtue of these discontinuities the latter technique was termed 'disc electrophoresis'. It should be noted, however, that the term has been used more loosely to describe an electrophoretic separation carried out in polyacrylamide gel rods where the separated and stained proteins appear as a series of 'discs' distributed along the axis of the rod.

The original technique of Ornstein and Davis utilized a conductivity jump across a moving boundary in order to concentrate the components to be separated into a relatively thin starting zone. As mentioned above the method involved a rather complex and rigid composition of gel, pH and buffer conditions. The author, along with many other workers, has found that equally satisfactory results can be achieved in simpler ways. Furthermore the technique of Ornstein and Davis was applicable to only a limited range of biological materials by virtue of the need to restrict pH conditions. The simplified procedures have the advantage that the great flexibility of polyacrylamide gel with respect to gel concentration, buffer and pH is not lost. The technique of Ornstein and Davis will not, therefore, be discussed further in its original form. For discussion of its theoretical basis the original paper should be consulted (*see* Whipple[2]).

It is now clear that to achieve satisfactory results it is essential that the particles to be separated must be concentrated into a sharp starting zone. Such sharpening can generally be achieved quite simply in two ways:

1. Initially the sample may be loaded in free solution on to the top of a polyacrylamide rod or onto a sample well formed in a slab of polyacrylamide gel. The migration velocity in free solution exceeds that in the gel and, therefore, the components will tend to 'pile up' at the gel buffer interface. In theory, therefore, the maxi-

mum degree of sharpening might be expected with the sample in free solution and with an initial gel layer of the highest possible concentration. In practice, however, this is impractical and undesirable. Inevitably, in free solution the particles to be separated are subject to convection effects which severely restrict the potential that can be applied before the proteins have entered the gel matrix. Also, with many mixtures, for example serum proteins, large molecular weight components will be present which will be excluded from any small pore gel and not detected by subsequent staining.

In practice, therefore, it is better to have an initial gel (usually referred to as a 'spacer' gel) of low concentration followed by a 'separation' gel of higher concentration where the molecular sieving effects of polyacrylamide will be fully exploited. When the components of the mixture have entered the gel of low concentration, and are therefore protected against distortion by convection effects, the potential can be increased, resulting in the components concentrating into a thin starting zone at the top of the 'separation' gel. It is vital that the top surface of the 'separation' gel be absolutely smooth.

2. Zone sharpening may also be easily achieved by giving the sample a lower conductivity than the buffer solution. This technique was first used by Haglund and Tiselius and applied by Hjerten to polyacrylamide gel electrophoresis.[2,3] The concentrating effect results from the fact that the rear (or top) of the component zone will migrate faster than the front. The effect is not, of course, a continuous one. When the conductivity discontinuity has passed the zone the latter migrates in a homogenous medium and will be steadily broadened by diffusion. The concentration that takes place in the more complex system of Ornstein and Davis is similarly a once and for all effect.

The *polymerization* of acrylamide and the incorporation of the crosslinking agent can be effected in a variety of ways. A commonly used system involves the initiation of polymerization by the formation of free oxygen radicals from ammonium, persulphate catalysed by the base TEMED (*N,N,N',N'*-tetramethyl ethylenediamine). A variety of other bases has been substituted.

Alternatively, free radicals may be produced by the action of UV light on riboflavin, which substitutes for ammonium persulphate. The usual laboratory fluorescent light tube is a suitable light source.

In outline, a stock solution containing the two monomers in the desired proportion is mixed with buffer, TEMED, and a solution of riboflavin or ammonium persulphate. Excess oxygen must be excluded as this impairs the polymerization process.

Hence the constituent solutions are 'degassed' by drawing them up into a syringe, capping the nozzle and drawing back the plunger to induce a strong negative pressure. All mixing must be conducted gently to avoid aeration, and as polymerization is inhibited by cooling the solutions should be warmed to room temperature before mixing.

The mixture is introduced into the mould in which it will set, which is almost invariably where the subsequent electrophoresis will be conducted. The mould is usually either a vertical glass tube or a vertical rectangular compartment of glass or perspex. During polymerization contact with air must be prevented, and this is done either by use of a closed mould or by placing a layer of water above the top surface of the gel. Water layering also produces the absolutely smooth gel top surface which is vital to obtain sharp bands.

Polymerization is not significantly inhibited by the presence of glycerol, sucrose, urea, or other additives such as SDS (sodium dodecyl sulphate). As, however, the reaction is an exothermic one, dissipation of the heat produced should be ensured by surrounding the glass tube or plates in which the gel is being cast with an adequate volume of buffer. Control of the temperature during setting is particularly important when gradient gels are being formed (*see* below).

Regrettably the catalyst systems used during polymerization may give rise to artifacts on subsequent electrophoresis. For example, residual ammonium persulphate has been implicated in the inactivation of enzymes. The mechanism of this is not certain. Ammonium persulphate migrates in the gel very much faster than proteins and, therefore, should not generally come into contact with them. Ornstein has suggested that persulphate may leave the gel in an oxygen rich state which may lead to the oxidation of the SH groups present in the protein molecules. Incorporation of anti-oxidants such as thioglycolate or mercaptoethanol may protect these groups, at the risk, however, of inducing other changes. The use of a riboflavin photocatalytic system has also been reported to cause artifacts in protein separation. In the author's experience, persulphate catalysis of polymerization is simpler and more reproducible than photocatalysis.

To explore the molecular sieving properties of polyacrylamide, a gel of the appropriate 'pore size' must be prepared. Pore size is not, however, simply related to the concentration of monomer present. The relative amounts of acrylamide and methylene-bis-acrylamide influence pore size and are also vital in determining the physical nature of the gel, i.e. its elasticity, toughness and transparency.

(In the description that follows the quantity of methylene-bis-acrylamide as a percentage of the total acrylamide present will be referred to simply as the 'percentage of bis'.)

The effect of varying the proportions of bis-acrylamide to acrylamide over a wide range of total monomer concentration was investigated by Fawcett and Morrison (summarized by Gordon[7]). They found that a minimum concentration of 2 g total monomer per 100 ml solution was required to allow gel formation. At any given concentration of total monomer the pore diameter was found to be a minimum at approximately 5% of bis-acrylamide. Therefore, depending on the quantity of bis present, it is possible for a gel of greater total monomer concentration to have a larger effective pore size than a gel of lower concentration. Although the conclusions of Fawcett and Morris were drawn from chromatographic studies using polyacrylamide gels, similar results using electrophoresis were reported by Hjerten.

Gels containing 5% of bis-acrylamide are widely used. However, to obtain optimum physical characteristics in the gel, the author has followed the recommendations of Davis to decrease the concentration of bis as the total monomer concentration is increased. A variety of formulae have been devised to achieve this end. That used by the author has been the formula of Richards. After the total concentration of monomer required has been decided the relative percentage of bis is calculated as follows:

$$\text{Per cent concentration of bis} = 6{\cdot}5 - 0{\cdot}3\,T$$

where T is the total monomer concentration in g/100 ml.

For the optimum separation of serum proteins a gel of concentration 7 g of total monomer per 100 ml buffer with bis calculated by the above equation has been found to be very satisfactory.

Although the modification has found little application, it is relatively simple to incorporate charged groups into the polyacrylamide gel. An anionic gel can be made by the incorporation of acrylic acid residues and a cationic gel by the incorporation of methacryl choline methyl sulphate. The incorporation of charged groups results in electro-endosmotic flow and problems of gel swelling and contraction.

Separation on unmodified polyacrylamide gel is dependent partly on the charge and partly on the size of the particle. It is possible to determine the molecular weight of particles by polyacrylamide gel electrophoresis, either directly or indirectly. It has been found that the logarithm of the electrophoretic mobility of a particle is linearly related to the gel concentration provided that the proportion of cross-linking agent is kept constant. If electrophoresis of proteins of different molecular weights is carried out in gels of different concentration, a series of straight lines of differing slopes will be obtained when the logarithm of the electrophoretic mobility of each protein is plotted against gel concentration. Mobility is used here in the sense of the distance (absolute, or relative to some marker dye) travelled by a particle under constant electrophoretic conditions and for a fixed time.

Proteins of identical molecular size but different charge, e.g. LDH isoenzymes, will give rise to parallel lines in such a plot. Proteins of different size but similar charge, e.g. polymers of albumin, will give rise to lines which intersect if extrapolated to the theoretical point where gel concentration is zero.

To calculate the molecular weight of a protein, the mobility of the protein relative to two proteins of known molecular weight should be observed under identical electrophoretic conditions in gels of two or, preferably, more concentrations. The mobilities of the proteins in the large pore gel and in the small pore gel are measured and the slope of the line relating mobility to gel concentration calculated. The slopes of the lines obtained are directly related to the molecular weights of the protein, allowing the molecular weight of the test protein to be calculated.

The relationship between charge, molecular size and electrophoretic mobility in polyacrylamide gel electrophoresis is such that the appearance of a single band on electrophoresis cannot be interpreted as unequivocal evidence of protein homogeneity. The separation should be repeated at different gel concentrations to eliminate the possibility that under the conditions initially used a large highly charged protein is migrating at the same rate as a small lightly charged protein.

Rather surprisingly perhaps, data at present available suggest that the shape of a protein molecule does not appear to have any very great effect on electrophoretic mobility, although certain proteins show anomalous behaviour for this reason. Such shape effects may be minimized by conducting the separation in the presence of a dissociating agent such as 8 M urea.

The separation of proteins purely on a molecular weight basis may be achieved directly by the incorporation of the detergent sodium dodecyl sulphate (SDS) in both gel and buffer systems. This, of course, gives another method of molecular weight determination. The technique was introduced by Shapiro and co-workers who found that in the presence of the detergent an inverse linear relationship existed between the relative migration distance of a wide variety of proteins and the logarithm of their molecular weights. It is postulated that SDS anions form a micellar complex with the proteins. The size of this complex is related to the molecular weight of the protein, but no significant charge difference exists between one protein/detergent complex and another. The author has found the method simple to carry out, although, as the detergent renders the gel extremely slippery, special precautions may have to be taken to prevent the gel slipping out of the glass tube or cell in which it is contained. Protein staining may also present difficulties and enzymes may be inactivated.

As mentioned above, the zone-sharpening achieved by voltage or gel discontinuities is a once and for all effect. Thereafter the zones will be constantly broadened as the electrophoresis proceeds.

This effect may in theory be obviated if the electrophoresis is conducted into a gradient of increasing gel concentration. Ultimately any particular protein should proceed until the pores present in the gel become too small to permit further progress. Hence electrophoresis in polyacrylamide gel gradients is sometimes termed '*pore limit*' electrophoresis. Gradients of linear, exponential, or convex form may be prepared, the incorporation of sucrose into the gel assisting in the production of smooth gradients. Gradients can be achieved by multi-channel pumps or by the use of simple gradient forming devices. Satisfactory gels are only obtained if gelation is arranged to start at the top of the gel and proceed downwards. This may be achieved by the incorporation of differential amounts of catalysts.

The author's experience has been that while such gradients are easily achieved in tubes, they are more difficult to achieve in rectangular cells. However, the inability to run reference preparations in the same tube as the test solution does mean that comparable results are highly dependent on absolute consistency of gel composition in each tube. This is difficult to achieve in non-gradient polyacrylamide gel systems and very much more difficult in gradient systems. The recent introduction of pumping systems controlled by inexpensive desk-top computers ensures greater uniformity and allows the rapid investigation of the usefulness of different gradient forms in a particular application.

In summary the technique can achieve separation on a molecular size basis with a useful zone-sharpening effect and in addition a single gradient gel can resolve mixtures of a wider range of molecular sizes than a gel of uniform concentration.

Polyacrylamide gel electrophoresis can be carried out either in *cylindrical glass tubes* or in a *flat bed apparatus* of one sort or another. Electrophoresis can also be conducted in thin layers of acrylamide on glass plates. However, this does not give a resolution equal to that achieved in vertical flat bed apparatus, and is reserved for polyacrylamide gel isoelectric focusing (*see* below), where the sample can be applied directly to the gel or via filter paper squares and where resolution does not depend on the establishment of a thin starting zone.

The use of thin slabs of polyacrylamide rather than cylindrical rods has many advantages. Temperature is easier to control, and comparison between one serum sample and another is possible as a dozen or more samples, including appropriate markers, can be run simultaneously, allowing very small differences in mobility between the protein or enzyme bands in different samples to be detected. Protein and enzyme staining is more even, and subsequent densitometry easier.

Only very simple apparatus is required to carry out either the cylindrical rod or flat slab technique. As far as polyacrylamide rods are concerned glass tubes of about 5 mm bore, 1 mm wall thickness and 75 mm or more in length are adequate as moulds and running tubes. Using as a basis sheets of glass of dimensions $1.5 \times 75 \times 200$ mm, obtained cheaply from any glass merchant, the author has devised several flat-bed devices involving the use of rubber tubing gaskets and Teflon® or perspex spacer strips. The two types of apparatus are illustrated in Fig. 7.

Many of the *buffer systems* introduced for other types of gel electrophoresis will also give satisfactory results with polyacrylamide gel. A comprehensive list of buffers that have been used in gel electrophoresis is to be found in Gordon.[7]

The considerations covering the choice of buffer for polyacrylamide are to a large extent similar to those for other media although an advantage of the technique is that a wider pH range is possible with this medium than with others. The pH should be that which maximizes the difference in mobility between the components it is desired to separate, and ideally the ionic strength should be as low as possible to minimize heat production to allow high potential gradients and rapid separation. However, strict limits are placed on this by the solubility of the proteins being separated.

Another factor that must always be borne in mind with high discrimination techniques is the possibility of interaction between the buffer and the component being separated. It is not always true that the presence of a band indicates the presence of a separate protein species. It is possible that complexes between component and buffer give rise to multiple bands from a single molecule species in the original mixture.

The use of discontinuous buffer systems and other 'zone-sharpening' techniques commonly used in polyacrylamide gel electrophoresis, but not specific to it, has been discussed in the theoretical section above.

Preparative Electrophoresis. For preparative purposes an electrophoretic technique must be able to handle much larger quantities of material than is necessary for analytical purposes. Simple scaling up of analytical electrophoretic procedures has rarely been fully successful. For example, although multiple layers of filter paper or thicker layers of starch or polyacrylamide gel have been used for preparative electrophoresis, the quality of separation has almost invariably been poor compared with the same medium used on an analytical scale. One reason for these poor results has been the difficulty of achieving even cooling in the thick layer of paper or gel.

Continuous electrophoresis for preparative purposes is fairly simple to conduct using paper. The paper is arranged vertically (Fig. 8) and has a serrated lower edge, the tip of each serration dipping into a sample container. Chromatographic effects do of course occur with this method but in theory, if the ratio of buffer flow and electrical potential is carefully

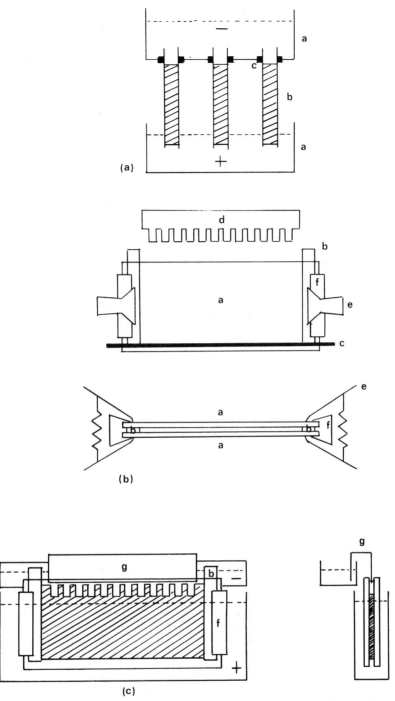

Fig. 7 Apparatus for polyacrylamide gel electrophoresis. Figure 7(a) apparatus using cylindrical rods of polyacrylamide (a) buffer reservoirs; (b) glass tubes; (c) gaskets. Polyacrylamide gel is indicated by the hatched area. Figure 7(b) apparatus for electrophoresis in thin vertical slabs of polyacrylamide assembled for casting of gel, and Fig. 7(c) in the running position: (a) glass plates; (b) teflon spacers; (c) silicon rubber tubing gasket; (d) teflon comb; (e) metal spring clip; (f) plastic binding bars (Denee-Bind); (g) filter paper wick. Note that the lower electrode compartment is deep, to allow the assembly to be surrounded by chilled buffer during the electrophoretic run.

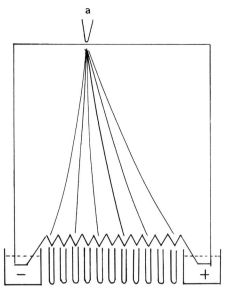

Fig. 8 Continuous preparative electrophoresis. The sample is applied at point a. The lines represent the path followed by the components of a mixture during separation.

adjusted and maintained constant during the course of the run, then reproducible separation should be achieved. However, it is difficult to keep these factors constant, particularly when the procedure is complicated by evaporation and heating effects.

Using flat bed polyacrylamide gel systems it is simple to stain a series of vertical marker strips across the width of a polyacrylamide gel slab to allow accurate location of separated components in unstained portions of the gel. Horizontal slices containing a purified component may be isolated. However, the quantity of material that can be obtained in this way is very small, and it is further reduced or diluted by any attempt to elute from the gel section. This may not be necessary for every purpose as, for example, macerated polyacrylamide gel containing purified protein has been injected directly into animals and an antiserum obtained to the protein component in the acrylamide.

After maceration of the gel sections, protein can be eluted by simple diffusion into buffer or by a further electrophoretic step. Various elution cells for the latter purpose have been described. The eluate can then be concentrated by freeze drying. Gel maceration may be achieved by forcing the gel through the needle of a syringe. However, to obtain the increased amounts of material necessary for preparative purposes either multiple gels have to be run, resulting in a highly dilute final sample, or alternatively thicker gel slabs have to be used with the drawbacks mentioned above.

Several preparative devices involving the use of column electrophoresis have been described. A variety of support media has been used in these or the electrophoresis may be conducted essentially in free solution by using a sucrose density gradient. Using this latter system the separated components may be isolated either by running off the gradient directly from the lower end of the column or alternatively by displacing the gradient from the top of the column by pumping a high density sucrose solution in from the bottom.

Preparative devices involving electrophoresis in free solution are limited by turbulence caused by convection and particle sedimentation. As experiments in the US Space Shuttle demonstrated, elimination of interference effects caused in part at least by gravity, allowed a free electrophoretic system to work at equal or higher degrees of purification at dramatically increased speed. Stabilization of electrophoretic conditions has also been achieved by use of a rotary separator in the Biostream system devised by Harwell Laboratory (UKAEA-CJB Developments Limited). Electrophoretic separation takes place in an upward flowing buffer stream in the annular space between an inner stationary cylinder and an outer rotating cylinder. The separated components form concentric bands and are isolated by multiple collection plates at the top of the device (Fig. 9).

The essential features of a device to collect separated components after electrophoresis in a solid or gel medium are shown in Fig. 10. Elution is achieved by means of a transverse flow of buffer at the lower end of the column. A membrane of some type is required which prevents the passage of the separated components from the elution chamber but allows unimpeded passage to the electrical current. The flow of eluting buffer must be adequate to avoid mixing of the components separated by electrophoresis, and similarly the eluting buffer must be collected in small enough fractions to avoid mixing one component with another. The elution of protein components may be monitored by the usual devices used to monitor the effluent from chromatography columns. The eluted protein will present as a series of peaks. The width of any peak will be inversely proportional to the mobility of the component. This is not solely a result of the time taken to enter the elution chamber but also results from the fact that components of lower mobility will have spent a longer period of time exposed to the various influences which, during an electrophoretic run, cause zone broadening. To ensure that the dilution of the eluted components is as uniform as possible the flow of eluting buffer may be steadily reduced as the separation proceeds.

Because of the relatively well-defined nature of the medium, and its capacity to handle substantial amounts of protein, this form of preparative electrophoresis in columns is often conducted using polyacrylamide gel. Annular columns of polyacrylamide gel, enclosed between two cooled surfaces, have been used to allow adequate cooling, and it is possible to handle several hundred milligrams of proteins on these.

In summary it can be said that as a general rule

Carrier input — — Migrant
mixture input

Migrant
fractions
outlets

Stator

Electrophoresis

Rotor

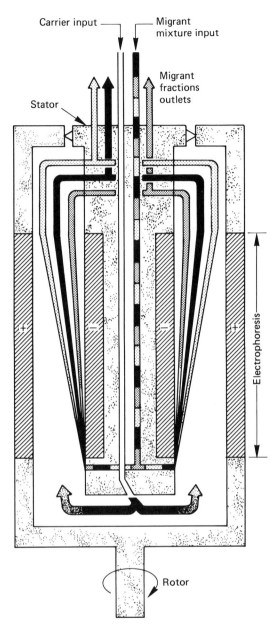

Fig. 9 Biostream Separator, CJB Developments Ltd (*courtesy:* Harwell Laboratory,
UKAEA).

the degree of resolution obtained with all these preparative techniques is considerably inferior to that
obtained with the same medium used for analytical
purposes. The contrast is of course particularly striking in the case of polyacrylamide gel.

Electrophoresis in a pH Gradient—Isoelectric Focusing

Zones containing separated protein fractions gradually broaden due to diffusion during the course
of most electrophoretic procedures. Electrophoresis
in an increasing concentration gradient of polyacrylamide can reduce this diffusion effect. A more powerful technique to minimize the effects of diffusion in

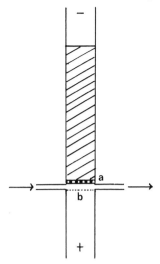

Fig. 10 Schematic representation
of elution chamber for recovery of
separated components in column
electrophoresis. The gel or other
stabilizing medium is indicated by
the hatched area, the flow of eluting buffer by the arrow, and the
column support and semi-
permeable membrane at (a) and
(b) respectively. The eluted components pass to a column monitor
and fraction collector.

the separation of proteins or other biological compounds is that usually known as 'isoelectric focusing',
where the electrophoretic migration of particles is
conducted in a pH gradient, and where the protein
zones sharpen as the separation proceeds.

Basically the apparatus used is similar to that used
for electrophoresis save that an increasing pH gradient is established from anode to cathode. Amphoteric
substances such as proteins present within the system
migrate under the influence of the electric current
until they reach their isoelectric point within the pH
gradient. The principles of the separation are outlined in Fig. 11.

A protein at a pH higher than its isoelectric point
will be negatively charged and will migrate towards
the anode, whereas at a pH below its isoelectric point
it will be positively charged and will move towards
the cathode. The presence of an acid at the anode
and a strong base in the cathode compartment in
place of the buffer systems used in electrophoresis
ensures that positively charged components are
repelled from the former and negatively charged particles from the latter.

A pH gradient can easily become disrupted due
to convection and to uneven field strength, and the
principal obstacle to be overcome before the technique could be effectively exploited was to find a
means of stabilizing the gradient.

The technique became a practical proposition in
the early 1960s after Svensson specified the qualities
necessary in the constituents of a stable gradient and

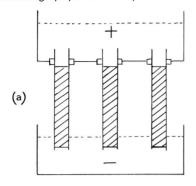

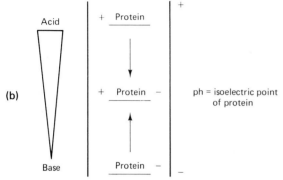

Fig. 11 Isoelectric focusing, apparatus (a) and principle (b). The apparatus (a) is similar to that used in 'disc' electrophoresis. The upper reservoir (anode) is filled with 0·2% H_2SO_4 the lower (cathode) with 0·4% diethanolamine.

Vesterberg synthesized suitable materials—known as ampholytes. The ampholytes (marketed as 'Ampholines' by LKB) were formed by reacting acrylic acid with the amino groups of a mixture of aliphatic polyamines. The general formula of these and the resultant ampholines is shown in Fig. 12. The result is a mixture containing a large number of polyamino polycarboxylic acids.

$$R_1.\overset{+}{N}H_2.(CH_2)_n.\overset{+}{N}H_2.R_2 + CH_2 = CH.COO^-$$

$$\rightleftharpoons R_1.\overset{+}{N}H_2.(CH_2)_n.\overset{+}{N}H.R_2$$
$$|$$
$$CH_2.CH_2.COO^-$$

Fig. 12 Formation and structure of Ampholines®, R_1 and R_2 = H or aliphatic radical with additional amino groups.

Subsequently a number of other manufacturers have introduced compounds of generally similar properties. The various commercial preparations have been synthesized in different ways and their exact composition is not known. However, it has been observed that certain products are considerably more effective in some pH regions than in others and it is possible therefore to blend the available products to give a mixture optimized for a particular purpose.

In order to achieve adequate stability in use, ampholytes need to be combined either with a sucrose density gradient or, even better, with polyacrylamide gel of low concentration, the latter technique generally being referred to as *gel isoelectric focusing*. The commercial materials in general meet Svensson's specifications for ampholytes suitable for the technique. First, their buffering power is adequate at the isoelectric point but does vary with change of pH. The presence of the ampholytes is responsible for the maintenance of the pH gradient and, therefore, the pH must not alter due to the presence of focused proteins or other amphoteric compounds. Secondly, they have adequate, but sometimes uneven, conductivity; low conductivity at the isoelectric point would lead to overheating and disruption of the pH gradient. Reasonable field strengths can be tolerated, and drifting of the pH gradient minimized, by the presence of the strong acid and base in the anode and cathode respectively. The ampholytes have a higher water solubility at the isoelectric point, and the fact that they have a lower molecular weight than the proteins which they are generally used to separate aids their subsequent removal. Although they absorb heavily in the low ultraviolet they do not absorb significantly at the wavelengths used to monitor the separation of proteins by the techniques commonly used in column chromatography. However, the ampholytes may interact with the components being separated, with complex metal ions necessary for enzyme activity and with some of the common protein stains.

With care, samples containing denaturing and solubilizing agents such as urea, non-ionic detergents and even ionic detergents such as sodium dodecyl sulphate (SDS) can be examined by isoelectric focusing. The review by Hjelmeland and Chrambach[8] should be consulted. Samples with a high salt concentration may need to be desalted.

Because of variations in conductivity during isoelectric separation, use of 'constant power' supplies is desirable, enabling voltage to be automatically increased as current decreases. Strict control of temperature is essential.

To illustrate the principles of the procedure short descriptions of the two methods of using ampholytes for separative purposes will be given.

pH Gradient Stabilized with a Sucrose Density Gradient. This technique is particularly useful for preparative work but is time-consuming and for satisfactory results requires special apparatus such as the electrofocusing column marketed by LKB. First, an appropriate ampholyte mixture covering the desired pH range is selected and two solutions of high and low density prepared, the former by mixing the ampholyte with sucrose and water, and the latter by simple dilution of the ampholyte solution. The sample is mixed with the solution of low density. These solutions are then added to the electrofocusing column using a gradient mixing device, or alternatively by adding small proportions of a mixture prepared from varying proportions of the high and low density solutions. The high density mixture is added to the bottom of the column and layers of decreasing density added on top by means of some capillary system. This results in a stepwise linear density gradient containing ampholyte and protein from bottom to top of the column. A strong base, usually ethanolamine, is added to the cathode electrode compartment and phosphoric acid or other strong acid added to the anode. Cooling water is passed through the cooling jacket and a potential applied across the electrodes. Both ampholyte and protein move in the electric field, the more acidic towards the anode and the most basic towards the cathode. The final arrangement of ampholytes and of proteins takes many hours, and one or two days are generally required to complete the process.

The proteins concentrate in zones which sharpen as time proceeds, although broadening as a result of diffusion may occur. When focusing is complete the current is shut off and the column contents passed through the measuring cell of any suitable chromatographic column effluent protein monitoring device, and may be collected in a fraction collector. The pH of the collected fractions may also be measured to give some idea of the regularity and completeness of the pH gradient. The isoelectric point of any separated components can, therefore, be determined.

pH Gradient Stabilized by Polyacrylamide Gel. The apparatus is similar to that used in polyacrylamide gel electrophoresis, and the procedure may be carried out either in gel rods or on a gel slab. A mixture is prepared containing ampholine, acrylamide, methylene-bis-acrylamide, and TEMED, with either riboflavin to act as a photo-catalyst or ammonium persulphate as a chemical catalyst. There have been many reports in the literature of the effectiveness or otherwise of these catalysts for a particular purpose, and the author can only suggest that both systems be investigated for any particular application.

In comparison with gel electrophoresis, a lower gel concentration is used so that the molecular sieving properties of polyacrylamide play little or no part in the separation achieved, the gel matrix merely being present in order to stabilize the pH gradient. The gel mixture is added to the glass tube or slab apparatus and water layered on the top surface to exclude air and to allow polymerization to take place. The protein-containing sample may either be dispersed throughout the gel mixture, or, if a reasonably concentrated solution such as serum is being fractionated, it may be mixed with 10% sucrose and applied to the top of the gel.

If a concentrated sample, mixed with 10% sucrose, is layered on top of the gel, it is desirable to protect the sample from contact with the strong acid in the anode compartment by adding the sample as a layer under a mixture of ampholyte and 5% sucrose. The

upper buffer compartment is then topped up with acid, and the lower buffer compartment with the strong base. A potential is then applied, generally considerably less than that used for polyacrylamide gel electrophoresis. It should be noted that it is possible to establish the pH gradient and to remove any of the breakdown products of the catalytic procedure by a preliminary period of 30 minutes application of current before the sample is added. A voltage of several hundred volts may be applied and it will be found that a period of several hours is necessary for the electrofocusing to take place. It is, of course, difficult to monitor the progress of the focusing, but it is generally satisfactory to add some haemolysed serum to one or other of the sample compartments and to observe the sharpening of the haemoglobin bands. The gel is then removed from the tube or slab apparatus by the usual rimming procedure with water introduced through a syringe and hypodermic needle.

Isoelectric focusing can also be carried out horizontally in ultrathin (typically 100–250 μm) polyacrylamide gels, using less ampholyte and allowing high voltage gradients and shorter focusing times. Acrylamide will only adhere effectively to glass under these conditions if the glass support plate is silanized. The result of this treatment is that the polyacrylamide gel is effective covalently bound to the glass, thus minimizing gel distortion and the risk of damage during handling.

The thickness of such gels is generally determined by the application of several layers of adhesive tape to the edges of the plate. Although the gel is allowed to set in a glass plate sandwich, the non-silanized top plate is removed before running and the sample applied to the middle of the gel directly or by filter paper squares. Use of glass fibre electrode wicks containing no charged groups is desirable and efficient cooling is essential. An advantage of these thin polyacrylamide layers is that after washing in a 3% glycerol solution they can be dried down for storage.

After focusing on polyacrylamide the regularity and completeness of the pH gradient may be checked by slicing the gel, eluting the sections with distilled water and measuring the pH of the eluant. Alternatively the pH gradient may be checked by running a mixture of proteins of known isoelectric point. Preparations of such calibration proteins are available in kit form from commercial suppliers. A frequent problem is drift of the gradient towards the cathode. The reason for this is not known with certainty, but is probably caused by electro-endosmosis induced by charges in the gel or on the walls of the glass support.

Gel isoelectric focusing illustrates the advantages that gel slabs enjoy over gel rods for separation purposes. With this technique the separated zones of protein are often very fine, but it is virtually impossible to get a regular and identical pH gradient in a series of gel rods to allow accurate comparison between the components in one sample with another.

pH Gradient Stabilized by Agarose Gel. The use of agarose as a support medium for isoelectric focusing has many attractions. The gel is easy to prepare, optically clear and its large effective pore size does not interfere with the free movement of the particles being separated. As no catalysts are required for gelation the risk of interaction between these and the carrier ampholytes is eliminated. As against this it is essential to use an agarose with the minimum number of charged groups to reduce the endosmosis responsible for drift of the pH gradient. A number of suitable commercial preparations are available.

The technique is simple and requires no special apparatus. One of the commercial ampholyte preparations is added to the agarose mixture when it has cooled to about 75 °C prior to addition to the support. As with agarose electrophoresis this may be a glass plate or hydrophilic polyester sheet. Wells or slots are not cut or cast in the gel, samples being applied to filter paper squares laid on the surface of the gel. Good contact between the gels and the electrode wicks and adequate control of temperature are essential if distortions are to be avoided. After completion of the run the gel is fixed, washed and dried by placing layers of weighted filter paper on top. The dried gel is then ready for application of location procedures.

The definition achieved by agarose isoelectric focusing is not generally as good as that obtained with polyacrylamide as a support, but the simplicity of the technique and its ability to handle larger molecular weight species makes it attractive for particular applications. Agarose is not suitable for use at extremes of the pH range.

The detection of proteins or of enzymes after gel isoelectric focusing requires special techniques (*see* section on Identification and quantitation). The principles and practice of isoelectric focusing have been reviewed by Latner[9] and Catsimpoolas.[10]

High-resolution Two-dimensional Electrophoresis

This involves separation in one dimension on the basis of one physical property of the particles being studied, followed by separation in a second dimension on the basis of an independent physical attribute. Smithies and Poulik in 1956 were among the first to appreciate the advantages such a procedure could bring, when separation on the basis of charge in one dimension was followed by separation on the basis of molecular weight in a second dimension.

The number of components that can in theory be separated by such a combination is equal to the product of the number of components resolved by each technique used in isolation. While such a degree of resolution is rarely achieved in practice, nearly 2000 peptides have been identified in a single two-dimensional analysis of cell constituents.

While many combinations of technique have been used, current approaches tend to follow the work of O'Farrell[11] in joining the two techniques currently capable of giving the highest resolution on the basis of charge and molecular weight respectively, namely, isoelectric focusing on polyacrylamide gel in the first dimension, followed by SDS or gradient polyacrylamide gel electrophoresis in the second dimension. There is of course no theoretical reason why these techniques have to be used in this sequence but in practice it is best and customary to conduct the isoelectric focusing first, to avoid possible interference from SDS residues, or difficult elution of protein from the small pore areas of a gradient gel.

The first dimension isoelectric focusing in acrylamide can be carried out in any of the ways mentioned above, but there seems little doubt that the best resolution and reproducibility is achieved with horizontal flat bed techniques. The method is applicable to both soluble and non-soluble proteins, dissolution generally being accomplished by use of urea and a non-ionic detergent. The protective effects of the latter may be lost in later stages of the process resulting in precipitation. Occasionally, SDS is added to assist dissolution and the amount of this must be carefully controlled to avoid interference with the focusing. When focusing is complete the separated 'track' is cut out from the rest of the gel and applied to the top of a vertical polyacrylamide SDS or gradient gel. Most workers find it desirable to seal the isoelectric focusing gel to the top of the second gel with agarose or with acrylamide. It may be desirable to equilibrate the isoelectric focusing track with SDS and buffer before placing on the second gel. However, considerable loss of protein or poor resolution may result.

Despite the rather unpromising geometry of this arrangement thin starting zones can be achieved. The relatively large pore isoelectric focusing gel acts as an anticonvection zone while allowing free movement of the separated components, and the particle zones are sharpened by the smooth top surface and small pore size of the second-dimension gel. It is usual to employ a discontinuous buffer system to improve resolution.

Two-dimensional electrophoresis is a technique requiring considerable skill if satisfactory resolution and reproducibility is to be achieved. In addition to the problems that may arise with each of the techniques (*see* above), difficulties may also result from the transfer of the isoelectric focusing track to the second dimension gel. The focusing gel must be of large pore gel to avoid molecular sieving effects and such gels are less stable dimensionally. It is therefore easy to stretch or distort the gel during transfer. The relatively recent introduction of gels bound to plastic supports may resolve this problem although the adhesion of gel to support may be much reduced in the presence of urea and non-ionic detergent used to dissolve tissue proteins.

Two-dimensional electrophoresis is a technique of great potential usefulness in the study of human disease. The technique approaches the degree of resolution required to document the many protein products of living cells and therefore to observe any alterations produced by disease.

However, it is doubtful whether the technique is of immediate application in the clinical laboratory for diagnostic purposes. Although the basic equipment required is quite simple the patterns produced are complex. Careful calibration is required to ensure reproducibility and computer-assisted pattern evaluation seems essential. There is the further difficulty that proteins such as albumin are present in very large relative amounts and their prior removal by affinity chromatography or some other procedure may be essential to avoid the masking of other important components. The technique therefore requires skill and must be considered relatively labour intensive.

The likely gains for the clinical laboratory have been considered by Young and Tracy[12] who conclude that the technique is more likely to be of value in identifying the presence or absence of a protein in diseased tissue, allowing its isolation, the raising of mono- or polyclonal antisera and the development of an assay for measurement of the protein in body fluids or tissues.

Affinity Electrophoresis

The term 'affinity electrophoresis' was introduced by Bøg-Hanson to describe any electrophoretic system in which interacting components are allowed to react during electrophoresis. Well established electrophoretic techniques such as Laurell's 'rocket' immunoelectrophoresis, counter immunoelectrophoresis, and crossed immunoelectrophoresis are particular examples of affinity electrophoresis involving reaction of an antigen with its antibody. More recently affinity electrophoretic procedures have exploited the selective carbohydrate binding properties of protein lectins of plant origin to detect and characterize the clinically important glycoproteins.

The theory of the technique has been elaborated by Takeo and by Horejsi and Ticha. A more practically orientated description of the different ways of exploiting these techniques using the interaction of lectins with glycoproteins as an example, is given by Bøg-Hanson.[13]

Interactions between a substance and an affinity ligand can be explored in a number of ways. The affinity ligand can of course be bound to the electrophoretic support but if the substance and its affinity ligand have opposite or greatly different electrophoretic mobility then interaction will take place when their paths cross or the faster component overtakes the slower. In this context it is useful that most immunoglobulins at the pH used for protein electrophoresis have a relatively low mobility and that plant lectins are also relatively immobile.

An example of interaction of a substance and an affinity ligand of opposite mobility is shown in Fig. 13 which illustrates the principle of counter-immunoelectrophoresis. In this case a negatively charged

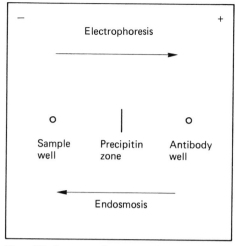

Fig. 13 Counter immunoelectrophoresis. Reaction of a negatively charged antigen of relatively high mobility with weakly charged antibodies carried in a cathodal direction by endosmosis.

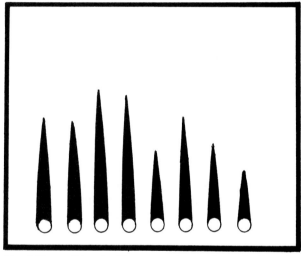

Fig. 14 Laurell 'rocket' immunoelectrophoresis. Protein migrates from point sources into gel containing uniform concentration of specific antiserum. Peak height is approximately proportional to amount of protein antigen present.

antigen placed in one well of an agar gel or on a point application to a cellulose acetate strip interacts with an antibody carried in the opposite direction by electro-endosmotic flow overcoming the weak negative charge on the immunoglobulins involved.

Similarly in Laurell 'rocket' immunoelectrophoresis protein migrates from a point application into a gel containing a uniform distribution of specific antibody (Fig. 14).

In crossed immunoelectrophoresis (Fig. 15) migration is at right angles to the axis of a first dimension electrophoretic separation, into a gel containing either specific antibodies or an antiserum raised against the protein population being separated.

methods which cannot be applied to the original support medium.

Examples of longer established transfer techniques are the conduct, subsequent to an electrophoretic separation on cellulose acetate, of immunodiffusion and enzyme detection reactions in agar gel. The reason for these manoeuvres will be found below.

Direct Absorptimetry

An example of this approach is the detection of separated proteins or nucleic acids by detection of their UV absorption using an ultraviolet microdensitometer operating at wavelengths around 260 nm. In practice all such direct photometric methods require a medium of high transparency; this limits their application to separations carried out on polyacrylamide gel although the absorbance of light by polyacrylamide gel increases quite rapidly in the UV. Evaluation must also generally be carried out immediately after separation, as the unfixed components will continue to diffuse. It may be necessary to transfer the gel to a quartz tube or cell capable of being mounted in the densitometer. Quantitation of separated proteins requires care, as the content of tryptophan and tyrosine largely influences the absorption in the UV and the content of these two amino acids does differ from one protein to another. Accurate quantitation of any protein is only possible when its specific absorbance at a particular wavelength is known.

Further problems arise in that unpolymerized acrylamide may show a significant UV absorbance. Generally a pre-run in the absence of sample is essential to remove this and any other UV-absorbing impurities. UV-absorbing buffers must, of course, be avoided.

Detection of separated nucleotides or a limited number of other materials, may be possible on paper or cellulose acetate by exposure of the paper or cellulose strip to UV light, when the position of the separated components will be revealed by the presence of dark spots or bands.

Chemical Detection—General Discussion

Only a very few substances of biological interest may be detected by virtue of their intrinsic colour, and the application of some chemical reaction is usually necessary. A staining reaction that detects all the members of a particular group of compounds, for example amino acids, may be followed by procedures designed to detect specific members of the group. Ninhydrin staining to detect amino acids or peptides may be followed by application of the Pauly reaction to detect the presence of histidine. For all forms of electrophoresis certain preliminary stages may be necessary. At the end of the electrophoresis the separated particles will still be capable of diffusion within the gel matrix. In order to minimize this it is usual either to dry the stabilizing medium, for example paper or agar, or in the case of protein separation, to denature the proteins by a 'fixative' either prior to or during the chemical staining. Not all detection procedures available for a particular compound can be applied to separations in all stabilizing media. As far as identification is concerned it is vital that reference materials and unknown samples are subjected to electrophoresis under similar conditions. Ideally, unknown and reference solutions should be run together in the same strip or gel. This is not always possible. In two-dimensional separation by electrophoresis followed by chromatography it is customary to run a reference solution containing the amino acids of clinical interest. It is not practicable to apply this to the same paper as the unknown.

As mentioned above polyacrylamide gel electrophoresis in cylinders of polyacrylamide (so-called 'disc' electrophoresis) is also difficult to control in this way. One solution of the problem is to insert a small spacer into the glass tube, thus splitting the gel cylinder effectively into two halves, the unknown solution being run in one half and the reference solution in the other.

Perhaps the most reliable method of quantitating components separated by electrophoresis is to elute them from the stabilizing medium and to apply a detection method identical to that which would normally be used to quantitate the component in solution. However, this process is invariably tedious. Recovery of the separated components from paper or cellulose acetate will generally be good, but recovery from starch or polyacrylamide gel is usually poor. As a general rule separated components which diffuse only poorly in the particular stabilizing medium will be the most difficult to elute from that medium. Elution inevitably means dilution and may necessitate a further concentration step before any chemical reaction can be applied.

Needless to say, before the elution of any invisible component can be carried out, it must first of all be located by reference to a marker run alongside the unknown or it may be possible to detect the separated component by chemical means, and to elute the resultant colour. For example, proteins separated by cellulose acetate electrophoresis and stained by the widely used dye, Ponceau S, may be quantitated by elution of the dye from the strip. The coloured spot or band is cut out of the strip, cut into small fragments, placed in a test tube and the colour eluted. The absorbance of the coloured solution is then read directly in a photometer. Quantitation by elution may be complicated if the components are not completely separated from one another.

As these direct and indirect methods are tedious, evaluation by densitometry is popular. The densitometry can be based either on the quantity of light reflected from the surface of the separating medium or by quantitation of the amount of light transmitted through the medium. Both methods, particularly the latter, require the stabilizing medium either to be relatively transparent, for example polyacrylamide gel, or agar, or to be capable of being cleared, for example, cellulose acetate. A variety of methods are available for clearing cellulose acetate membrane, for example immersion in oil or decalin. Not all clearing procedures are applicable to the products of every firm. The reasons for this are obscure but reflect variation in the chemical and physical nature of the product.

A number of qualifications must be borne in mind in quantitating separated components either by elution of stained bands or by densitometric evaluation. Using the detection of proteins as an example, it would be surprising if equal amounts of every separated protein component bind equal amounts of stain. Furthermore, the proportion of dye bound to any particular protein may vary as the concentration of protein varies. Particular problems may be caused in serum protein electrophoresis by differences in the dye-binding properties of albumin and the globulins and by the great preponderance of albumin relative to the various globulin components.

Eluted dye may not be in true solution and any turbidity may cause deviations from Beer's Law. Densitometers may not give a linear response to a linear increase in dye concentration. Problems are likely to result from the fact that several well-known protein stains are polychromatic, and that one batch of stain may exhibit different properties from another. In addition, particularly with polyacrylamide gel electrophoresis carried out in gel rods, staining may be very uneven due to poor penetration of the stain to the centre of the rod.

As a general rule better results will be obtained from densitometric scanning if gel electrophoretograms are dried down to a thin layer prior to evaluation. This is easily achieved with agar gels but can be more difficult with polyacrylamide. Prior washing of the latter gels in glycerol-containing solutions usually renders them sufficiently flexible to allow drying if the original gel is sufficiently thin.

In order that the standard of the location and quantitation can match the high discrimination produced by electrophoresis in polyacrylamide gel, it may be necessary to use a special densitometer employing microscope optics or the 'flying spot' principle to detect and integrate the narrow stained bands. Such high discrimination densitometers are usually expensive and devices to document the results of two-dimensional electrophoresis even more so. However, the increasing availability of low-cost personal computers allows more reliable identification of the separated bands or spots as 'adjustment' of the observed pattern can be made on the basis of the positions of known components. This eliminates some but not all of the inevitable irregularities between one gel and another.

Silver Staining. The large increase in resolution of protein mixtures obtained by the application of poly-acrylamide electrophoresis and subsequently by the development of high resolution two-dimensional techniques, prompted the search for protein stains of greatly improved sensitivity to match the improved resolution available. Increased sensitivity could be achieved by autoradiography but this technique could not be satisfactorily applied to all problems. Detection of proteins by fluorescent methods involving reaction with fluorescamine for example, also gives increased sensitivity but the special illumination conditions required has restricted the application of this technique.

In 1979 Merril and his co-workers introduced a silver staining method which with subsequent modifications has shown a sensitivity approaching that of autoradiography and some 200 times greater than the most sensitive stain previously available, Coomassie Blue.

The chemistry of this stain is ill-understood and many variations of the basic procedure have appeared claiming advantages of sensitivity, lower cost, lower background staining or improved protein identification through the production of particular colours with individual proteins. An attempt at diagrammatic classification of the many varieties of stain has been made by Dunn and Burghes[17] (Fig. 18).

As more sensitive stains have appeared it has become clear that the formerly widely used method of 'fixing' proteins in gels, by use of various alcohol, water and acetic acid mixtures is very ineffective. It is generally agreed that fixing in 20% trichloroacetic acid gives much better recovery of the separated pro-

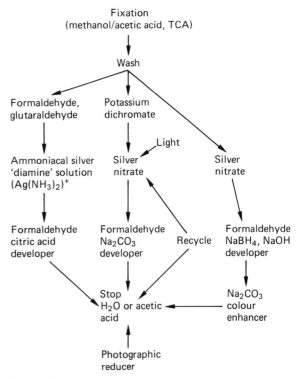

Fig. 18 Steps involved in silver staining procedures. (From Dunn and Burghes.[17])

tein. Following fixation the published silver stain methods recommend treatment either with an aldehyde solution or with dichromate or other oxidizing agent. The effect of these treatments is obscure but they may increase the number of aldehyde groups on the protein which may convert silver ions into metallic silver in the next stage of the process, which is the addition of ammoniacal silver or silver nitrate.

Silver stains are of undoubted sensitivity but have a number of disadvantages. Common problems are heavy and variable background staining, silver deposition on the surface of the acrylamide gel and poor staining in the denser regions of gradient polyacrylamide gels. The stains cannot be successfully applied to agarose gels and tend to be less satisfactory with gels less than 1 or 2 mm thick. There is also considerable doubt as to whether the stain intensity bears a linear relationship to the amount of protein present and it is clear that all proteins do not show the same sensitivity. It will be appreciated that many of these reservations have been voiced with respect to longer-established protein stains such as Coomassie Blue and it must be remembered that it is only with the greatly improved sensitivity of silver stains that the resolving power of two-dimensional electrophoresis in particular can be exploited.

Affinity Detection

The use of affinity binding ligands during the course of an electrophoretic separation has been discussed above. It has also been mentioned that affinity chromatography involving antibodies or other affinity binding agents can be used to 'clean up' serum prior to electrophoresis by removing a protein such as albumin.

Such affinity location reagents can often be tagged in some way, e.g. by radioactive tracers or by enzymes, to improve the sensitivity of detection. The sensitivity of enzyme labels may be further improved by enzyme amplification procedures, where the primary enzyme label is used to provide an initiator for an enzyme cascade to generate a larger quantity of coloured product.

The term affinity reaction has no exact meaning but is usually applied to potentially reversible reactions between biological components which do not involve covalent binding. Examples are the reaction of lectins with glycoproteins, substrates with enzymes, antibodies with antigens and single-stranded nucleic acids with their complementary base sequence.

Lectin Probes. The well-established periodic acid–Schiff (PAS) reaction is a fairly sensitive but general stain for glycoproteins and more discrimination may be introduced by exploiting the ability of an individual lectin to bind to a particular carbohydrate group. One approach is to use a fluorescein isothiocyanate (FITC)-conjugated lectin, the other to react the separated glycoproteins with a lectin/horseradish peroxidase conjugate followed by washing and application of a stain consisting for example, of diaminobenzidine and hydrogen peroxide.

Enzyme Location. Enzymes may be separated from other proteins by electrophoresis, and their presence detected by virtue of their particular catalytic properties. In addition multiple molecular forms of enzyme proteins having the same basic catalytic properties (isoenzymes) may also be separated by electrophoresis. The separation and quantitation of isoenzymes in blood has attained considerable importance in clinical biochemistry, as a particular isoenzyme or isoenzyme pattern may be characteristic of a particular organ of the body, an elevation in the blood levels indicating the involvement of that organ in the disease process.

Although the technique is essentially one of protein separation a number of particular precautions may have to be taken in order to discover how much of an elevated total enzyme activity is contributed by each of the various isoenzyme fractions. It is essential that all fractions enter the medium and are detected by the location process. High molecular weight isoenzymes, such as those of alkaline phosphatase, may not penetrate polyacrylamide gel unless a large pore spacer gel is used and their presence may go unnoticed, or their activity underestimated. It has also been found both with polyacrylamide and agar electrophoresis that the slow-moving isoenzymes of lactic dehydrogenase often appear to be underestimated unless certain precautions are taken. For reasons that are not entirely clear, the addition of protein supplements either permits the isoenzyme to enter the gel or protects its activity.

The preservation of enzyme activity and isoenzyme distribution in the specimen to be examined is of primary importance. Special precautions may have to be taken during the separation and subsequent storage of the serum or plasma. Deep freezing may be satisfactory to preserve some enzyme species but may have a damaging effect in others. For example, the total activity and isoenzyme pattern of alkaline phosphatase is relatively stable when deep frozen but the LDH isoenzyme pattern is disrupted by such treatment. Investigation of the stability of total activity and isoenzyme pattern during storage at different temperatures is an essential preliminary to the clinical use of isoenzyme fractionation. Strict temperature control is also necessary during the electrophoretic run.

The buffer used for the electrophoretic separation of proteins can be simply that producing the maximum separation of the protein bands. However, for isoenzyme separation it is essential that the buffer does not cause significant inhibition of the enzyme activity. For example, buffer containing glycine may cause inhibition of alkaline phosphatase activity. It cannot be assumed that the inhibition caused by such electrophoretic buffers will be overcome in the staining process even if the stain is made up in a different buffer.

The use of detergents such as SDS may be expected to disrupt lipoprotein complexes, a form in which a variety of enzymes, particularly those bound to subcellular particles may well exist. Whereas the total enzyme activity may be satisfactorily measured in the original serum without the addition of supplementary co-factors, this may no longer be true when the serum specimen has been subjected to electrophoresis. It is frequently necessary to add to the location solution co-factors and trace metals which are required for enzyme activity.

The metal-complexing ability of ampholytes causes particular difficulty with enzymes which require metals as co-factors or which are metallo-proteins, e.g. after isoelectric focusing or gel isoelectric focusing of alkaline phosphatase, it is necessary to add both zinc and magnesium to the location reagent. However, supplementation must be performed with care, as zinc inhibits alkaline phosphatase at higher concentrations. Any attempt to measure isoenzymes after isoelectric focusing requires a thorough preliminary investigation into all of these factors. As the exact conditions at the site of enzyme protein cannot be known, such a study must be conducted empirically.

With media such as polyacrylamide gel a preliminary electrophoretic run may be valuable to ensure the removal of any of the polymerization products.

The location process differs from most protein location techniques in that the protein is not 'fixed' in any way during or before the staining process. Fixation procedures such as the acetone/ethanol, formaldehyde and glutaraldehyde procedures used prior to histological enzyme staining have not been generally used after isoenzyme electrophoresis. The degree of inhibition caused by these procedures certainly varies widely, from the relatively small to the near total. Clinical biochemists will not generally find it necessary to use fixation procedures but should be aware that they can be carried out without completely destroying enzyme activity and may, therefore, be valuable in certain circumstances.

Ideally, the separated enzyme protein in the form of a thin zone or 'disc' should be held securely during incubation with the location reagent. The degree of protein diffusion which occurs during staining is, of course, very dependent upon the electrophoretic medium that has been used. Protein will diffuse readily out of cellulose acetate strips but more slowly out of polyacrylamide gel; the rate of diffusion is reduced as the concentration of polyacrylamide is increased. The rate of diffusion will, of course, be inversely proportional to the size of the protein molecule and directly proportional to the temperature of incubation. A consequence is that enzyme location after polyacrylamide gel electrophoresis can be performed simply by placing the gel in a solution of the appropriate location reagent, whereas a more elaborate approach is generally necessary after a cellulose acetate electrophoresis.

The commonest approach is to place the cellulose acetate strip containing the separated proteins on top of a gel (usually agar) containing the location reagent. Enzyme diffuses from the cellulose acetate into the agar as the location reagents diffuse from agar onto the strip. The final product of the staining reaction will also diffuse, leading to staining in both gel and strip. An alternative approach is to soak another strip of cellulose acetate in the location reagent and place this on top of the original strip, incubating both in a well-sealed moist box. It has been the author's experience that spreading location reagents directly on cellulose acetate strips does not give satisfactory results.

It is important that the substrate and the capture reagent, i.e. the reagent that reacts with a product of the initial reaction, must penetrate rapidly into the electrophoretic medium. The substrate and the capture reagent should, therefore, be reasonably soluble to allow a high concentration in the incubation medium and should also be of low molecular weight to allow quick and easy penetration.

Ideally the kinetics of the enzyme reaction should be zero order, i.e. the substrate concentration should be high relative to the enzyme concentration so that the rate of reaction is proportional to the enzyme concentration and independent of the substrate concentration. Low concentrations of substrate at the site of enzyme protein, which may result from the use of a thick gel slab or gel rods or a substrate that penetrates slowly into the gel, will make zero order kinetics less likely, and quantitative comparisons uncertain. Studies to ensure that the reaction is linear within the relevant range of enzyme activity should be carried out before any quantitative deductions are made.

The first product of an enzyme reaction may diffuse very rapidly and it is desirable, therefore, that the capture reagent be present in excess so as to trap the initial product of the reaction immediately. Location is precise when the diffusion of the enzyme protein and of the primary and secondary reaction product is minimal.

With respect to hydrolytic enzymes such as alkaline phosphatase, a variety of techniques is theoretically possible. A possible approach is to use a substrate which is both coloured and soluble but which is rendered insoluble by action of the enzyme. Clearly this method is of limited application. An alternative is to use a substrate which is colourless but which is acted upon by the enzyme to give a coloured product. A well-known example in clinical enzymology is the action of alkaline phosphatase on the colourless substrate, p-nitrophenol phosphate to give p-nitrophenol which in alkaline solution has a yellow colour. However, the rate of diffusion of p-nitrophenol is so rapid that only very imprecise location is obtained on incubation of separated isoenzymes with *p*-nitro-phenol phosphate.

More generally applicable techniques for the detection of alkaline phosphatase and other hydrolytic enzymes are the 'post incubation' and 'simultaneous coupling' azo-dye methods. In outline and using alkaline phosphatase as an example, a substrate such as α- or β-naphthylphosphate is acted upon by the enzyme to give α- or β-naphthol, which then reacts either in a subsequent reaction or simultaneously with an azo-dye. As far as post-incubation coupling is concerned the product of the primary reaction must be sufficiently insoluble to remain in place without significant diffusion during the initial enzyme reaction and the subsequent staining reactions. In general the post-incubation technique has two advantages. The enzyme is not in contact with the azo-dye during the hydrolysis stage and this is desirable as these dyes certainly have some inhibiting effect. The technique can also be used to detect enzymes having optimum activity at an acid pH, where most diazonium salts are unstable and efficient coupling is impossible.

Both substituted and unsubstituted naphthols have been used with the simultaneous coupling azo-dye methods. Hydrolysis of the phosphate group from unsubstituted naphthols and the immediate coupling with a suitable azo-dye forms an insoluble coloured product at the site of enzyme activity. More insoluble substituted naphthols were introduced later, and although the diffusion of the coloured product is certainly reduced, the advantage is in many cases outweighed by the relative insolubility of the substrate which results in only low concentrations of substrate at the site of enzyme activity.

It must be appreciated that isoenzymes may show different activities with different substrates, and that therefore caution must be exercised in drawing conclusions as to the distribution of enzyme activity among the isoenzyme fractions on the basis of a single location procedure.

It is regrettable that innumerable recipes for detection reagents exist for any enzyme of importance. This testifies both to the fact that no one recipe has been found ideal and also to the rarity of any rigorous examination of the optimum conditions for the determination of a particular enzyme. Most published papers include a favourite recipe without any justification of the choice. A rare example of an attempt to examine critically the various factors important in the separation and detection of isoenzymes is the paper by Rosalki[18] which although dealing with LDH illustrates many of the principles that have to be borne in mind for any enzyme detection method.

Immunochemical Methods. Immunochemical methods of detection and quantitation are based on the reaction of components separated by electrophoresis with an antibody directed against them.

Where the detection involves immunodiffusion in the electrophoretic support the technique is known as immunoelectrophoresis. This can be conducted in agar or agarose gels and on cellulose acetate but not in polyacrylamide gel as the matrix presents too great an obstacle to free diffusion of antigen and antibody.

Agar and agarose are ideal media for the conduct of immunodiffusion reactions, as the gel allows relatively free diffusion of antigen and antibody while holding the immunoprecipitate relatively firmly during washing procedures to remove unprecipitated protein. The media are also optically clear allowing the development of the immune precipitate to be observed. Although the basic discrimination of the electrophoretic process is poor the subsequent immunodiffusion process can reveal the presence of many more proteins than can be resolved by chemical staining.

The technique was introduced by Graber and Williams in 1953, and subsequently miniaturized by Scheidegger in 1955.

In outline, electrophoretic separation is carried out in a 1–1·5 mm thick layer of 1–1·5% agar in buffer on a $3\frac{1}{4}$ in × $3\frac{1}{4}$ in glass plate or a microscope slide. A circular well is punched in the agar to hold the sample which in the case of serum protein electrophoresis is 2–5 μl and troughs are cut 0·5–1 cm from the axis of electrophoretic migration. These troughs are about 1 mm wide and approximately 60 mm long (Fig. 19). At the end of the electrophoretic separation the slide is removed from the apparatus and 20–50 μl of antiserum are added evenly to the troughs from a Hamilton or similar syringe. The plate is transferred to a moist box overnight to allow diffusion to occur and specific precipitation to take place. Specific precipitation lines will be seen as white lines against the translucent agar, and can be more clearly visualized in simple, indirect light, viewing boxes (*see* Fig. 20). The precipitation lines can be preserved indefinitely by drying and staining. It should be noted that an

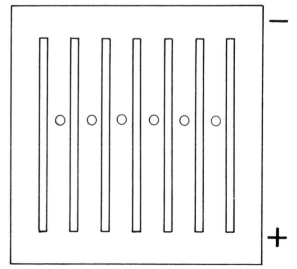

Fig. 19 Arrangements of antiserum troughs and sample wells cut in agar layer on glass plate.

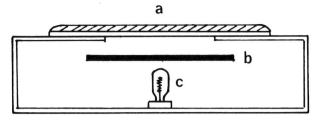

Fig. 20 Indirect-light viewing box. (a) Immunoelectrophoresis plate; (b) black shield; (c) light bulb.

antigen may complex with antibody but may not produce a visible aggregate although the complex may be detected by autoradiography or by the enzymic activity of the complexed antigen.

With care the position, sharpness and strength of the precipitin line may be used to obtain quantitative as well as qualitative information. However, if one precipitin line is stronger than another it must not be assumed that the antigen concerned is present in greater amount in the fluid being examined. It may be that the ratio of antigen to antibody for that particular component is closer to the optimum for precipitation.

The precipitation arcs formed in immunoelectrophoresis have to be interpreted in much the same way as those formed in double-diffusion techniques such as that of Ouchterlony. The distribution of the separated antigen component in the gel influences the shape of the precipitin arc formed by antibody diffusing against it. At the end of the electrophoretic stage in the commonly used technique of immunoelectrophoresis in agar, the separated antigens may be conceived as diffusing radially from a series of point sources, whereas the antibody molecules will diffuse as a straight front from the antibody troughs (Fig. 21). The lower the rate of diffusion of any anti-

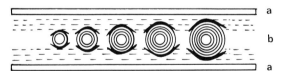

Fig. 21 Diffusion of antigen and antibody at the immunodiffusion stage of immunoelectrophoresis. (a) antiserum troughs; – – – – indicates diffusion of antibody; (b) separated antigens diffusing radially. The slower the diffusion of antigens, the sharper the radius of the precipitin arc.

gen component with respect to the antibody, the smaller the radius of the precipitation line formed. The formation of a long smooth arc of large radius such as that produced by immunoglobulins after immunoelectrophoresis in agar suggests the presence of an electrophoretically heterogenous group of molecules with basic antigen similarities.

Some serum proteins become less soluble in the absence of the protective effect of other proteins and this may give rise to irregular non-specific precipitation. Although the author has generally conducted

immunoelectrophoresis in agar using a barbitone buffer at the pH of 8·6, which is optimum for the electrophoretic separation, it must be borne in mind that some specific precipitation reactions may be inhibited if the pH is greater than 8·2. It must be emphasized that the buffer has to be suitable both for efficient electrophoretic separation and for the subsequent precipitation reaction. It is very desirable that the efficiency of the buffer for the former purpose is checked from time to time by conventional chemical staining.

During the immunodiffusion process precipitation bands may appear and disappear as an antigen/antibody complex may redissolve in antigen excess and be forced into the antiserum troughs. It may, therefore, be necessary to make frequent observations of the developing pattern. This is easily done in agar immunoelectrophoresis as the precipitation lines are shown as white arcs in a relatively clear medium. In clinical work frequent observation is particularly necessary when the detection of small molecular weight compounds, such as Bence–Jones proteins, is the major interest. It is important to maintain a constant temperature during the immunodiffusion stage, as otherwise artifacts such as multiple precipitation lines may form.

Although agar is the most commonly used medium for immunoelectrophoresis it is also possible to conduct both stages of the process in cellulose acetate. A conventional electrophoresis on cellulose acetate membrane is followed by an immunodiffusion stage where the membrane is kept in a moist environment and thin strips of filter paper soaked in antiserum are placed a short distance from the axis of the electrophoretic migration. The sample is best applied as a point source. The inability to observe the development of the precipitation lines is a disadvantage. As the membrane is very thin there is also a danger of washing out specific precipitates when the strip is washed to remove unprecipitated protein.

To avoid such problems it may be advantageous to carry out the immunodiffusion reaction in agar. A thin strip is cut from the cellulose acetate electrophoretic track and transferred to an agar gel. Troughs are cut out a short distance from the strip and filled with antiserum.

To examine an individual separated component, sections can be cut from the cellulose acetate, placed on agar and their reactions against specific antiserum observed by classic Ouchterlony gel-diffusion techniques.[19] Such an approach can be very economical when expensive antisera are involved.

However, for the identification of specific proteins after electrophoresis on agarose or cellulose acetate, *immunofixation techniques* have rendered many of the earlier gel immunodiffusion procedures described above obsolete. Fixation procedures were pioneered in the 1960s by Alfonso and by Alper and Johnson but current techniques derive from the procedures of Ritchie and Smith for agarose, and Kohn and

Riches[20] for cellulose acetate. The procedure for agarose involves the placing of cellulose acetate soaked in antiserum over the electrophoretic track, or the portion of the track containing the proteins of interest. After incubation for one hour the cellulose acetate strip is discarded, the agarose gel is dried down by a weighted filter paper pad, washed, and the immunoprecipitate stained.

The cellulose acetate procedure is even simpler. The strip or an appropriate portion of it is immersed for a few minutes in a diluted antiserum containing 4% polyethylene glycol (mol. wt. 6000) which increases the intensity and speed of formation of the precipitate. The strip is then rinsed in tap water and finally washed in an electrophoretic buffer containing 0·1% Triton X 100. Staining with Ponceau S or Nigrosine is usually adequate but increased sensitivity can be achieved by use of enzyme, fluorescent- or isotope-labelled antibodies.

Nucleic Acid Probes. The use of DNA hybridization techniques for the diagnosis of inherited or malignant disease entails the detection of small alterations in DNA sequence. In outline the genome is fragmented by treatment with an appropriate bacterial restriction endonuclease and the digest subjected to gel electrophoresis to separate the components on a molecular weight basis.

The fragments are denatured to single strand fragments and transferred, by the blotting techniques described above, to a nitrocellulose membrane. The separated DNA is then reacted with a probe consisting of ^{32}P-labelled single-stranded DNA of base sequence complementary to the alteration being looked for. Hybridization of the probe and any homologous genome fragment takes place and is detected by subsequent autoradiography (*see* below). The technique is often termed the Southern blot technique after its originator, E. M. Southern.[21]

Radioisotope Methods

The incorporation of isotopic tracer into the components being separated by electrophoresis allows the subsequent detection of the components. The attractions of this approach are high sensitivity and the unique capacity to evaluate metabolic pathways. It must be appreciated that it is the presence of the isotope which is detected and not any particular compound. At its simplest the use of isotopes involves the technique of autoradiography which may be useful in itself or as a preliminary to a more exact evaluation. In outline the procedure involves the placing of a film in contact with the electrophoretogram for as long as is necessary to detect the radioactive components. It is important that an even pressure be applied on placing the film over the paper or other separation medium. It should be remembered that due to decay of the radioisotope attempts to increase sensitivity by leaving the film in contact with the

medium for longer periods of time will be subject to the law of diminishing returns. In general, exposure for periods longer than twice the half life of the isotope will be found to be unprofitable. Subsequently the exposed film may be evaluated densitometrically.

A more rigorous approach is to cut the separation medium into sections and to measure the radioactivity either by gamma or liquid scintillation counting as appropriate. Elution of the separated material is usually desirable. Methods are, however, available to dissolve polyacrylamide gels to facilitate their evaluation in this way.

SUMMARY

Electrophoresis has emerged as a powerful separative tool in clinical biochemistry. Over the last few decades techniques of greatly increased resolving power have been developed and matched with detection systems of dramatically improved sensitivity. Fortunately this has not been accompanied by increased sophistication and cost of apparatus. It is true, however, that quantitation and standardization of the technique is less satisfactory and may require expensive subsidiary equipment.

REFERENCES

1. Sklar J. (1985). DNA hybridization in diagnostic pathology. *Human Pathol*; **16**: 654–8.
2. Whipple H. E. (1964). Gel electrop-horesis. *Ann. NY Acad. Sci*; **121**: 305.
3. Maurer H. R. (1971). *Disc Electrophoresis and Related Techniques of Polyacrylamide Gel Electrophoresis*, 2nd edn. Berlin and New York: Walter de Gruyter.
4. Serwer P. (1983). Agarose gels: properties and use for electrophoresis. *Electrophoresis*; **6**: 375–82.
5. Smith I. (1976). *Chromatographic and Electrophoretic Techniques. Vol. II, Zone Electrophoresis*, 4th edn. London: William Heinemann Medical Books.
6. Crowle A. J. (1961). *Immunodiffusion*. New York and London: Academic Press.
7. Gordon A. H. (1975). *Electrophoresis of Proteins in Polyacrylamide and Starch Gels*. Revised enlarged edition. Amsterdam and Oxford: North-Holland Publishing Co.
8. Hjelmeland L. M., Chrambach A. (1981). Electrophoresis and electrofocusing in detergent containing media: A discussion of basic concepts. *Electrophoresis*; **1**: 1.
9. Latner A. L. (1975). Isoelectric focussing in liquid and gels as applied to clinical chemistry. *Adv. Clin. Chem*; **17**: 193–250. San Francisco: Academic Press.
10. Catsimpoolas W. (1973). Isoelectric focussing and isotachophoresis of proteins *Separation Sci*; **8**: 71.
11. O'Farrell P. H. (1975). High resolution two-dimensional electrophoresis of proteins. *J. Biol. Chem*; **250**: 4007.
12. Young D. S., Tracy R. P. (1983). Two-dimensional electrophoresis in the development of clinical laboratory tests. *Electrophoresis*; **2**: 117.

13. Bøg-Hansen T. C. (1981). Affinity electrophoresis of glycoproteins. In *Solid Phase Biochemistry: Analytical and Synthetic Aspects* (Scouten W. H., ed.), pp. 223–251. New York: Wiley.

14. Rosalki S. B., Ying Foo A. (1984). Two new methods for separating and quantifying bone and liver alkaline phosphatase isoenzymes in plasma. *Clin. Chem*; **30**: 1182.

15. Haglund H. (1970). Isotachophoresis. *Science Tools*; **17**: 2.

16. Holloway C. J., Pingoud V. (1981). The analysis of amino acids and peptides by isotachophoresis. *Electrophoresis*; **3**: 127.

17. Dunn M. J., Burghes A. H. M. (1983). High resolution two-dimensional polyacrylamide gel electrophoresis. i. Methodological procedures; ii. Analysis and application. *Electrophoresis*; **2**: 97; **3**: 173.

18. Rosalki S. B. (1974). Standardisation of isoenzyme assays with special reference to lactate dehydrogenase isoenzyme electrophoresis. *Clin. Biochem.*; **7**: 29.

19. Ouchterlony O. (1958). Diffusion-in-gel methods for immunological analysis. In *Progress in Allergy* (Kallos P., ed.), Vol. V, pp. 1–77. Basel and New York: S. Karger.

20. Kohn J., Riches P. G. (1978). A cellulose acetate immunofixation technique. *J. Immunol. Meth*; **20**: 325.

21. Southern E. M. (1975). Detection of specific sequences among DNA fragments separated by gel electrophoresis. *J. Mol. Biol*; **98**: 503.

Recent Monographs

Allen R. C., Saravis C. A., Maurer H. R. (1984). *Gel Electrophoresis and Isoelectric Focusing of Proteins, Selected Techniques.* Berlin and New York: Walter de Gruyter.

Andrews A. T. (1981). *Electrophoresis, Theory, Techniques and Biochemical and Clinical Applications.* Oxford: Clarendon Press.

Deyl Z., with Chrambach A., Everaerts F. M., Prusick A. (1983). Electrophoresis, A survey of techniques and applications. *Journal of Chromatography Library*; Vol. 18A—Techniques; Vol. 18B—Applications. Amsterdam, Oxford, New York: Elsevier.

SECTION 4
BIOLOGICAL MEASUREMENTS

27. Theoretical Enzymology: Enzyme Kinetics and Enzyme Inhibition

Donald W. Moss

INTRODUCTION

Enzymes are proteins with catalytic activity: that is, in the presence of enzymes, chemical reactions which would otherwise proceed at low or even immeasurable rates become significant. More than 1000 distinct enzymes are now known to exist, differing principally in the nature of the reactions for which they act as specific catalysts. Nevertheless, in spite of this great variety of enzymes, certain generalizations can be made with regard to the effects of several factors on the rates of enzyme-catalysed reactions *in vitro*.

Estimations of the amount of an enzyme present in a particular system, e.g. in a sample of blood taken for diagnostic purposes, are essentially synonymous at the present time with estimations of catalytic activity. Therefore, an understanding of those factors which influence the rates of enzymic reactions is fundamental to the use of enzyme tests in clinical biochemistry.

PROGRESS OF ENZYMIC REACTIONS

The progress of the transformation of the substrate (the substance on which the enzyme acts) into products in the presence of an enzyme can be followed by measuring the decreasing concentration of the substrate or the increasing concentration of a product. Measurement of product formation is preferred where possible in practice, because determination of the increase in concentration of a substance above an initially zero or low level is analytically more reliable than that of a fall from an initially high level, although several clinically important determinations measure decrease in substrate concentration.

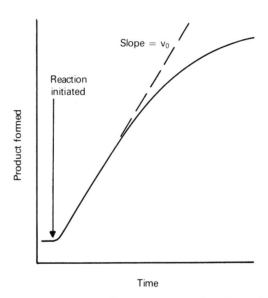

Fig. 1 Progress curve of an enzyme-catalysed reaction.

The progress curve of an enzyme-catalysed reaction typically has the form shown in Fig. 1 when excess substrate is initially present. Although the time-scale of the changes varies with the reaction conditions several distinct phases can be recognized as making up the progress curve. Immediately following the initiation of the reaction by the introduction of enzyme or substrate there is a period of equilibration or induction before pronounced changes become established: this 'lag phase' often lasts only for a few seconds but may extend to several minutes, and can be influenced by the experimental conditions. It is followed by a phase during which the concentration of product increases linearly with respect to time; i.e. the rate of product formation is constant. This is the most useful portion of the curve from the point of view of enzyme-activity determination and the rate of formation of product during this phase is usually referred to as the *initial rate* of reaction v_0, or simply v. As will be seen later, the rate of the reaction during this phase is independent of the concentration of substrate; in other words, the reaction is zero-order with respect to substrate.

E and *S*. For many years the substrate concentration at which the observed velocity of reaction is half the maximum velocity has been referred to as the Michaelis constant and given the symbol K_m. The significance of K_m determined experimentally was assumed to be synonymous with that of K_s in the Michaelis–Menten derivation. Determination of the rates of the separate forward and backward reactions between *E* and *S* has shown, in some cases, that equilibrium is not set up between them; i.e. K_m is not an equilibrium constant. The term Michaelis constant and its symbol K_m are now reserved for the experimentally determined substrate concentration at which *v* is half *V*. When an equilibrium constant is implied, as in discussions of reaction kinetics, K_s (substrate constant) is used.

A derivation of the relationship between the velocity of an enzymic reaction and the substrate concentration which does not assume that an equilibrium is established between *E*, *S* and *ES* was published by Briggs and Haldane in 1925. They assumed that the concentration of *ES* is constant over the short period needed for measurement of *v* because the rates of formation and breakdown of the complex are equal; i.e.

$$k_{+1} \times [E][S] = k_{-1} \times [ES] + k_{+2} \times [ES]$$

and therefore,

$$\frac{k_{-1} + k_{+2}}{k_{+1}} = \frac{[E][S]}{[ES]}$$

If $(k_{-1} + k_{+2})/k_{+1}$ is given the symbol K_m, an expression relating *v* and [S] can be derived exactly as for the equilibrium conditions of Michaelis and Menten, such that

$$v = \frac{V[S]}{K_m + [S]}$$

Although the Briggs–Haldane steady-state equation has the same form as the Michaelis equation, K_m only reduces to $K_s (= k_{-1}/k_{+1})$ when k_{+2} is very small compared with k_{-1}, or in other words when the breakdown of *ES* into products is insufficiently rapid to disturb the equilibrium between *E*, *S* and *ES*.

The relationship between *v* and [S] found experimentally almost always conforms to the shape required by the equation of the form

$$v = \frac{V[S]}{K_m + [S]}$$

in which K_m is the substrate concentration at which $v = V/2$. It is not possible to determine whether K_m is equivalent to K_s, as required by the Michaelis–Menten derivation, or whether it has the meaning $(K_s + [k_{+2}/k_{+1}])$ assigned to it by Briggs and Haldane, from the usual measurements of overall rate of reaction. This can be done only when the properties of the intermediate complex and the availability of suitable techniques for following rapid reactions

enable the rates of formation and breakdown of the *ES* complex to be measured individually.

The value of the Michaelis constant is, in most cases, independent of the amount of enzyme used in determining it. However, any change in conditions which affects the binding of substrate by the enzyme will alter the observed value of K_m. These changes may involve permanent alterations in the structures of binding groups in enzyme or substrate (i.e. changes in covalent linkages), reversible variations in distribution of ionic charge (i.e. effects of pH changes), or changes in enzyme conformation which affect the orientation or accessibility of binding groups. In addition, substances present in the reaction mixture other than the enzyme and its substrate may interfere with the formation of the enzyme–substrate complex. The kinetics of competitive inhibition arising in this way are discussed in a later section.

Enzyme Concentration and Reaction Rate

As well as accounting for the relationship between *v* and [S], the formation of the *ES* complex, the concentration of which determines the rate of appearance of products, also explains the direct relationship between initial reaction velocity (*v*) and enzyme concentration. This relationship is the basis for comparing amounts of (active) enzymes by their relative rates of reaction.

At either high or low substrate concentration, raising [E] increases the concentration of *ES* and, therefore, *v*. When the concentration of substrate is such that all the enzyme already present is saturated (i.e., is in the form of the *ES* complex), addition of more free enzyme is the only way in which [ES] can be increased and, with it, *v*. Under these conditions the reaction is zero-order with respect to substrate concentration but first-order with respect to enzyme concentration. As the concentration of substrate is reduced the dependence on [E] remains, but *v* becomes increasingly dependent on [S] also, until, when [S] is low compared with K_m, the reaction is essentially first-order with respect to substrate concentration. Thus, although *v* is directly proportional to [E] throughout the range of concentrations of substrate, measurement of enzyme activity is preferably made at high substrate concentration: not only is *v* ($\rightarrow V$) greatest under these conditions, but also complications introduced by variation in [S] during measurement are avoided.

The region of substrate concentration over which *v* shows a first-order dependence on [S] is useful in the enzymic determination of substances which can act as substrates for a suitable reagent enzyme.

Deviations from Michaelis–Menten Behaviour

In practice the relationship between *v* and [S] may depart from the predicted form at high substrate concentrations, although agreement between the observed and theoretical curves is close at lower values of $[S]$. Because both in theory and practice the velocity–substrate curve is nearly parallel with the abscissa at high substrate concentrations, deviations from predicted behaviour are more easily seen if a transform of the Michaelis–Menten equation is used which gives a straight line when plotted.

Several alternative linearized equations are available. The best-known is the plot of $1/v$ against $1/[S]$ (Lineweaver and Burk) which gives a straight line of slope K_m/V and intercept on the ordinate at $1/V$ since

$$\frac{1}{v} = \frac{K_m}{V} \cdot \frac{1}{[S]} + \frac{1}{V}$$

The intercept on the abscissa is at $-1/K_m$ (Fig. 4a). This method of plotting has been widely used, and almost as widely criticized since the double-reciprocal method of plotting gives values of v obtained at low concentrations of S a disproportionate influence on the slope of the line and its intercepts, although these values are least reliable from an experimental point of view. However, computer programs are now available which weight each experimental point according to its reliability, removing this particular objection to the double-reciprocal plot.

An alternative linear plot (Hanes) is of $[S]/v$ against $[S]$, with slope $1/V$ and intercepts of K_m/V and $-K_m$ on the ordinate and abscissa, respectively (Fig. 4b). The equation of the line is

$$\frac{[S]}{v} = \frac{K_m}{V} + \frac{[S]}{V}$$

The linear transformations of the Michaelis–Menten equation make the derivation of values of V and K_m from experimental data much simpler than in the case of the original hyperbolic relationship. As well as showing up deviations from typical Michaelis–Menten kinetics, they are useful also in interpreting the kinetics of enzyme inhibition, as will be seen later.

If the Michaelis–Menten equation is obeyed strictly, V is only reached at infinite substrate concentration. The effective limiting value reached by v is therefore usually considerably less than the value of V calculated from the linear plots of the Michaelis–Menten equation. In some cases the observed value of v reaches a maximum with increasing $[S]$, from which it declines as $[S]$ is increased still further (Fig. 3). This phenomenon of inhibition by excess substrate is probably due in many cases to formation of catalytically ineffective ES complexes in which more than one substrate molecule combines with the active centre of the enzyme. Competition between the first substrate and a second substrate involved in a two-substrate reaction may account for some examples of inhibition by excess substrate: water is the second reactant in hydrolytic reactions, for example, and its effective concentration may be reduced at high substrate concentrations.

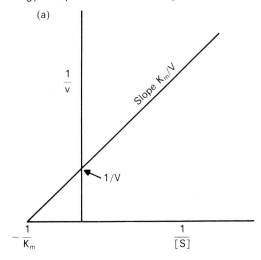

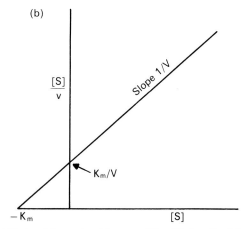

Fig. 4 Plots of linearized forms of the Michaelis–Menten equation. (a) Lineweaver and Burk; (b) Hanes.

In a few instances an enzyme may be activated by increasing concentrations of its substrate, i.e. v may be greater at high values of $[S]$ than predicted from the Michaelis equation. Instead of the hyperbolic dependence of v on $[S]$ typical of Michaelis–Menten kinetics, some enzymes show a sigmoid relationship between these two variables. Sigmoid kinetics are now recognized to be important in regulation of the activity of certain enzymes and their significance is discussed more fully in a later section.

Two-substrate Reactions

Most reactions catalysed by enzymes are of the type:

$$A + B \rightleftharpoons C + D$$

When one of the substrates is water (i.e. when the process is one of hydrolysis) with the reaction taking place in aqueous solution, only a fraction of the total number of water molecules present participates in the reaction. The small change in the concentration of water has no effect on the rate of reaction, which is thus *pseudo*-unimolecular with respect to the other effect of pH-changes on v is reversible, except after exposure to extremes of pH at which denaturation of the enzyme may occur. There is a great deal of variation between enzymes with regard to the pH at which activity is at a maximum and in the width of the zone of pH over which the enzyme is active. Also, some of the effects of pH on v are due to changes in ionization of the substrate, rather than of the enzyme. Nevertheless, certain generalizations can be made from the study of the effects of pH on enzymic reactions.

Since enzymes are proteins, they possess a large number of radicals which are capable of existing in different ionic forms. Some of these groups are on the outside of the molecule and respond to pH changes in the aqueous environment by changes in ionization. The relative proportions of the ionized and un-ionized forms of each group at a given pH are given by the equation

$$pH = pK_a + \log \cdot \frac{[\text{ionized form}]}{[\text{un-ionized form}]}$$

in which pK_a is the negative logarithm of the ionization constant of the group concerned.

The existence of a fairly narrow pH-optimum for most enzymes suggests that one particular ionic form of the enzyme molecule, out of the many that can potentially exist, is the catalytically active one. Changes in the ionization of groups remote from the active centre of the enzyme would not be expected to affect the rate of reaction greatly, although other properties of the enzyme molecule would be affected, such as solubility or electrophoretic mobility. Therefore, changes in activity in response to pH changes are more probably due to alterations in the ionization of groups responsible for substrate binding and catalysis, and the probable identity of active groups has been inferred from a study of pH–activity relationships for a number of enzymes.

For an enzyme, E, in which one of two ionizable groups is unprotonated and the other protonated in the catalytically active form of the enzyme, changes in pH have the following effects:

$$HEH \underset{}{\overset{K_1}{\rightleftharpoons}} EH' + H^+ \underset{}{\overset{K_2}{\rightleftharpoons}} E'' + H^+$$

Both groups protonated (more acid than optimum pH)	Active form	Both groups unprotonated (more alkaline than optimum pH)

K_1 and K_2 are the acid dissociation constants for the two groups. The total enzyme concentration E_0 is the sum of the concentrations of the various ionized forms, i.e.

$$[E_0] = [HEH] + [EH'] + [E'']$$

By the Law of Mass Action,

$$K_1 = \frac{[EH'][H^+]}{[HEH]} \text{ and } K_2 = \frac{[E''][H^+]}{[EH']}$$

Elimination of E'' from these three equations gives

$$[EH'] = \frac{[E_0]}{1 + ([H^+]/K_1) + (K_2/[H^+])}$$

pH is equal to $-\log [H^+]$. Therefore, the denominator of this equation varies with pH. It is known as a Michaelis pH function (f^-). Dividing the total

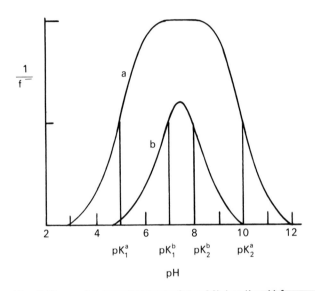

Fig. 7 Plots of the reciprocal of the Michaelis pH function, f^-, against pH. Values of pK_1 and pK_2 of 5 and 10 have been assumed for curve a, and values of 7 and 8 for curve b.

enzyme concentration by the appropriate value of f^- gives the concentration of enzyme in the active form at that pH. When $[H^+]$ is high (at low pH) the dominant term in the function is $[H^+]/K_1$, whereas when $[H^+]$ is low (at high pH) $K_2/[H^+]$ becomes dominant. (pH functions of a similar form can be derived which express the concentration of enzyme in the forms E'' and HEH.)

A plot of $1/f^-$ against pH gives a bell-shaped curve (Fig. 7), with inflexions corresponding to pK_1 and pK_2. Since the overall velocity of the catalysed reaction is directly proportional to the concentration of active enzyme this curve should have the same shape as the pH–activity curve of the enzyme if the correct values for K_1 and K_2 have been assumed in calculating f^-.

When deducing values for K_1 and K_2 from plots of experimental data, e.g. of the variation of V with pH, it is usual to plot log V against pH. This is equivalent to plotting pf^- (i.e. the negative logarithm of f^-) against pH, and the plot is made up of three linear portions which intersect at pK_1 and pK_2 (Fig. 8).

In plotting velocities against pH in this way it is actually the acid dissociation constants K_1 and K_2 of the enzyme–substrate complex (EHS) which are obtained since it is changes in the ionization of this complex which affect the observed rate of reaction. Values of K_1 and K_2 may not prove to be identical with those applying to the free enzyme, EH'.

Michaelis-type pH functions can be extended to show how the concentrations of various ionic forms of the enzyme, substrate, and enzyme–substrate complex depend on pH and, therefore, how K_s varies

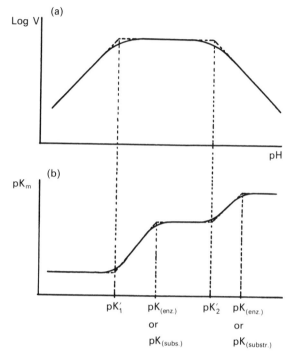

Fig. 8 Plots of (a) log V against pH, and (b) pK_m against pH. Bends at pK_1' and pK_2' are due to ionizations of groups in the enzyme–substrate complex; other bends may represent ionizations in either the free enzyme or the free substrate.

with pH. Plots of pK_s ($= -\log K_s$) against pH consist of linear segments intersecting at points which correspond to pH values of ionizations affecting the enzyme and substrate, as well as the enzyme–substrate complex. When pK_s (or, strictly speaking, pK_m since this is the quantity usually determined experimentally) is plotted against pH, upward bends (increases of positive slope) in the line correspond to pK's of ionizations in the enzyme–substrate complex and downward bends to pK's of free enzyme or free substrate (Fig. 8). The changes in slope due to ionization of the substrate can usually be identified from its known characteristics of dissociation.

Caution is needed when deducing the probable identity of essential ionizing groups in the active centre of the enzyme from the values of K_1 and K_2 derived from velocity–pH or K_m–pH relationships. Combination of amino acids into polypeptide chains,

with the proximity of other groups influencing ionization, almost certainly alters acid dissociation constants of groups in amino acid side-chains compared with the values determined by titration of the free acids.

The variation of K_m with pH is often very marked. Since K_m reflects the shape of the Michaelis curve, this also shows a pronounced variation with pH in these cases. Consequently, when pH–activity curves are determined at different concentrations of substrate the observed optimum pH is found to vary with substrate concentration. This is the case for human alkaline phosphatase and provides an example of the interdependence of the several variables which affect enzyme activity (Fig. 6).

Modification of the activity of enzymes by substances other than the enzyme and its substrate (activators and inhibitors) is usually pH-dependent, also. The effects of pH changes on activation and inhibition can be analysed in a similar manner to effects on interaction with substrate.

Effect of Temperature on Enzyme-catalysed Reactions. The rate of an enzymic reaction increases with increasing temperature. Although there are significant variations from one enzyme to another, the rate approximately doubles, on average, for each 10 °C rise in temperature; i.e. Q_{10} is of the order of 2. A difference in 1 °C between two measurements of enzyme activity thus causes a difference of about 10% in observed rates, emphasizing the need for close control of temperature in all such measurements.

In theory, the initial rate of reaction measured instantaneously at saturating substrate concentrations goes on increasing with rising temperature. In practice, however, a finite time is needed in all methods to allow the components of the reaction mixture, including the enzyme solution, to reach temperature equilibrium and to permit the formation of a measurable amount of product. During this period the enzyme is undergoing thermal inactivation and denaturation. This process, which is one of the factors contributing to non-linearity of reaction progress curves, has a very large temperature coefficient for most enzymes and thus becomes virtually instantaneous at temperatures in the region of 60°–70 °C.

The counteracting effects of the increased rate of the catalysed reaction and more rapid enzyme inactivation as the temperature is raised, account for the existence of an apparent 'optimum temperature' for enzyme activity often referred to in the older literature of enzymology. The apparent optimum temperature depends on the time at which measurements of activity are made (Fig. 9). With older methods of assay, requiring lengthy periods of incubation of enzyme and substrate, enzyme inactivation takes effect at lower temperatures and the phenomenon is more easily seen.

Thermal inactivation of enzymes is influenced by other factors as well as duration of exposure to a particular temperature. These include the presence of substrate and its concentration, and the pH, nature and ionic strength of the buffer. The presence of other proteins, as in serum samples, may help to stabilize the enzyme.

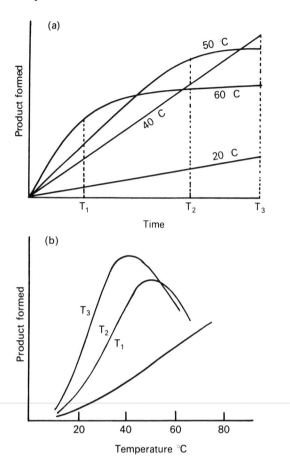

Fig. 9 Relationship between product formed in an enzymic reaction and (a) time of incubation at various temperatures, and (b) temperature of incubation for various times. The apparent optimum temperature depends on the duration of incubation.

The rate of a chemical reaction is related to the absolute temperature by the empirical equation of Arrhenius:

$$2\cdot303\frac{d(\log k)}{dt} = \frac{A}{RT^2}$$

in which k is the rate constant for the reaction, T the absolute temperature and R the gas constant (1·987 calories per degree per mole). A is also a constant for the particular reaction, called the Energy of Activation.* Integrating the Arrhenius equation,

$$\log k = \frac{-A}{2\cdot303RT} + \text{constant}$$

* Energy of activation is usually given the symbol E. A has been chosen here to avoid confusion with E used to denote 'enzyme'.

Since the maximum velocity, V is given by $k\,[E]$ at a fixed enzyme concentration $[E]$, a plot of $\log V$ against $1/T$ is linear, of slope $-A/2\cdot303R$. The energy of activation of the reaction can thus be calculated.

Plots of V against $1/T$ are linear for most enzymes, but breaks in the line do occur in some cases, indicating that A is not constant over the whole range of temperature. This may be due in some instances to irreversible inactivation of the enzyme. Comparison of the values of A obtained for an enzymic reaction in the presence and absence of the catalyst (if the reaction proceeds at a measurable rate without the enzyme) shows that the energy of activation is much lower when the enzyme is present. Therefore, the enzyme increases the rate of reaction by lowering the energy barrier which otherwise separates the reactants and the products.

INHIBITION OF ENZYME ACTIVITY

Modification of Enzyme Activity

The rates of enzymic reactions are affected by changes in the concentrations of substances other than the enzyme or substrate. These modifiers may be activators, i.e. they increase the rate of reaction, or their presence may inhibit the enzyme, reducing the reaction rate. Activators and inhibitors are usually small molecules, or even ions. They vary in specificity from modifiers which exert similar effects on a wide range of different enzymic reactions at one extreme, to substances which affect only a single reaction at the other. Reagents such as strong acids or multivalent anions and cations, which denature or precipitate proteins, destroy enzyme activity and so may be regarded as extreme examples of non-specific enzyme inhibitors. However, these effects, which depend on the properties of enzymes as proteins rather than catalysts, are not usually included in discussions of enzyme inhibition.

Inhibitors are divisible into reversible and irreversible types. Reversible inhibition implies that the activity of the enzyme is fully restored when the inhibitor is removed from the system in which the enzyme acts by some physical separative process such as dialysis, gel filtration or chromatography. An irreversible inhibitor, on the other hand, combines covalently with the enzyme so that physical methods are ineffective in separating the two. For example, certain organophosphorus compounds are extremely potent inhibitors of esterases, including acetylcholinesterase, with which they form phosphoryl compounds. In some cases enzymes which have combined with irreversible inhibitors can be reactivated by a chemical reaction which removes the blocking group: e.g. the phosphoryl enzymes formed with organophosphorus compounds can sometimes be reactivated by treatment with oximes or hydroxamic acids.

Kinetics of Irreversible Inhibition

An irreversible inhibitor is not in equilibrium with the enzyme. Its effect is progressive with time, becoming complete if the amount of inhibitor present exceeds the total amount of enzyme. The rate of the reaction between enzyme and inhibitor is expressed as the fraction of the enzyme activity which is inhibited in a fixed time by a given concentration of inhibitor. The velocity constant of the reaction of the inhibitor with the enzyme is a measure of the effectiveness of the inhibitor.

When the inhibitor is added to the enzyme in the presence of its substrate, combination of the enzyme and inhibitor may be delayed because a proportion of the enzyme molecules will be combined with the substrate and therefore protected from reacting with the inhibitor. However, as the substrate molecules are broken down the active centres become available for combination with the inhibitor. Thus, inhibition will eventually become complete even though an excess of substrate may initially be present, compared with the inhibitor concentration. Furthermore, addition of more substrate is ineffective in reversing the inhibition, in contrast to its effect on reversible competitive inhibition discussed below.

Kinetics of Reversible Inhibition

Reversible inhibition is characterized by the existence of an equilibrium between enzyme and inhibitor:

$$E + I \rightleftharpoons EI$$

The equilibrium constant of the reaction, K_i, given by

$$K_i = \frac{[E][I]}{[EI]}$$

is a measure of the affinity of the inhibitor for the enzyme, the smaller the value of K_i, the greater being the proportion of enzyme combined as the EI complex.

Competitive Inhibition. The inhibitor is usually a structural analogue of the substrate and binds to the enzyme at the substrate-binding site but, because it is not identical with the substrate, breakdown into products does not take place. When the process of inhibition is fully competitive the enzyme can be combined with either the substrate or the inhibitor, but not with both simultaneously. Two equilibria are therefore possible:

$$E + S \underset{k_{-1}}{\overset{k_{+1}}{\rightleftharpoons}} ES \overset{k_{+2}}{\longrightarrow} E + \text{Products}$$

and

$$E + I \underset{k_{-3}}{\overset{k_{+3}}{\rightleftharpoons}} EI$$

The concentrations of S and I are usually large compared with the total enzyme concentration, $[E_t]$, so that the amounts of S and I combined with the enzyme are negligible and the concentrations of free S and I are essentially equal to their total concentrations.

The rate of change of the concentration of ES is given by

$$\frac{d[ES]}{dt} = k_{+1}([E_t] - [ES] - [EI]) \times \\ [S] - (k_{-1} + k_{+2}) \times [ES]$$

Under steady-state conditions, when the rates of formation and breakdown of ES are equal, $d[ES]/dt = 0$. Therefore,

$$k_{+1} \cdot ([E_t] - [ES] - [EI]) \times [S] = (k_{-1} + k_{+2}) \times [ES]$$

For equilibrium between E and I,

$$k_{+3} \cdot ([E_t] - [ES] - [EI]) \times [I] = k_{-3} \cdot [EI]$$

The velocity of reaction, v, is given by

$$v = k_{+2} \cdot [ES]$$

Eliminating $[ES]$ and $[EI]$ from the last three equations shows that

$$v = \frac{k_{+2} \times [E_t][S]}{K_m(1 + (k_{+3} \cdot [I]/k_{-3})) + [S]}$$

But $k_{-3}/k_{+3} = K_i$, the inhibitor constant (the equilibrium constant for the reaction between E and I), and $k_{+2}E_t = V$, hence

$$v = \frac{V[S]}{K_m(1 + ([I]/K_i)) + [S]}$$

This is the Michaelis–Menten equation, but with K_m modified by a term including the inhibitor concentration and inhibitor constant. V is unaltered. Therefore, curves of v against $[S]$ in the presence and absence of inhibitor reach the same limiting value at high substrate concentrations, but, when the inhibitor is present, K_m is apparently greater. Plots of $1/v$ against $1/[S]$ with and without inhibitor cut the ordinate at the same point, but have different slopes and intercepts on the abscissa (Fig. 10a).

Non-competitive Inhibition. A non-competitive inhibitor is usually unlike the substrate in structure. It is assumed to bind at a site on the enzyme molecule distinct from the substrate-binding site; thus, there is no competition between inhibitor and substrate and a ternary enzyme–inhibitor–substrate complex can form. Attachment of the inhibitor to the enzyme does not modify the affinity of the enzyme for its substrate, but the enzyme–inhibitor–substrate complex does not break down to give products.

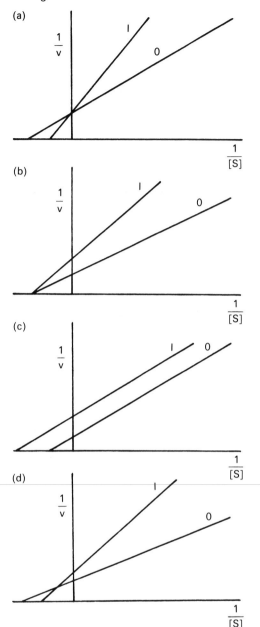

(a)

(b)

(c)

(d)

Fig. 10 The effects of different types of reversible inhibitors (I) on plots of $1/v$ against $1/[S]$, compared with plots in the absence of inhibitor (0). The types of inhibition are: (a) competitive; (b) non-competitive; (c) uncompetitive, and (d) mixed.

The following equilibria are therefore possible:

$$E + S \underset{k_{-1}}{\overset{k_{+1}}{\rightleftharpoons}} ES \overset{k_{+2}}{\longrightarrow} E + \text{Products}$$

$$E + I \underset{k_{-3}}{\overset{k_{+3}}{\rightleftharpoons}} EI$$

$$EI + S \underset{k_{-1}}{\overset{k_{+1}}{\rightleftharpoons}} EIS$$

$$ES + I \underset{k_{-3}}{\overset{k_{+3}}{\rightleftharpoons}} EIS$$

Since S and I do not interfere with the binding of each other, the rate constants for the combination of S with EI are the same as those for the binding of S with E. Similarly, the same rate constants apply to the reaction of I with ES as with E.

Derivation of an expression for v as for the competitive case gives the following:

$$v = \frac{V[S]}{(K_m + [S])(1 + ([I]/K_i))}$$

The effect of a non-competitive inhibitor is therefore to divide V by a factor of $(1 + [I]/K_i)$. Plots of v against $[S]$ have the same shape when the inhibitor is present as when it is omitted, but do not reach the uninhibited value of V, however great the substrate concentration. Double-reciprocal plots are altered in both slope and intercept on the ordinate by the presence of the inhibitor (Fig. 10b).

Uncompetitive Inhibition. In this rather unusual type of inhibition parallel lines are obtained when plots of $1/v$ against $1/[S]$ with and without the inhibitor are compared (Fig. 10c), i.e. the slope remains constant but the intercept on the ordinate is altered by the presence of the inhibitor.

Uncompetitive inhibition is rare in single-substrate reactions. It can occur in such reactions when the inhibitor binds to the ES complex, but not to the free enzyme. A ternary complex can form, but only after the enzyme has combined with the substrate:

$$E + S \underset{k_{-1}}{\overset{k_{+1}}{\rightleftharpoons}} ES \overset{k_{+2}}{\longrightarrow} \text{Products}$$

$$ES + I \overset{K_i}{\rightleftharpoons} ESI$$

The rate equation is

$$v = \frac{V \cdot ([S]/(1 + [I]/K_i))}{(K_m/(1 + [I]/K_i)) + [S]}$$

V and K_m are both divided by $(1 + [I]/K_i)$ when the inhibitor is present, compared with the reaction without inhibitor. In the double-reciprocal plot of $1/v$ against $1/[S]$, therefore, the inhibitor alters the intercept on both axes by the same factor, giving rise to parallel lines at different concentrations of I (Fig. 10c).

Uncompetitive inhibition is more common in two-substrate reactions. For an enzymic process in which A and B are converted into products C and D which follows the route

$$E + A \rightleftharpoons EA \overset{+B}{\rightleftharpoons} EAB \rightleftharpoons C + D$$

an inhibitor (I) which is similar in structure to B can compete with B for its binding site on EA. Therefore, at constant concentrations of A, plots of $1/v$ against $1/[B]$ with and without the inhibitor will be characteristic of competitive inhibition. With the same inhibitor but with $[A]$ varied and $[B]$ fixed, however, uncompetitive inhibition results because I binds to the enzyme–substrate complex EA, as in the single-substrate case of uncompetitive inhibition just described. Because in bi-substrate reactions the uncompetitive inhibitor of the first substrate is a competitive inhibitor of the second substrate and therefore related to the latter in structure, it is easier to postulate possible inhibitors and to test them than is the case with single-substrate reactions, where there is usually no obvious structural relationship between the substrate and an uncompetitive inhibitor.

Mixed Inhibition. Plots of $1/v$ against $1/[S]$ for the inhibited and uninhibited reactions are often found not to fit any of the three patterns described above. Instead, the lines intersect to the left of the y-axis but above the x-axis (Fig. 10d). These cases are usually interpreted as implying that the inhibitor interferes with both the binding of the substrate to the enzyme and its catalytic breakdown.

As with two-substrate reactions, further information about the process of inhibition can sometimes be obtained by re-plotting the slopes and intercepts of $1/v$ against $1/[S]$ plots, obtained at different inhibitor concentrations, against $[I]$. For fully competitive inhibition, the slope of the double-reciprocal plot varies linearly with $[I]$ (the intercept is not affected by the presence of the inhibitor), while in non-competitive inhibition both slope and intercept are linearly related to $[I]$. However, replots may have a hyperbolic or a parabolic form instead of being straight lines. These curves may arise if the inhibitor can combine with more than one form of the enzyme, or if the enzyme–inhibitor complex can break down by a pathway other than the reverse of that by which it was formed, thus diverting the reaction along an alternative route.

Other Ways of Plotting Inhibitor Data

The effects of inhibitors on plots of $1/v$ against $1/[S]$ allow changes in K_m and V to be readily seen. However, in some cases it is impracticable to vary substrate concentration over a sufficiently wide range, or, when the substrate is a large molecule of ill-defined molecular weight such as a polysaccharide or protein, to prepare substrate solutions of known molarity. An alternative method suggested by Dixon is to vary the inhibitor concentration at each of two known concentrations of the substrate. The reciprocals of v are then plotted against $[I]$.

For competitive inhibition, the equation for v can be rearranged to

$$\frac{1}{v} = \frac{[I] \cdot K_m}{K_i \cdot V[S]} + \frac{1}{V}\left(1 + \frac{K_m}{[S]}\right)$$

showing that $1/v$ is linearly related to $[I]$. For two substrate concentrations $[S_1]$ and $[S_2]$, the two

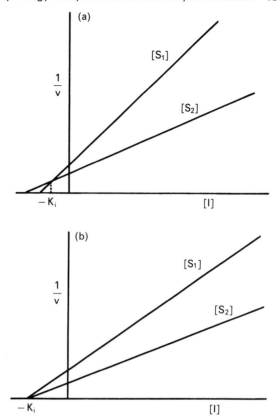

Fig. 11 Plots of $1/v$ against inhibitor concentration, $[I]$, at different substrate concentrations, $[S_1]$ and $[S_2]$, for (a) competitive and (b) non-competitive inhibition.

straight lines will intersect at the point at which both give the same value of $1/v$. Then

$$\frac{[I] \cdot K_m}{K_i \cdot V[S_1]} + \frac{1}{V}\left(1 + \frac{K_m}{[S_1]}\right) =$$
$$\frac{[I] \cdot K_m}{K_i \cdot V[S_2]} + \frac{1}{V}\left(1 + \frac{K_m}{[S_2]}\right)$$

so that

$$\frac{[I]}{K_i}\left(\frac{1}{[S_1]} - \frac{1}{[S_2]}\right) = \left(\frac{1}{[S_2]} - \frac{1}{[S_1]}\right)$$

or

$$[I] = -K_i$$

Therefore, plots of $1/v$ against $[I]$ at different values of $[S]$ intersect at a point at which $[I] = -K_i$ (Fig. 11). It is not necessary to know exactly the values of $[S_1]$ and $[S_2]$ to derive the value of K_i but they should be sufficiently different to ensure a marked difference in slope and consequently a clear crossing of the two lines.

In the case of a non-competitive inhibitor the re-arranged rate equation is

$$\frac{1}{v} = \frac{K_m + [S]}{V[S]} + \frac{[I] \cdot (K_m + [S])}{K_i \cdot V[S]}$$

Again, $1/v$ plotted against $[I]$ gives a straight line, and the lines for substrate concentrations $[S_1]$ and $[S_2]$ cross at the point at which $[I] = -K_i$. However, for non-competitive inhibition, substitution of $-K_i$ for $[I]$ in the equation for $1/v$ shows that this value of $[I]$ occurs when $1/v$ is zero; in other words, the two lines for non-competitive inhibition meet on the abscissa at $-K_i$, not above it as for a competitive inhibitor (Fig. 11).

For an uncompetitive inhibitor,

$$\frac{1}{v} = \frac{K_m}{V[S]} + \frac{1}{V} + \frac{[I]}{V \cdot K_i}$$

The slope of the plot of $1/v$ against $[I]$ is $1/V \cdot K_i$. Since both K_i and V are constants for a given amount of enzyme the slope is independent of $[S]$, but the intercept on the ordinate, $(K_m/V[S] + 1/V)$, is not. Thus, parallel lines are obtained at different substrate concentrations, and K_i cannot be obtained from measurements of the variation of v with $[I]$ at two substrate concentrations unless K_m and V are already known.

Inhibition by Reaction Products

Accumulation of reaction products can contribute in two ways to the fall in velocity of an enzymic reaction with time. First, the increasing concentration of products will tend to drive the reaction backwards, if it is freely reversible. Second, a product may itself be an inhibitor of the forward reaction so that, even if the reaction is not readily reversible, it proceeds against a rising concentration of inhibitor. A familiar example is the release of the competitive inhibitor, inorganic phosphate, by the action of alkaline phosphatase on its substrates. In this case both organic phosphates and inorganic phosphate bind to the active centre of the enzyme with similar affinities; i.e. K_m and K_i are of the same order of magnitude.

Complex effects of product inhibition can arise in two substrate reactions and are influenced by the order of binding of the substrates by the enzyme as well as by the order of release of the products.

ACTIVATION OF ENZYME ACTIVITY

Activators are considered to increase the rates of enzyme-catalysed reactions by promoting formation of the most active state of the enzyme itself or of other reactants such as the substrate. This generalization probably covers a wide variety of mechanisms of activation.

Activators with a Structural Role

Many enzymes contain metal ions as an integral part of their structures, e.g. zinc in alkaline phosphatase and carboxypeptidase A. The function of the metal may be to stabilize tertiary and quaternary protein structure, and removal of the metal ions by treatment with concentrated EDTA solution is often accompanied by conformational changes with inactivation of the enzyme. The enzyme can often be reactivated by dialysis against a solution of the appropriate metal ion. This process may take some time, because rearrangement of the polypeptide chains into the active conformation is not instantaneous.

The metal-ion component of many enzymes appears to play a direct part in catalysis, possibly in addition to any structural role it may fulfil. A metal ion may function in catalysis by providing an electropositive centre in the enzyme with which negatively charged groups in the substrate can form coordinate links.

When the activator ion is an essential part of the functional enzyme molecule, whether as a purely structural element or with an additional catalytic role, it is usually incorporated firmly into the enzyme molecule. It is usually not necessary, therefore, to add the activator to reaction mixtures; indeed, to do so may in fact have an inhibitory effect, as when even a slight excess of Zn^{2+} ions is added to alkaline phosphatase assay mixtures. The ion need only be added, and excess removed by dialysis, when the enzyme has been depleted of it by partial denaturation (e.g. during purification). On the other hand, activators which are not part of the molecule produce their effects when added to enzyme–substrate reaction mixtures.

Combination of Activator with Substrate or Product

For some enzymes combination of the apparent substrate with a metal ion may be necessary before full, or even any, catalytic activity is observed. In these cases the true substrate of the enzyme is the metal–substrate complex, and it is the concentration of this complex which determines the rate of reaction. For reaction between a metal, M, and substrate, S:

$$M + S \underset{\longleftarrow}{\overset{K}{\longrightarrow}} MS$$

followed by

$$E + MS \rightleftharpoons EMS \rightarrow Products$$

the concentration of MS is related to the concentrations of M and S by the equilibrium constant, K. If this is known, the concentration of MS can be calculated for given values of $[M]$ and $[S]$ and used in the equation for v, since

$$v = \frac{[MS] \cdot V}{[MS] + K_m}$$

Thus K_m and V can be determined in terms of the concentration of the true substrate, MS.

In many reactions catalysed by ATPases, and also in some inorganic pyrophosphatase reactions, there seems to be obligatory formation of complexes between the substrate and magnesium ions. In these and other cases the metal ion may act as a bridge between the substrate and the enzyme, or it may alter the configuration of the substrate, or it may neutralize ionic charges in the substrate which would otherwise hinder the approach of the substrate to the active centre.

Removal of a product may activate an enzymic reaction which is freely reversible, or one in which the product is a potent inhibitor of the forward reaction. The activating effect of Ca^{2+} ions on lipase activity has been explained as the removal of the inhibitory free fatty acids, produced as a result of the action of lipases, by the formation of insoluble calcium soaps.

Reversible Combination of Activator and Enzyme

Some enzymes possess activator-binding sites which are separate from the site at which the substrate is bound. The effects of combination with the activator are transmitted through the protein to produce an effect on the substrate-binding site, either facilitating binding (i.e. affecting K_m), or increasing the rate of breakdown of the ES complex into products (i.e. increasing V). Both K_m and V may be affected. Co-operative effects, in which the binding of one molecule of ligand facilitates the binding of additional molecules, are characteristic of allosteric enzymes discussed in a later section but, when these effects are not present, activation by binding to a separate activator site is kinetically similar to non-competitive inhibition, except that V is increased rather than decreased in the former case. Catalysis may not take place at all in some instances unless the activator is bound to the enzyme.

When v is plotted as a function of the concentration of a reversibly combining activator A, at a fixed value of $[S]$, a hyperbola is usually obtained from which a value for K_A can be derived, representing the concentration of A at which v is half the maximum velocity observed at high values of $[A]$. The simplest interpretation of the meaning of K_A is that it is the dissociation constant of the equilibrium between E and A. However, this is only true when the combination of enzyme and activator is independent of the reaction between E and S; i.e. the same value for K_A is obtained at all concentrations of the substrate. If the free enzyme and the enzyme–substrate complex have different affinities for the activator the value for K_A varies with $[S]$. The kinetics are further complicated when the activator and substrate combine with each other.

Activation of salivary and pancreatic amylases by chloride ions (one of the rare examples of activation by anions as distinct from cations) probably involves a reversible combination of chloride with the enzyme. Addition of 5 mmol/l Cl^- increases amylase activity almost threefold, at the same time shifting the pH optimum from 6·5 to 7·0. The chloride ion may combine with a positively charged group in the enzyme and change the ionization constant of a group important in catalysis. However, other anions such as bromide or iodide are less effective activators of amylase, so that some degree of specificity is involved in the process of activation.

Coenzymes

Some coenzymes fill the roles of second substrates in two-substrate reactions and their effect on the rate of reaction follows the Michaelis–Menten pattern of dependence on substrate concentration. This is the case with oxidized and reduced NAD and NADP, for example.

A number of coenzymes are more or less permanently bound to the enzyme molecules, where they form part of the active centre and undergo cycles of chemical change during the reaction. An example of this kind of prosthetic group is pyridoxal 5′-phosphate, a component of aspartate and alanine transaminases. Prosthetic groups, like activators with a structural role, do not usually have to be added to elicit full catalytic activity of a sample of the enzyme unless previous treatment has caused the prosthetic group to be lost from some molecules.

ALLOSTERIC MODIFIERS OF ENZYME ACTIVITY

A number of enzymes have been shown to exhibit a sigmoid dependence of v upon $[S]$, instead of the more usual hyperbolic relationship (Fig. 12). When

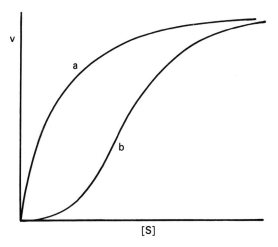

Fig. 12 Sigmoid relationship between v and $[S]$ (b) contrasted with the more usual Michaelis–Menten hyperbolic relationship (a).

the v against $[S]$ curve is S-shaped, the increase in v for a given increase in $[S]$ is lower than that predicted by the Michaelis–Menten equation at low values of $[S]$, but greater than predicted at higher values of $[S]$. The initial flat portion of the sigmoid curve essentially constitutes a threshold of substrate concentration, below which v is low and is little affected by changes in [S]. At a critical concentration of substrate the enzyme responds markedly to changes in [S], switching from very low to pronounced activity. Not surprisingly, therefore, enzymes which occupy rate-limiting positions in metabolic reaction sequences are often found to exhibit sigmoid kinetics.

Not all examples of an apparently sigmoid relationship between v and [S] imply an anomalous interaction of the enzyme with its substrate. When the added substrate interacts with a third component of the system, i.e. an inhibitor or an activator, so that either the inhibitor is removed or the true substrate is formed, the observed value of v is lower than expected until favourable relative concentrations of added substrate and inhibitor or activator have been reached. Further addition of substrate then produces a Michaelis type of dependence of v on [S].

Apart from exceptions such as these, the existence of a sigmoid curve for v against [S] is taken to imply that more than one molecule of substrate binds to each molecule of enzyme and that binding of the second molecule is affected by the presence of the substrate molecule already bound, and so on until all the substrate-combining sites are filled. When, as for the sigmoid relationship between v and [S], the attachment of succeeding molecules is facilitated by those bound earlier, the interaction between them is described by the term cooperativity. Activators and inhibitors can also exhibit cooperative effects in their binding to enzyme molecules, shown as sigmoid inhibition or activation curves.

The degree of sigmoidicity of the curve relating v and [S] may be altered by the presence of an appropriate modifier. An inhibitor tends to make the curve more sigmoid, increasing the concentration of substrate needed to produce a significant increase in v. On the other hand, an activator may bring the curve to a more hyperbolic shape (Fig. 13). These modifiers

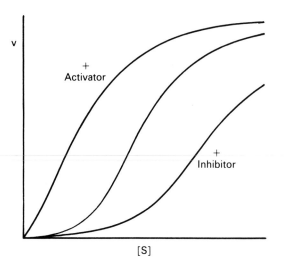

Fig. 13 Alterations in the relationship between v and [S] for an enzyme exhibiting sigmoid kinetics in the presence of an activator or inhibitor.

do not combine with the substrate-binding site and have been termed allosteric modifiers by Monod, Changeux and Jacob to emphasize their supposed effects on the conformation of the enzyme molecules. The existence of different binding sites, with its implication of different specificity requirements for substrate and modifiers, has obvious advantages for the operation of a regulatory enzyme in a metabolic sequence. The modifier need not resemble the substrate of the enzyme in structure, as a competitive inhibitor would have to do, for example, and so could be the product of a later enzyme in the same sequence or even a molecule produced in a different sequence of reactions. Allosteric modifiers thus offer increased possibilities for control of metabolism.

Although the modifier need not be an analogue of the substrate, the site at which the modifier binds to the enzyme has its own specificity requirements. Therefore, analogues of the modifier may be found which compete with the modifier itself for its own binding site. If these analogues are without action on the enzyme their effect will be to prevent the activation or inhibition which follows combination between the enzyme and the true modifier. However, some analogues of the modifier may themselves have effects on the activity of the enzyme similar to those of the true modifier with which they act cooperatively.

The existence of separate binding sites for substrate and modifier is supported by evidence that, in some cases, treatments which abolish the effects of the modifier leave the ability to bind the substrate unchanged. Thus, when some regulatory enzymes are heated for a short period of time the shape of the curve of v against [S] changes from sigmoid to hyperbolic, without a change in V.

Cooperative effects in the binding of substrate imply that more than one molecule of substrate is bound to each molecule of enzyme at separate but identical sites. For an enzyme with n binding sites per molecule for the ligand S, if equilibrium is rapidly attained between the free enzyme and the enzyme with all the sites filled, ES_n, then

$$E + nS \underset{k_{-1}}{\overset{k_{+1}}{\rightleftharpoons}} ES_n$$

and the dissociation constant for the reaction is

$$K = \frac{k_{-1}}{k_{+1}} = \frac{[E][S]^n}{[ES_n]}$$

For the reaction to reach equilibrium the degree of cooperativity must be high, i.e. each bound molecule of substrate increases the affinity of the remaining sites so much that partly filled enzyme molecules have only a transient existence. The rate of the catalysed reaction is then virtually entirely accounted for by the breakdown of the ES_n complex. Therefore,

$$v = k_{+2}[ES_n]$$

At equilibrium, the total concentration of enzyme is given by

$$[E_t] = [E] + [ES_n]$$

hence

$$[E] = [E_t] - [ES_n]$$

Since

$$V = k_{+2}[E_t],$$
$$V - v = k_{+2}[E_t] - k_{+2}[ES_n]$$

or

$$V - v = k_{+2}[E]$$

Eliminating $[E]$,

$$V - v = k_{+2}\frac{[ES_n] \cdot K}{[S]^n}$$

Substituting for $[ES_n]$, $= v/k_{+2}$, and rearranging:

$$\frac{v}{V - v} = \frac{[S]^n}{K}$$

or

$$\frac{v}{V} = \frac{[S]^n}{K + [S]^n}$$

The rate of reaction thus depends on the nth power of the substrate concentration. When $n = 1$, the equation reduces to the Michaelis–Menten equation but, when n is greater than 1, plots of v against $[S]$ take on an increasingly sigmoid appearance. In order to determine the value of n, the log of $v/V-v$ is usually plotted against $\log[S]$ to obtain a straight line of slope n and intercept on the ordinate at $-\log K$, since

$$\log \frac{v}{V - v} = n \log[S] - \log K$$

Values of n of greater than one indicate the existence of cooperative effects in the binding of successive substrate molecules, and values of less than one that the ligands behave anticooperatively, i.e. that binding of the first molecule reduces affinity for further binding. If n is found to be unity it does not necessarily imply that only one molecule of substrate is bound to each molecule of enzyme, but that binding of the first molecule of substrate neither helps nor hinders the attachment of any further substrate molecules to the same molecule of enzyme. Similarly, n will only correspond to the number of binding sites of an enzyme when the fully saturated enzyme molecules are the only ones which give rise to products at a significant rate.

Cooperativity in substrate binding implies that more than one separate but presumably identical sites exist on the enzyme molecule to accommodate the several substrate molecules. Similarly, the existence of cooperative effects between molecules of a modifier implies the existence of a further set of identical sites specific for the modifier molecules. The various sites could be distributed along a single polypeptide chain, which would involve repeated sequences of amino acids in the primary structure. More easily envisaged is a set of protein subunits, called monomers or protomers, which associate with each other to form the active enzyme oligomer and each of which carries a substrate binding site, as well as activator and/or inhibitor binding sites. All the enzymes exhibiting cooperativity which have so far been investigated have been found to be oligomeric and the models proposed for the action of allosteric enzymes have assumed the existence of quaternary structure.

ENZYMES AS ANALYTICAL REAGENTS

The use of enzymes as analytical reagents offers the advantage of great specificity for the substance being determined, which typically removes the need for preliminary separation or purification stages. Enzymes with absolute specificity for the substance being estimated are preferable for analytical use, e.g. uricase (urate oxidase), urease and glucose oxidase. However, this ideal cannot always be achieved in practice, and a knowledge of the substrate specificities of reagent enzymes is therefore essential to allow possible interferences with the assay to be anticipated and corrected. Coupled reactions are often used to construct an enzymatic analytical system for determining a particular compound and the specificity of the coupled reactions may modify the specificity of the overall process. An example of this is the determination of glucose by the hexokinase reaction. Hexokinase will convert sugars other than glucose into their 6-phosphate esters; however, the indicator reaction used to monitor this change is catalysed by glucose-6-phosphate dehydrogenase, an enzyme that is highly specific for its substrate, so that the overall process is highly specific for glucose.

The principle that is most widely used to determine the amount of a substance enzymatically is to allow the reaction to go to completion, so that all the substrate has been converted into a measurable product. These methods are called 'end-point' or, more correctly, 'equilibrium' methods, since the reaction ceases when the equilibrium is reached. Reactions in which the equilibrium point corresponds to virtually complete conversion of the substrate are obviously preferable for this type of analysis. However, unfavourable equilibria can often be displaced in the desired direction by additional enzymatic or non-enzymatic reactions that convert or 'trap' a product of the first reaction; e.g. in measuring lactate with lactate dehydrogenase, the pyruvate formed can be trapped by the addition of hydrazine with which it forms a hydrazone.

The time required to transform a fixed quantity of substrate into products is inversely proportional to the amount of enzyme present. Equilibrium methods may therefore require the use of appreciable amounts of enzyme for each sample to avoid inconveniently long incubation periods. As the substrate concentration falls, the reaction enters a phase of first-order dependence on [S]. Under these conditions, the rate equation approaches

$$v = \frac{V \cdot [S]}{K_m}$$

This is the rate equation of a first-order reaction with rate constant equal to V/K_m. Enzymes with high affinities for the substrates (low K_m values) are, therefore, most suitable for equilibrium analysis. Equilibrium methods are largely insensitive to minor changes in reaction conditions. It is not necessary to have exactly the same amount of enzyme in each reaction mixture, or to maintain the pH or temperature absolutely constant, provided that the variations are not so great that the reaction is not completed within the fixed time allowed.

The amount of reagent enzyme required for each analysis can be reduced and the time shortened by the use of kinetic methods, i.e. methods in which the rate of change is measured. As already mentioned, the rate of an enzyme-catalysed reaction which with initially high substrate concentration at first follows zero-order kinetics, passes into a first-order kinetic phase as the substrate concentration declines.

For any first-order reaction, the substrate concentration [S] at a given time t after the start of the reaction is given by

$$[S] = [S_0] \times e^{-kt}$$

where $[S_0]$ is the initial substrate concentration and k is the rate constant.

The change in substrate concentration $\Delta [S]$ over a fixed time interval t_1 to t_2 is related to $[S_0]$ by the equation

$$[S_0] = \frac{-\Delta [S]}{e^{-kt_1} - e^{-kt_2}}$$

That is, the change in substrate concentration over a fixed time interval is directly proportional to its initial concentration. This is a general property of first-order reactions.

Methods in which some property related to substrate concentration (such as UV absorbance) is measured at two fixed times during the course of the reaction are known as 'two-point' kinetic methods. They are theoretically the most accurate for the enzymatic determination of substrates. However, these methods are technically more demanding than equilibrium methods. Since reaction rate is being measured in the two-point methods, all the factors that affect reaction rate such as pH, temperature, and amount of enzyme must be kept constant from one assay to the next, as must the timing of the two measurements. A standard solution of the analyte (substrate) must be used for calibration. To ensure first-order reaction conditions the substrate concentration must be low, of the order of less than $0.2 \times K_m$. Enzymes with high K_m values are therefore preferred for kinetic analysis to give a wider usable range of substrate concentration. Introduction of a competitive inhibitor has been suggested as a way of increasing the apparent K_m of a reagent enzyme. The low substrate concentrations needed for kinetic analysis also require the measurement of small changes.

28. Bioassay
J. Chayen and Lucille Bitensky

FUNCTIONAL VERSUS ANALYTICAL ASSAYS

In this review we will concentrate on the main current use of bioassay namely that of polypeptide hormones. However, the same basic principles are applicable to the assay of any biologically active material.

A hormone, like any other biologically active molecule, is characterized and defined by its biological activity. It is therefore appropriate to assay it by one or other of its biological effects in living matter, which may be the whole body, the target-tissue or the target-cells. This is the purpose of bioassay which is a 'functional assay'. In contrast, following the advent of saturation assay techniques, and more recently of refined physicochemical analytical procedures including high-pressure liquid chromatography,[1] there has been a swing towards 'analytical assays'. These are based on the argument that since hormones are chemically definable entities, they should be assayable by the same procedures used for any other chemical entity. These two approaches have been discussed in some detail (e.g.[2,3]).

Superficially there seemed to be good reason for discarding bioassay (which is always likely to be cumbersome since it depends on living organisms or cells) in favour of analytical assays, like radioimmunoassay, which can be rapid and automated; many require little skill on the part of the operator. But there are major drawbacks, the main being that often analytical assays do not give a comprehensive analysis of the molecule: they give only an approximation. Yet it has now become apparent that minor modifications in the structure of a peptide can totally alter its biological activity. For example, as regards parathyroid hormone (PTH), whereas 1–34 PTH is fully active both on bone and on kidney, desamino 1–34 PTH has only 1% of this activity in the renal adenylate cyclase assay and only 50% activity in the *in vivo* bone hypercalcaemic assay.[4] The 3–34 PTH has no biological activity[4] and may even act as an antagonist of PTH activity.[4] Even minor modifications at the 'biologically inert' region of the molecule, such as aspartate instead of asparagine at position 76, can cause virtual loss of the biological activity. Though current analytical assays are becoming increasingly sophisticated, they are not yet sufficiently comprehensive in their analysis to discriminate such modifications. A recent example, concerning the radioimmunoassay of osteocalcin, lends weight to this conclusion. This peptide, of 49 amino acids, has been much investigated because of its possible involvement in calcification. It is generally conceded that its significance resides in the fact that three glutamate (Glu) residues, at positions 17, 21 and 24, are carboxylated by the vitamin K cycle,[5] to γ-glutamate (Gla); it is the Gla that binds calcium or hydroxyapatite. The investigation of this peptide in bone disease should have been greatly advanced by the development of a radioimmunoassay for osteocalcin. In fact, it has been retarded by the fact that the 'osteocalcin' measured by RIA cannot discriminate between the biologically active osteocalcin (with Gla residues) and the totally inactive peptide (with Glu residues).[6]

WHY DO WE NEED BIOASSAYS?

Are All Requests for Assay Justifiable?

It may be salutary to consider whether in clinical biochemical practice we really require so many assays, of any sort, of polypeptide hormones. It may be argued that the diagnosis and management of most patients with hormonal disorders, based on standard clinical and clinical biochemical assessments, was no less efficient in the era prior to the mass production of assays of polypeptide hormones than it is now. Fundamentally, there is a case for saying that most simple assays (as contrasted with supression–stimulation tests) that are done currently are suppor-

tive, rather than decisive: they are indeed decisive in particular conditions and, ideally, they could be restricted to such conditions. For example, measurement of circulating levels of corticosteroids provides sufficient biochemical evidence of Cushing's syndrome, but an assay of the adrenocorticotrophic hormone (ACTH) is needed to differentiate it from Cushing's disease. A busy clinical endocrinology laboratory may meet only six such cases each year. Another relatively rare example is the need for an assay of renin in Conn's syndrome, to distinguish between patients with high or low renin values in the presence of elevated aldosterone: assays of aldosterone are necessary but only rarely is it necessary to assay for renin. On the other hand, there is a clear need for assay when tumours of the pituitary may be involved, especially in hyperprolactinaemia (with the current possibility of treatment). Another example of such need relates to the assay of luteinizing hormone (LH) and follicle stimulating hormone (FSH) to discriminate ovarian or testicular failure and for conditions of male and female infertility.

There is clearly a need for the assay of polypeptide hormones when provocation tests of the responsiveness of endocrine organs are essential for diagnosis. Examples of these are the pituitary suppression test of growth hormone (GH) in acromegaly and the GH-stimulation test in conditions of short stature. Although the early detection of myxoedema may be best achieved by a simple thyrotrophin (TSH) assay, the real province of TSH assays may be mainly in relation to tests of the thyroid–pituitary axis, with the use of the TSH-releasing hormone (TRH) and the subsequent measurement of the TSH released.

These few examples have been selected to suggest that, while there is indeed a genuine role for such assays, it is doubtful whether the current massive demand for assays of polypeptide hormones is justified. Perhaps the problem is that, because RIA can cope with such large numbers the assays are being requested whether or not they can materially contribute to the diagnosis and management of the patient.

The Real Need for Bioassays

The requirements for a bioassay seem to be mainly the following.

Standardization of international standard preparations and reference preparations of polypeptide hormones. It may not generally be recognized that the World Health Organization (through the WHO Expert Committee on Biological Standardization) is responsible for establishing international standard (and reference) preparations of polypeptide hormones and their unitage.[7] To conform rigorously to standard practice, any assay of a polypeptide hormone should be recorded in International Units, not in 'ng/ml'. Suitable reference standards are available (e.g. from the National Institute for Biological Standards and Control, London) against which the various national or laboratory standard preparations should be calibrated. The need for bioassay comes from the fact[7] that 'a limitation on the use of immunoassays for evaluating hormonal bioactivity is that the methods measure a composite of antigenic activity, which is not necessarily related to the bioactivity of the hormone'. Several standard preparations, labelled 'for immunoassay' may have virtually no biological activity. For these reasons the WHO Expert Committee called for the development of bioassays which would have at least the same sensitivity as the equivalent RIA: this was the stimulus for the cytochemical bioassays which are discussed in this chapter.

When clinical assessment and immunoassay are discrepant. Fundamental to all discussion on assay of hormones is the fact that a hormone is a biological entity that has a biological function, by which it can be recognized. Consequently it is reasonable to assay it by a functional assay (bioassay) in terms of units of its biological activity. It is convenient to argue that it is also a specific molecule, which can be assayed by an analytical assay, such as RIA, in terms of so many ng/l of this specific peptide. Very frequently, these assays will produce the same results and it is more convenient to use RIA. But there are many instances where the results obtained by RIA are in discord with clinical assessment. This may come about for a number of reasons: RIA may be detecting forms of the hormone that are relatively inactive biologically, such as 'big gastrin' or 'big ACTH'; RIA may be measuring biologically inactive fragments of the hormone that have a relatively long life in the circulation, as occurs with assays of parathyroid hormone in secondary hyperparathyroidism. These discrepancies have been discussed elsewhere.[2]

Where there is no 'pure' hormone. This is a major function of bioassay at present.[8] It is still the most decisive way of assaying the long-acting thyroid-stimulating immunoglobulin of Graves' disease. It is the only way of detecting the thyroid-growth-stimulating immunoglobulins associated with goitre; the immunoglobulins associated with blockade of thyroid-function in myxoedema; the anti-parietal cell immunoglobulins of pernicious anaemia; and some, as yet uncharacterized natriuretic factors.[8] In all these, and in similar cases, the factors can be assayed decisively only by their biological function.

For the study of the actual effect of the hormone. This is largely of value in research: detailed study of the biochemical mode of action of a hormone, acting on its target-cells, may elucidate functions of that hormone other than those by which the hormone was first recognized. The cytochemical bioassay system is of especial value in this respect.

For the assay of such hormones where immunoassay is as yet insufficiently sensitive or discriminatory. In spite of the great advances made in the various forms of immunoassay, some that are in current use are still too insensitive to measure low normal circulating levels adequately. One of the special advantages of the cytochemical bioassays (CBA) is that they are at least 10^3 times more sensitive than the equivalent RIA, as practised generally. Consequently they can measure low-normal and subnormal circulating levels. In this context it may be pertinent of comment on what is meant by 'sensitivity'. This is not a measure of the sensitivity of the final detection mechanism, for example the scintillation counter or the counts per minute detectable in the final sample; this term should be restricted to the lowest concentration in the plasma or serum that can be measured adequately (above 'background').

Perhaps the best example of this requirement for bioassay is the assay of PTH. It is now well established[4] that the normal circulating level of this hormone is from about 5 pg/ml up to, perhaps, 20 pg/ml. Most current RIAs cannot detect such levels and give values of at least ten-times this concentration due, to some extent at least, to the measurement of biologically inactive fragments. Consequently RIA is often of little value in detecting primary hyperparathyroidism (which is readily discriminated by CBA). Moreover, in certain conditions such as pseudohypoparathyroidism type I (and possibly nutritional vitamin-D deficiency) there is evidence that the huge discrepancy between the results of RIA and of CBA may be related to the presence, in the plasma, of material that inhibits the biological activity of the hormone acting on its target tissue.[9] RIA has not been able to discriminate between the biologically active PTH and its inhibitory material.

WHAT CONSTITUTES A BIOASSAY?

Although it must be conceded that there is no general agreement on what constitutes 'a biological assay',[10] we argue that it must involve a response that can be achieved only by intact cells. This excludes assays done on isolated receptors, on receptors in isolated membranes, or on cell fragments. The fact that receptors can bind a hormone does not constitute a bioassay of that hormone: the same receptors will bind inhibitors of the hormone. Equally, the response by adenylate cyclase in isolated membranes, or in cell fragments, consequent to hormone-binding is equally unconvincing. It should be construed simply as a chemical response, in that no living system is involved: in essence it is no different from an assay in which the enzyme was sequestered into artificial liposomes with the receptor (and regulator protein) in the surface of the liposome.

Thus the lowest level of organization required for a bioassay is the isolated cell bioassay. These seem acceptable for assaying bioactivity and are of considerable value in clinical endocrinological practice. However, there are good reasons for believing that the metabolic response induced by a hormone on isolated cells can be quite different from that which pertains when these cells occur within an organized tissue.[11] Hence for *studying* the biological activity of a biologically active molecule (in contrast to assaying it against a standard preparation in the same assay system) it is necessary to use a tissue assay, as in the cytochemical bioassays, or an *in-vivo* bioassay.

WHAT INFORMATION IS SUPPLIED BY BIOASSAY?

Over the past fifteen years there has been much concern over 'problems' of bioassay. For example, different *in vivo* bioassays may give different results depending on the route of administration. Another example is the argument[3] that *in vitro* bioassays are inadequate because they do not necessarily distinguish between sialated and desialated hormone that may have equal potencies on the target organ (or isolated cells) but different half-lives in the circulation. These 'worries' arise from ignorance of the purpose of bioassays and of what can legitimately be derived from them.

In our view,[1,2] the function of a bioassay is to measure the relative potency of the hormone preparation, or plasma sample (compared with that of a standard reference preparation) acting directly on the target cells. How it becomes diluted, or metabolized, when administered by different routes, is the subject of physiological studies, and these cannot be done on a laboratory animal when the effect of the hormone preparation is to be assessed in man in which the rates of metabolic conversion might be very different from that in, for example, the rat. Such studies have been discussed in detail, particularly in relation to long-acting hormone preparations.[2]

EXAMPLES OF BIOASSAYS

In this section we outline some representative bioassays of polypeptide hormones that illustrate the range of techniques employed. For full details, the original publications should be consulted.

The basic criterion of the usefulness of a bioassay[2] is the index of precision (designated as λ). This is compounded of the slope (b) of the dose–response graph (as in Fig. 1) and the standard deviation (s) of the values, obtained in the normal way of subtracting each value of y from its calculated value y_c (as given by the calculated regression line), namely

$$s = \frac{\Sigma(y - y_c)^2}{n - 1}$$

where n is the number of readings.

Then

$$\lambda = s/b.$$

(It may be noted that in some publications, the value s_{yx} is used instead of s, as above.)

In general it can be said that when $\lambda = 0.3$, in practice, the log dose estimated from a single observation has a standard error of 0.3. So within the limits of a single standard deviation, sd, (68% confidence limits), this single observation would be in error to $\pm$ antilog 0.3, that is 2 times or half the value (50% to 200%) produced by the assay. In practice, this is often adequate in bioassay. However, most bioassayists would work to a λ of 0.1 where a single observation has a 68% chance (i.e. to 1 sd) of being from 79% to 126% of the correct value (or, using 2 sd, to give the 95% confidence limits, and therefore antilog of $2 \times \lambda$, it would give 63%–158% of the true value, i.e. antilog of 100 ± 0.2).[2]

The fiducial limits of a complete assay is a more precise indicator of the precision of the bioassay, and is generally done on at least two dilutions of the test material and two or three dilutions of the standard reference preparation (as in Fig. 1). Such calculations[12] take into account the parallelism of the

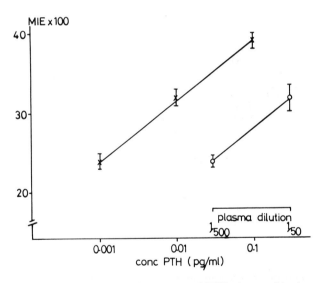

Fig. 1 A cytochemical bioassay of PTH, done with the bone bioassay (and kindly provided by Dr Jane Dunham). The assay depends on the stimulation of glucose 6-phosphate dehydrogenase (G6PD) activity in the growth plate of rat metatarsals maintained *in vitro* for 5 h prior to the assay. Different bones have been exposed either to one of three concentrations of a standard reference preparation of the hormone (crosses) or to one of two dilutions of a plasma (circles). After 8 min exposure, the bones were chilled to $-70\,°C$; sectioned; reacted for G6PD activity; and the activity, in individual cells (mean integrated extinction, MIE $\times$ 100) was determined by microdensitometry. The results are given as mean $\pm$ SEM for 20 cells in each preparation. The results from the standard preparation and from the plasma give parallel dose-response graphs. The slope of the graphs (change in MIE $\times$ 100 with each log dose of assayed material: b) and the deviation of each point from the calculated regression-line ($y - y_c$) can readily be determined.

response of the test as against the standard and give 95% confidence limits of that particular assay.

In vivo Bioassay of ACTH

The method of Lipscomb and Nelson[13] has been taken as representing an ideal *in vivo* bioassay.[1] The rats (150–200 g body weight) are hypophysectomized 2–4 h prior to assay. The standard preparation of ACTH, or the test preparation, is then injected retrogradely into the left adrenal vein. After 90 s adrenal vein blood is collected into the same syringe. The blood is then analysed for corticosterone content by a standard fluorimetric procedure. A 2×2 design is usually employed (two concentrations of the standard preparation, one four times the other, and two dilutions of the test material), with four to six animals for each point. The response is linear against the log dose. Values of λ have been reported to be as low as 0·02, but there have been reports of very variable degrees of precision.

This assay can be used to assay ACTH in plasma but it can detect levels only at the very upper end of the normal range and elevated levels. The point to be noted is that the hormone is presented direct to the target organ, so obviating physiological effects that have been discussed above.

In vivo Bioassays of TSH

The most widely used of these bioassays are variants of the McKenzie[14] assay which is based on the discharge of radioactive iodine from the mouse thyroid.

The method has been considerably modified, but the general procedure is as follows. Female mice weighing 15 g are given a low-iodine diet for about a week, following which they are injected intraperitoneally with 5–8 μCi of ^{131}I. Subcutaneous injections of thyroxine, 10–15 μg, are given 4, 24 and 48 h after the radioactive iodine, and 24 h after the last thyroxine injection the TSH standards and unknowns are injected into a tail vein. In some of the modifications thyroxine is also added to the feed or drinking water. Blood samples are taken for the determination of radioactivity at the time of TSH injection and 2 h later. The percentage increase in radioactivity is plotted against log-dose and is linear over a useful range. The method detects 0·25 mU of TSH activity and λ ranges from 0·17 to 0·29. It is insufficiently sensitive to assay plasma levels in the normal range. By counting the radioactivity of a blood sample 9–24 h after injection of the assay material the long-acting thyroid stimulating immunoglobulin (LATS) may also be assayed.

Both 2×3 and 2×2 designs have been used, with from 6 to 12 mice at each dosage point.

In vivo Bioassays of FSH

These depend mainly on the ability of FSH to augment the action of HCG in increasing the weight of the ovaries or uterus of intact or hypophysectomized rats or mice.

In the assay described by Lamond and Bindon[15] mice 18–21 days old (10–12 g) are hypophysectomized, and 5 h later are injected at separate sites with 4·5 iu of HCG and the standard or unknown FSH dose. Two days later the animals are killed and their uteri weighed. The precision of the assay is satisfactory, λ ranging from 0·07 to 0·29. Designs vary, but three to six mice are usually used at each dosage point. One group may be given HCG only as control. The method permits determination of urinary FSH in normally menstruating women.

In vivo Bioassays of LH

These depend on the depletion of cholesterol or ascorbate from the ovaries of immature intact female rats, or the increase in weight of the rat ventral prostate.

In Schmidt-Elmendorff and Loraine's[16] modification of Parlow's ascorbate depletion procedure, immature female rats (40–50 g, 25–27 days old) are treated with PMS-G and HCG. As a result their ovaries become heavily luteinized. About one week later, standards or unknown LH solutions are injected intravenously. Four hours following the injection the animals are killed and their ovaries removed. These are cleaned, weighed and homogenized and the ascorbate concentration determined by a standard chemical technique. There is a linear log dose-response relationship over a rather narrow range. The design is usually 2×2 with five animals at each point. The log dose interval is usually five or tenfold, and λ values should be less than 0·3.

In vivo Bioassays of GH

The most satisfactory bioassay of GH is that based on increase in width of the proximal epiphysis of the rat tibia.[17]

Female rats, about 4 weeks old, are hypophysectomized. Two weeks later the animals are injected with standard or unknown GH intraperitoneally once daily for 4 days and are killed 24 h after the last injection. A tibia is removed, cleaned, split between the condyles at the proximal end and stained with silver nitrate. The calcified bone turns dark brown so that the epiphyseal cartilage stands out clearly. The width of the cartilage is measured with a low-power microscope having a calibrated micrometer eye piece.

A 2×3 design is usual with four animals at each point, and a group of saline-injected controls is desirable. Standards are used in a ratio of 1:3:9, with similar dilutions of unknown. The response is linear when plotted against log dose and λ values average 0·16. The assay is valuable for calibrating standard preparations, but is too insensitive for clinical use.

Isolated Cell Bioassays

Techniques have been devised for isolating cells from

many organs, including the pituitary, adrenal and thyroid glands, the testis and corpus luteum and for using these cells, without additional culture, for assaying the relevant hormones. The two most commonly used will be considered as examples of this type of bioassay.

In the ACTH assay[18] adrenals from a group of rats are cleaned and quartered and immersed in a flask containing ice-cold Krebs–Ringer bicarbonate and trypsin. The flask is then warmed to 37 °C and mechanically agitated with an electrically driven paddle for 20 min. This process is repeated two or three times with fresh buffer-trypsin. The cells are then centrifuged and washed with fresh buffer containing trypsin inhibitor. The deposit of cells is resuspended and aliquots of the suspension used for the assay.

Doses of standard or unknown ACTH are added to these suspensions and incubated at 37 °C for 2 h. The suspensions are then extracted with dichlormethane and the corticosterone produced is determined by a standard fluorimetric technique. The log dose–response curve is sigmoid, but linear over a sufficient range to be useful and the assay is sensitive and precise. Unfortunately, however, ACTH cannot be assayed in plasma without extraction, as plasma, for some ill-understood reason, alters the shape of the dose–response curve.

In the LH assay[19] Leydig cells from mouse testis are isolated mechanically in Eagle's medium containing 2% calf serum. No enzyme is used to assist dispersal, as it was found that this reduced sensitivity. LH standards and unknowns are added to the suspensions and incubated for 3 h. The testosterone produced is then measured by radioimmunoassay. A 2×3 design is used, with four suspensions at each dose level and a log dose interval of 1.5. The log dose–response curve is linear when the square root of the testosterone produced is used as the response metameter. The assay is precise (mean λ value 0.044) and sensitive enough to allow estimations of LH activity in plasma.

A feature of this type of assay is that the direct exhibition of the hormone to the target cells avoids problems which may be caused by penetration and diffusion of the hormone through tissue. In addition, each dose of hormone is added to an aliquot of cells derived from a homogeneous pool. Thus sensitivity and precision are far greater than in most assays.

Cytochemical Bioassays

These bioassays have been reviewed extensively recently.[2,8] They are the most sensitive assays of polypeptide hormones currently available, being 10^3 times more sensitive than the equivalent RIAs. Consequently they readily assay normal circulating levels; discriminate subnormal levels; and, being so sensitive, require very little plasma: the ACTH assay has been done on heel-pricks from neonates. They are also very specific[1] in that (1) they depend initially on the specificity by which the hormone is recognized by the receptor at the surface of the target-cells; (2) secondly on the provocation of the relevant 'second messenger' which (3) must induce the particular metabolic response within the target cells that will give rise to the biochemical (and physiological) response by which the hormone is normally identified. Part of the increased sensitivity of these assays is the fact that they are 'within-animal' assays, so obviating the great variability found in conventional *in vivo* bioassays which require the use of many animals. Other factors that increase sensitivity are (1) the hormone is not diluted into a large volume but applied directly to the target tissue; (2) the metabolic activity of the target cells is allowed to reach basal level before it is stimulated by the hormone; and (3) the activity is not measured by the accumulation of a reaction product but by measuring the *rate* of altered metabolic activity.[2]

Cytochemical Segment Bioassays. In these assays, segments of the target organ, for example of the thyroid gland for assaying TSH, of a suitable animal (normally the guinea pig) are maintained separately in non-proliferative organ maintenance culture, in contact with a synthetic culture medium, for 5 h. This allows the cells to recover from the trauma of excision and from any stimulation of the hormone that may have occurred in life. It therefore allows the metabolic activity of the target cells to revert to basal level. Then, for four of these segments, the culture-medium is replaced by fresh medium containing one of four graded concentrations of the standard reference preparation of the hormone, normally 5 fg/ml to 5 pg/ml. These will provide the reference dose–response graph, as in Fig. 1. At least two of the other segments are exposed to fresh medium containing one of a graded dilution of the plasma (or other test material) to be assayed, usually at dilutions of $1:10^2$ and $1:10^3$. (It may be noted that unextracted plasma is used for these assays: there is too much danger of degradation of the polypeptide hormones during the separation of serum, and also the possibility of biologically active moieties, such as polyamines, being released from the circulating blood cells.) The time of exposure to the hormone is measured in minutes: 4 min for the assay of ACTH; 8 min for assaying PTH. The tissue is then chilled to -70 °C. Sections are cut in a cryostat with an automatic cutting device (to ensure uniform thickness of the sections), with the cabinet temperature about -25 °C and the knife cooled further with solid carbon dioxide. The sections are flash-dried on to glass slides and are then reacted for the appropriate biochemical activity associated with the biological action of the hormone (Table 1). The reaction is measured, solely in the target cells, by microdensitometry.

Cytochemical Section Assays. Although the segment assays benefited from the fact that all the segments

TABLE 1
THE RANGE OF APPLICATION OF CURRENT CYTOCHEMICAL BIOASSAYS (CBA)

Biological activity	Target cell	Biochemical activity affected	Biological function	Sensitivity (per ml)	Index of precision
ACTH	Adrenal zona reticularis	Ascorbate depletion	Steroidogenesis	5 fg	0.076 ± 0.002
LH	Corpus luteum	Ascorbate depletion	Steroidogenesis	10^{-4} mU	0.12 ± 0.01
TSH	Thyroid follicle cells	Lysosomal activation	Production of T_3, T_4	4×10^{-5} µU	0.13
Gastrin	Gastric parietal cells	Carbonic anhydrase	Acid secretion	5 fg	0.1 ± 0.05
PTH	Renal distal convoluted tubules	G6PD*	Calcium resorption	5 fg	0.12 ± 0.07
PTH	Epiphyseal osteoblasts	G6PD*	Calcium movement	5 fg	0.14 ± 0.015
Antidiuretic hormone	Renal thick ascending limb of loop of Henle	Na^+-K^+-ATPase	Sodium transport	2 fg	†
Angiotensin II	Renal zona glomerulosa	Ascorbate depletion	Steroidogenesis	0.5 fg	0.065
TRH	Pituitary	Production of TSH‡			
CRF	Pituitary	Production of ACTH‡			
Thyroid-stimulating immunoglobulins	Thyroid follicle cell	Lysosomal activation (long course of action)	Production of T_3, T_4		
Thyroid growth-stimulating immunoglobulins	Thyroid follicle cell	DNA synthesis	Goitre		
Thyroid blocking immunoglobulins	Thyroid follicle cell	Inhibition of TSH action	Thyroid atrophy		
Gastrin-blocking immunoglobulins	Gastric parietal cells	Inhibition of gastrin effect	Hypochlorhydria		

* G6PD: glucose 6-phosphate dehydrogenase
† Inter-assay coefficient of variation = 6·4%
‡ Measured in the culture-medium by the appropriate CBA

were derived from one animal, so that they were 'within-animal' assays, they had the drawback that only relatively few segments were available. Since four were required for establishing the dose–response graph for that animal, only few samples could be assayed, each at two dilutions. To improve the 'through-put', some of these (for ACTH, TSH, LH and gastrin) have been converted into section bioassays. In these, the target organ is cut into relatively large segments (e.g. half a thyroid gland) and these are maintained in the normal culture conditions for 5 h. They are then chilled to −70 °C and relatively thick sections, that enclose whole cells (e.g. 20 µm), are cut. It is these sections, in contrast to whole segments, that are exposed (under suitable stabilizing conditions) to the hormone. The response is now a matter of tens of seconds rather than of minutes. The cytochemical reactions and their measurement are the same as for the segment assays. The sensitivity and the response is identical to that of the segment assays. It will be appreciated that this indicates that the precise procedures used in these assays for producing sections do not apparently vitiate the biological function of the cells in the sections. These section assays permit the assay of very many samples, based on the same calibration graph.

CONCLUSIONS

For general, routine purposes, it is probably acceptable to use an analytical type of assay, such as RIA since, as argued above, the results of these assays are generally supportive, rather than critical for diagnosis. However, when the results of the assay are critical, there is increasing evidence for the contention that such analytical assays do not analyse the complete molecule. Consequently grossly misleading results may be produced by long-lived, biologically inactive fragments of the hormone, by modified hormone, such as 'big' varieties, or by inhibitory molecules that may have similar molecular structure. Thus when the results of the analytical assay are in discord with the clinical findings, recourse must be made to bioassay.

Bioassay is enjoying a resurgence of importance also in respect of immunoglobulins that have endocrine influence, such as those that affect the thyroid gland (as discussed above), and it is becoming of increased value for detecting inhibitory influences.[9] The latter are readily detected by including 'recovery' studies in the standard bioassay.[9] These were used originally, in standard bioassay practice, for determining the 'accuracy' of the bioassay.[2] Thus a known concentration of a standard preparation of the hormone was added to two dilutions of the test material (or plasma) and the amount 'recovered' by the assay was determined: if the test material contained inhibitory factors, the recovery of the known concentration of the standard preparation would be considerably less than normal for this assay.

Although it must be conceded that bioassays are more tedious and labour intensive than analytical assays, and therefore have a low 'through-put', it has been argued (above) that the number of such assays actually required, for any large laboratory, is quite small, and therefore within the capacity of bioassay. The cytochemical bioassays have the additional advantage of utilizing the same expertise and equipment for assaying the biological activity of a wide range of polypeptide hormones, and for determining the presence of endocrinologically significant immunoglobulins and inhibitory factors. Thus it seems reasonable to argue, that, in view of the relatively few essential assays that must be done, and the versatility (and sensitivity) of the cytochemical bioassays, it would be prudent to establish a few centres where such assays can be done.

REFERENCES

1. Chayen J. (1982). In *Hormone Drugs* p. 48. Rockville, Maryland: United States Pharmacopeial Convention.
2. Chayen J. (1980). *The Cytochemical Bioassay of Polypeptide Hormones*. Berlin: Springer.
3. Ekins R. P. (1976). In *Hormone Assays and their Clinical Application*, 2nd edn, p. 1. London and Edinburgh: Livingstone.
4. Kent G. N., Zanelli J. M. (1983). In *Cytochemical Bioassays: Techniques and Clinical Applications*, (Chayen J., Bitensky L., eds), p. 255. New York and Basel: Marcel Dekker.
5. Hauschka P. V., Lian J. B., Gallop P. M. (1978). Vitamin K and mineralization. *Trends Biochem. Sci*; **3**: 75.
6. Price P. A., Lothringer J. W., Nishimoto S. K. (1980). Absence of the vitamin K-dependent bone protein in fetal rat mineral: evidence for another γ-carboxyglutamic acid-containing component in bone. *J. Biol. Chem*; **255**: 2938.
7. WHO Report (1975). *WHO Expert Committee on Biological Standardization*, 26th Report, WHO Tech Rep Ser 565.
8. Chayen J., Bitensky L. (eds) (1983). *Cytochemical Bioassays: Techniques and Clinical Applications*. New York and Basel: Marcel Dekker.
9. Loveridge N., Fischer J. A., Nagant de Deuxchaisnes C., Dambacher M. A., Tschopp F., Werder E., Devogelaer J.-P., De Meyer R., Bitensky L., Chayen J. (1982). Inhibition of cytochemical bioactivity of parathyroid hormone by plasma in pseudohypoparathyroidism type I. *J. Clin. Endocrinol. Metab*; **54**: 1274.
10. Bangham D. R. (1983). In *Cytochemical Bioassays: Techniques and Clinical Applications*. New York and Basel: Marcel Dekker.
11. Vinson G. P., Hinson J. P., Raven P. W. (1985). The relationship between tissue preparation and function: methods for the study of control of aldosterone secretion. *Cell Biochem. Function*; **3**: 235.
12. European Pharmacopoeia (1971). In *European Pharmacopoeia*, vol. II, p. 441–98. Maisonneuve: Paris.
13. Lipscomb H. S., Nelson D. H. (1962). A sensitive biologic assay for ACTH. *Endocrinology*; **71**: 13.
14. McKenzie J. M. (1958). The bioassay of thyrotrophin in serum. *Endocrinology*; **63**: 372.
15. Lamond D. R., Bindon B. M. (1966). The biological assay of follicle-stimulating hormone in hypophysectomised immature mice. *J. Endocrinol*; **34**: 365.
16. Schmidt-Elmendorff H., Loraine J. A. (1962). Some observations on the ovarian ascorbic acid method as a test for luteinising hormone activity. *J. Endocrinol.*, **23**: 413.
17. Wilhelmi A. E. (1973). In *Methods in Investigative and Diagnostic Endocrinology*, Vol. 2A, (Berson S. A., Yalow R. S., eds). Amsterdam and London: North-Holland.
18. Sayers M. A., Swallow R. L., Giordano N. D. (1971). An improved technique for the preparation of isolated rat adrenal cells. A sensitive, accurate and specific method for the assay of ACTH. *Endocrinology*; **88**: 1063.
19. Van Damme M. P., Robertson D. M., Diczfalusy E. (1974). An improved *in vitro* bioassay for measuring luteinising hormone (LH) activity using mouse Leydig cell preparations. *Acta Endocrinol. (Kbh.)*; **77**: 655.

29. Antigens and Antibodies

R. Hubbard

ANTIGENS

Introduction

Antigens are complex chemical molecules recognized as foreign (non-self), by immunocompetent cells. When introduced into a vertebrate animal, antigens activate two effector arms of the immune system; they stimulate the production of immunoglobulin molecules, i.e. antibodies, and they also lead to the sensitization of certain lymphoid cells. Both these cells and the antibodies can react specifically with the antigen.

The term *antigen*, which actually means in Greek 'to generate against', is used in two ways: first, to mean a substance which elicits an immune response, either the production of antibodies, or a cellular response; secondly, to mean a substance which reacts with an antibody. The first meaning relates to immunogenicity, and the term *immunogen* simply means the ability to induce an immune response.

Antigenic Determinants

The antigen must possess certain chemical structures that differ from those normally encountered, thus enabling the non-self recognition. Antigenic determinants may vary in size, but usually possess a surface area ranging between 500 and 700 $Å^2$. This surface area is approximately equal to about five or six amino acids. Thus, in a protein antigen the antigenic determinant may be composed of either a linear sequence of five or six amino acids, or a similar grouping derived from adjacent folds of the polypeptide chain. Certain antigenic determinants which are present may provoke a stronger immune response to themselves and are described as 'dominant' compared to the other determinants which are present. The number of antigenic determinants are large and rise according to the molecular weight of the antigen. To each antigenic determinant there is a specific antibody produced, and the immunological specificity depends upon the degree of perfection with which the determinant matches the cavity of the antibody.

The simple polysaccharide antigens are represented by polymers of glucose, the most studied of which, from the immunological point of view, is dextran. Kabat studied the degree of inhibition of the dextran–antibody reaction by oligosaccharides, which allowed the measurement of the maximum size of binding site of the antibody. The maximum inhibition was found to be with hexo- or hepto-oligomers indicating that the maximum size of the antibody binding site is about $34 \times 12 \times 7$ Å. Information obtained with synthetic polypeptides confirms this maximum size and produces an answer of five to six amino acid residues.

Antigen Classification

Antigens are divided into three classes: natural, artificial and synthetic.

Natural antigens originate, for example, from micro-organisms, animals, and plants. Examples include, viruses, bacteria, blood cells, plant cells, and animal cells, and include soluble chemical material, such as proteins, carbohydrates, glycoproteins, and lipoproteins.

Artificial antigens consist of natural antigens which have been chemically modified; examples of these include iodinated proteins and hapten–protein conjugates.

Synthetic antigens are chemically synthesized molecules. For example, these include amino acid co-polymers and polypeptides.

Haptens

Haptens are small, chemical molecules which are non-immunogenic. They are, however, able to induce an immune response when covalently linked to 'carrier' molecules (proteins). In the hapten–

protein carrier, the 'conjugate' as it is called, the hapten becomes immunogenic and antibodies are produced against it. A hapten is able to bind to an antibody which has been made against itself in this way. Examples of haptens include steroid hormones, simple aromatic molecules and small peptides.

Investigations with haptens have led to our present knowledge of the B-cell/T-cell co-operation in the antibody response to certain antigens called T-dependent antigens. The majority of proteins are T-dependent antigens, whereas most of the polysaccharides are T-independent antigens. The difference is due to the fact that globular proteins lack repeating antigenic determinants and fail to induce B-cell proliferation without T-helper (T_H) cells, whereas polysaccharides, having identical repeating antigenic determinants, can act independently to stimulate B-cells.

The use of haptens conjugated to carrier molecules has provided the ability to study antibody specificity and the basic principles of antigen/antibody interactions. There is a wide range of reactions that are commonly used to couple haptens to carrier proteins, including diazotization, and the use of isocyanates, isothiocyanates, carbodiimides, and even azides.

The protein in the hapten carrier is actually covalently linked to the hapten, and is involved in the regulation of the antibody response to the hapten. It has been shown that in the secondary, or memory, antibody response only re-challenge with a hapten carrier conjugate containing the carrier to which the animal had been previously sensitized, can produce a secondary, anti-hapten, response. Further, if an animal is immunized with the carrier alone, and is then immunized with a hapten–carrier conjugate, a secondary anti-hapten response occurs. Therefore, immunological memory is determined to a significant extent by the carrier molecule. The hapten–carrier concept is important in explaining how drugs and chemicals in the environment can bind to body proteins and cause immunological responses, such as the allergic reaction involving IgE antibodies.

Antigen Characteristics

Antigens are characterized by their size, foreign recognition and their precise chemical structure.

Simple substances of low molecular weight are normally not immunogenic. Chemicals or biochemicals with a molecular weight of less than about 10 000 are usually non-immunogenic or, at best, weakly immunogenic. It can be appreciated from the above discussion that small molecules can become immunogenic once bound to a carrier protein, and so the fact that small molecules such as drugs do elicit antibodies to themselves, sometimes of IgE class, leading to an allergic reaction, is due to the formation of a conjugate molecule of the drug bound to an endogenous protein.

Antibodies are produced against antigens which are recognized as foreign. Thus antigens derived from different species produce antibodies. However, there are many examples of antibodies being produced against components of members of the same species. This is the case in alloimmunization and occurs, for example, in maternal fetal incompatibility for antigens of different blood groups, and also in the rejection of allografts (transplantation alloantigens). Antibodies can also be produced which are capable of reacting with components of self-tissue, and these antibodies are called *autoantibodies*. Normally, the lymphocytes which are self-reactive are repressed by the immune regulatory system and such autoantibodies or autoreactive cells are not produced. There is a variety of mechanisms and diseases which may lead to the production of autoantibodies.

The precise chemical structure of the antigen is extremely important. Not only is the chemical composition of the antigen vital, but also its three-dimensional conformation. Antibodies are very specific reagents, and they can distinguish between two antigenic determinants which have extremely small differences. They can, for example, identify a single amino acid change in a peptide, distinguish between cis- and trans-isomers or optical isomers, and detect changes in molecular conformational structure very readily.

Certain substances with relatively low molecular weight have been found to be immunogenic, e.g. bacitracin and angiotensin, but the general rule of large molecular weight and chemical complexity applies. Studies in immunogenicity show that homopolymers of one amino acid are not immunogenic, whilst polymers of two, three or four amino acids are usually very immunogenic. Ring structure, provided for example by phenylalanine and tyrosine residues aid immunogenicity. Conformations are easily distinguished from one another, for example, random coil and α-helix structures can be distinguished from one another by differences in binding to antibodies despite the same amino acid sequences being present. In terms of the electrical charge on an antigen, there seems to be an inverse relationship between antigens and antibodies, i.e. basic antigens induce acidic antibodies and vice versa. Antibodies are also able to distinguish between optical configurations of their antigens. There is a very high degree of specificity of the antibody with the optical centres of the antigen.

The influence of optical configurations can be illustrated by studying the antibody specificities of the proteins conjugated to the optical isomers of tartaric acid. Each antiserum reacts strongly with the immunizing antigen without there being appreciable cross-reaction between the levo- and dextro-tartaric acids. The antiserum against the meso-tartaric acid, however, exhibits some cross-reactivity with both levo- and dextro-acids. A further example of this antibody specificity, is the capability of an antiserum to distinguish specifically between glucose and galactose which differ only in the configuration at one carbon atom.

Immunogenicity of Natural Substances

Protein Antigens. Protein antigens are generally immunogenic. They are highly complex molecules which are readily obtained in a pure state from plants, animals and microorganisms. Nevertheless, there is still little information on the antigenic nature of these molecules. The immunogenicity of a range of smaller polypeptides, such as insulin, glucagon, calcitonin, adrenocorticotrophic hormone, and growth hormone has been studied; it can be increased either by immunization with adjuvants, or by chemical coupling to natural or synthetic carrier molecules. The investigation of antigenic regions on the surface of proteins and viruses has become much easier with the production of monoclonal antibodies, and also the rapid methods of peptide synthesis. For the smaller proteins of known sequence and conformation, such as cytochrome C, insulin, myoglobin, and lysozyme, the immunogenic sites are described as surface domains made up of amino acid side-chains, which may actually be distant in sequence, but close in three-dimensional space. These domains are probably overlapping and cover most of the protein surface.

Carbohydrates. Many bacteria have carbohydrates in their cell walls. These carbohydrates react with antibody raised to the bacteria, but are not always themselves immunogenic. In other cases isolated carbohydrates such as those from group A and group C, meningococci and the pneumococcal polysaccharides are immunogenic in man. Dextrans, levans and teichoic acids are also immunogenic in man. Immunogenicity of carbohydrates is dependent on their molecular weight as well as their sugar composition. Many polysaccharides have extensive side-branching and exhibit a secondary and tertiary structure and this type of conformation contributes to their immunogenicity, especially when they are found as substituent groups on proteins, for example, glycoproteins. The immunogenicity of substances with repeating antigenic determinants, such as the dextrans, polymers of D-glucose, have been widely studied and it has been shown that dextrans of molecular weight less than 50 000 are far less immunogenic in man than those of molecular weight greater than 90 000.

Lipids. Lipids are normally non-immunogenic and it appears that in order to produce antibody to a lipid molecule it is necessary to conjugate it to a larger molecule or structure, such as a protein or red blood cell, so that the lipid acts as a hapten.

Nucleic Acids. The nucleic acids are normally non-immunogenic in their native state. However, immunization of animals with denatured or single-stranded DNA coupled to carrier molecules results in the production of antibodies specific for single-stranded DNA. Antibodies can also be produced against nucleic acid fragments such as bases, nucleosides and nucleotides, as haptens and these antibodies react with the immunizing antigen and with single-stranded DNA. Denatured nucleic acid can be immunogenic even in the same animal. There is evidence indicating that antibodies induced by a denatured nucleic acid can cross-react with the normal form of the nucleic acid. Systemic lupus erythematosus is an autoimmune disease in which the serum of the patients contains antibodies which react with their own DNA. These antibodies react to single- and double-stranded DNA, RNA, ribosomes, RNA proteins, histones and to synthetic polynucleotides. The formation of these autoantibodies is an interesting problem since the antigens with which they react are, in general, poor immunogens.

Cross-reactivity

If two antigens possess common or structurally very similar antigenic determinants, the antibodies produced to one of these antigens may well react with the other antigen. These interactions are called cross-reactions.

There is more than one type of cross-reactivity. For example, genuine or true cross-reactivity by two antigens for the same antibody describes the situation in which both antigens bind the same antibody binding site but with different affinities. Genuine cross-reactivity applies to monoclonal antibodies reacting with two different antigens, which have at least one antigenic determinant with the same, or very similar, chemical structure. Another example is the cross-reactivity exhibited by the haptens, dinitrophenyl (DNP) and trinitrophenyl (TNP) which bind to anti-DNP antibodies, but with different avidities. Similarly, it is possible for a peptide fragment containing all the amino acids of an antigenic determinant to cross-react with the same antibody raised against a similar determinant in a three-dimensional conformation on a protein. Nevertheless, the avidity of binding to the peptide may well be lower because the conformation is different.

In conventional antiserum preparations the antibody populations are heterogeneous, showing heterogeneity with respect to the antigenic determinants which are recognized and heterogeneity of affinity within the subpopulation of antibodies reacting with each determinant. If a protein has antigenic determinants which are common to another protein, then antiserum raised to either protein will partially cross-react with the other, and sometimes this phenomenon is termed 'shared reactivity'. This type of partial cross-reactivity, which can also be called 'antigenic determinant sharing', is dependent on the use of heterogeneous antibodies to different determinants on the immunogen. If a monoclonal antibody is used, i.e. an antibody raised against a single determinant, then only genuine cross-reactivity can be observed.

An example of cross-reactivity between unrelated antigens is that of the Forssman antigen, which is a structure encountered in many animal species and in bacteria. When sheep erythrocytes are used as immunogen, two types of antibodies are produced, those which are species specific, recognizing only the determinants of the species, and others which are specific for the Forssman antigen, which therefore cross-react with a wide range of animal and bacterial cells.

Adjuvants

Materials or protocols which augment the immunogenicity of antigens are termed *adjuvants*. Many substances are known to be capable of adjuvant activity, for example, alum, aluminium hydroxide, aluminium phosphate, beryllium sulphate, saponin, alginate of calcium, mineral oil emulsions, guanidine, silica, double-helix synthetic nucleic acids, and lipopolysaccharides obtained from numerous gram negative bacteria, such as *S. typhii*, *B. pertussis* and *E. coli*. The mechanism of action of adjuvants is poorly understood, although it is generally accepted that they operate in three ways: (1) by continuous liberation of the antigenic material (depot effect), (2) by stimulating phagocytosis, and (3) by non-specific activation of the lymphocytes (mitogenicity).

One of the most commonly used adjuvant mixtures is Freund's adjuvant (FA). This consists of an aqueous solution of the immunogen in an oil emulsion. This mixture is called Freund's incomplete adjuvant (FIA). The same mixture containing dead mycobacteria in suspension, such as *M. tuberculosis*, or *M. butyricum*, is termed Freund's complete adjuvant (FCA). The adjuvant activity of the mycobacteria is attributed to various substances which have been extracted from them, e.g. peptidoglycolipid, which is composed of mycolic acid esters with different polysaccharides bound by an amide linkage to a heptapeptide.

Gram-negative bacteria also have strong adjuvant effects due largely to endotoxins. Endotoxins in cell walls are often extremely toxic, pyrogenic, immunogenic, and produce an adjuvant effect. These substances are composed of polysaccharides, lipids and proteins. Lipopolysaccharide (LPS) has a toxic and an adjuvant effect. LPS is a T-cell-independent antigen and is also a specific mitogen of the B-lymphocytes. Mitogens are substances which stimulate the proliferation of a wide range of clones of B- or T-lymphocytes. The mitogenic effect of LPS is doubtless related to its notable adjuvanticity.

Some adjuvants appear to favour the induction of particular classes of antibodies, in preference to others. For example, in guinea pigs, Freund's complete adjuvant (FCA) administered with ovalbumin induces IgG$_1$, while Freund's complete adjuvant (FCA) tends to produce IgG$_2$ antibodies. *B. pertussis*, when used as an adjuvant, tends to produce IgE

antibodies in mice and rats. It seems clear that many adjuvants act at the cellular level and that the type of cell which is affected determines the class of antibody which is induced in the immune response.

ANTIBODIES

Introduction

Antibodies are large glycoprotein molecules which are made by an animal in response to the invasion by foreign material, whether it be molecular, cellular, or microbiological. The antibodies produced are specific to the invader antigen and can bind it noncovalently, leading to a number of physiological consequences normally inactivating or killing the antigen.

Antibodies are secreted by plasma cells which have been produced by differentiation of B-lymphocytes and are transported in the blood, and can both recognize the antigen and lead to its elimination. The immune system is able to distinguish between self and non-self components, and it must be clear that antibodies are very highly specific reagents. The success of the antibody molecules, therefore, depends on them being highly sensitive to minor structural changes in the antigens which they recognize and combine with. A vast number of antibody molecules can be produced by the vertebrate animal to interact with a virtually unlimited number of antigens. The antibody molecule has evolved a number of discrete globular domains to carry out certain functions. The antibody domains are able not only to bind the antigen, but also to mediate certain immune effector functions.

The ability of the immune system to recognize self tissue is vital since breakdown of this principle leads to the production of antibodies which will attack self tissue, leading to autoimmune diseases. Antibodies produced in this manner are called autoantibodies.

Antibody Structure and Class

Antibodies are large glycoprotein molecules, having some 1300–1400 amino acids in a monomeric antibody, arranged as four polypeptide chains linked by disulphide bonds. These are two identical heavy chains and two identical light chains (*see* Fig. 1), and the molecule has regions of amino acids which are relatively constant and regions which are relatively variable in sequence, when compared with a range of other antibody molecules. The elucidation of the structure of antibody molecules is largely due to the research of Porter and Edelman; in recognition of their work, they shared the Nobel Prize in 1972.

The Five Immunoglobulin Classes. There are five distinct classes of antibody or immunoglobulin molecule, and these are present in most higher mammals,

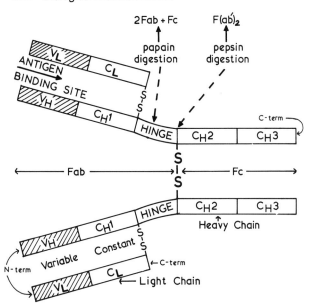

Fig. 1 IgG antibody structure. Immunoglobulin G consists of two identical heavy (H) chains and two identical light (L) polypeptide chains linked by disulphide bonds. The antigen-binding sites are located at the variable (V) regions of amino acid sequence shown as the shaded areas. The structure was elucidated by enzymic digestion using pepsin and papain, which gave the characteristic antibody fragments shown. Papain digestion of IgG produces three fragments (2 Fab + Fc) whilst pepsin produces a larger divalent antigen-binding fragment designated F(ab')$_2$. The disulphide bridges between the chains may be reduced and stabilized by alkylation, and then the light and heavy chains can be isolated, separated and characterized. H = heavy chain; L = light chain; C = constant region, V = variable region, in respect of amino acid sequence studies. Numbers on chains refer to the globular domains in the structure. Fab = Fragment antigen-binding, monovalent; F(ab')$_2$ = Fragment antigen-binding, divalent; Fc = Fragment crystallizable; C-term., N-term., amino acid terminal end. (Reproduced with permission from Gibson G. G., Hubbard R., Parke D. V. (eds) (1983). *Immunotoxicology, Proceedings of the 1st International Symposium on Immunotoxicology*. London: Academic Press.

namely: IgG, IgA, IgM. IgD and IgE (see Fig. 2). These classes differ from each other in structure, charge, size, amino acid sequence and carbohydrate content. Each class is also heterogeneous and electrophoretically the immunoglobulins show a range of heterogeneity which extends from the γ to the α fractions of normal serum.

Antibody Function. One region of the antibody molecule is concerned specifically with binding to the antigen, while other regions mediate a number of immune effector mechanisms, e.g. binding to phagocytes and binding to the first component (Cl_q) of the classical complement system. The physiological

properties of antibodies are encoded in the constant regions of the heavy chain, and each class (or subclass) has characteristic properties, for example, IgG is able to cross the placenta and provide sensitized antibodies to the baby at birth. IgA owes some of its properties to the secretory component which is attached to the dimeric form of the antibody and allows it to be secreted onto external surfaces. It is present in the upper respiratory tract, in saliva, tears, sweat, nasal, lung and gastrointestinal secretions. The structural form of an antibody is clearly very significant. Human IgM is a pentamer and is largely confined to the blood, being very effective against blood-borne infections. Tables 1 and 2 show some of the major functions and properties of the different classes of antibody.

Antibody Structure. Originally, one of the main difficulties in studying antibody structure was the fact that samples of antibodies were mixtures. It was not until pure homogeneous antibodies were obtained from patients with multiple myelomatosis, that significant advances were made. Multiple myeloma is a neoplastic proliferation of a single plasma cell line of the bone marrow. The cancerous B-cell line produces a single antibody which is therefore monoclonal. Thus the patient produces large amounts of structurally identical antibody and is a source of pure material. Often, patients have Bence-Jones proteins in their urine as well. These urinary proteins were first observed by Henry Bence-Jones at Guy's Hospital in London, in 1847. The proteins precipitate on heating urine to 60°C and redissolve at 90°C. They have been found to contain light chains which are actually part of the immunoglobulin molecule. The Bence-Jones proteins are, in fact, present in the urine as light-chain dimers. Bence-Jones proteins were obtained easily from the urine of such patients without the need to draw blood and as such, provided the first immunoglobulin components which were analysed for their amino acid sequence. The homogeneous antibody produced from a proliferating clone of neoplastic plasma cells is usually called a 'myeloma protein' or a 'paraprotein', and shows up as a single sharp band in the serum electrophoretic pattern.

As described, the antibody molecule is composed of four polypeptide chains with two identical heavy chains and two identical light chains joined by disulphide bonds. Two major lines of research led to these conclusions. First, the separation of the chains after treatment with reducing agents, and secondly, the digestion of the immunoglobulin molecule using enzymes.

Chain Separation. Edelman, in 1959, attempted to reduce the disulphide bridges of the peptide chains of the antibody molecule. He showed that the molecular weight of the immunoglobulin fell from 150 000 to 50 000, and also that another sub-component of

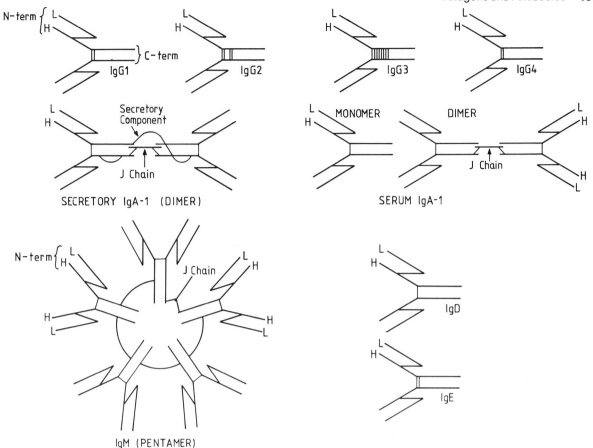

Fig. 2 Structure of human immunoglobulins. There are five basic classes of human immunoglobulin: IgA, IgG, IgM, IgD and IgE. All the IgG subclasses, IgD and IgE are monomeric. IgA may be a monomer, dimer or trimer. Secretory IgA is dimeric and contains a polypeptide J-chain which is involved in the polymerization process and a chain called secretory component which aids secretion. IgM is a large pentameric molecule also containing the J-chain.

TABLE 1
PHYSICAL PROPERTIES OF HUMAN IMMUNOGLOBULINS

Class designation (WHO)	IgG	IgA	IgM	IgD	IgE
Subclass	1,2,3,4	1,2			
Heavy chain class	γ	α	μ	δ	ε
Heavy chain mol. wt. (approx.)	50 000	55 000	70 000	60 000–70 000	65 000–70 000
Number of heavy chain domains	4	4	5	5	5
Light chain types	κ or λ	κ or λ	κ or λ	κ or λ	κ or λ
Immunoglobulin mol. wt.	150 000	$(160\,000)_n$	900 000	185 000 or larger?	180 000 200 000
Sedimentation	7S	7S,9S,11S	19S	7S	8S
Molecular formula	$\gamma_2\kappa_2$	$J(\alpha_2\kappa_2)_{1-3}$ $J(\alpha_2\lambda_2)_{1-3}$	$J(\mu_2\kappa_2)_5$	$\delta_2\kappa_2$	$\varepsilon_2\kappa_2$
	$\gamma_2\lambda_2$	$JS(\alpha_2\kappa_2)_2$ $JS(\alpha_2\lambda_2)_2$	$J(\mu_2\lambda_2)_5$	$\delta_2\lambda_2$	$\varepsilon_2\lambda_2$
Carbohydrate content (%)	2–3	7–11	9–15	12	12
Valency for antigen binding	2	2+	5(10)	?	2

J = J chain in polymers.
S = Secretory piece in IgA dimers.

(Reproduced with permission from Hubbard R. (1983). Monoclonal antibodies: production properties and applications. In *Topics in Enzyme and Fermentation Biotechnology*, no. 7 (Wiseman A., ed.). Chichester: Ellis Horwood.)

TABLE 2

BIOLOGICAL PROPERTIES AND FUNCTIONS OF HUMAN IMMUNOGLOBULINS

	IgG	IgA	IgM	IgD	IgE
% of serum Ig.	80	13	6	1	0·002
Concentration range in normal serum (mg/ml)	8–16	1·4–4·0	0·5–2·0	0–0·4	0·00017–0·0004
Serum half-life (days)	23*	6	5	3	4
Complement fixation (classical)	Yes	No	Yes	Probably No?	No
Binding to macrophages and polymorphs	Yes	No	No	No	No
Binding to mast cells	No	No	No	No	Yes
Placental transfer	Yes	No	No	No	No
Physiological role	Defence against bacteria viruses, and bacterial toxins. Most abundant Ig in the serum. Very important in the secondary immune response. In extra vascular fluids it combats micro-organisms and toxins. Crosses placenta to give sensitized IgG to baby at birth.	Defends external body surfaces especially in the upper respiratory tract. Very important in secretions, present in saliva, tears, sweat, nasal, lung and gastrointestinal secretions. Particularly effective against viruses. Less important in blood. Possesses a 'secretory piece' in the secreted dimer molecule for enzyme protection.	Important in primary immune response. Mainly confined to blood stream due to M.Wt. and is very effective against blood-borne infections, e.g. bacteraemia. Excellent complement fixation and effective agglutinator. Structure of human and mammal IgM is a cyclic pentamer.	Largely unknown. Found to be present on lymphocyte surfaces (mouse and human blood) frequently with IgM. Very low concentration in serum and very short half-life (2–3 days).	Raised levels in parasitic infections and may be involved in defence vs. parasites. Synthesized in submucosa of gastrointestinal and respiratory tract and in nasopharynx. Present in nasal and bronchial secretions. Firmly fixes to the surface of cells especially mast cells and is responsible for symptoms of immediate-type allergy, e.g. Hay fever, asthma.

* Excluding IgG$_3$ (10 days).

(Reproduced with permission from Hubbard R. (1983). In *Topics in Enzyme and Fermentation Biotechnology*, no. 7 (Wiseman A. ed.). Chichester: Ellis Horwood.)

lower molecular weight (25 000) was produced. This work was done on rabbit immunoglobulin and Edelman suggested that there were four polypeptide chains, two with a molecular weight of about 50 000, and two with a molecular weight of about 25 000. The experiments were conducted in the presence of urea or guanidine, which led to the uncoiling of the peptide chain and the exposure of the intra-chain disulphide bridges, and hence products were produced which lacked biological activity. Porter overcame this when, in 1962, he used mercaptoethanol at pH 8·2 for the reduction, and followed this by alkylation with iodoacetamide in order to avoid the further oxidation of the SH groups. The experiment was done in the presence of organic acids to prevent chain re-association, by providing them with positive charges. Gel filtration using dextran (Sephadex G-75) equilibrated with acetic or propionic acid resulted in the separation of the two chains, the heavy chain and the light chain. The heavy chain represented 70% of the total material, and the light chain, 30%. Since the molecular weight of the heavy chain was known to be around 50 000 and that of the light chain, around 25 000, that the stoichiometry of H to L was one to one, that IgG is divalent and has a molecular weight of 156 000, the minimum structure was shown to contain two heavy and two light chains.

Antibody Fragmentation by Enzymes. In 1959, Rodney Porter subjected rabbit IgG antibodies to enzymic degradation with papain. Fragments were obtained and these were separated by ion-exchange chromatography. Porter isolated one fragment which was capable of binding the antigen, but only in a monovalent way. This fragment was called the Fab fragment, standing for Fragment antigen binding (see Fig. 1). This fragment did not precipitate with the antigen and it was concluded that it was monovalent since precipitation requires cross-linking and multivalency. The other fragment which Porter obtained was a crystallizable fragment and he called this the Fc fragment. The Fc fragment did not bind the antigen.

Nisonoff, in 1960, digested rabbit IgG with pepsin (see Fig. 1). In the absence of cysteine, Nisonoff showed that the main fragment produced still had the capacity for precipitation, and was clearly a divalent antibody fragment, and Nisonoff called this the $F(ab')_2$. If this fragment was reduced, it produced two fragments which bound the antigen without precipitation and were monovalent. These, of course, were very similar to the Fab fragments isolated by Porter but had slightly greater molecular weight and were termed the Fab' fragments. The results of these enzyme fragmentations by papain and pepsin led to the conclusion that the two enzymes attack to the left and to the right of the main disulphide bridge that unites the heavy chains (see Fig. 1).

The five immunoglobulin classes differ in the type of heavy chain which they carry, of which there are five types, γ, μ, α, δ and ε. There are also immunoglobulin subclasses, which are determined by the heavy chain type which an antibody molecule carries. Thus, there are four human IgG subclasses (IgG$_1$, IgG$_2$, IgG$_3$ and IgG$_4$) having heavy chains called γ_1, γ_2, γ_3 and γ_4; they differ only slightly from one another, so that differences between the various subclasses are marginal compared to the differences between the actual classes. The human IgG subclasses occur in approximate proportions of 66, 23, 7 and 4% respectively in human serum. Human IgA is also known to have subclasses (IgA$_1$ and IgA$_2$), but none have definitely been described for the other classes. The Fc region of the heavy chain of different antibodies is largely responsible for the physiological properties of that particular antibody.

There are only two types of antibody light chain κ or λ, and all antibody molecules possess either two κ or two λ chains and therefore are represented for example, $\gamma_2\kappa_2$ or $\gamma_2\lambda_2$.

Amino acid sequence studies of the light chains, heavy chains and whole molecules reveal that there are constant region domains and variable region domains (see Fig. 1) (C = constant, V = variable, H = heavy chain, L = light chain, and numbers represent the number of the constant region domains). Each domain has around 60 to 80 amino acids present and is an independent globular structure stabilized by one disulphide bond. Detailed amino acid sequence studies showed that there were some relatively constant parts in the V-region domains, whilst there were some very variable regions in the V-regions. These very variable segments were called the hypervariable regions, and it is now known that

these are the parts of the molecule which form the antibody binding site. The antibody molecule also has a hinge region which allows a degree of flexibility, so that it can bind to antigenic determinants which are different distances apart. The antigen binding site is formed between the variable region of the heavy and the variable region of the light chains and hence each monomeric antibody structure has two antigen binding sites. The antibody molecule is a Y-shaped molecule and indeed the electron micrograph of a crystal of human IgG from a multiple myeloma patient shows a Y-shaped antibody molecule, lined up in regular fashion (antibody molecules are often represented simply as a Y-shaped molecule).

Amino acid sequence studies on Bence-Jones proteins confirmed the fact that there were only two different light chains. It was also shown that the variable sequence extended to 108 amino acids of a total of 214 of the whole light chain. Similar studies on heavy chains derived from myeloma patients showed, of the total of around 440 amino acids, the variable sequence, or domain, consisted of between 108 and 125 amino acids starting at the N-terminal end.

X-ray diffraction studies on Fab crystals showed that each domain is an independent and cylindrical unit consisting of two β-pleated sheets of three- and four-stranded chains which run anti-parallel and are held together by disulphide bonds. The antigen-binding site is confirmed to be at the end of the V-region and the hinge region is shown to be present and allows flexibility of the molecule. X-ray diffraction studies also confirmed that Bence-Jones proteins were dimers of the light chain and had a similar conformation to the Fab fragment.

The Genetic Basis of Antibody Heterogeneity

The variability of antibodies can be divided into three types which depend on the amino acid sequences that are present.

Isotypes. The genes for the isotypic variants of antibodies are present in all healthy individual members of a species, thus in man, the genes for γ_1, γ_2, γ_3, γ_4, μ, α_1, α_2, δ, ε, κ and λ chains are all present. Isotypes therefore cover the classes, subclasses and types of antibody which involve the constant regions of the heavy or light chains. There are also subtypes and subgroups which are isotypes. The subtypes involve amino acid sequence variations found in the constant regions of the λ light chain. There are two markers, one at position 152, termed the Kern marker, and one at position 190, designated the Oz marker. This polymorphism represents isotypes coded by at least four Cλ genes present in every individual. The subgroups are coded within the framework parts of the variable region of the heavy chain. There are at least four of these subgroups, V$_{HI}$, V$_{HII}$, V$_{HIII}$ and V$_{HIV}$.

Allotypes. Allotypes involve genetic variation within a species, involving different alleles at a given locus. These are not present in all individuals (compare the allelic forms in blood groups). Thus, the variant of IgG_3 called G_{3m} (an allotype having phenylalanine at position 436 of its heavy chain) is not found in all humans and is therefore an allotype. Allotypes occur most frequently as variants of the constant regions of the heavy or light chain.

Idiotypes. Different amino acid sequences in the variable domains, especially in the hypervariable regions, produce idiotypic antibodies. Idiotypes are normally specific for the individual antibody clone. The precise genetic basis of idiotypic variability is only partly understood but corresponds to an individually specific amino acid sequence present in the hypervariable regions of the heavy and light chains.

Antibody Domains and their Functions

Edelman originally suggested that immunoglobulin molecules had domains on the basis of the presence of homologous regions. The domains of the antibody molecule consist of comparable regions of as many as 110 amino acids which are stabilized through disulphide bonds and engage in one or more specific functions.

Clearly, the overwhelming evidence is that the V_H and the V_L domains interact to form the antigen-binding surfaces of the antibody molecule and, as discussed above, x-ray crystallography has confirmed that prediction. The other domains also mediate certain effector functions of the antibody molecule. Exact structural location of these sites has still to be elucidated (*see* Table 3).

TABLE 3
FUNCTIONS OF IgG DOMAINS

Domains	Function
V_H and V_L	Antigen binding.
$C\gamma_1$	Binds complement C4b fragment.
$C\gamma_2$	Binds complement component Cl_q, i.e. complement fixation, and control of catabolic rates.
$C\gamma_3$	Binding to the Fc receptor on macrophages and monocytes.
$C\gamma_2$ and $C\gamma_3$	Binding to staphylococcal protein A and the Fc receptor on placental tissue, neutrophils and K cells.

Structure in Relation to Antigen Binding

It is now well established that certain short polypeptide segments show considerable variability in the V-region domains, and are termed hypervariable regions. The hypervariable regions in the κ and λ light chains are located around positions 30, 50 and 95. These are directly involved in the formation of the antigen binding site. Hypervariable regions are now sometimes referred to as Complimentarity Determining Regions (CDR), and the intervening peptide segments as Framework Regions (FR). There are four FRs and three CDRs in both the light and heavy chain variable regions. It has been suggested that the antigen binding site is therefore produced from these hypervariable regions, which in the V_L domain correspond to positions 24–34, 50–56 and 89–97, and in the V_H domain to positions 31–35, 50–65 and 95–102.

The exact chemical structure of the combining site of the antibody cannot be defined. It must await a full x-ray crystallographic study to establish its spatial makeup. However, the maximum size of the combining site can be gauged from its accommodation of molecules with dimensions of a hexapeptide or a hexasaccharide. This is similar in size to the molecules of the lysozyme substrate. In this case there are about 15–20 contact amino acids and the same is presumably true for the antibody combining site. If any amino acid can occupy one of these 15–20 positions then the number of possible combining sites is extremely large.

It is possible to define some of the amino acids in the combining site by the technique known as 'affinity labelling'. In this technique a labelled, chemically modified, hapten containing a highly reactive group such as diazonium, bromoacetyl, or azide grouping is capable of forming a covalent bond at the combining site, and is therefore bound permanently to one or more amino acids. The amount of labelled hapten in the peptides is then studied by hydrolysis of the antibody. The results of such experiments with different antibodies and labelling reagents suggest that tyrosine and lysine residues in the hypervariable regions of V_H and V_L play an important role in the specific binding of the antigen.

The factors which determine the high specificity of an antibody are related to the antibody combining site. The shape of this site is complementary to that of the antigen, and is concave in order to expose a large surface area to the antigen. The amino acid side-chains within this cavity are precisely positioned to take full advantage of electrostatic forces, hydrogen bonding, hydrophobic and Van der Waals forces. These forces require close approach of the interacting groups but form very strong non-covalent bonds between the antibody and antigen. It is important to realize, however, that the antibody/antigen interaction is always reversible (this is further discussed below).

Antibody Biosynthesis

Antibodies are secreted by mature plasma cells, which are formed by the differentiation of normal B-lymphocytes. The rate of antibody secretion is quite substantial, amounting to an output of 2000 to 3000 molecules per second. The plasma cell, like most secretory cells, has a highly organized endoplasmic reticulum, consisting of both rough and smooth membranes. The rough membrane has ribosomes on the cytoplasmic surface while the smooth (often called the Golgi zone) is a mass of vacuoles. The plasma cell represents a terminal differentiation stage and the immunoglobulin which it secretes is homogeneous and contains the identical V_H/V_L pair expressed on the original precursor lymphocyte. Hence, the antibody specificity of the lymphocyte is preserved in the daughter cells which is consistent with the clonal selection theory (see below). Each plasma cell expresses only one C_H and C_L but it is possible for cells to undergo a switch in immunoglobulin gene expression during the development of such clones. For example, it is possible to produce a genetic switch from IgM and/or IgD to plasma cells secreting IgG or IgA. Administration of antibodies against IgM *in vivo* can abolish the appearance of IgG and IgA, and this suggests the existence of this type of switching mechanism.

Synthesis and Assembly of 4-Chain (H_2L_2). The immunoglobulin heavy and light chains are synthesized independently on polyribosomes in immune tissue and myeloma cells. The genes for the heavy and light chains are not linked. The synthesis of heavy and light chains in virtually all cases is balanced so that the only secretory product of plasma cells is fully assembled immunoglobulin. The immediate event after the completion of the synthesis of heavy and light chains is their assembly into the four polypeptide chain structures. For IgA and IgM biosynthesis this is followed by the addition of the J-chain (see Fig. 2), and the formation of polymeric molecules, whilst for IgA found in mucosal secretions, another polypeptide, the secretory component, is added. The secretory component is synthesized by the epithelial cells rather than by the plasma cells and the addition of the component takes place after secretion of dimeric IgA from plasma cells. Assembly is accompanied or followed by ordinary addition of carbohydrate residues at various points along the polypeptide chain.

The 4-chain structures are held together by both covalent disulphide bridges and non-covalent links. The first disulphide-linked product formed in the assembly of an H_2L_2 structure could be either H_2 or H-L. Formation of the 4-chain molecule then occurs either by addition of light chains to H_2 or by dimerization of H-L. Covalent assembly to the H_2L_2 structure, like the synthesis of the polypeptide chain, is relatively rapid, taking 5–15 min (shown using pulse–chase experiments). In the mouse, most IgG is produced by the H_2 intermediate, whereas IgM is assembled from H-L sub-units.

Polymeric Immunoglobulins. The major immunoglobulin observed on the surface of B-lymphocytes is IgM, perhaps indicating its importance in terms of ontogeny and phylogeny. IgM therefore functions as a receptor for antigens on these lymphocytes and is secreted from plasma cells as a large cyclic pentameric molecule. The polypeptide J-chain is known to be involved in the assembly of polymeric immunoglobulins. Both IgA and IgM can be polymerized from sub-units which have been prepared by reduction of the polymeric forms and from intracellular or secreted monomeric units. IgM monomer is converted into the cyclic pentamer whilst IgA monomer is converted into the dimer. Polymerization is complete and there is no residue of the monomeric form, but polymerization only occurs when the J-chain and the purified disulphide interchange enzyme are available. The J-chain is not simply a catalyst, because all the J-chain released from IgM by reductive cleavage is incorporated into the reassembled polymer. Overall, it is clear that the J-chain appears to be an essential structural requirement for polymeric immunoglobulins.

Secretory IgA is held in the dimeric configuration by the J-chain, and is secreted by submucosal plasma cells, which actively bind secretory component as it traverses epithelial cell layers. Bound secretory component may both facilitate transport of secretory IgA into the secretions and protect the molecule from proteolytic attack.

Antibody Characteristics in the Immune Response. The principles which underlie immunological defence mechanisms include, (1) recognition of self and non-self, (2) specificity, and (3) memory. These principles can give rise to certain other immunological phenomena, for example, breakdown of recognition leads to the production of autoantibodies. Cross-reactivity of an antibody with different antigens may occur because of identical antigenic determinants on different antigens, or it may be because of a very similar chemical structure for different determinants. Memory cells are the basis of immunization and long-term immunity against various pathogens, and these cells are formed during the differentiation of the B- and T-lymphocytes.

Memory cells ensure that the secondary response to an immunogen occurs quickly and produces higher levels of antibody, something like a 100- to 1000-fold increase in antibody concentration. The major antibody of the primary immune response is IgM, whilst that in the secondary immune response is IgG. The secondary response is more rapid and longer lasting than the primary response. Specificity is also held in that a secondary response is only ever produced if the animal has memory cells for that immunogen. The development of the primary immune response to an immunogen usually takes around ten days to produce sufficient quantity of antibody, whilst in the secondary immune response, the production of large quantities of IgG in particular may only take three to four days.

Antibody Formation at the Genetic Level. Antibodies

must provide enough different combining sites to recognize the millions of antigenic shapes in the environment, and also to provide the different physiological effector properties required. It has been estimated that an individual can produce at least 10^7 different antibody specificities. This means an individual produces more different forms of antibody than all the other proteins of the body put together and indicates that we produce more types of antibody than there are genes in our genome. This question has been of fundamental importance and one of great fascination to immunologists.

From an historical point of view, the theories on antibody formation were for many years of the instructive type. These maintained that the antibody specificity was acquired after the antigen entered the responding animal, and that the antigen acted instructively in influencing the antibody-synthesizing cells to produce new antibodies. The instructive theories assume that any antigen could direct any B-lymphocyte to produce the appropriate antibody. There was a direct template hypothesis which involved an antibody protein wrapping itself around the antigen, and an indirect template hypothesis in which DNA was involved in wrapping itself around the antigen and that DNA then made the antibody. Clearly, these theories are untenable and have been discarded, because they do not account for much of modern immunological knowledge, and are inconsistent with the basic concepts in molecular biology.

During the 1950s and early 1960s there was significant progress in molecular biology and Jerne and Burnett independently put forward the Clonal Selection Theory. Each lymphocyte only produces one type of immunoglobulin specificity and the antigen selects and stimulates the cells which carry that immunoglobulin type on their surface. The clonal selection theory is the most popular theory at present and is accepted by most immunologists. It is a selective theory and antigens act selectively by activating an innate ability to produce the required antibody. The antigen makes contact with the cell, switches on genetic equipment, and an immunoglobulin molecule is made with an individual primary amino acid sequence which subsequently folds spontaneously in the absence of antigen to give a specific antigen-combining site. Each lymphocyte has the genetic information available to make one particular antibody specificity and molecules of that antibody are built into the cell surface membrane as receptors. The essentials of the clonal selection theory can be summarized as follows:

1. Precursors of the cells that form antibodies are made up of a vast number of clones.
2. The clones capable of reacting with self tissue are eliminated or suppressed during fetal development.
3. The remaining clones specific for foreign substances react by the antigen binding to the cell surface receptor, leading to the proliferation and differentiation of that clone to produce a colony of identical cells.
4. There are specific receptors which are present on the surface of the cells (B- and T-lymphocytes).
5. All possible receptor structures are already represented in the body.
6. Receptor specificity on the B-lymphocyte is the same as the specificity of the secreted antibody from the plasma cell.
7. Each individual B- or T-cell is committed to one specificity.
8. This specificity commitment exists prior to antigenic stimulation and the progeny of the cells remain committed to that specificity.

The concept of memory is explained by the fact that memory cells are formed during the differentiation process of B- or T-lymphocytes. Therefore the clonal selection theory accounts for a number of important immunological concepts. The main problem for proponents of the clonal selection theory was how to explain the extreme diversity of the immune system, and in particular, the extremely large number of antibody specificities that can be made. This aspect of immunology is called the Generation of Diversity.

There is a great deal of experimental evidence for the clonal selection theory. In particular, it is now very well established that B-lymphocytes have immunoglobulins on their cell surface acting as receptors. This can easily be demonstrated using fluorescent or radioactively labelled anti-immunoglobulin antibodies. Similarly, the T-cell antigen receptors have now been identified and their structures established. Use can be made of these different receptors in terms of enumeration of B-cells or T-cells in a lymphocyte population, and they can also be used in order to separate B-cells from T-cells, for example, by affinity chromatography or differential adsorption, or by using fluorescently labelled cells in the fluorescence-activated cell sorter. Evidence for the clonal selection theory also comes from the fact that myeloma antibodies and monoclonal antibodies show precise amino acid sequences. There is commitment and retention of specificity in hybridomas, plasma-cell tumours, and isolated B-cell clones. There is also indirect evidence of pre-commitment to antibody specificity. Overall, there is very little experimental evidence against the clonal selection theory, but what little there is, does not carry much weight.

The Genetic Basis of Diversity

The genetic origin of antibody diversity has been a controversial subject for many years and it is still one of the most fascinating problems in immunology today. The antibodies show a number of unique characteristics including an enormous diversity in their primary structure. The immune system has the potential to mount a response with great specificity to an almost limitless array of antigens. How many different antibody molecules can the system produce? And how many genes are needed to do it?

It can be shown, by injection of a fluorescent or radiolabelled antigen into mice and counting the number of tagged cells, that the number of cells binding one antigen is about 1 in 10^4 lymphocytes. A largish protein like bovine serum albumin (BSA) has, say, ten antigenic determinants, and thus each individual can therefore produce 10^5 specificities. Such figures represent the minimum and values are certainly larger than this, and most probably reach at least 10^6 and probably 10^7 specificities. It has been shown that a mouse can make 30–100 different antibodies to a particular antigen and that different antibodies are made by different mice; for the antigen, NIP (nitroiodophenyl), the antibody repertoire of a particular strain of mice was estimated to be 5000–10 000 antibodies. If each mouse, let us say, makes 100 different anti-NIP antibodies and assuming no cross-reacting antibodies and 10^3 or 10^4 haptens, then each mouse must be able to make at least 10^5 or 10^6 different antibodies. One to ten million antibody specificities may seem a very large number, but it is the antibody combining site which dictates the molecular specificity and this is made up of the hypervariable regions of the heavy and light chains which can be occupied by between 10 and 15 different amino acids. Then there can be at least 10^{10}–10^{15} different hypervariable regions possible per chain, thus giving rise to a figure of 10^{20}–10^{30} different antibody molecules. Such an enormous figure has never been postulated but it is generally agreed that somewhere between one and ten million different antibodies are needed for an individual to face up to the antigenic universe.

How does this antibody repertoire originate? It has been suggested that to do so requires a Generator of Diversity (G.O.D.), hence introducing a theological element and a little mystery. However, this does not solve the problem!

If all the antibodies were coded in the normal way, one gene for each in the DNA, then we should need 10^6 genes to be present. This represents an impossibly large quantity of DNA. In fact the immune system has a strategy for maintaining this diversity in a way that does not need such an enormous number of genes. It side-steps the problem of carrying millions of separate genes by having a relatively modest number of separate genes that are juggled and recombined in successive steps (see below). There were originally two main theories postulated to explain the generation of diversity. These are as follows.

The Somatic Mutation Theory. The somatic mutation theory postulates a minimum number of germ-line genes which mutate rapidly during embryonic life to produce many different antibody-forming cells. The genes originally present are those that produce antibodies vital to the survival of the animal in early life

and each stem cell supports one of a few basic antibody molecule genes. This means that diversity is generated anew in each individual rather than being inherited. During differentiation these few genes undergo random somatic mutation, especially in the hypervariable regions. This would mean starting off with a number of cells having identical DNA sequences and then hypervariable mutations would occur leading to a very large number of cells having different DNA sequences from each other and coding for different antibodies. This theory would need perhaps only 20 to 50 genes to start with. Additional diversity may be generated by recombination processes during the development of the immune system.

There are modified versions of this somatic theory called *somatic combinatorial models* which propose that each hypervariable region is coded by a distinct gene and that the relatively constant remainder of the V region (framework portion) is coded by other genes. It proposes that during the differentiation of an antibody-secreting cell, the hypervariable region genes are inserted into the framework gene at certain positions to yield a V-gene. This combination model would amplify enormously the number of antibody genes that could be produced from a limited number of framework and hypervariable region genes.

The ordinary *somatic mutation model* suggests that the average antibody family has around 100–200 germ-line variable region genes and that additional V-region diversity arises from the somatic mutations which occur in the division of the cells. This, therefore, involves an extensive antigen-independent proliferation of lymphoid cells which give rise to a large variety of V-region genes in the lymphocyte population.

The *hypermutation model* proposes that the V-region diversity arises from several hundred germ line V-genes, by a special super-mutational mechanism. This would depend on there being frequent errors made in the DNA repair mechanism process.

The *somatic recombination model* suggests that V-region diversity again arises from a few hundred germ-line V-genes which during proliferation and differentiation of the lymphoid cells, undergo extensive somatic crossing-over between the chromatids. This mechanism might generate a virtually unlimited number of V-genes and is similar to the somatic combinatorial model, except that it will allow recombination to occur anywhere within the V-gene.

The Germ-Line Theory. This theory postulates that most, if not all, the V-region genes are encoded in the germ-line of the organism. Such genes are postulated to have arisen by mutation, selection and gene duplication during vertebrate evolution. Thus, the diversity of the V-region genes exists before the differentiation of each individual and antibody production requires the activation of three existing antibody genes in each individual lymphocyte. An individual lymphocyte expresses only one specificity. Thus, in the germ-line theory all the genes necessary are present in every cell and code for the 10^6 or 10^7 different antibody specificities and these are transmitted to the offspring through the germ-cell line.

The germ-line theory cannot be rejected on the basis of the argument that there is insufficient DNA in the germ-line to encode the diversity of the V-regions. In fact, the total DNA in a human sperm cell could possibly code for about 10^7 V-genes. It is probable that combinatorial association of heavy and light chains is applicable and then 10^4 V_L genes and 10^4 V_H genes could generate 10^8 different specific antibody molecules. This would mean that the fraction of the genome required to code for this information would be less than 0.1%, which appears fairly reasonable for a function as important as antibody immunity.

The advances in the study of genetic mechanisms have led to the proposal that the real situation is, in fact, somewhere between the two theories and involves an extensive number of germ-line genes, plus a number of somatic mechanisms which operate. It is clear that separate diversification mechanisms exist for each of the chains of the antibody molecule since they are coded for on separate chromosomes (*see* Table 4).

TABLE 4
CHROMOSOME LOCATIONS OF ANTIBODY GENES

Peptide chain	Mouse	Human
H	12	14
λ	16	22
κ	6	2

If we consider the way in which diversity arises in the heavy chain, for example, we will see what mechanisms operate. It seems that the key to the strategy is that diversity is achieved by a relatively modest number of separate genes that are juggled about and recombined in successive steps. Thus, for the V-region genes in each individual for the heavy chain there appears to be somewhere around 200 to 500 V-region genes available. Each of these V-region genes may be combined with one of about 10 diversity-region genes (D) and about four or five joining-region genes (J), thereby generating at least 10 000 possible genes. In reality this 10 000 is an underestimate because there are a number of mechanisms which are superimposed upon this situation. For example, the V-, D- and J-gene segments of each heavy chain of an antibody molecule can be brought together at slightly different joining points. Still further diversity is introduced into the variable region by the mechanism which most likely involves mutation at the cellular level after much of the immune system has undergone development. Further to this, once any new single combined heavy chain gene has been produced from the segments, V-, D-, J- and

the constant-region gene (C), then the heavy chain polypeptide product is presumably free to combine with any light chain polypeptide which has been generated by a very similar diversity-guaranteeing mechanism to form a complete antibody protein (see Fig. 3).

The mechanisms which operate for the light and for the heavy polypeptide chains differ very little. The light chain polypeptides, as we know, belong to two main families called κ and λ, but there is only one family of heavy polypeptide chains. The other major difference is that light chain genes contain no diversity-region genes, although they contain V, J- and C-regions that are comparable to those found in the heavy chain gene repertoire.

It is thought that there is a highly precise, developmentally regulated control of the expression of antibody genes and these are mediated by specific proteins. The control involves a one-way differentiation or developmental process during which the thousands of V-, D-, J- and C-gene regions are stitched together to produce the antibody-forming cells of the immune system. When these gene segments are spliced together in such cells, the original DNA, with its almost endless possibilities of synthesis, is lost, and thus such cells are terminally differentiated and each carries only one specialized message for making one particular antibody specificity.

The mechanisms described above for generating antibody diversity provide, at the very least, 10 million different antibody specificities. There are two other interesting genetic phenomena which need to be mentioned but will not be discussed in detail.

Allelic Exclusion. It appears that during the development of the B-lymphocytes, antibody gene families are rearranged sequentially. First, the heavy chain family to produce pre B-cells and then a light chain family to produce B_μ cells. The κ gene family is rearranged first, and then, if it appears that no κ rearrangements are productive, the λ gene family is rearranged. The ordered sequential rearrangement of antibody gene families during development suggests a carefully regulated process. Regardless of the mechanism of how these gene family rearrangements are initiated, their termination must be extremely carefully regulated because functional B-lymphocytes never express more than one rearranged V_H gene and V_L gene. This phenomenon is known as allelic exclusion. Thus, in an animal which is heterozygous for genetic markers on light and heavy chains, a given lymphocyte clone expresses only one L-chain and one H-chain allele. This behaviour contrasts to that of all other common mammalian proteins studied, such as allelic forms of haemoglobin which are produced co-dominantly in such cells of a heterozygous individual. Although the precise molecular basis of allelic exclusion is not known, it could be a consequence of the subtle genetic translocation mechanisms which operate.

The Organisation and Assembly of the Heavy Chain Gene

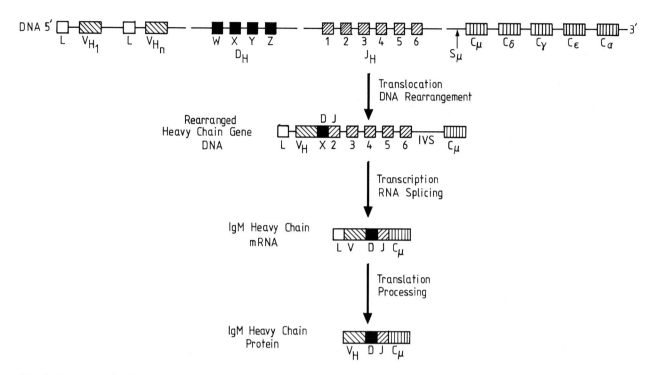

Fig. 3 The organization and assembly of the human heavy chain gene coding for IgM. In the human heavy chain gene there are multiple variable sequences (V_H) with their leader sequences (L), six joining segments (J_H) and a number of diversity segments (D_H). The recombination of the V_H, D_H and J_H gene segments occurs at the DNA level. Splicing occurs at the RNA level where intervening sequences (IVS) are removed. The constant region gene segments function individually (S = switch regions for constant sequences) and code for the different classes of antibody. There is one exception to this when the B-cell splices the RNA at a special site which incorporates C_μ and C_δ and allows simultaneous production of IgM and IgD. Light chain coding is similar except there are no D segments and the genes that code for the complete κ or λ chains are on different chromosomes.

Heavy Chain Class Switching. The light chains only have one C-region gene for each set of V-regions. However, each human heavy chain V-gene may be expressed with any of eight different heavy chain constant genes which produce the different classes of immunoglobulin molecules. All V_H genes are first expressed with the μ-constant gene, but upon differentiation of lymphocytes into plasma cells, the V_H region may associate with any of the other C-region genes, and this is called 'the heavy chain class switch'. Heavy chain class switches occur by genetic recombination between switch regions that lie from two to three kilobases in front of each C_H gene, with the possible exception of the $C\delta$ gene. These switch regions are quite large but are composed of many copies of short repeated elements. These sections appear to be the active sites for the switching process, because all the recombination events studied in the S-region have occurred within one of the 80 nucleotide repeats. It appears, therefore, that in class switching an assembled V_H region gene has been transferred from in front of a C_μ gene to one of the

other C_H genes with an accompanying removal and deletion of the intervening DNA sequence.

ANTIBODY–ANTIGEN INTERACTION

The primary function of any antibody is to bind to its antigen. The variable-region domains are primarily concerned with antigen binding while the constant-region domains are concerned with the physiological properties of the different immunoglobulins, to interact with various cells and host tissue. As discussed above, x-ray crystallography shows that particular amino acid sequences called the hypervariable regions actually make contact with the antigen, and although the remaining framework sequences of the variable-region do not come into direct contact with the antigen, they are essential in producing the correct stereochemistry of the V-region domains, and maintain the shape of the binding site.

The Antibody Combining Site. Antigen molecules bind to a concave cleft formed by the antibody variable-regions and the antigen makes contact with about 15 amino acids of the hypervariable regions of both heavy and light chains.

Antibody–Antigen Binding

The binding of antibody to antigen is always reversible, despite the fact that the bonding force may be very strong. The intermolecular attractive forces which bind antigen to antibody are: (1) hydrogen bonding, which results from the formation of hydrogen bonds produced between appropriate atoms; (2) electrostatic forces, which are due to the attraction of oppositely charged groups located on the side-chains of the protein, the force is proportional to $1/d^2$ for these forces (d = distance); (3) Van der Waals forces, which are generated by the interaction of the electron clouds and which are proportional to $1/d^7$, and (4) hydrophobic interactions, which rely on the association of non-polar, hydrophobic groups so that contact with water molecules is minimized. The hydrophobic forces may actually contribute up to half the total strength of the antigen–antibody binding. The interacting functional groups must come into close contact in molecular terms before these non-covalent forces become significant. There should be suitable atomic groups on the antigen and the antibody which interact, and it is essential that the shape of the combining site fits the antigen so that many of these non-covalent bonds can be formed. If the interaction between the antigen and antibody is such that there is steric hindrance between the groups, then repulsive forces between the electron clouds will be produced. These will lead to a fall in the binding energy of the antibody and antigen through increased repulsion and decreased attraction and hence, in the end, determine the specificity of the antibody molecule for a particular antigen.

Antibody Affinity

The antibody affinity is the strength of the non-covalent single antigen/antibody bond, and it is produced by the sum of the attractive and repulsive forces described above. The affinity of a single combining site is the binding energy to a monovalent antigen. As noted above, the interaction of the antigen and antibody is reversible, and the law of mass action can be applied to the reaction to determine the equilibrium constant. This is the affinity constant:

$$Ab + Ag \rightleftharpoons Ab\,Ag$$

$$K = \frac{[Ab\,Ag]}{[Ab]\,[Ag]}$$

where K = equilibrium constant or the antibody affinity constant (K must be calculated at equilibrium).

Affinity and Avidity. Each antibody unit has two antigen-binding sites and antigens can be monovalent or multivalent, and so the antibody–antigen reaction is normally of a multivalent type. Hapten–antibody binding is always a monovalent interaction.

Multivalent binding between the antigen and antibody is termed the 'avidity' or the 'functional affinity', and this results in a considerable increase in stability compared with the monovalent interaction (affinity or intrinsic affinity). This is often described as the 'bonus effect' of multivalency. The equilibrium constant, or affinity, for a monovalent antigen–antibody interaction, such as with the Fab fragment, and IgG, is 10^4 l/mol whereas the equilibrium constant for an IgG multivalent interaction with an antigen may be around 10^7 l/mol, and indeed, the equilibrium constant for a multivalent interaction between IgM, which has an effective antibody valency up to 10 with a multivalent antigen, can be around 10^{11} l/mol. These higher equilibrium constant values in multivalent interactions are therefore called 'avidity' and we can see that there is a 1000-fold increase in the binding energy of IgG when both valencies are utilized, and a 10^7-fold increase when IgM binds antigens in a multivalent mode.

Clearly, in the more normal physiological situations, it is avidity which is the relevant term, since naturally occurring antigens, like microorganisms, are multivalent. Nevertheless, the measurement of hapten–antibody reactions gives us an insight into the immunochemical nature of the antigen–antibody reaction.

Antibody Specificity. Antibody specificity results from the action of particular antibody molecules with particular antigenic determinants. In a polyclonal antiserum, there is a population of individual antibodies which react against different determinants on a particular antigen. If one or more of these react with antigenic determinants on another antigen, then there will be a cross-reaction with that antigen. With a monoclonal antibody, clearly the antibody will only normally react with one antigenic determinant, and so a cross-reaction will be genuine. In some cases, it is possible to get, with a polyclonal antiserum, an irrelevant antibody reacting with an antigenic determinant, and this is not a genuine cross-reaction. Cross-reactivity depends on the precise chemical configuration of a molecule. The three-dimensional shape of the molecule and its electron clouds can be the most important factors involved, and cross-reactions can be due to this three-dimensional shape. Antibodies are able to discriminate between three-dimensional shapes, such as α-helical structures, in contrast to non-helical structures, and they may also distinguish between optical isomers of particular compounds. Indeed, antibodies can be highly specific and react with only one isomer in a group. For example, the antiserum to p-aminophenyl-β-galactoside is specific to this compound and does not react with p-aminophenyl-α- or β-glucoside. Configurational specificity is also shown in the reaction of antiserum to the enzyme 'lysozyme'. This enzyme possesses an intra-chain disulphide bond which produces a loop in the peptide chain. Antiserum may be raised against either the whole enzyme, or the isolated loop peptide. These preparations are found to distinguish between the two and do not react with the isolated loop in its reduced state. This highlights the importance of tertiary structure in determining antibody specificity.

Determination of Affinity and Avidity. There are several methods available for the determination of affinity and avidity. It is necessary in each procedure to set up a reaction in which antigen and antibody are allowed to come to equilibrium. The quantities of free antigen and bound antigen are then determined without disturbing the equilibrium. Free antigen may be separated from the bound antigen by a number of physical methods such as dialysis, gel filtration, centrifugation, selective precipitation, or by studying changes in the fluorescence properties of the bound antigen or antibody. The data produced from such· a study are then analysed by using the law of mass action, as described above, to give the affinity constant, K.

Antibody Affinity Heterogeneity. A pure antibody, such as a monoclonal antibody, shows only one value for the antibody affinity, either high, or low. For a polyclonal antiserum, we actually determine the average affinity, or 'avidity'. For even a simple antigen, many antibodies are raised against different parts of the molecular structure, and the binding of these antibodies depends upon the number and type of secondary bonds formed between antigen and antibody. The antigen presents many different chemical configurations to the antibody-producing cells, and thus many different antibodies are produced to a given antigen. It is not only the antibody affinity which is important in antigen binding, because it must be remembered that many properties of the antibody are determined by its class and subclass.

Physiological Significance of Antibody Affinity. Affinity and avidity of antibodies affect their physiological and pathological properties. High-avidity antibody is better than low-avidity antibody in a number of biological reactions, such as complement fixation, haemolysis, haemagglutination, membrane damage, virus neutralization, protective capacity against bacteria, and immune elimination of antigen. There is also an immunopathological significance since, in experimental animals, immune complexes, containing low-avidity antibody, persist in the circulation, localize in the glomerular basement membrane of the kidney and lead to impaired renal function. High-avidity immune complexes, however, are more rapidly removed from the circulation, and generally have little effect on renal function.

The Antibody Response

The antibody responses in primary and secondary exposure to an antigen differ quite considerably. In the primary antibody response, there are four phases which can be identified: (1) a lag phase, when no antibodies are detected, (2) a log phase, in which the antibody concentration rises logarithmically; (3) a plateau phase, in which the level of antibody stabilizes, and (4) a decline phase, in which the antibody is cleared or catabolized. The major antibody of the primary immune response is of IgM class, while in the secondary immune response, the major antibody is IgG (see Fig. 4). In the secondary immune response, the antibody appears more quickly and persists for a longer period of time, and reaches a much higher concentration. In terms of antibody affinity, the antibodies of the secondary response have much greater affinity constants; this is referred to as 'affinity maturation'. The primary immune response leads to antibody production after about 5–7 days, while the secondary immune response can occur very rapidly, after 2 or 3 days.

Affinity Maturation. Antibodies produced in a secondary response to a T-cell-dependent antigen have higher average affinity than those produced in the primary immune response. Affinity maturation involves the selective expansion of clones of high affinity antibody-producing cells and this must be in association with the IgM to IgG switch, because there is no maturation in the affinity of the IgM response. The degree of affinity maturation is dependent on the antigen dose given. High antigen doses lead to a lower affinity response than do low antigen doses. It appears that low antigen concentrations lead to the stimulation of B-cells with high affinity receptors, whereas, in the presence of high antigen levels, there is sufficient material to bind and trigger high and low affinity B-lymphocytes. In summary, the affinity of the IgM response is constant throughout, whereas the maturation of the IgG response depends on the dose of antigen, lower doses producing antibodies with higher affinity.

ANTIBODIES AND DISEASE

There are many disease states in which there are changes in the levels of the immunoglobulin classes especially infective illness, liver disease, coeliac disease, rheumatic diseases, neurological diseases, autoimmune and hypersensitivity states. In a vast range of acute and chronic bacterial infections immunoglobulin levels are raised. Generally, immunoglobulin levels are also raised in autoimmune disease, cirrhosis of the liver, and sarcoidosis. A number of acute viral infections such as glandular fever, and infective hepatitis, lead to raised IgM levels. In certain situations, decreased immunoglobulin levels are

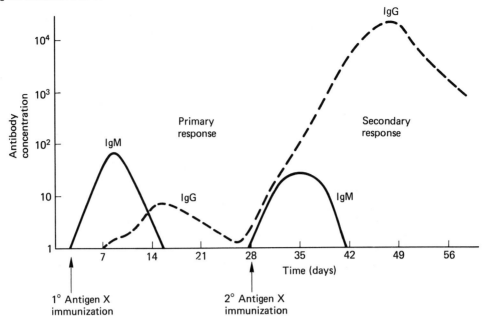

If antigen Y is injected at 28 days a *primary* response is produced

Fig. 4 Studies of antibodies produced in primary and secondary immune responses. The major antibody class formed in a primary immune response is IgM, while that in the secondary response is IgG. In the more rapid secondary response, antibody levels are considerably higher and longer lasting than in the primary response. Specificity is shown by the primary response produced against antigen Y. (Antibody concentration units are arbitrary and are comparative only.) (Reproduced with permission from Gibson G. G., Hubbard R., Parkes D. V. (eds) (1983). *Immunotoxicology, Proceedings of the 1st International Symposium on Immunotoxicology*. London: Academic Press.)

observed, for example, nephrotic syndrome, malabsorption, malnutrition and immunodeficiency.

There are a range of plasma cell abnormalities which lead to changed levels. The most common is multiple myeloma, which is a neoplastic change in a committed clone of plasma cell precursors, leading to the production of a homogeneous (monoclonal) antibody with excess free light chains (Bence-Jones proteins). In this disease, the other antibody class levels are normally decreased. The clinical effects observed include spontaneous fractures, hypercalcaemia, and renal failure. Macroglobulinaemia is also a plasma cell abnormality involving a neoplastic change in a committed clone of IgM-producing cells. This produces a homogeneous IgM, the clinical effects being similar to multiple myeloma, but showing an increased hyperviscosity syndrome. Heavy chain disease, which is rare, is also associated with a neoplastic change in the cells of the reticulo-endothelial system and involves production of part of the heavy chain which appears in the urine and serum of the patient. Cryoglobulinaemia is a neoplastic or reactive hyperactivity of the plasma cells and is associated with the reversible aggregation and precipitation of immunoglobulins, either homogeneous or mixed at temperatures below 37°C.

Changes in the immunoglobulin levels are very often characteristic for particular diseases. For example, in chronic bacterial infections, the immunoglobulin classes, G. A and M levels, all increase, while in SLE, chronic active hepatitis or Hashimoto's disease, immunoglobulin A and M levels remain normal, while the IgG levels increase substantially. Immunoglobulin E levels may be studied in order to investigate allergic individuals. The immunoglobulin class levels in cerebrospinal fluid may also be investigated and related to the diagnosis of a patient.

Immunological Tests for Antibodies

There is a vast range of suitable tests to detect antibodies; non-specific or specific, which are immunological in nature, and many of them are described in the current volumes. The most common include precipitation reactions in gels, such as double immunodiffusion, which may be quantitated in single radial immunodiffusion. The electrophoretic methods include immunoelectrophoresis, counter-current electrophoresis, and rocket electrophoresis. Further tests include haemagglutination, complement fixation, and immunofluorescence tests involving the direct, indirect, and indirect complement-amplified immunofluorescence. Tests for IgE levels involve the use of, for antigen-specific IgE, the radio-allergosorbent test (RAST) and the test for total serum IgE level is the radioimmunosorbent test (RIST). The other immunological tests which are very commonly used, include radioimmunoassay and enzyme-linked immunoadsorbent assay (ELISA), followed by a whole range of assays based on differently labelled antibodies or antigens.

IN VITRO USES OF ANTIBODIES

Antibodies have a vast number of applications, including use as analytical, diagnostic and therapeutic agents. This is largely because they can be highly specific and can be produced to react with almost any chemical, biochemical microbiological or cellular material. They may also be labelled, (e.g. radio-labelled, fluorescent, enzyme-labelled), and can be used to detect, localize and measure quantitatively any of the above materials. The applications of antibodies therefore run across the biological and chemical sciences since they may be produced against, for example, drugs, hormones, enzymes, proteins, receptors, cell surface markers such as ABO and HLA, viruses, bacteria, parasites, fungi and tumour cells.

Production of Conventional Antibodies

An essential prerequisite to the study of any antigen is the production of antibodies or 'antiserum' (immune serum), i.e., serum that reacts specifically with the antigen. To produce conventional antiserum, it is necessary to immunize an animal, normally several times, with the antigen or immunogen. In laboratory experiments, small animals, such as the rat or rabbit, can be used for the production of antiserum. However, when it is necessary to produce large quantities for diagnostic or therapeutic use, larger animals are necessary, such as sheep, goats, donkeys, or horses. Antiserum produced by injecting animals with antigens obtained from a different species is termed 'xeno-antiserum', whereas an intraspecies immunization is termed 'allo-antiserum'.

The techniques and schedules for immunization vary substantially according to the nature of the antigen and the manner of inoculation. Different workers prefer different methods and there is an understandable tendency to stick to one particular method which has been found to be successful. There are a number of steps which are, nevertheless, common to most schedules. An aqueous solution of the immunogen is first emulsified with an oily adjuvant in the ratio one volume of aqueous solution to one or two volumes of adjuvant. The mixture is emulsified and the emulsion then injected into one or more experimental animals. After two weeks or more the animal is given a second injection of the immunogen, usually of smaller quantity than the first. A sample of blood is taken about a week later, allowed to clot, and the serum is investigated to ascertain specific antibody content. The immunizing schedule raises a number of important questions, for example, what species and sex of animal should be selected for injection? What mass of immunogen should be given? What emulsion volume should be utilized? Which route of injection should be used? How many injection sites? How often should the injections be given? When should the animal be bled? How should the specific antibody in the serum samples be assayed? All these factors should be carefully considered before embarking on the production of a sample of conventional antiserum.

When one is satisfied that sufficient specific antibody in suitable concentration has been produced, a large blood sample may be taken from the animal and the serum produced and purified.

Antibodies are also called 'immunoglobulins' and are serum proteins. The first classification of serum proteins was by their solubility in ammonium sulphate. Thus, ammonium sulphate solutions precipitate globulins but leave albumin in solution.

Serum proteins can be separated by an electrical field, as in electrophoresis, a technique that depends largely on the charge and size of the proteins (see Chapter 26). Most proteins have a negative charge at pH 8 and migrate towards the anode. This procedure serves to separate albumin from the α, β and γ-globulins. Most antibodies are in the γ-globulin fraction, and this can be demonstrated when the serum is first adsorbed with the antigenic material used to produce it. Since antibodies are large glycoprotein molecules, they may be purified by protein separation techniques. Normally a combination of techniques is used; initially fractional precipitation with ammonium sulphate, followed by ion-exchange chromatography with, for example, diethylaminoethyl (DEAE) cellulose. Additional techniques include gel filtration, e.g. Sephadex G-200, electrophoresis e.g. zone electrophoresis on cellulose, starch or acrylamide gel, or gradient ultracentrifugation on sucrose or salt gradients. The purified immunoglobulins isolated in these ways are still highly heterogeneous with regard to their antibody composition. They may be further purified by immunological methods in which certain antibodies are adsorbed out with the antigen, often on a solid matrix. Production of conventional antiserum for use in an immunoassay should produce a non-precipitating antibody of the highest possible avidity. It is also an advantage if the antiserum has a high titre, since this can be used to perform a large number of assays.

Properties of Conventional Antibodies

A conventional antiserum contains a mixture of different antibody molecules. The antibody composition will vary from batch to batch, even from the same animal, and as such the specificity and the avidity of the material is not exactly reproducible. The antiserum will contain a certain amount of irrelevant immunoglobulin and other serum proteins will also be present. The antiserum will bind to all the antigenic determinants of all the components of the immunogen. The class and subclass of the immunoglobulin will be a typical mixture and the physical properties of the conventional antiserum will be an average of the properties of the antibodies present. Clearly, some of these properties are disadvantageous and some have distinct advantages.

Production of Monoclonal Antibodies

The production of monoclonal antibodies was pioneered by Köhler and Milstein, and the arrival of these pure antibodies has revolutionized immunology and enabled the investigation of many new areas of biological science. Köhler and Milstein showed that cell fusion could be used to produce a hybrid cell line, producing a single molecular type of antibody. The basic principle involved taking B-lymphocytes from a mouse which had been immunized with the desired antigen, and these were fused with a suitable mouse-derived plasmacytoma or myeloma line. The cell fusion of a specific antibody-producing lymphocyte of B-cell lineage with the mouse cancer cell produces a hybrid cell (hybridoma) which possesses both parental properties. Thus, it is a malignant cell which can be grown indefinitely, continuously secreting a

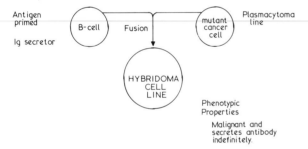

Fig. 5 Basic principle of monoclonals. Hybridoma cells secreting a single antibody of one specificity are the result of the fusion of an antigen-primed immunoglobulin-secreting B-cell with a suitable plasmacytoma line. The cell fusion is carried out in 50% polyethylene glycol mol. wt. 1500 to 4000 at 37°C, but its precise mechanism is unknown. Culture supernatants are screened for the required specific antibody to isolate the desired hybridomas. The excess infused B-cells die after 3 to 4 days, whilst the excess plasmacytoma cells could survive indefinitely in culture. They are thus killed selectively using hypoxanthine, aminopterin, thymidine (HAT) medium which prevents nucleic acid biosynthesis in cells lacking hypoxanthine-guanine-phosphoribosyl-transferase (HGPRT) or thymidine kinase (TK) enzymes. (Reproduced with permission from Gibson G. G., Hubbard R., Parke D. V. (eds) (1983). *Immunotoxicology, Proceedings of the 1st International Symposium on Immunotoxicology.* London: Academic Press.)

specific antibody against the desired antigen. Since one B-lymphocyte or plasma cell is committed to produce only one antibody specificity, this technique produces a pure antibody of the desired specificity (see Fig. 5). This led of course, to the production of homogeneous monoclonal antibodies against a wide variety of pre-defined antigens which could be used as pure, very specific, reagents in pure and applied research.

The procedure for the production of monoclonal antibodies is illustrated in Fig. 6, and is compared with the production of polyclonal antibodies in Fig. 7.

Immunization. Mice are the most convenient animals to use because the appropriate tumour lines are available and suitable for fusion (see below). However, one can use rats, since there is also a suitable myeloma cell line available. Normally the mice are of Balb/c type, because the myeloma cell lines are derived from Balb/c mice. Mice are usually immunized two or three times intraperitoneally and finally one immunization is given via the tail vein. The immunizations are at least two weeks apart. Often an adjuvant such as Freund's complete adjuvant can be used, although there are a wide variety of protocols which may be utilized in an immunization procedure. The serum of the mice may be examined to establish that an adequate antibody response has been made. A mouse is then killed and the spleen used as a source of lymphocytes. A cell suspension is produced from the spleen and used for the fusion experiment.

Cell Fusion Partners. The most popular mouse cell lines are the NSI line, which is a non-antibody secreting tumour line, but one which does synthesize the kappa (κ) chain, and the other is the SP2 line which is a non-secretor and a non-synthesizer. Both these lines fuse very well with mouse Balb/c lymphocytes. Rat myeloma cell lines are available, the most commonly used is Y3-Agl.2.3 which produces a light chain only. There are human myeloma lines available for cell fusion and the common ones are the Ludwig line L1CR/LON/HMy2, SKO-OO7, and GM15006TGA12. Human myeloma lines all produce immunoglobulin and the experiments that have been done with human fusions have led to human hybridomas but their growth and secretion rates are not very satisfactory.

Conditions of Cell Fusion. Cell fusion itself is not experimentally difficult and it is possible to carry it out in polyethyleneglycol (PEG) (chemical fusion) or by an electrical fusion technique. There are a variety of protocols for the chemical and the electrical methods. The first fusions were done using Sendai virus as the fusing agent but most hybridomas are now produced with polyethyleneglycol (PEG) which is commercially available and its use results in an adequate fusion frequency and greater reproducibility. The electrical cell fusion can be done on much fewer cells and eventually will probably get down to only a few cells at a time. In the chemical fusion, about 10^8 mouse spleen cells and 10^7 myeloma cells are fused in polyethyleneglycol (PEG), of molecular weight 1000–4000 in a concentration of 35–50%. The fusion is commonly performed with plasma cells from the spleens of immunized donors three to four days after the last intravenous antigen injection. The myeloma plasma cell mixture is incubated for several minutes with 0·2–0·5 ml of PEG, which is then diluted out with about 30 ml of culture medium. The cells are then washed and distributed in the culture wells of microtitre plates.

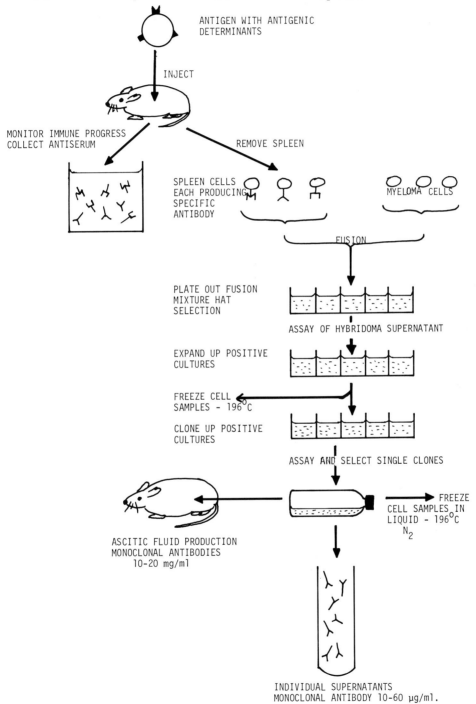

Fig. 6 Production of monoclonal antibodies. Monoclonal antibody production involves (a) producing lymphocytes which are immune to the antigen, (b) fusion of these cells with a suitable myeloma line, (c) hybridoma selection using HAT, (d) supernatant antibody screening, and (e) cloning and final monoclonal antibody growth *in vitro* or *in vivo*.

Removing Excess Myeloma Cells. The excess myeloma cells will compete with the hybridomas which have been produced since both cells lines are tumour lines. The myeloma lines derived from Balb/c mice cells used for the production of monoclonal antibodies were selected for certain enzyme deficiencies, that is thymidine kinase (TK) and/or hypoxanthine–guanine–phosphoribosyl-transferase (HGPRT) deficiency. The reason for this is as follows. When the cells are grown after the fusion, they are grown in HAT medium which contains hypoxanthine, aminopterin and thymidine. This is a biochemical selective medium, the aminopterin blocking the main synthetic

pathway of pyrimidines and purines because aminopterin is a folic acid antagonist. However, the cells may still use the salvage pathway to these nucleic acid precursors. This necessitates using the provided hypoxanthine and thymidine, and the enzymes mentioned above. Since the myeloma cells do not possess these enzymes they are now incapable of producing the necessary nucleic acid by either pathway and so die in HAT medium. The unfused B-lymphocytes do not survive in culture more than a few days and so do not interfere. The hybridoma cell lines, however, do not die because they are provided with both HGPRT and TK enzymes by virtue of the fusion with

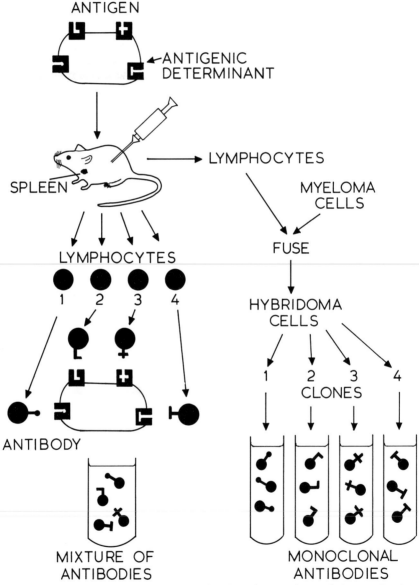

Fig. 7 Monoclonal and polyclonal antibodies. Comparison of the production of monoclonal and polyclonal antibodies shows the crucial differences between the antibody samples. Polyclonal antiserum consists of a mixture of antibodies to all the determinants of the antigen, whereas, because of cell fusion and cloning, each monoclonal antibody is pure and directed to only one antigenic determinant.

the B-lymphocyte line. Thus the myeloma cells will die usually after five to seven days, and the hybridoma cells can grow on in the culture medium.

Screening of Supernatants: Selection of Hybridomas. The supernatants of the cell cultures are investigated after about two weeks of growth and are assayed for specific antibody secretion. A wide range of antibody antigen tests are available, such as radioimmunoassay, enzyme-linked immunosorbent assay, haemagglutination, and complement-dependent cytotoxicity. The positive cultures are selected, the cells are cloned and assayed again. The cloning is usually done by limiting dilution methods but some workers prefer physically to select a cell under the microscope. Often a second or third cloning is carried out and assayed to confirm the selected desired antibody specificity. At any stage, the positive cultures may be frozen in liquid nitrogen at −196°C. The clones finally selected are always stored at −196°C and the samples may be thawed out and viable cells obtained to grow in cell culture again.

Growth of Hybridomas. These single cell lines may be propagated *in vitro* to produce mass cell culture and involves no further use of animals. Alternatively, they may be grown *in vivo*, by injecting the cells into Balb/c mice to produce tumours, the antibody being obtained from the ascitic fluid. The *in vitro* method produces, in the supernatant fluid, about 5–50 µg/ml, whereas the *in vitro* method produces significantly more, in the range 1–20 mg/ml of specific antibody. The monoclonality of the secreted antibody is confirmed by the use of isoelectric focusing (IEF).

Hybridoma technology allows the production of specific antibodies, even when highly complex antigens, molecular or cellular, are used, or even when the antigen of interest cannot be purified from contaminating substances.

Advantages of Monoclonal Antibodies. The properties and disadvantages of conventional antiserum as compared with monoclonal antibodies are shown in Tables 5 and 6.

There are several other reasons which increase the utility of monoclonal antibodies. Since the hybridoma technique produces monoclonal cell lines to individual components of a mixture, it becomes possible to detect, assay and purify (by affinity chromatography) antigens which may even be completely unknown to us. This often occurs when using cells as immunogens, when antibodies are produced against all the cell surface molecules, whether they are known or unknown to the researchers. There is also the possibility of isolating a rare or inaccessible antibody against an extremely weak immunogen, although great effort will be required because the statistics of the cell fusion process would make this difficult. A monoclonal antibody is relatively easy to produce in a pure state and gives low backgrounds

TABLE 5
PROPERTIES AND DISADVANTAGES OF CONVENTIONALLY PRODUCED ANTISERUM

1. A pure immunogen is needed or the antiserum must be purified for specificity.
2. Consists of a heterogeneous mixture of antibodies.
3. Can never be reproduced exactly with respect to specificity or binding.
4. Cross-reactions are not necessarily genuine.
5. A mixture of antibody classes and subclasses.
6. Physical properties are an average.

TABLE 6
ADVANTAGES OF MONOCLONAL ANTIBODIES

1. Pure material consisting of one molecular species only.
2. Specific for one antigenic determinant only.
3. Cross-reactions do mean shared determinants.
4. High or low avidity antibodies may be produced.
5. An impure immunogen can be used.
6. Reproducible with respect to avidity and specificity.
7. One class and subclass of immunoglobulin.
8. Unlimited amounts can be produced *in vitro* or *in vivo*.
9. Further animals and the use of a 'farm' are not needed for immunization and bleeding.
10. Hybridomas are immortal cell lines.
11. Monoclonal antibodies can act as worldwide standard reagents with identical specificities and constant properties.

in staining and assay reactions. It is easily radiolabelled or conjugated with fluorescent or enzyme markers. Incorporation of radiolabels such as ^{14}C, ^{3}H or ^{35}S into monoclonal antibodies can be done by simply growing the hybridomas in medium containing appropriately labelled amino acids. Quality control with monoclonal antibodies is much easier than with conventional antiserum, since they are precisely reproducible.

Limitations of Monoclonal Antibodies. There is no doubt that monoclonal antibodies are expensive to produce and characterize. Hybridoma technology is time-consuming and has its own difficulties. Nevertheless the cost of continued production of monoclonal antibodies will decrease as *in vitro* technology for their production improves.

The fact that monoclonal antibodies recognize a single antigenic determinant is often an advantage but in certain cases it can be a problem, for example, where there is heterogeneity of the antigen, a labile antigenic determinant, or the chance occurrence of a similar determinant on an unrelated molecule. Table 7 lists the common disadvantages of monoclonal antibodies.

A monoclonal antibody has a definite energy of binding to its antigen, whereas the conventional antiserum has an average energy of binding. The antibody avidity may be high or low for a monoclonal

TABLE 7
DISADVANTAGES OF MONOCLONAL ANTIBODIES

1 May not form a precipitate unless used as mixtures.
2 Do not necessarily react with protein A.
3 May be of low affinity.
4 May not fix complement.
5 May have unusual physical properties, e.g. sensitivity to iodination or pH.

antibody and may be a disadvantage or an advantage depending on the application required. In immunoassay procedures a high avidity antibody is desirable, whilst for purification using affinity chromatography, with a solid-phase antibody, the preference is for a low avidity antibody.

Applications of Monoclonal Antibodies. It is possible to use monoclonal antibodies in much the same way as conventional antiserum but they will have certain advantages, particularly specificity and reproducibility. They may therefore be used to detect, localize and measure most biological molecules and cell-surface antigens. The applications of monoclonal antibodies can be classified in three main areas: (1) analytical, (2) diagnostic, and (3) therapeutic (Table 8).

TABLE 8
APPLICATIONS OF MONOCLONAL ANTIBODIES

1 ABO and rare blood groups.
2 HLA antigens, tissue typing, disease association.
3 Classification of cells, cell subpopulations and their function.
4 Cell separation, cell–cell interactions and differentiation, biochemistry of cell surfaces.
5 Tumour-associated antigens and tumour cells.
6 Immunoassays of drugs, hormones, enzymes, proteins, receptors, etc.
7 Structural investigation and classification of viruses, bacteria, and parasites.
8 Purification of complex mixtures.
9 Diagnosis of infections.
10 Radiolabelled monoclonal antibodies can be used as imaging agents, e.g. for tumours.
11 Toxin-labelled monoclonal antibodies can be used as therapeutic agents to kill particular cell lines, e.g. tumours.

Anti-idiotype Antibodies

The structural determinant of an antigen which elicits antibodies is normally called an 'epitope', and this structure leads to the production of a complementary antibody-combining site, which is often called a 'paratope'. Antibodies can be made against antibody molecules, and so antibodies themselves present epitopes to produce complementary paratopes. Epitopes which are located on the constant parts of the framework of antibodies are called 'allotypes', whereas those epitopes formed by the variable part of the antibody molecule are called 'idiotypes'. Thus,

an idiotype denotes a set of epitopes (idiotopes); the location of the epitope is at the antigen-binding site of the antibody.

Animals can be stimulated to make antibodies to the idiotope of an antibody molecule and these antibodies are called 'anti-idiotype' antibodies. Hence, the immune system has a complex network of paratopes and idiotopes, and antibody molecules can occur both in the free state and as receptor molecules on B- and T-cells, leading to a network which intertwines cells and molecules. In this antibody network, there are possibilities for on-off switches, leading to the suppression of an immune response by an anti-idiotype antibody, and this has been demonstrated. In 1974, Jerne proposed a theory of an antibody network for the regulation of the immune response.

One of the important points about anti-idiotypic antibodies is that they carry the image of the foreign antigen as part of their structures. This means that an injection of the anti-idiotype antibody may well be equivalent to injecting the antigen itself, and lead to the production of the same type of antibodies. In the case of a pathogen, it may be possible to vaccinate without actually using pathogenic material, and this represents an important possible application.

Similarly, it may well be possible to make an antibody that will interact with a cellular receptor without having to isolate the receptor itself.

Anti-idiotypic antibodies have also been investigated in terms of turning off the production of particular antibodies. For example, in autoimmune diseases, where autoantibodies are produced, it may be possible to produce an anti-idiotypic antibody to the autoantibody which will lead to the suppression and turning-off of the production of the autoantibody and hence lead to control of the autoimmune disease.

Chimeric Antibodies

Monoclonal antibodies of mouse origin have been used for therapeutic purposes. However, mouse antibodies can lead to a hypersensitivity reaction in man, and hence, destroy their effectiveness. There is some evidence of an immune reaction against mouse monoclonal antibodies used in the treatment of patients with leukaemia. A new method of making antibodies may help to solve this antigenicity problem. By utilizing monoclonal antibody and recombinant-DNA technologies, immunologists have produced novel antibodies by combining portions of one antibody gene with segments of another, thus designing molecules to have whatever features the researcher requires. Of the new antibodies, the more interesting ones are chimeric antibodies in which the antigen-binding variable regions of mouse antibodies are connected to the constant regions of human antibodies. These chimeric antibodies should be less likely to produce a hypersensitivity response in man than the all-mouse monoclonal antibodies. Chimeric antibodies have a large number of potential applications in addition to cancer therapy, for example, the treatment of autoimmune diseases such as multiple sclerosis and systemic lupus erythematosus. Here, the antibodies may be able to destroy the specific immune cells required for mounting the attack on the bodies' own tissues. Similarly, the antibodies of this type may also be used for specific immune suppression in individuals who require organ transplantation. The new technology should also be able to help in dissecting out the contribution of the various regions of antibody proteins to their functions.

SUGGESTIONS FOR FURTHER READING

Arnzel L. M., Poljak R. J. (1979). Three-dimensional structure of immunoglobulins. *Ann. Rev. Biochem*; **48**: 961.

Bier O. G., Dias da Silva W., Gotze D., Mota I. (1980). *Fundamentals of Immunology*. New York: Springer-Verlag.

Capra J. D., Edmundson A. B. (1977). The antibody combining site. *Sci. Am*; **236**: 50.

Edelman G. M. (1970). The structure and function of antibodies. *Sci. Am*; **223**: 34.

Glynn L. E., Steward M. W. (eds) (1981). *Antibody production*. Chichester: Wiley.

Glynn L. E., Steward M. W. (eds) (1981). *Structure and function of Antibodies*. Chichester: Wiley.

Hahn G. S. (1982). Antibody structure, function and active sites. In *Physiology of Immunoglobulins. Diagnostic and Clinical Aspects* (Ritzmann, S. E., ed.). New York: Alan Liss.

Holborow E. J., Reeves W. G. (eds) (1983). *Immunology in Medicine: A Comprehensive Guide to Clinical Immunology*, 2nd edn. London: Academic Press, and New York: Grune and Stratton.

Hubbard R. (1983). Monoclonal antibodies: Production, properties and applications. In *Topics in Enzyme and Fermentation Biotechnology* (Wiseman A. ed.), Vol. 7, pp. 196–263. Chichester: Horwood.

Kabat E. A. (1976). *Structural Concepts in Immunology and Immunochemistry*, 2nd edn. New York: Holt, Rinehart and Winston.

Milstein C. (1980). Monoclonal antibodies. *Sci. Am*; **243**: 56.

Nisonoff A. (1973). *The Antibody Molecule*. New York: Academic Press.

Nisonoff A. (1982). *Introduction to Molecular Immunology*. (Sinauer Associates) Oxford: Blackwell Scientific Publications.

Porter R. R. (1967). The structure of antibodies. *Sci. Am*; **217**: 81.

Roitt I., Brostoff J., Male D. (eds) (1985). *Immunology*. London and New York: Gower.

Sela M. (ed.) (1973). *The Antigen*, Vol. 1. New York: Academic Press.

Steward M. W. (1977). In *Immunochemistry, An Advanced Textbook* (Glynn L. E., Steward M. W., eds) Chichester: Wiley.

Steward M. W. (1983). *Antibodies: Their Structure and Function*. London: Chapman and Hall.

Turner M. W. (1977). Structure and function of immunoglobulins. In *Immunochemistry: An Advanced Textbook* (Glynn L. E., Steward M. W., eds). Chichester: Wiley.

30. Turbidimetry and Nephelometry

J. T. Whicher and C. P. Price

INTRODUCTION

When a beam of light is directed through a gas or liquid containing a suspension of particles some of the light will be scattered, a very small amount will be absorbed while the remainder will be transmitted through the medium. Tyndall in 1854 first drew attention to the fact that particles of all sizes, including molecules, will scatter and absorb light. Thus even pure liquids and dust free gases are very slightly turbid.

The interaction of light with particulate matter may be used to measure the concentration of particles in suspension by the measurement of the decrease in light transmitted (turbidimetry) or of the light scattered (nephelometry). In addition, as large particles scatter more light than small ones, the amount of light scattered by a known concentration of particles

may be used to measure their average molecular mass.

In clinical chemistry laboratories nephelometry and turbidimetry are most widely used to measure the concentrations of proteins after reaction with specific antibodies to form light-scattering complexes. More recently immunochemical techniques using the agglutination of particles coated with antibody or antigen have given rise to the so-called particle-enhanced light-scattering immunoassays. The techniques may also be used to measure total protein in body fluids after precipitation with denaturing reagents and total mucopolysaccharides after forming complexes with organic compounds. In the past nephelometry was used to measure the concentration of light-scattering lipoprotein particles in plasma.

PRINCIPLES OF NEPHELOMETRY AND TURBIDIMETRY

All molecules scatter light to some extent. Light, in common with other forms of electromagnetic radiation, will induce oscillation of electron clouds within a molecule in synchrony with the wavelength of the incident radiation. This results in the re-radiation of electromagnetic energy of the same wavelength from the particle in all directions. For very small particles of greatest dimension less than 1/20 of the wavelength of the incident radiation the re-radiated light waves are in phase and reinforce each other resulting in a symmetrical, though not spherical, envelope of scattered light (Fig. 1). A particle of greater size acts

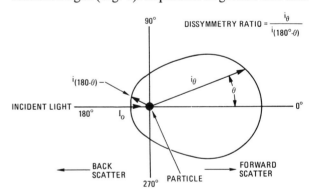

Fig. 1 The angular distribution of light scattered by a particle of a diameter similar to or less than the wavelength of the incident light. (From Kusnetz J., Mansberg H. P. (1978). Optical considerations: nephelometry. In *Automated Immunoanalysis*, Part 1 (Ritchie R. F., ed.) p. 1. New York: Marcel Dekker.)

as a number of randomly spaced point sources and destructive interference between light arising from different sites within the particle will occur resulting in maxima and minima of re-radiated light. As the particle increases in size more light is scattered at a forward angle and the asymmetric re-radiation of light may be used for measuring particle dimension.

Rayleigh in 1881 and 1910, Debye in 1915 and Mie in 1908 derived the mathematical basis for the light scattering of particles of any size and shape. For small particles of size less than $1/20$ of the wavelength of the incident light the intensity I_θ of the scattered light conforms to the following relationship.

$$I_\theta = I_0 \frac{8\pi^4\alpha^2}{\lambda^4 r^2}(1 + \cos^2\theta)$$

where I_θ, intensity of scattered light; I_0, intensity of incident light; λ, wavelength of incident light; θ, angle at which scatter is measured; α, polarizability (ease with which electron cloud will oscillate upon excitation); r, distance at which the light intensity is measured.

The most important feature of the concepts are that the intensity of the scattered light is low relative to the incident light intensity and is dependent on the angle at which it is measured and the wavelength of the incident light. For a suspension of particles the total amount of scattering depends on these characteristics and also on the concentration of particles, the scattering of solvent molecules and absorption of re-radiated light. Since the intensity of scattered light is proportional to $1/\lambda^4$ then blue light ($\lambda = 450\,nm$) is scattered much more than red light ($\lambda = 650\,nm$). It is for this reason that when white light is scattered by dust or smoke it appears blue (that is why the sky is blue); red light will be transmitted through such suspensions resulting in the characteristic colour of a sunset.

The light transmitted through a suspension of particles is the incident light energy less the radiation consumed in inducing oscillation of electron clouds and by reflection from particle surfaces. Energy is also lost by conversion to electromagnetic radiation of other wavelengths (Raman Shift). Thus, in turbidimetry, the light transmitted through the particulate suspension is measured and compared with the light transmitted through the solvent alone; the difference, i.e. the light 'absorbed', is related to particle concentration.

APPLICATIONS OF NEPHELOMETRY

Molecular Mass Measurement

If the dimension of a scattering particle is less than $\lambda/20$ then the scattered light waves arising from any part of the particle cannot be more than $\lambda/10$ out of phase and are then additive. The total amplitude of the scattered light is proportional to the number of point sources and thus to the volume and hence mass of the particle. For a random dispersion of n particles of mass M the total amount of light scattered is proportional to nM^2.

Light scattering measurements become easier as particle size increases up to $\lambda/20$. It is thus a useful technique for measuring particles of size 20–25 nm

(using light of $\lambda = 600\,nm$). Much larger particles can in fact also be studied by current techniques but scatter light much more at a forward angle. This dissymmetry ratio may in itself be used to study particle size and characteristics.

Particle Concentration Measurement

A random suspension of particles creates incoherent scattering with no definite destructive or reinforcing interferences. The total amplitude of the scattered light is proportional to the square root of the number of scattering particles. Since the intensity of a light wave is proportional to the square of its amplitude the total intensity of the scattered light is proportional to the number of particles. This relationship holds true only if there are sufficiently few particles in the suspension to avoid self-absorbtion and reflection and if the particles are of approximately constant size and shape.

The measurement of scattered light, nephelometry, may thus be used as a method of measuring particles in very dilute suspensions. Under these conditions the relationship between the concentration of particles and the intensity of scattered light is linear over a very wide range but the intensity of light scattered is very low (about 10^{-4} of the incident light intensity). Such systems require high incident-light intensity, preferably of short wavelength (scattering is proportional to $1/\lambda4$), sensitive photodetectors and cuvettes designed to minimize reflected light from glass air interfaces. As most of the particles which we are interested in measuring are in the region of between 35–50 nm in diameter, about $1/10$ of the wavelength of the incident light, they scatter much more light at forward angles, requiring suitable optics. The major problems of nephelometry for the measurement of particles present in, or generated within, biological fluids are the presence of endogenous light-scattering molecules such as proteins and lipids. In addition reagents must be dust-free as large particles of this type produce enormous amplitudes of scattered light from the many point sources within them. It is this background or blank scatter that limits the sensitivity of nephelometry.

APPLICATIONS OF TURBIDIMETRY

Particle Concentration Measurement

The decrease in light transmitted through a suspension of particles, turbidimetry, may similarly be used for the measurement of their concentrations. As the amount of light 'absorbed' is very small the major problem arises in the ability to detect a small change in intensity of light over a high background level. In recent years this has been overcome by the use of microprocessors which are able to subtract the high intensity of background light while retaining sensitivity. The optimal particle concentrations for turbidimetry are higher than for nephelometry as self absorption of scattered light and reflection contribute usefully to the total light absorbed. Not surprisingly the relationship of absorption to concentration of particles is not linear and typically the absorbance ranges used in assays are from 0·005 to 0·3 absorbance units.

OPTICAL IMMUNOASSAYS

Macromolecular antigens may be measured by their ability to complex with specific antibody directed against them and to form complexes which, because of their increased size, scatter or 'absorb' much more light than antibody or antigen alone. Alternatively antigen or antibody may be attached to particles or protein cores which are agglutinated causing increased light scattering or 'absorption'—the particle-enhanced immunoassays.

The Antibody–Antigen Reaction

Protein antigens have a large number of antigenic determinants which, when injected into animals, result in the production of polyclonal antiserum containing a wide range of antibody species in the blood. The spectrum of antibodies produced determines the specificity of the antiserum prepared from this blood and represents the characteristic set of determinants for a given macromolecule. Cross-reactivity will of course occur if any of the antigenic determinants are shared with another substance. In addition each determinant will elicit a spectrum of antibodies which bind with varying degrees of tightness (affinity). The overall binding constant (avidity) for all the antibody molecules in the antiserum determines the speed with which the reaction will occur and the net amount of complex formed. This is because there is continuous association and disassociation of antibody molecules and their respective antigens. At any moment more high-affinity antibodies will be bound to their antigenic determinants than low affinity ones.

When antigen is added to a solution of antibody in excess, complexes will be formed beginning with simple binary complexes of antibody and antigen leading to one antigen molecule surrounded by several antibody molecules. For protein antigens of molecular weight less than 10^6 daltons it is unlikely that more than 2–5 antibody molecules will bind to the antigen owing to steric exclusion (IgG has a molecular weight of 150 000 daltons). For a given antibody–antigen system, complexes are of a relatively constant size, in the region of 35–50 nm. Such complexes scatter more light than unreacted antibody and antigen and, because they have a particle size : wavelength ration of between 0·13 and 0·4, show a high dissymmetry ratio with much more forward scatter.

As more antigen is added to the solution more free antibody molecules will be consumed and there will be crosslinking between the complexes forming larger lattices. As the size of complex grows less light will be scattered; the decrease in light scattered that is seen with increasing size of complex will depend in part on the angle of measurement. Furthermore there is a different relationship seen between light absorbed and complex size compared with light scattered. The increasing signal obtained by adding antigen to antibody will thus plateau; addition of further amounts of antigen will lead to dissociation of the lattice-complex due to competition from excess antigen. The antigen concentration at which this plateau occurs will not necessarily be the same when the complex is monitored by the measurement of turbidity or light scattered at a given angle. Eventually small complexes are formed of one antibody and two antigen molecules which, owing to their small size, scatter less light. This phenomenon gives rise to the characteristic appearance of the precipitin curve which is seen both for the formation of antibody–antigen precipitates and for the formation of light-scattering complexes (Fig. 2). It is worth noting that at the anti-

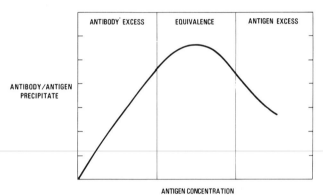

Fig. 2 The precipitin curve generated by adding increasing amounts of antigen to a solution of antibody and measuring antibody–antigen complexes by nephelometry. (From Whicher J., Blow C. (1980). *Ann. Clin. Biochem*; **7**: 170.)

gen concentration associated with maximum lattice formation (the plateau or 'equivalence point') the lattices are prone to aggregation with the formation of a visible precipitate and a greater tendency to sediment.

It is clear that in order to measure antigen in a solution and to obtain a positive dose–response relationship there must be an excess of antibody in the system. Antigen excess must be avoided, if possible, as it may provide a comparable signal at a high antigen concentration to that of a low concentration and thus invalidate the assay.

The formation of antibody–antigen complexes progresses rapidly on initiation of the reaction with the peak rate of increase of light scattering or absorption occurring between 20 s and 1 min (Fig. 3). The rate of reaction will depend upon the avidity of the antiserum, high-affinity antibodies binding much more rapidly than those of low affinity.

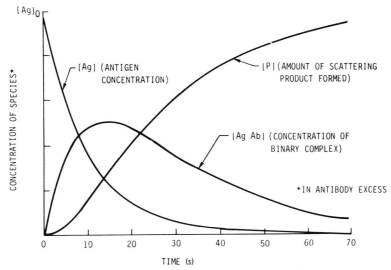

Fig. 3 Time-dependent changes in concentration of antigen, binary antigen–antibody complex, and large light-scattering complexes in an immunoprecipitin reaction. (From Anderson R. J., Sternberg J. C. (1978). A rate nephelometer for immunoprecipitin measurement of serum protein. In *Automated Immunoanalysis* Part 2 (Ritchie R. F., ed.) p. 409. New York: Marcel Dekker.)

After a period of time, when the light-scattering signal has apparently reached equilibrium, there is a balance between continuing formation of complexes, decreasing sensitivity of detection due to growth of larger complexes, and a loss of complex from solution due to precipitation. After extended periods of time there is a gradual formation of larger complexes due to non-specific agglutination with sedimentation from the suspension and decreased light scatter (Fig. 4).

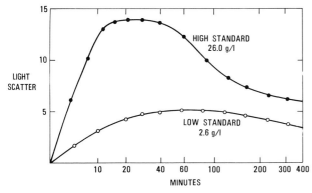

Fig. 4 Time course for the development and disappearance of light scattering complexes in a nephelometric IgG assay. (From Whicher J., Blow C. (1980). *Ann. Clin. Biochem*; **7**: 170.)

It has been shown that when the reactants in a fluid-phase antibody–antigen reaction are identical the rate of complex formation is apparently faster when monitoring the light scattered at 90° than when measuring the light passing through the solution, namely the turbidity. Monitoring the light scattered at an angle such as 90° is thought to favour smaller

complexes; destructive light scattering gradually increasing as the complexes grow in size. Turbidimetric monitoring favours larger complexes, with sensitivity to complex size increasing with the wavelength of the incident light.

Studies have shown that the peak rate of formation of optically interactive complexes relates to antigen concentration in a very similar way to the relationship between the amount of complex formed after a fixed period of time. This produces the so-called 'kinetic' precipitin curve and forms the basis for rate-of-reaction, optical immunoassays.

Time Frame for Monitoring the Antibody–Antigen Reaction

Antigen concentration may be measured in three ways.

1. Kinetic assays depend upon the measurement of peak rate which is related, though not linearly, to antigen concentration. The kinetic 'precipitation curve' is similar to that of end-point measurement but has a shorter antibody-excess time, a narrower peak of equivalence and a steeper antigen-excess slope. There is a lag phase before peak rate of reaction occurs which varies with antigen concentration (Fig. 5), thus necessitating continuous monitoring of the reaction with electronic differentiation to identify and record peak rate whenever it may occur.
2. Two-point or fixed-interval assays utilize a first absorbance reading, taken immediately after mixing the reactants (to give a blank reading), and a second reading taken after a precisely

such particles by prior treatment with polymers followed by centrifugation (thus increasing assay time and cost). Nevertheless it is usually necessary to measure blank scattering or turbidimetry though this is obviated in kinetic and two-point assays.

Detection of Antigen Excess

It is desirable that optical immunoassays are designed in such a way that antigen excess does not occur. For the majority of proteins the range of concentrations encountered in test samples is sufficiently small that, given antisera of good titre and affinity, an assay can be designed that allows all samples to fall on the antibody-excess side of the curve. This is shorter in kinetic assays and provides a somewhat narrower assay range for these systems.

Monoclonal immunoglobulins, C-reactive protein and β_2-microglobulin in urine are examples of proteins which span such a wide range of concentration as to present difficulties. The simplest approach to antigen-excess detection in both kinetic and endpoint systems is to assay samples at two dilutions when the absence of a positive dose–response relationship indicates antigen excess. Another commonly used method is to add more antibody or antigen to the reaction mixture and to look for an increment in signal, either immediately in a kinetic system, or after a further period of incubation in an endpoint system. Antigen-excess detection may be time consuming and costly in reagents but is aided by automatic reassay of samples in some analytical systems. It may be possible in some systems to detect antigen excess by computer analysis of the rate curve.

INSTRUMENTATION FOR NEPHELOMETRY

The design of instruments to obtain sensitive immunonephelometric assays has depended on an understanding of the physics of light scattering. Very simple instruments designed primarily for fluorimetry have been successfully used, though with limited sensitivity, whereas purpose-built instruments have attained sensitivities of 0·5 mg of antigen/l for both endpoint and kinetic assays.

A sensitive nephelometer must measure scattered light of very low intensity, if possible at a forward angle (due to the high dissymmetry ratio of antibody–antigen complexes), with a minimal interference from transmitted light and light reflected from surfaces within the cuvette compartment. Collimated high-intensity light is required as the proportion of incident light scattered is very small and stray light must be avoided. Conventional light sources such as tungsten bulbs, mercury discharge lamps and xenon arcs require slits and lenses of varying complexity to minimize stray light. Photomultiplier tubes are used for light detection and usually employ filters to remove spurious light generated by fluorescence within the sample. The helium neon laser provides a cheap source of light of high intensity without the problems of cooling. Unfortunately the long-wavelength red light, produced at 632·8 nm, is not scattered as much as short-wavelength light. The optimal wavelength for scatter of antibody–antigen complexes is about 460 nm, and a xenon arc is a suitable source with its peak emission at 467 nm. In general little attention has been paid in nephelometer design to optimizing incident light wavelengths; in kinetic immunoassays it has been shown that the optimally scattered wavelength of the incident light changes as the immune complexes grow during the first seconds and minutes of reaction. This makes monochromatic light undesirable and light over a broad waveband provides more reproducible peak rates.

The angle at which the scattered light is measured has, however, received more attention and a considerable increase in sensitivity can be achieved by measurement at forward angles near to 180° to the source of incident light. Commercial nephelometers use angles between 5 and 90° to the axis of transmitted light. Another advantage of the laser is that the highly collimated beam of light allows measurement at far forward angles as the narrow beam of 0·5–0·8 mm in diameter can pass through the cuvette into a very small light trap.

A number of nephelometers employ refinements to obviate the scatter produced by large particles such as dust. These range from the use of two photomultipliers at right angles to each other which correct for the assymetric scattering of very large particles to electronic filtration capable of removing the large amplitude scatter they produce.

Kinetic nephelometers tend to be more complex than endpoint instruments. Microprocessors may be used to differentiate the scatter signal and to identify and measure the peak rate. In addition, in order to monitor the early phase of the reaction, measurement must be initiated precisely at the time of addition of antibody to antigen.

The optimal design for nephelometric measurements has been embodied in several centrifugal analysers ranging from forward angle scatter in research instruments to 90° angle scatter in commercially available instruments. The particular advantage of the centrifugal analyser includes the reproducible and rapid mixing of reactants, the ability to monitor reactions immediately after mixing and the opportunity to monitor a reaction continuously. The centrifugal analyser rotor incorporates from 20 to 39 cuvettes depending on the model; this enables several assays to be undertaken simultaneously, tests and standards being treated in an identical fashion.

Automated sample dilution, antiserum addition and antigen excess-checking are features of modern instruments. In practice, for large batches of analyses, kinetic assays tend to be rather slow owing to the delay before the peak rate occurs.

INSTRUMENTATION FOR TURBIDIMETRY

In theory any spectrophotometer can be used to measure turbidity; however, in view of the relatively small absorbance changes achieved, it is important that the instrument is capable of precise measurement with a low signal to noise ratio. The need to take an early absorbance reading after mixing and the cost of reagents have in practice led to the use of automated photometric instruments with small reaction cuvettes.

The optical systems will typically comprise a tungsten or quartz halogen light source producing a narrow light beam, an interference filter (band pass of about 10 nm) and photomultiplier. The monitoring wavelength offering maximum sensitivity is 340 nm, or lower, depending on the capabilities of the light source and the material of the reaction cuvette.

The majority of turbidimetric immunoassays have been developed on automated analysers capable of 'two point' measurements. The ideal instrument is one in which the first absorbance measurement can be made within 5 s of mixing of the reactants. The second absorbance reading is typically made between 2 and 5 min after initiating the reaction.

Early methods were developed on so-called kinetic enzyme analysers which were designed to measure small absorbance changes very precisely. These instruments were superseded by the development of the centrifugal analyser which enabled the simultaneous initiation of several reactions; furthermore centrifugal analysers were capable of absorbance measurements immediately after mixing, enabling automatic correction for sample and reagent blanks. The development of the so-called discretionary analyser has facilitated continuous reaction monitoring (kinetic assay) but instrument design has delayed the time for the first absorbance measurement. Consequently, it has been necessary in some instances to perform a separate sample blank determination.

PRACTICALITIES OF TURBIDIMETRIC AND NEPHELOMETRIC IMMUNOASSAYS

Nephelometry or Turbidimetry?

A considerable proportion of the literature on optical immunoassays has used the terms nephelometry and turbidimetry synonymously. It has been pointed out earlier in this chapter that the methods do not detect aggregates of equal size and furthermore are susceptible to different interferences. Thus, for a given set of reactants the apparent rate of reaction is quicker when monitored by measuring the light scattering at 90° than by turbidimetric monitoring. It is not surprising therefore that factors affecting the reaction rate, the equivalence point, and the method sensitivity exert their effects to a different extent in each of the systems. It is therefore important that assays are individualized both for an instrument and for the anti-

TABLE 1

FACTORS TO BE CONSIDERED WHEN ESTABLISHING A LIGHT-SCATTERING ASSAY

Position on the precipitin curve of the antigen–antibody rate range used in the assay
Assay sensitivity and range
    Instrument sensitivity
    Problem of sample blanks
    Values likely to be encountered in patient samples
Time course of the reaction
Need for polymer enhancement
Suitability of the antiserum
Economy of antiserum consumption

Source: Whicher J. T., Price C. P., Spencer K. (1983). Immuno-nephelometric and immunoturbidimetric assays for proteins, *CRC Crit. Rev. Clin. Lab. Sci.*; **18**: 213.

gen and antibody preparations. The factors to be considered when establishing assays in the laboratory are shown in Table 1.

In practice nephelometry, requiring more dilute solutions of reactants, is more economical in antiserum consumption than turbidimetry. It is also slightly more sensitive. Despite these considerations the need for specialized instruments for nephelometry and the ability of turbidimetry to be performed on many automated analysers makes nephelometry the less attractive technique.

ASSAY DETAILS

Antigen–Antibody Ratio. It is essential to establish the shape and characteristics of the precipitin curve for a given antibody–antigen system. This is generally done by taking a series of dilutions of antibody and assaying a range of antigen concentrations in each. It can be seen in Fig. 7 that the curve for antiserum at a dilution of 1/320 passes into antigen excess at 25 units of antigen concentration. As would be

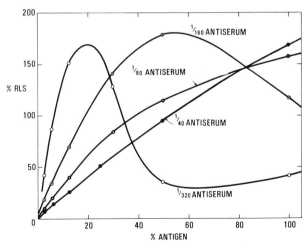

Fig. 7 Nephelometric assay for prealbumin showing reference curves for a series of dilutions of antigen performed in different concentrations of antibody. (From Whicher J., Blow C. (1980) *Ann. Clin. Biochem*; **7**: 170.)

This is a laser technique that monitors the Brownian movement of particles in a medium and is sensitive to the change in particle size. As the particle size increases due to antibody–antigen reaction the spectral line width of the scattered laser light is broadened. The measurements are based on the temporal fluctuations about the mean value rather than the intensity of the scattered light. As in the case of particle counting, a dedicated piece of equipment is required for this type of method.

Application of Enhanced Immunoassays

At the present time enhanced light-scattering immunoassay principles have been employed for the measurement of proteins at sample concentrations in the range 1–2000 $\mu g/l$, and for the measurement of haptens and small peptides.

Direct agglutination techniques monitoring at 340 nm have been described for several proteins; an assay range of 0·1–10 mg/l can be readily attained. The detection limit of the approach has been shown to be in the region of 10 $\mu g/l$.

The light-scattering inhibition assays have been described using nephelometric and turbidimetric monitoring. The single particle systems are capable of measuring free hapten levels in the concentration range upward from 1 $\mu mol/l$. Dual-particle reagent systems are capable of detecting hapten levels down to a sample concentration of 0·25 nmol/l.

Particle-counting techniques employ longer incubation periods but demonstrate similar sensitivity to the enhanced light-scattering assays. Similarly quasi-elastic scattering immunoassay techniques employ lengthy incubation periods but demonstrate similar sensitivity.

OTHER QUANTITATIVE ASSAYS BASED ON NEPHELOMETRY AND TURBIDIMETRY

Measurement of Macromolecular Precipitates

The turbidity produced by precipitation of proteins with denaturing agents such as sulphosalicylic acid and trichloroacetic acid has been used for many years for measuring the total protein content of urine and CSF. Particle size is very variable and depends upon the concentration of denaturant, ionic strength and the type of proteins present in the solution. In general such systems operate better in the presence of high ionic strength giving more constant particle size. It is, however, for these reasons that such methods show poor precision and accuracy. In recent years these tests have been modified to allow nephelometric measurement of the precipitates by using much more dilute solutions of protein. Under these conditions the precipitated protein particles are more constant in size and aggregation does not occur as rapidly.

Several turbidimetric techniques have been devised for the detection of abnormal quantities of globulins, particularly immunoglobulins; such tests include zinc and thymol turbidity procedures. Most of these tests have been superseded by more specific immunoassay techniques.

The level of fibrinogen in plasma may be determined using a salt precipitation technique with ammonium sulphate or sodium sulphate as precipitant.

The total serum lipids may be measured by turbidimetry following extraction with solvent and subsequent reaction with dioxane and sulphuric acid. Alternatively, the serum can be diluted with a low concentration phenol solution causing precipitation of the lipid with proteins remaining in solution.

Mucopolysaccharides may be precipitated from serum by complex formation with such substances as cetyl pyridinium chloride. Assays for total mucopolysaccharides based on this have been developed utilizing both nephelometry and turbidimetry.

Lectin–Protein Complexes

A number of lectins complex to the oligosaccharide side-chains of proteins forming macromolecular particles which may be measured by nephelometry and turbidimetry. Concanavalin A has a specific affinity for α-D-glucose residues on a number of proteins and has been used to measure acute-phase glycoproteins. Though these methods now have little direct clinical application they provide useful research tools in the study of such interactions.

Lipoprotein Particles

Both chylomicroms and VLDL scatter light and nephelometric assays have been used to determine their concentrations in plasma. By passing samples through graded filters it is possible to isolate particles that approximate to chylomicroms, VLDL and LDL. Thorpe and Stone made use of a simple nephelometer, together with cholesterol and triglyceride measurements to develop a comprehensive system for identifying different types of hyperlipidaemia. It is however no longer widely used, as most of the clinically relevant abnormalities can be recognized by simple quantitation of cholesterol and triglycerides followed by visual examination of the samples. After storage overnight the chylomicra rise to the surface and appear as a cream; VLDL produce a turbidity throughout, while LDL do not produce visible turbidity.

Other Assay Types

Total sulphur and sulphates in urine can be determined by conversion into barium sulphate. The barium sulphate precipitate is stabilized with polyethylene glycol 6000 to improve method performance characteristics.

The measurement of lysozyme is based on its action on bacterial cell membranes, the disruption of the membrane and lysis of the bacteria being monitored turbidimetrically.

Enzymes such as lipase and amylase have been measured by their ability to decrease the turbidity of suspensions of lipids or starch. Bacterial sensitivity testing has been done by measuring bacterial growth using turbidimetry.

SUGGESTED REFERENCES AND FURTHER READING

Cambiaso C. L., Leck A. E., de Steenwinkel F. *et al.* (1977). Particle counting immunoassay (PACIA). I. A general method for the determination of antibodies, antigens and haptens. *J. Immunol. Methods*; **18**: 33.

Deverill I., Jefferis R., Ling N. R., Reeves W. G. (1981). Monoclonal antibodies to human IgG: reaction characteristics in the centrifugal analyser. *Clin. Chem*; **27**: 2044.

Galvin J. P. (1983). Particle enhanced immunoassays—a review. In *Diagnostic Immunology: Technology Assessment and Quality Assurance*, pp. 18–30. Skokie, Illinois: College of American Pathologists.

Price C. P., Spencer K., Whicher J. T. (1983). Light scattering immunoassay of specific proteins: A review. *Ann. Clin. Biochem*; **20**: 1.

Ritchie R. F. (ed.) (1978). *Automated Immunoanalysis.* New York: Marcel Dekker, two volumes.

Whicher J. T., Price C. P., Spencer K. (1983). Immunonephelometric and immunoturbidimetric assays for proteins. *CRC Crit. Rev. Clin. Lab. Sci*; **18**: 213.

31. Radioimmunoassay
J. D. Teale

INTRODUCTION

There can be few analytical techniques to have made a greater impact on clinical biochemistry than radioimmunoassay (RIA) and its variants. During the 10 years since the appearance of the first edition of this volume, there has been a continuing expansion of the number and diversity of analytes subjected to measurement by some type of immunoassay. It has been estimated that in 1975 the annual number of RIA tests performed worldwide was approximately 50 million. A decade later that figure has increased tenfold.

In theory, RIA may be used for the measurement of any substance to which an antibody can be raised. More than 400 compounds of various types have been subjected to quantitative analysis by RIA, mainly in the areas of clinical diagnosis and research. Approximately 100 assays are considered to have important routine diagnostic uses in the measurement of peptide hormones, non-peptide hormones and drugs. Historically, RIA owed its success to its discovery at a time when progress in hormone assay development was limited to bioassays which, whilst providing a measure at least of biological activity, are time consuming, technically demanding and poorly reproducible. The first RIA, published by Yalow and Berson in 1960, was a sensitive and specific technique for measuring insulin levels.

The basis of the techniques involves the use of a saturable binding agent, an antibody, which is incubated in a restricted quantity sufficient to bind a fraction of added labelled antigen. The introduction of unlabelled antigen will, by competitive inhibition, reduce the amount of antibody-bound label to a degree relative to the concentration of unlabelled antigen. The specific nature of the antigen–antibody interaction permits the direct measurement of a particular antigen in a complex mixture of proteins such as is present in serum. Most other techniques require tedious and exhaustive preliminary extraction and purification procedures. Since the early assays, sensitivity has increased with improvement of the production of reagents, particularly antibodies. Following the production of antibodies to naturally immunogenic peptides, steroids were used as haptens by attachment to carrier proteins. This broadened the scope of RIA to include many other non-protein compounds for which antibodies could thereby be produced.

The quality of each antiserum predetermines assay characteristics, and methods of immunization have evolved which are aimed at raising antibodies of high avidity. The avidity constant of the binding reagent can be regarded as the reciprocal of the sensitivity potential of the assay, when optimized for the available reagents, so that an avidity constant of 10^{-12} l/mol is equivalent to a detection limit of 10^{-12} mol/l. In this usage sensitivity is defined as the minimal detection limit of an assay—the least amount of antigen that is statistically distinguishable from zero antigen. Receptor sites used as binding agents have a high avidity for a hormone, so conferring great sensitivity on an assay. Binding proteins used in competitive binding protein assays tend to have lower avidity constants (10^7–10^8 l/mol) than immunoglobulins so giving a minimum detection limit of 10^{-7}–10^{-8} mol/l.

The development of isotope labelling techniques has meant the availability of labelled compounds with high specific radioactivity that are suitable for RIA. The most important single contribution in this respect was the description by Hunter and Greenwood in 1962 of a safe and simple peptide iodination technique involving an oxidizing agent, chloramine T. Variations on this method have since been introduced, aimed mainly at reducing the damage which occurs during exposure of the antigen to the oxidizing agent whilst maintaining the high incorporation of isotope.

Both advantages and disadvantages of RIA derive from the radioactive nature of the tracer. Objections to the use of radioisotopes may influence the future development of RIA as much as any other factor, although the action on living tissue by ionizing radiation from nuclear decay is of minor significance to operatives performing routine assays, because very small quantities of radioactivity are involved. However, for those who prepare iodinated compounds the risks are potentially more severe and cumulative. These dangers have prompted restrictive laws and regulations for the distribution, use and disposal of radioactive substances.

The shelf-life of RIA reagents is limited solely by the physical half-life of the isotope incorporated into the label and by label degradation induced by radioactive decay. However, radioactivity can be detected with great sensitivity even though for every 100 disintegrations of ^{125}I that occur in a minute, $1 \cdot 25 \times 10^7$ atoms remain unchanged. A minimum of the order of 10^5–10^7 atoms are needed to produce a signal which is distinguishable from the background count. Therefore, although radiolabels are relatively inefficient in only producing a detectable signal from such a potentially large source, they do provide a signal which cannot have arisen from any other source. Unlike the majority of non-isotope labels the activity of radiolabels is unaffected by the physico-chemical environment imposed by such mixtures as serum, plasma, urine, saliva and amniotic fluid. This property of RIA, probably above all others, makes it applicable to the measurement of almost any hormone, drug or protein found in any of the above-mentioned fluids.

Very often developers of immunoassays opt initially for radiolabelling for antiserum assessment and subsequently in the establishment of assay procedures. These then become quoted as reference methods in many reports describing the production of alternative (non-radioisotopic) immunoassays. Most alternative-label immunoassays have taken much longer to become established in routine clinical biochemistry than did the original RIA methods. Even current practice sees almost the sole use of non-isotopic immunoassays in the field of low-molecular-weight drug and steroid measurement and for this purpose reliance has been placed on the availability of many commercial kits rather than on the development of in-house methods. To date RIA has remained the first choice option for the measurement of many peptide hormones.

PRINCIPLE OF RIA

The term radioimmunoassay usually implies competitive (saturation) analysis as distinct from excess reagent systems which are termed immunoradiometric methods. The following equation represents the fundamental reaction on which the RIA technique is based.

$$Ag + Ag^* + Ab \underset{k_2}{\overset{k_1}{\rightleftharpoons}} AgAb + Ag^*Ab + Ag + Ag^*$$

The antigen (Ag) component will be either in the form of a pure standard preparation or part of the biological sample under analysis. To these is added a fixed aliquot of radiolabelled antigen (Ag*) which should display immunoreactive characteristics similar, but not necessarily identical, to those of the native compound. Following the introduction of labelled material, the immunoreactive components (Ag + Ag*) are incubated with a limited amount of binding reagent which, in the case of RIA, will be an antiserum containing specific antibodies (Ab).

The reaction, which obeys the Law of Mass Action, is usually allowed to reach equilibrium and the time taken to achieve this state will depend both on the avidity constant ($K_{av} = k_1/k_2$) of the antiserum and on the molecular characteristics of the antigen. Experimentally determined optimum incubation conditions also facilitate the attainment of equilibrium and for most assays high avidity antibodies are available.

Two species of labelled material will be present in the incubate when equilibrium has been reached.

Since total antigen concentration is greater than antibody binding site concentration, all binding sites should be occupied by antigen, a proportion of which is labelled. The antibody-bound fraction is thereby distinct from the free (non-antibody-bound) fraction. The final assay requirement is to devise a method of separating these two fractions by a procedure which will not interfere with the established equilibrium.

Once complete physical isolation of the free and antibody-bound fractions of label has been achieved, the amount of radioactivity present in either fraction can be measured. This value, as well as being related to the antibody concentration and the avidity constant, will be related to the amount of antigen present. Since the concentrations of antibody and labelled antigen are kept constant the amount of label bound will vary only through changes in the ratio of labelled to unlabelled antigen, brought about by changes in the concentration of antigen from standard or unknown samples. When the antibody-bound label is measured the response will have an inverse relationship with the added dose of antigen.

By the construction of a dose–response curve, in which increasing amounts of standard antigen are introduced into the optimized incubation system containing fixed amounts of label and antibody, the decrease in antibody-bound label may be plotted against standard antigen concentration in the incubate. Treatment of unknown samples under similar conditions will yield a value for antibody-bound label for each sample. It is then necessary to read off the amount of standard antigen corresponding to that value.

In summary, the four basic requirements for an RIA system are an antibody to the compound to be measured, the availability of a radioactively labelled form of the compound, a method whereby antibody bound tracer can be separated from unbound tracer, and standard unlabelled material.

LABEL PRODUCTION

Types of Radioactivity

Radioisotopes are used for labelling compounds to be detected by RIA. The incorporation of atoms emitting either β or γ-radiation have been the most widely developed techniques. The availability of counting equipment which can detect accurately small amounts of radioactivity has facilitated these procedures. Since a minute amount of a compound can be labelled to a high specific radioactivity, it is possible to measure picogram amounts of label accurately.

Several radioactive nuclides have been tried for this purpose, mainly isotopes of iodine, although others such as cobalt, selenium and indium have been used successfully. ^{131}I was used originally for insulin labelling but ^{125}I is now preferred, mainly because

of its longer half-life (60 days compared with 8 days) and because of the higher efficiency with which it can be counted. The counting procedure for γ-emitting isotopes is relatively simple. Samples are brought in close proximity to a sodium iodide crystal detector and the disintegrations counted electronically as flashes of light emitting from the crystal. Several automatic machines are available which are capable of handling several hundred samples. Multi-head gamma-counters permit the simultaneous processing of 12 or 16 samples.

In general γ-emitting labels can be counted with greater ease than β-emitters. Drugs and steroids, often difficult to iodinate, have been labelled by the incorporation of either ^3H or ^{14}C atoms. Such labels have half-lives of several years and do not suffer radiation damage. β-counting is, however, much more laborious and prone to error than γ-counting.

A further disadvantage of β-emitting labels is that they have relatively low specific radioactivities, so that in order to achieve low assay sensitivity much longer counting times are necessary. One atom of ^{125}I provides 25 times the detectable count rate given by four atoms of ^3H. For reasons of stability this is the maximum number of ^3H atoms which can be introduced into a molecule.

Iodination of Peptides

One of the key factors contributing to the rapid progress that RIA has made in its wide applicability is the relative ease with which a radiolabel can be produced. The incorporation of iodine atoms into a peptide can be simply achieved in the presence of an oxidizing agent. Equally important is that this reaction can be performed on a few μg of protein. Pure preparations of newly discovered peptide hormones may be available only in amounts barely sufficient to raise antibodies and therefore iodination methods requiring only μg amounts are necessarily advantageous.

Ideally an antigen should not suffer change in affinity for its antiserum through being iodinated. Some peptides may be iodinated to high specific radioactivity without affecting their immunoreactivity, others exhibit extreme lability in the presence of the more vigorous iodination reagents and alternative methods have been assessed.

There are two basic types of iodination procedure, either atoms of isotopic iodine are incorporated directly into a peptide, or a molecule, which itself may be already iodinated, is conjugated to the antigen. Some of the more commonly used examples of these methods are shown in Table 1 and will be considered in more detail.

Oxidation Methods
Chloramine T. The most frequently used oxidizing agent has been chloramine T. A typical reaction mixture contains 5 μg of peptide and 1 mCi of Na^{125}I in

TABLE 1
IODINATION METHODS

Direct

Oxidizing reagent	Reaction inhibitor
Chloramine T	Metabisulphite, cysteamine (1)
Lactoperoxidase/peroxide	Azide (2)
Iodogen	None required
N-bromosuccinimide	Dilution
Hypochlorite	Metabisulphite, cysteamine

Conjugation

Bolton–Hunter reagent (3)
Histamine, tyramine (3)

(1) Reducing agents
(2) Enzyme inhibitor
(3) Conjugation before or after iodination.

50 μl phosphate buffer, pH 7·4. The addition of 50 μg chloramine T to initiate the reaction is followed almost immediately by 120 μg sodium metabisulphite, which neutralizes the chloramine T and reduces any unreacted atomic ^{125}iodine back to ^{125}iodide.

Several variations now exist on this basic method. An important disadvantage of chloramine T is the damage it can inflict upon a hormone even during the few seconds of reaction time. Equally disruptive may be the effect of the reducing agent. The labelled peptide is exposed to an excess of reducing agent for a much longer period than the few seconds of reaction time. Less damaging alternatives to metabisulphite are cysteine and cysteamine.

Lactoperoxidase. A frequently used alternative to chloramine T has been an enzyme-mediated iodination. Oxidation by lactoperoxidase with peroxide has proved as efficient in ^{125}I incorporation as chloramine T. The reaction can be controlled by sequential additions of peroxide and although this system initially seemed to yield labelled proteins of high immunoreactivity no obvious improvement in deterioration during storage has been observed when compared with chloramine T preparations. Use of solid-phase lactoperoxidase is viewed as beneficial in facilitating the removal of the iodinated enzyme generated during the iodination reaction. The reaction is terminated by the addition of azide to inhibit the enzyme activity.

Iodogen. The compound 1,3,4,6-tetrachloro-3,6-diphenyl glycouril is water-insoluble and therefore has minimal effects on peptide integrity. The procedure involves coating the interior of the reaction vessel by introduction of a solution of Iodogen dissolved in an organic solvent. After drying, iodinations proceed by addition of peptide and radioiodide. The reaction may be stopped by removal of the mixture from the vessel.

N-Bromosuccinimide, hypochlorite. These compounds are mild oxidizing agents found to be beneficial under certain conditions and for some peptides, but incorporation may be low.

Comparative studies which have examined the effectiveness of the various oxidizing iodination reactions indicate that under optimum conditions each reagent will promote sufficient radioiodine incorporation into any peptide. Some peptides are more susceptible to damage than others but in all cases labels tend to deiodinate on storage. Repurification may be required if it is desirable to maintain maximum immunoreactivity.

Conjugation Methods. These techniques eliminate contact between hormone and oxidizing or reducing agents. There are also indications that radioiodine can be as noxious as oxidizing agents in causing peptide damage. The principle therefore is to preiodinate another compound which can be readily attached to the hormone in a stable covalent link. One compound which fulfils the requirements is 3-(*p*-hydroxyphenyl)propionic acid *N*-succinimide ester. Following chloramine T iodination the labelled ester is extracted into solvent, evaporated to dryness and the simple reaction of hormone with the residue results in the formation of peptide bonds between amine groups on the hormone and the ester. The immunoreactivity of these labelled preparations has been shown to be higher than those produced by direct chloramine T iodination. Of additional importance is that this technique permits the iodination of peptides which lack tyrosine residues.

Critical Factors

All the previously described iodination procedures have been concerned with reactions in which iodine is incorporated into tyrosine residues of the peptide. Mono- or di-iodotyrosine may be formed although labels contain almost entirely the mono-iodinated form. The iodine atoms substitute in the ortho-position to the phenolic hydroxyl group of tyrosine. The physical size of the iodine atom, being approximately equivalent to a benzene ring, may alter the configuration of a hormone, particularly when overiodination has occurred. This may result in a loss of immunoreactivity, especially if a tyrosine residue is part of an immunoreactive site (antigenic determinant). Under different conditions of ionic strength and pH, histidine, tryptophan or sulphydryl groups may be iodinated. The specific activities of these preparations may, however, be relatively low.

Specific radioactivity may vary according to the iodination method employed but values greater than 100 μCi/μg can be achieved for most peptides using chloramine T. Achieving a high radioiodine incorporation for the benefits of low counting times and low detection limits should be weighed against the stability of the resultant label. Many published methods involve a molar ratio of hormone to oxidizing agent approaching 1:1000. However, data from a study optimizing radioiodination conditions for a glycoprotein hormone using chloramine T suggest that the molar ratio of hormone to oxidizing agent should not exceed 1:20. A higher ratio resulted in diminished immunoreactivity probably as a result of oxidative effects on the hormone. Disulphide bonds will be particularly susceptible to oxidation, resulting in disruption of the peptide molecule. At lower molar ratios of reagents specific radioactivities may be kept below $100\,\mu Ci/\mu g$. At higher specific activities some labelled preparations may exhibit decreased stability on storage.

Although a label with high specific activity may increase assay sensitivity, the avidity of the antiserum has a greater influence on this parameter. As a guide to specific activity it may be remembered that the concentration of label in an assay should be approximately the same as that of unlabelled antigen at the detection limit and that a minimum amount of radioactivity should be added to each tube in order to minimize counting errors. These requirements apply to competitive assays in which labelled and unlabelled antigens are added simultaneously. For a disequilibrium assay in which the label addition is delayed, the label concentration may be much higher than that of unlabelled antigen at the detection limit. Therefore the specific activity of the label can be correspondingly lower. On average one atom of ^{125}I incorporated per mole of hormone results in a specific activity of about $100\,\mu Ci/\mu g$ for a peptide of 20000 daltons. Since most hormones are smaller than this, the specific activities are usually much lower. Incorporation of iodine may be less than 10 atoms/100 molecules of peptide but adequate assay sensitivity is still achievable.

Purification of Labelled Peptide

Adsorption. After termination of the iodination reaction the labelled peptide can be separated from the other reactants by various means (Table 2). One of

TABLE 2
METHODS FOR THE PURIFICATION OF IODINATED PEPTIDES

Adsorption onto silica

Chromatography by gel filtration
                ion exchange
                hydrophobic interaction
                high pressure liquid separation
                affinity for specific antibodies

Electrophoresis on polyacrylamide gel

the simplest methods is to adsorb the hormone onto a solid phase such as silica. After centrifugation the supernatant, containing low-molecular-weight reactants, is discarded and the hormone eluted from the silica with an acid-alcohol wash. A similar procedure involves ion-exchange gels instead of silica.

Chromatography. Purification on molecular sieve or ion-exchange columns produces labelled preparations initially of high purity. Materials such as Sephadex or Ultrogel are often used. The grade of gel should be selected so that the hormone is eluted at the void volume (complete exclusion from gel permeation) in a sharp peak and the unreacted iodide eluted later or retained on the gel. The eluting medium should contain carrier protein to reduce glassware adsorption of the hormone. Ion-exchange media sequester inorganic ions such as free iodide. Such gels have also been used in attempts to fractionate mono- and di-iodinated peptides. The physical properties of peptides with low molecular weight will be changed to a greater degree by the incorporation of iodine atoms and therefore will be more readily separated through differences in surface charge.

Hydrophobic interaction chromatography exploits the differences in hydrophobicity between the immunoreactive iodinated peptide and its non-immunoreactive contaminants. The labelled peptide is applied to a column of substituted Sepharose and interacts with alkyl side chains. After washing off contaminants the authentic label is eluted with an aqueous buffer/organic solvent mixture.

The availability of column packing materials capable of exploiting the high resolution capacity of HPLC now means iodination mixtures can be purified in a matter of minutes and, under ideal conditions, isolation of the different iodinated species can be achieved. Even the larger pituitary peptides have been fractionated by this procedure, although the broader use has been in the purification of labelled haptens and small peptides.

Affinity chromatography holds the attraction of producing the truly immunoreactive species of label. Purified antibodies (from polyclonal or monoclonal preparations) are covalently attached to a solid matrix. The iodination mixture is reacted with the matrix and after a suitable incubation period impurities are washed free. The tracer bound to the immobilized antibodies may then be eluted by high pH, low pH, high salt or detergent solutions. Denaturation of the label may occur under the conditions required to break the antigen–antibody complex. The resultant labelled preparation may also be contaminated with antibody lost from the solid matrix during elution.

Electrophoresis. Polyacrylamide gel electrophoresis provides a system whereby bulk preparation of chemically and immunologically pure labelled peptides may be achieved. A satisfactory method of eluting the product from the gel is required.

In efforts towards greater assay sensitivity the purity of labelled hormone preparations can have beneficial influence. Originally it was acceptable simply to iodinate under optimum conditions the purest hormone preparations available. A rapid Sephadex or silica purification produced preparations at least free

tions has been derived from the production of enzyme labels in non-isotopic immunoassay development. The availability of such information facilitates the choice of alternative points of conjugation on an antigen thereby enabling potential antigenic determinants to remain exposed.

Site of Conjugation. Through the use of the many available reactions, conjugates may be produced which will influence antiserum specificity. It is well established that an antibody will recognize the part of a hapten which is furthest from the site of conjugation to the carrier. If therefore this site is part of the only point of distinction between two molecules the resultant antibodies would be raised to common determinants and could not be expected to discriminate between the compounds. The most notable example of this has been antiserum production against steroid conjugates. Originally the expedient of using the reactive groups at the 3 and 17 positions of the steroid nucleus permitted the simple formation of conjugates. However, the antisera produced did not discriminate between steroids differing in structure at the point of conjugation. Use of alternative linkage points resulted in the production of more specific antisera.

The problem of absolute specificity is greater in the case of small molecules since the antigenic determinant may be two or three times the size of the hapten molecule. Correct orientation and maximum exposure of the hapten to receptors on the antibody-producing cell membrane is, therefore, a critical influence on antibody specificity.

Type of Carrier. The most popular carriers have been albumins, together with larger protein molecules such as γ-globulins. Bovine thyroglobulin has proved highly immunogenic; because of its very high molecular weight it has the capacity to allow hundreds of haptens to be linked onto it without impairing its natural immunogenicity.

The chances of successful antibody production are higher if a protein carrier that is foreign to the species to be immunized is used for conjugation. Carriers from the same species (homologous) have proved immunogenic because of the introduction of new antigenic determinants by hapten conjugation. Response to the conjugate with homologous protein carrier is slow initially because of lack of cooperation in antibody production from carrier determinants, but subsequent boosts will raise the titre to similar values produced by foreign protein conjugates. These 'helper' determinants are found normally with heterologous carriers.

Homogeneous carriers such as poly-L-lysine or poly-L-glutamic acid have been examined in attempts to reduce antibody production against the carrier to interfere and thereby to increase production to the hapten. Such carriers appear on the whole to be much less immunogenic than random proteins.

It has been shown necessary to use the same hapten–carrier conjugate for booster immunizations, particularly when a heterologous carrier is used.

Electrostatic complexes have been formed by reaction of hapten with, for example, acetylated bovine serum albumin. Their ability to provoke antibody production to the hapten moiety remains in doubt but their usefulness in the formation of a complex between a carrier and a relatively inert hapten may be the only method available for immunogen production.

Adjuvants

The most successful, and therefore the most popular, mixture has been Freund's complete adjuvant. When adjuvant is mixed with an aqueous solution of immunogen in a ratio of greater than 2 : 1 a stable water-in-oil emulsion is formed. The optimum ratio for maximum stability can be checked by emulsifying mixtures and allowing to stand for long periods. Unstable emulsions will separate out relatively quickly. Adequate mixing of aqueous solution and adjuvant is important in creating a stable emulsion and has been assisted by the use of double-hubbed syringe connectors.

The adjuvant ingredients consist of a stabilizing emulsifier and a mineral oil, together with inactivated bacteria in the complete type. A stable emulsion permits slow release of immunogen into the sytemic circulation and continuous stimulation of the reticuloendothelial antibody-production system. The inclusion of bacteria also stimulates initial response. The type of mineral oil used in Freund's adjuvant often produces ulceration on or under the skin of laboratory animals. Ulceration will create isolation of the depot of adjuvant mixture and prevent release of the immunogen. For this reason alternative medical oils, notably the Marcol series, have been used in adjuvant mixtures. Ideally the adjuvant should provoke local inflammation without ulceration.

Partial denaturation or insolubilization of the immunogen appears to be beneficial in increasing immunogenicity. This can occur during conjugation, as already described, or can be brought about directly by mild acid hydrolysis. Emulsification in adjuvant produces further denaturation. Adsorption of an immunogen onto insoluble particles offers an alternative form of adjuvant mixture. Materials that have been used are carbon particles, aluminium hydroxide gel and polyacrylamide gel.

Route of Immunization

Intramuscular routes are the most appropriate for emulsified immunogen, particularly when using Freund's complete adjuvant.

Subcutaneous routes are often used for booster doses of emulsion but absorption into the circulation is slow and complete adjuvants often cause abcess formation.

Intradermal routes offer several advantages. The low immunogen doses permit conservation of precious material. It is reported that animals require only primary immunizations by this route, boosters having no effect on titre. Antibody production requires several months to build up to a maximum. In theory because of continuous stimulation with minute quantities of immunogen, the resultant antibodies should be of high avidity. This theory has yet to be firmly established in practice.

Other routes of immunization have been less used. Intravenous injections are the most appropriate for particulate immunogens. Intra-lymph node, intra-articular or foot pad injections are either difficult to administer or result in severe discomfort to the animal without any real advantage over other routes in antiserum quality.

Dose Levels and Schedules

A single primary immunization followed by boosters at monthly intervals has been the simplest, most successful schedule followed. Dose level may depend largely on the immunogenicity of the immunogen. Microgram quantities of peptides have produced antisera of high avidity and titre. Low, infrequent doses in general appear to have the most beneficial influence on avidity, although the antisera take time to harvest. It has been suggested that if large amounts of immunogen are injected it is quite probable that the high avidity antibodies will be selectively removed from the circulation leaving a population of mainly low avidity antibodies.

Frequent doses would produce a quicker response and may be useful in testing the immunogenicity of hapten conjugates. However, as well as avidity being adversely affected, this type of schedule results in earlier decrease in titre after several boosters. Recovery in antiserum titre may sometimes be brought about by resting the animal for several months before boosting again.

The size of each dose will depend upon the immunogen and the required quality of antiserum. In general the more immunogenic the material the smaller the dose. Hapten conjugates are usually given, therefore, in mg doses compared with μg amounts for peptides. In addition the larger animal can be given slightly larger doses.

Bleeding

Animals are usually bled between 7 and 14 days following a booster injection. Guinea pigs are bled by heart puncture, rabbits from a lateral ear vein and larger animals, such as goats and sheep, by jugular vein cannulation. The blood is allowed to clot at room temperature and the serum separated off.

Storage of Antiserum

Many serum preparations have been found to be stable for several months either frozen (at about $-22°C$) or liquid (at $4°C$). Occasionally antibodies are unstable at $-22°C$ and it may be necessary to exceed the eutectic point of saline ($-26°C$) as an added precaution. Neat serum may be frozen and thawed several times without loss of activity but, once diluted, serum should only be thawed once after freezing. When kept at $4°C$ serum should be treated with a bacteriostatic agent such as azide, merthiolate or puromycin. Freeze-drying allows diluted serum to be stored indefinitely although some loss of activity may occur during the process.

Assessment of Antiserum

Early reports suggested that it is important, especially in the development of antibodies to haptens, that individual collections of serum, particularly those following booster doses of immunogen, should be assessed primarily for specificity. It is claimed that this is necessary since specificity for the priming hapten increases during immunization. Data from other reports, however, have not confirmed this observation. Apparent changes in specificity are more likely to be caused by an increase in the titre of high avidity antibodies which will be manifest in an assay as an increase in specific binding of hapten when in competition with potentially cross-reacting derivatives. The properties of individual collections of serum from the same animal nevertheless require to be assessed.

STANDARDIZATION

The preparation of standard antigen solutions of accurate concentration represents the one factor which affects results of sample analysis more than variation in any other RIA reagent. Since label binding in the presence of sample antigen will ultimately be related to that in the presence of a known standard concentration, the accuracy of the standard concentration is the only absolute factor in the system, since the concentrations of the other assay components may vary within certain limits from assay to assay (providing they are the same in each incubate of any one assay). Factors such as specific radioactivity of label, antibody-binding capacity or phase-separation efficiency may be subject to slight variation without affecting assay performance but variation in standard solution concentration will directly alter sample values.

Reference Preparations

The preparation of pure standard solutions may appear to be a relatively simple matter in the case of steroids and drugs which are available in pure form and in large quantities, but accuracy in dispensing must still be observed. A primary solution of a compound with low molecular weight can be calibrated by the use of an independent physicochemical technique such as spectrophotometry. These solutions will be necessarily of relatively high concentration; for use in assays much lower concentrations are required. The dilutions involved may be a further source of calibration error. Serum calibrators have been accurately assessed by gas chromatography-/mass spectrometry but only in limited areas and producing limited supplies for short-term use. Such techniques are not yet widely available.

Reference preparations for many peptides and protein hormones have been painstakingly assembled and assessed by national and international organizations such as NIBSC and WHO. International Reference Preparations (IRP) are needed because of the heterogeneity of purified protein preparations. RIA methods involving antisera often of uncertain or even unknown specificities require a common calibrant which has been independently assessed and assigned a potency value. Independent assessment involves data from bioassays (when available), from ligand binding assays which use some type of biological receptor instead of antibodies, as well as from individual RIA methods.

Logistical problems of subdivision into a large number of aliquots whilst maintaining potency have been the subject of rigorous attention. Careful checks of stability under different storage conditions result in recommendations aimed at maintaining the viability of preparations. Reconstitution of the lyophilized material in an ampoule of IRP and subsequent storage of working dilutions are further potential sources of deterioration. The ultimate interpretation of RIA results, particularly measurements of peptide hormones, requires familiarity with IRP heterogeneity. With the increasing availability of recombinant-DNA techniques peptide preparations of high purity are minimizing doubts over standardization.

Matrix Preparation

For almost all RIA methods the protein concentration in each incubate exerts some degree of influence on assay performance parameters. For this reason it is essential for almost all RIA systems that the standard preparation is diluted in a matrix with similar properties to those of the medium in which the analyte will be present during analysis, such as serum, plasma, urine, saliva or CSF.

Several artificial fluids have been described for this purpose, e.g. high concentrations of a single protein (albumin, gelatin, immunoglobulins) in a buffer at the pH and ionic strength of serum. Few of these solutions have proved suitable under all circumstances. Animal serum may be adequate for some assays. The preferred procedure is the use of analyte-free human serum. The removal of endogenous analyte presents certain problems. Physiological suppression in volunteer donors may be used in some cases. Usually, however, only normal serum will be available and must be stripped of the analyte in question. Components of low molecular weight may be readily removed by adsorption onto such materials as charcoal, silica or ion-exchange resins. Care must be taken to ensure that both analyte and adsorptive medium are removed from the serum, either of which will interfere in subsequent assays. Adsorption will remove other endogenous serum constituents and therefore the product will only be approximately representative of whole serum, although in most applications it will function satisfactorily.

An alternative may be required for peptide hormones of high molecular weight which are not adsorbable by physical means. Immunoadsorption using antibodies linked to a solid-phase is the principal alternative. This system is beset with the problem of free antibodies being lost from the solid-phase and contaminating the serum leading to erroneous assay results. The efficiency of immunoadsorption is dependent upon the cross-reactivity of the antibodies. Some related peptides may not be removed and could react with an assay antiserum of different specificity.

Assessment of analyte-free serum preparations is not easily achieved. Label binding levels observed in incubates containing samples from patients known to be hormone-deficient or undergoing suppressant therapy should not be significantly different from binding in the presence of the analyte-free preparation. The data from such observations may be slow to accumulate, depending on the availability of the appropriate type of patient.

PHASE SEPARATION TECHNIQUES

The final critical stage in any RIA method is the separation of the antibody-bound fraction of antigen from that remaining free in solution. All methods involve the insolubilization of either fraction of label (free or antibody-bound) followed by sedimentation (by centrifugation, magnetism or gravity) of the insolubilized fraction. The soluble supernatant is usually then discarded by decantation or aspiration allowing the isolated sedimented pellet to be counted. The requirement for a method defining a sharp and accurate physical separation, without disruption of the antigen–antibody equilibrium, is of paramount importance if a correct determination of the relative distribution of label is to be made. Variable contamination of one fraction with label from the other will result in poor assay performance. Such errors constitute a major source of assay imprecision and bias.

Selection and testing of several separation systems is therefore needed for each RIA before it is acceptable for routine use. Differences in composition of the incubation medium, due for example to variation in protein content of each sample under analysis, may

TABLE 3
PHASE SEPARATION TECHNIQUES

Basis of method	Material used
Adsorption	
of free antigen	Coated charcoal
	Ion-exchange resin
Precipitation	
of bound antigen	
(a) chemical	Sodium sulphate
	Polyethylene glycol 6000
(b) immunological	Precipitating double
	antibody
Solid phase	
First or second antibody	Assay tubes, dextran gels
coupled to a solid matrix	glass beads, cellulose

affect the phase separation adversely and to different degrees.

Separation may also be affected by time, temperature, pH and, most significantly, technical expertise. Some non-antibody-bound antigen may be adsorbed on to the assay tube or may be trapped in the sedimented antibody-bound fraction. Radioactive impurities in the label or incomplete physical separation following adequate insolubilization and sedimentation of the antibody-bound fraction are also factors affecting efficient separation.

The alternative methods listed in Table 3 are those used currently in routine analysis and are therefore practical options in being simple and cheap and, in most cases relatively quick to perform. There are three types of system: *adsorption* of the free antigen fraction (applicable only to compounds with low molecular weight, such as drugs, steroids and peptides), *immunological precipitation* and *solid-phase sedimentation* (in which first or second antibody is linked to an inert matrix).

Adsorption

Adsorption methods are usually simple and rapid and have the capacity therefore for routine use. Particulate charcoal has been by far the most widely used type of material, finding application particularly in the RIA of smaller compounds. There are available many grades of charcoal based on particle size, but activated Norit A has been found to be almost universally acceptable. It is unusual for a simple, untreated charcoal suspension to be used, since very often a certain amount of antigen–antibody complex will adhere to untreated charcoal as well as small amounts of label non-specifically bound to other proteins. In order to ensure that only the free fraction of label is adsorbed the particulate charcoal is coated with a dextran, of molecular weight between 10 000 and 250 000 daltons, depending on the size of the antigen to be adsorbed. In theory the dextran acts as a reverse molecular sieve, permitting the smaller antigen to penetrate into and be adsorbed by the inner core

of charcoal whilst excluding the much larger antigen–antibody and non-specific antigen–protein complexes.

Most important of the pitfalls in the use of charcoal is the propensity for stripping or removal of antigen which has already bound to antibody. This problem is aggravated when a low avidity antiserum is being used. The stripping effect is partially alleviated by dextran-coating and also by maintaining the serum protein (particularly globulin) concentration in the incubate at a sufficiently high level. Furthermore, it is advisable to perform separation stages at 4°C. This should include cooling the incubates to 4°C if the reaction has not been carried out at this temperature and maintaining the incubates and the charcoal suspension at 4°C. Refrigerated centrifugation is also beneficial in this respect.

Chemical Precipitation

Several salt and solvent solutions have been used for differential precipitation of higher-molecular-weight protein components of any assay incubate. Most suffer the disadvantage of difficulties with ease of dispensing and, in the case of tritium labels, interference with liquid scintillation counting. The only compound to find general use has been polyethylene glycol (PEG) 6000 which, when added in equal volume as a 20% solution, will precipitate immunoglobulins. Partial precipitation of other proteins to which label or labelled contaminants may be bound produces high non-specific binding and therefore lower assay precision and sensitivity. PEG precipitation can be useful in assay systems which use a low titre antiserum and which cannot therefore be readily immunoprecipitated.

Double Antibody

In contrast to chemical techniques of separating free and antibody-bound fractions, there are in use several variations of an immunologically based procedure. This involves a second (double) antibody raised against IgG protein from the species in which the first antibody was produced. When used originally, the requirement was for a second antibody capable of producing an insoluble matrix after reaction with the first antigen–antibody complex. The antibody-bound fraction of label could then be isolated by centrifugation. Whilst the precipitating type of second antiserum is still in widespread use, there are now alternative procedures involving second antibodies linked to an inert solid matrix; or precipitation can be accelerated by the addition of PEG at low concentrations. These alternatives make use of second antibodies of the non-precipitating type.

Precipitating antibodies are usually raised in larger animals (donkeys, goats or sheep) by immunization with purified IgG fractions from the species in which first antiserum was produced (guinea pigs, rabbits or sheep). Titration of the second antiserum against the concentration of IgG contributed by the first antiserum must first be performed in order to establish whether relative concentrations can be achieved which are conducive to insoluble matrix formation. In the case of a first antiserum with very high titre there will be insufficient IgG present for this to occur. In this instance normal (non-immune) carrier serum must be added to facilitate the formation of a complex capable of sedimentation and subsequent isolation from its supernatant without contamination of one fraction with the other. It may sometimes be necessary to wash the insoluble pellet to remove any free labelled antigen which may be trapped within the matrix, but in most cases pellet formation can be arranged to minimize this effect and obviate the need for such a time-consuming procedure.

When the IgG concentration is at an optimum level in the incubate titration with varying amounts of second antiserum is performed. If insufficient second antiserum is added precipitation will not occur since first IgG molecules will combine with the limited number of anti-IgG molecules on a one-to-one basis. In addition, preparations of second antiserum from certain animals exhibit a so-called *pro-zone effect* which also results in non-precipitation. This phenomenon is due to an excess of second antibody compared with first antibody; when all first IgG antigenic determinants are saturated with anti-IgG molecules complexes of the non-precipitating type and of relatively low molecular weight are produced. In order for precipitation to occur therefore the correct relative concentrations of first IgG and anti-IgG must be determined by titration. At the correct relative concentrations crosslinking occurs, each first IgG molecule containing at least two antigenic determinants reacting with each of two sites on each anti-IgG molecule to form a very high-molecular-weight matrix, resulting in precipitation.

Once a satisfactory procedure has been developed this type of phase separation has wide application, particularly (1) for assays of hormones with higher molecular weight, for which the adsorptive type of separation is inappropriate; or (2) where the first antiserum is of low avidity and a less rigorous means of separation is required in order not to disturb the equilibrium between hormone antigen and antibody. A disadvantage is that the system is relatively time-consuming, involving a second incubation period. In addition second antisera are often of low titre, requiring the use of larger volumes. There may be problems with substances contained in unknown samples. Serum proteins and anticoagulants may affect precipitation and different batches of second antisera should be assessed for this type of interference.

The combined addition of double antibody and PEG is a procedure which can overcome many of the errors arising in the use of a double antibody alone. The efficiency of the double-antibody precipitation is enhanced by the addition of PEG to a final concentration of 4%. This has the effect of precipitating the soluble complexes of first and second antibodies which have not formed the insoluble complexes owing to the presence of interfering substances. Not only will this procedure improve assay performance but will permit the use of low-titre or non-precipitating second antibody which would otherwise not be considered.

Non-precipitating second antibodies can also be employed in other types of separation system. These involve chemical attachment of the anti-IgG antibody protein to inert solid matrices. Amongst the solid-phase materials used have been cellulose, cross-linked dextran gels, and glass beads. This type of reagent is relatively cheap to produce since it uses smaller amounts of second antibody than would be used for precipitation purposes and can make use of non-precipitating antiserum. However, problems may arise of a similar nature to those encountered with the simple precipitating method, namely non-specific trapping of labelled antigen by the insoluble matrix. Fortunately, with this type of stable phase, repeated washing of the pellet can be introduced (and automated) to remove non-antibody-bound contamination.

Solid Phase

The concept of this type of phase separation is similar to that for the double-antibody solid-phase system in that the antibody, in this case the first antibody, is covalently attached to a solid matrix. The insoluble materials used are those mentioned above as well as the plastic tubes in which assays are incubated. In the latter system plastic tubes are coated by simply dispensing aliquots of antiserum into them and pouring out the surplus. The protein adhering to the walls of the tubes is then incubated with the other RIA reagents. Binding to the antibodies occurs and the tubes are again drained of fluid. After the washing stage, antibody-bound label can be measured by simply counting the drained tubes for radioactivity. The main disadvantage is that batches of tubes vary in quality and must therefore be carefully selected and prepared before use. Coated-tube techniques are also limited by the relatively small surface areas of adsorbed antibody.

Larger surface areas can be produced through the use of particulate solid-phase materials. Ideally particle size should permit a large surface area for conjugation of antibody which will not sediment rapidly, but will remain in suspension for a sufficient period of time to allow the antigen–antibody reaction to proceed as near as possible to the equilibrium point. In practice there are few materials which permit this balance to be achieved and some solid-phase first antibodies will require continual mixing. Double-antibody solid-phases which are added in excess may not need prolonged mixing. After reaching equilibrium the solid-phase is sedimented to a dense pellet by centrifugation.

An alternative non-centrifugation system involves magnetizable particles. These consist of a core of iron oxide coated with various polymers to which antibodies can be readily attached. At equilibrium the incubates are simply positioned on a tray containing a magnet. After a few minutes the solid-phase is held in a sufficiently tight pellet for the tubes to be inverted and the supernatant decanted off. Several washing steps may also be rapidly and simply performed. The use of antibodies attached to insoluble particles can greatly simplify an assay procedure providing that the linked antibodies retain their viability. Often some immunoreactivity is lost during the conjugation reaction and this could be wasteful of an antiserum which may be valuable and in short supply.

ASSAY DESIGN

Theory

Theoretical concepts underlying the optimization of an RIA procedure are often secondary to practically derived data for this purpose. Computerized models have become available, themselves based on experimental data, for the establishment of optimum assay conditions. By these means the most beneficial use of the available reagents is made, in terms of maximum sensitivity, selectivity, precision and speed of analysis.

The raison d'etre of an RIA is to operate as closely as possible to its limit of detection. As a result of the availability of extremely sensitive RIA methods peptide hormones can be quantified with reasonable accuracy. In theory the most sensitive RIA is achieved as the antibody concentration tends to zero. It has also been proven mathematically that the detection limit of an assay is relatively independent of the specific radioactivity of the labelled antigen, being a function of antibody avidity and the precision with which zero (standard) ligand is measured (incubation of tracer with antiserum only). The zero precision component can be subdivided into errors arising from technical manipulations (pipetting, efficiency of separation) and from statistical counting errors.

In practice the minimum level of label which can be detected with acceptable precision will depend not only upon the antibody concentration (in turn dependent on K_{av}) but also on the specific activity of the label. This situation is particularly relevant to assay systems when labelled ligand and unlabelled ligand compete for antibody binding sites. Label concentration must be kept minimal in order that a significant degree of displacement can be detected. Specific activity then dictates the minimal level to permit counting times that are not impractically long for routine use. It is noteworthy that the introduction of multi-head gamma-counters has made a significant contribution in facilitating the increased throughput of samples and thereby permitting longer counting

times without an overall increase in the total counting time required.

It has been traditionally accepted that in the absence of unlabelled antigen, a combination of label and antibody be used at concentrations sufficient to restrict the label binding to antibody to approximately 50%. In this way antigen will always be present in excess and quite often the adoption of this system has yielded sensitive assays. It may be necessary to push the detection limit lower and there are certain procedures for achieving this end. Delayed addition of label is frequently used, particularly in a system where there is disparity in immunoreactivity between native and labelled antigens or when the specific activity of the latter is low. Hapten assay sensitivity usually does not improve by delaying label addition because equilibrium is reached more rapidly.

In the technique employing delayed addition of label two incubations are involved. The first is the reaction between unlabelled antigen (standard or unknown) and antibody. Labelled antigen is then added followed by a second, often much shorter, incubation period. The amount of label can be much greater than that which would be used for the previously described simultaneous reagent addition system for which a 50% binding label was required. In the delayed addition system the total percentage binding of the label will be much lower, but precise counting can be achieved because of the larger amount added. Although assay precision and sensitivity benefit, the delayed addition of label increases the number of manipulations involved in performing the assay resulting in longer assay times. This may be less acceptable in practical terms at a time when an important emphasis is placed on speed of availability of results.

Practice

Incubation Conditions. The association rate of antigen and antibody during incubation can be influenced by factors other than their respective concentrations. These factors include temperature, pH, ionic strength and contaminants. Incubations are usually performed in a dilute buffer medium at physiological pH. When measuring a range of antigen concentrations it is important to ensure that the ionic strength of the incubate is not affected by the addition of serum samples. Likewise assay of an extremely alkaline or acid urine sample should not produce an alteration in assay pH.

The extreme dilution of reagents, aimed at maximum assay sensitivity, can result in longer incubation times during which reagent damage can arise, particularly in label preparations. Dilute protein solutions can cause problems of adsorption to the walls of the incubation tubes. This can be alleviated in most cases by the addition of a solubilizing agent to the incubation buffer. The incubation system should therefore be designed to counteract these potentially disruptive factors.

Dilutions of reagents are made in assay diluent buffer. This consists, for example, of phosphate buffered saline at a pH between 7 and 8. Azide, or other bacteriostat, should be added to prevent bacterial contamination during prolonged incubation. A variety of proteins (bovine or human serum albumins, animal serum, γ-globulins, gelatin) have been used as carriers to prevent reagent adsorption to vessel walls. Low concentrations of detergent (Triton, Tween) have also been employed to similar effect.

Conditions of incubation such as time, temperature and incubate volume may be chosen initially on an arbitrary basis from experiences reported for similar RIA methods. The incubation temperature for most peptide RIA methods is 4°C to minimize incubation damage. Most hapten RIA methods can be carried out at room temperature. Incubate volume is kept to a workable minimum (usually less than 1 ml) since this will aid antigen–antibody interaction. Optimum incubation time can be determined by allowing the equilibrium between label and antibody to reach a plateau. Incubation time will be affected by a number of factors such as antiserum dilution and avidity, antigen concentration and molecular weight and incubation temperature.

Reagent Assessment. Having selected initial assay conditions, the first incubation system can be attempted. This is the assessment of an antiserum for antibody content by titration of the antiserum preparation with labelled antigen, from which can be constructed an antiserum dilution curve. This involves a series of incubation systems containing increasing (often doubling) dilutions of antiserum together with a constant amount (mass) of labelled antigen. The mass of label should be of the order of magnitude of the expected assay sensitivity, where possible, though early bleeds of antisera of low avidity may not permit this to be achieved initially. After phase separation, the amount of label (in terms of radioactivity) bound to antibody can be measured and expressed as a percentage of the total amount added (%B/T). The %B/T value for each dilution of antiserum is plotted against antiserum dilution to produce the type of curve shown in Fig. 1. Also shown in Fig. 1 are several other dilution curves which result from incubates containing varying amounts of label with the same successive dilutions of antiserum. It can be seen that, as the label concentration decreases (provided that the radioactivity is not limiting and can be measured precisely even at the lowest concentration) the curves begin to merge. This indicates the optimum concentration for the batch of label used and the antiserum dilution which binds 50% of label at that concentration. From Fig. 1 it can be seen that a 1:80 K dilution of antiserum will bind 50% of 10 pg of labelled antigen. The dilution of an antiserum in the solution added to the incubate, or the final dilu-

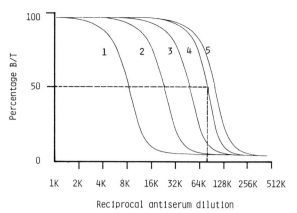

Fig. 1 Antiserum dilution curves. Increasing dilutions of antiserum incubated with decreasing amounts of labelled antigen 1, 10 ng; 2, 1 ng; 3, 100 pg; 4, 10 pg; 5, 2 pg.

tion in the total incubate volume, is referred to as the *titre* (at which 50% of the label is antibody-bound).

Some information on the immunoreactivity of the label preparation can also be gained from Fig. 1. In the presence of excess antiserum 100% of the label should be antibody-bound. Less than 100% binding will indicate the presence of radioactive, non-immunoreactive material and further purification of the label may be necessary.

Further assessment of a label preparation for damage may be achieved by construction of *standard curves*. First the normal assay standard curve is produced by the addition of increasing amounts of unlabelled antigen to a series of incubates, each of which contains label at its previously determined optimum amount (10 pg) and antiserum at a dilution (1:80 K) sufficient to bind 50% of the label. A second series of tubes, containing the same dilution of antiserum, will contain increasing amounts of label. After calculation of %B/T for each concentration of added antigen (labelled or unlabelled) curves can be plotted (Fig. 2). If the two curves are superimposable, label (Ag*) and native antigen (Ag) have identical antibody-binding characteristics. If the curve from incubations of Ag* and antiserum alone exhibits a flatter slope than that for Ag additions, a loss of affinity, probably due to alterations during labelling, is indicated. A further comparison of affinities of Ag* and Ag for antibody binding sites can be carried out as displayed in Fig. 3. This shows three series of antiserum dilutions to each of which has been added (1) a low amount of Ag*, (2) a high amount of Ag* and (3) a low amount of Ag* plus sufficient Ag to make the total (Ag* + Ag) equal to the high amount of Ag* in (2). If curves 2 and 3 are superimposable Ag* and Ag have equal affinities for the antibody.

The specific activity of the label (radioactivity/unit mass) can be assessed by relating in Fig. 2 the fall in %B/T produced by the addition of an unknown amount of label with the amount of unlabelled antigen producing the same decrease in %B/T. Thus,

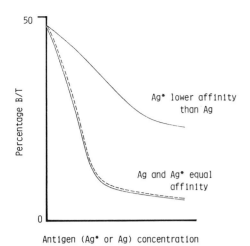

Fig. 2 Standard curves. Decrease in percentage label binding with increasing concentrations of labelled or unlabelled antigen.

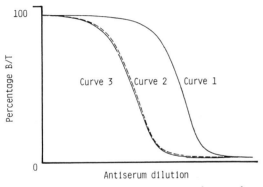

Fig. 3 Antiserum dilution curves. Increasing dilutions of antiserum incubated with 0·1 ng labelled antigen (curve 1), 1·0 ng labelled antigen (curve 2) or 0·1 ng labelled and 0·9 ng unlabelled antigen (curve 3).

the mass of antigen in that aliquot of label can be calculated and since the radioactivity in the aliquot can be accurately measured it is then a simple matter to determine the specific activity.

Partial assessment of the antiserum in terms of titre has already been carried out by use of the antiserum dilution curve (Fig. 1). The potential *avidity* of the antibodies for the antigen will be apparent from the sensitivity displayed in the same figure, in which a displacement in titre is still observed even at the smallest reduction in antigen concentration. The *sensitivity* can be estimated from a standard curve (Fig. 2) in which the smallest detectable displacement of label can be related to the smallest detectable amount of unlabelled antigen. Sensitivity has been defined in this chapter as the least amount of antigen that can be distinguished (with precision) from zero. It, therefore, depends on the accuracy of measurement of the difference in radioactivity between such incubates, as well as the accuracy of the concentration of the standard antigen solution. From a series of

standard curves constructed under similar conditions of the assay sensitivity can be calculated from:

$$\frac{2 \times \text{standard deviation of } B_0}{\text{initial slope of the curve at } B_0}$$

where B_0 is the label binding in the absence of unlabelled antigen.

The effect on assay sensitivity of delaying the addition of label is illustrated in Fig. 4. Curve C repre-

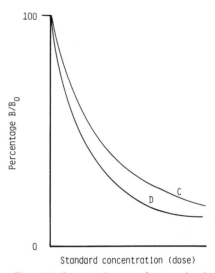

Fig. 4 Comparison of standard curves produced under conditions of simultaneous reagent addition (C) and delayed addition of label (D).

sents the dose–response obtained from a competitive RIA system (simultaneous reagent addition). Curve D represents the dose–response to a delayed label addition, all other conditions remaining the same. It is assumed that both systems are subject to the same experimental errors. Using the above equation therefore the increase in initial slope of the standard curve represents an increase in assay sensitivity.

From a standard curve constructed under optimum competitive assay conditions can be produced a *Scatchard plot* (Fig. 5), the slope of which offers a measure of the antiserum avidity constant (K_{av}). From the standard curve data, calculation of B/F ratios for each datum point is made and plotted against the corresponding total antigen (labelled and unlabelled) concentration. For this purpose an accurate value for the specific activity of the label is required.

It is usually the case that Scatchard plots produced using RIA data are of a non-linear nature. This is an indication of the heterogeneity of the assay antiserum, in that it contains several binding sites of different avidities. The initial slope of the plot is a measure of the avidity constant of the high avidity antibodies. Values of up to 10^{12} litres/mole have been achieved for high avidity antibodies. The intersection of the asymptote with the abscissa (where B/F = 0)

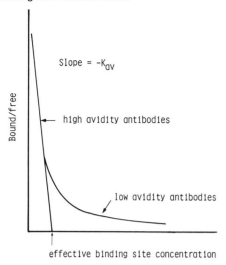

Total antigen (Ag + Ag*) concentration

Fig. 5 Scatchard plot for the determination of the avidity constant (K_{av}) and the effective binding site concentration of high avidity antibodies.

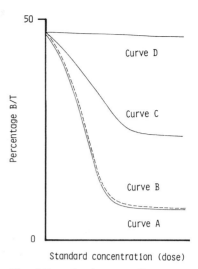

Fig. 6 Standard curves. Decrease in percentage label binding with increasing concentrations of compounds possessing varying cross-reactivities (affinities) for the antiserum.

gives a value for the effective concentration of such high avidity binding sites.

The *specificity* of the antiserum is of equal importance to avidity when considering the practical applications of an RIA. The specificity, or lack of it, means that an RIA is dependent on the immunoreactivity of antibodies with certain antigenic determinants. Often the immunoreactivity of an antigen is different from its biological activity. In addition any compound containing the particular antigenic determinant will react with the antibody. This results in false measurements of, for example, a peptide hormone, when determinant-containing fragments may be detected as intact molecules. Improvement in the assay specificity may be brought about by immunization of several more animals or, in the case of a hapten, by using an alternative site of conjugation.

An example of the detection of cross-reacting material is shown in Fig. 6. Curve A is a normal standard curve of label displacement from antibody-binding sites by increments of unlabelled antigen. Any superimposable curve (B) indicates material of similar immunoreactivity (affinity) for the antibody. Curve C represents material cross-reacting with antibody but of lower affinity. Curve D indicates non-cross-reacting material.

Having established the viability of the principal reagents (label immunoreactivity and specific activity; antiserum titre, avidity and specificity) further validation of the assay should be undertaken to assess its clinical usefulness. Essential factors to consider are not only sensitivity but also precision and working range. Each are interrelated and each can therefore be evaluated simultaneously from data generated under the optimum conditions already established.

From the replicate response determinations of bound label at each standard concentration dose estimates (d) can be derived and the standard deviation (SD) of the dose estimates calculated. Figure 7 (after Ekins) represents examples of *precision-dose profiles* constructed from standard curve data manipulated in this way. From a plot of SD against d (Fig. 7A) the assay sensitivity can be obtained from the SD value at zero dose. To derive the assay sensitivity this value is modified depending on the degree of significance required (multiply by 2 for 95% confidence) and the number of assay replicates used (divide by the square root of 2 for duplicates).

From the associated plot of coefficient of variation (SD/d) against d (Fig. 7B) the working range of the assay can be defined as the range within which dose estimates display an acceptable precision. The practical use of precision–dose profiles is illustrated by Fig. 8 (after Ekins) which displays data from two assay systems. Assay A is more sensitive than B but B has higher precision over the analyte concentration range of clinical interest. In this example where maximum sensitivity is not necessary, reagent concentrations can be adjusted to provide more precise measurements; these will therefore carry more weight in clinical decision-making and diagnosis. Conversely, where maximum sensitivity is required due regard must be given to the less precise nature of these measurements and their consequent clinical validity.

Calculation of Results. Increasing demands on RIA have produced various responses from technologists. While higher quality reagents and their more efficient use have shortened assay times and improved analytical performance equal attention has been paid to more flexible methods of assay data reduction. This includes conversion of raw counts into sample analyte

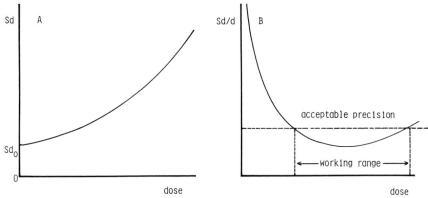

Fig. 7 A. Error profile of standard deviation (SD) in replicate determinations of each dose against dose level. The variability at zero dose (SD_0) is related to assay sensitivity. B. Precision profile over the assay standard range measurements with acceptable precision indicating the working concentration range.

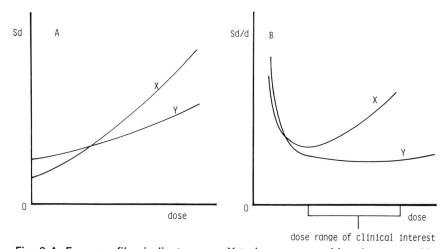

Fig. 8 A. Error profiles indicate assay X to be more sensitive than assay Y. B. Precision profiles indicate assay Y to be more capable than assay X of acceptably precise measurements over the clinically important concentration range.

values together with the production of information on the consistency of assay performance parameters.

The trend to multi-head γ-counters has increased the rate of data production. In order to maintain the advantages afforded by this rapid availability of counts automated procedures for their reduction to sample results have superseded laborious manual calculation methods that were often prone to error and inconsistency.

The initial function of data processing is the construction of a standard curve which relates the measured response to standard analyte concentration. There are several alternative methods for producing dose–response curve plots. The principal manual methods necessarily employ simple plots of raw count data and standard values on linear scales, usually antibody-bound counts against standard concentration (see Fig. 2). A manually drawn 'best-fit' curve or linear interpolation (straight line connection of adjacent points) are two options for establishing the relationship between response and dose.

Several procedures exist for converting assay data into straight-line plots but require some degree of computing capacity. The symmetrical sigmoid curves often encountered in RIA can be linearized by logit transformation of the antibody-bound counts plotted against the logarithm of the standard concentration. Some curves are asymmetrical and will produce a non-linear transformation. A much favoured curve-fitting system is the use of spline functions. By a series of polynomial equations adjacent points on the standard curve are joined so that the slope of the curve for each section is carried over to the next. By weighting the dose responses depending on their replicate variance a smoothed curve may be obtained by repeated recalculations of the spline until a best fit is reached. The flexibility of this option enables the computation of the equivalent of a manually drawn plot in that aberrant points are assigned less significance. Goodness of fit may be expressed numerically by measurement of the differences of each observed point from the equivalent point on the calculated plot. These error differences may then be used to construct a precision envelope around the smoothed dose–response curve.

In the use of any curve-fitting procedure account should be taken of the errors in both standard concentration and the measured response. Replicate determinations at each dose, whether from standards or samples, can yield information on the magnitude of the errors at different points on the dose–response curve. Such errors will contribute to the computation of the precision of sample values.

Internal Assay Quality Assurance

Reagents. Each RIA reagent is subject to variation in quality as a result of inconsistencies in production or deterioration during use and storage. In view of these variations continual re-assessment of the routine systems should be maintained. Immediate and simple examination of standard curve parameters such as the percentage binding at zero standard and the doses required to decrease the binding by 20%, 50% and 80% should remain relatively stable within the overall variability of the assay. Statistical comparison of successive dose–response curves and their respective error envelopes represents the first option in the diagnosis of assay error. For occasional checks on reagent variability and assay performance precision profiling (see Fig. 7) can yield valuable information since the data can be derived from sample analysis as well as from the dose–response curve.

Sample analytical validity. Analysis of data from control material is the most commonly used and reliable method of monitoring between-assay variability. Important guidelines should be followed to maximize the effectiveness of this form of control. The material used should be similar to the unknown samples. At least three levels of analyte should be used to cover the working range of the assay. Sufficient material for long-term use will provide continuity and minimize continual re-establishment of target values. The optimal storage conditions should be assessed to ensure stability. The optimum number of control tubes should be equal to the square root of the total number of tubes in the assay and should be distributed at regular intervals throughout, as a check on drift.

At least 10 estimates of each control pool are required to establish the target mean and its standard deviation. The simplest use of the resultant data is in the establishment of control charts consisting of plots of each target mean with their upper and lower 1 and 2 SD limits. For each subsequent assay the mean of each control pool is plotted on the chart. This simple visual display of assay performance can indicate the acceptability of the batch under consideration. Rejection criteria may be based on the mean of one pool being greater than 3 SD from its expected value; or 2 pool means greater than 2 SD (in the same direction); or all 3 more than 1 SD and in the same direction. Consistent bias of all three pools suggests incorrect standardization. Inconsistent bias (two pools high, one pool low, etc.) suggests high assay variability which may also be observed from high sample replicate variability. Progressively increasing (or decreasing) control sample values is an indication of within-assay drift, a phenomenon which is often time-related.

The use of control charts may, however, lead to a false sense of security in assay assessment. In the initial establishment of target mean values an inadequately validated and imprecise assay will produce wide limits of acceptability. Consequently, few subsequent batches will be rejected. However, internal control guidelines should be adopted with due consideration to the ultimate clinical objectives of any particular assay.

External Quality Assurance.

The principal objective of external quality assessment is to make interlaboratory comparisons of results in order to derive target values for each sample distributed. Patterns of bias from such values can then be accumulated for individual laboratories. Consistent bias can indicate systematic errors due, for example, to incorrect standardization or, at low analyte concentrations, to sample matrix interference (background 'noise').

Accurate assessment of bias is made difficult when assay reproducibility is poor. Variability of bias is indicative of imprecision although the latter is more properly measured by the redistribution of samples from the same pool. A method may appear to be highly biased, for no known cause, but if the system is proved to be rugged and precise its diagnostic value can be quite acceptable when based on knowledge of performance and reference data.

The infrequent checks afforded by external control procedures can only be representative of the coarse adjustments required to maintain participating laboratories in general agreement. The fine control necessary for daily or weekly between-batch consistency should be based on rigorous internal control procedures.

Sources of Error.

Virtually every manipulation in an RIA procedure is susceptible to imprecision, the cumulative effect of which is to produce a sample value which may be inaccurate but precise or accurate but imprecise. Contributions to assay error can arise from incorrect reagent assessment, reagent instability, incorrect assay design, non-specific binding effects, sample matrix effects, inefficient phase separation, inaccurate and/or imprecise pipetting and counting errors. Such errors may be conveniently divided into within-batch and between-batch types.

The main source of within-batch error is experimental, arising almost exclusively from imprecise pipetting. This includes the preparation of working standard solutions as well as the dispensing of standards and samples. The addition of reagent solutions is less susceptible to error due to the availability of repeating dispensers.

Phase separation is the second most important cause of imprecision, as well as bias. Such errors may be limited by meticulous attention to correct optimization of the separation system; for example: correct titration of double-antibody reagents to form a sedimentable matrix; or the time in contact with an adsorptive medium such as charcoal.

Counting errors can assume significant proportions when the total activity falls to low levels. In general, however, such errors are relatively small and there is little benefit to be gained by increasing counting times in attempts to minimize them, particularly when the experimental error is already high.

Other minor causes of within-batch error can arise from the sample dilution required when a result falls beyond the assay working range and from minor calculation errors (manual and automated).

Between-batch errors can be assigned more usually to variation in reagent type or quality. Inevitably changes in standard preparation will affect results. It cannot be assumed that control or unknown samples will not vary in composition particularly during long-term storage or if storage conditions change. Different batches of label can produce subtle changes in assay specificity, leading to bias. Similar changes may result from the use of different antiserum. Incubation conditions may vary when, for example, buffer media deteriorate or temperature varies. Inconsistencies in data calculation can occur particularly in manual methods but should be minimal when automated. Finally, the almost inevitable clerical transcription and major calculation blunders are unforeseen sources of error.

Automation. Many of the errors described above can be reduced to acceptable proportions, if not completely eliminated, through assay automation. However RIA methods have been notoriously difficult to automate because of the relatively long incubation times and the phase separation requirement. The latter has posed particularly difficult technical problems.

In general there have been two main developments in automated RIA procedures; one based on continuous-flow concepts and the other on discrete modules. Continuous-flow methods are reliant on reactions reaching equilibrium relatively quickly and are suitable therefore for analysis of small molecules, such as thyroid or steroid hormones. Modular systems are more flexible but longer incubation necessitates off-line intervention following sampling and reagent dispensing. Phase separation in both types of system usually involves filtration for removal of a precipitated or solid-phase pellet of antibody-bound label. Automated washing stages can be introduced with consequent improvement in assay precision. Computerized data handling, quality control and generated sample results also contribute to improved assay performance by minimizing errors.

The capital costs of most automated RIA systems are high and unless a large throughput of samples is anticipated such an investment is not justified for most laboratories.

FURTHER READING

Butt W. R. (ed.) (1984). *Practical Immunoassay*. New York: Marcel Dekker.

Gray C. H., James V. H. T. (eds) (1983). *Hormones in Blood*. Vols. 4 and 5. London: Academic Press.

Hunter W. M., Corrie J. E. T. (eds) (1983). *Immunoassays for Clinical Chemistry*. Edinburgh: Churchill Livingstone.

Jeffcoate S. L. (1981). *Efficiency and Effectiveness in the Endocrine Laboratory*. London: Academic Press.

Marks V., Mould G. P., O'Sullivan M. J., Teale J. D. (1980). Monitoring of drug disposition by immunoassay. In *Progress in Drug Metabolism* (Bridges J. W., Chasseaud L. F., eds) vol. 5, pp. 255–310. Chichester: Wiley.

Sonksen P H. (ed.) (1974), Radioimmunoassay and saturation analysis. *Br. Med. Bull*; **30**.

32. Immunometric Assays
R. Goodburn

INTRODUCTION

Immunometric assays comprise a group in which two antibodies are used to detect and quantitate an analyte. One antibody is immobilized on a solid matrix and effectively extracts the analyte from the test serum, while the second is tagged with a label to quantitate the bound analyte. A variety of labels have been used, and the type of label determines the nomenclature of the assay.

IMMUNORADIOMETRIC ASSAYS

The original immunoradiometric assay was described by Miles and Hales,[1] and used [125]iodine as the label. The two-site Immuno-Radio-Metric Assay (IRMA) was developed from the original assay by Addison and Hales.[2,3] The term was coined in order to differentiate the IRMA method from conventional Radio-Immuno Assays (RIA), since the principles underlying the two assays were totally different. Other variants of the immunoradiometric assay were also developed by this group, but have not been widely adopted, and will not be discussed here.

Basic Immunoradiometric Assay Procedure

In summary, the two-site immunoradiometric assay consists of the following steps:

1. Diluted antiserum is immobilized on a suitable solid phase such as the wall of a test tube, or cellulose particles. Unattached antibody is removed by washing. Large batches of immobilized antibody are normally prepared, in order to maintain long-term assay stability.

2. The immobilized antiserum is incubated with diluted standard or test serum for a predetermined period.
3. After removing the serum and washing, the immobilized antibody and bound antigen are incubated with a second antiserum, also directed against the antigen and labelled with [125]iodine.
4. After again removing unreacted material and washing, the immobilized antibody with its trapped antigen and labelled antibody are subjected to gamma counting, and the results calculated.

These basic principles are illustrated in Fig. 1.

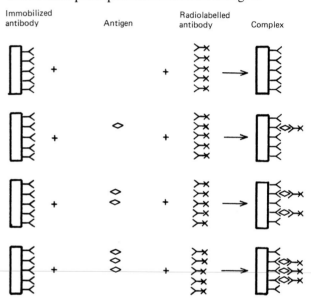

Fig. 1 Schematic representation of the immunoradiometric assay procedure. From top to bottom, the sequence of events is shown with increasing amounts of antigen added into the assay system. As more antigen is added, an increasing amount of radiolabel will be detected.

Preparation of Labelled Antibody

Batches of the second antiserum are prepared by labelling and purifying the antiserum while it is bound to a specific immunoadsorbent (antigen coupled to a solid phase). The antibody may be retained on the immunoadsorbent for storage, with elution of sufficient label for each assay. Products of radiological damage are first washed from the immunoadsorbent followed by elution of the label by an appropriate strength acid. The more avid antibodies are eluted by stronger acid. This practice ensures that the antiserum is specific for the antigen, and of relatively high specific radioactivity.

Solid Phases

Since the introduction of the IRMA technique, a wide range of immobilization supports has been used.

At present the most popular are particulate materials such as cellulose powder, agarose derivatives and synthetic resins, and plastic surfaces such as test tubes, microtitre plate wells and beads. The major requirement is for high antibody density on the matrix in order to maintain antibody excess. Particulate materials require centrifugation for separation of bound and free fractions, although this may be avoided by the use of magnetizable particles, and separation by magnetic means.

Immobilization Methods

In order to maximize antibody density on the solid phase, the efficiency of immobilization procedures is of great importance. When chemically applicable, cyanogen bromide activation of the matrix is suitable. Physical adsorption of antibody to the matrix is simple and inexpensive, but is inefficient and wasteful of antibody.

Two important factors differentiate the IRMA method from RIA. First, the antigen is detected by means of a labelled antibody rather than labelled antigen, and secondly the assay is not competitive. Both of the antisera are required to be in excess in relation to the antigen in order for the assay to be effective. Since the assay is not competitive, the response is directly proportional to the concentration of analyte, as shown in Fig. 2.

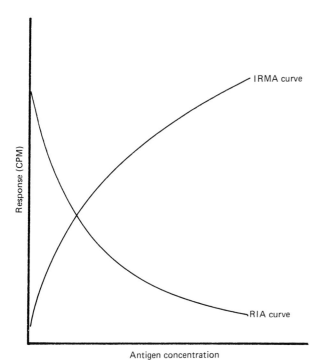

Fig. 2 Typical standard curves for radioimmunoassay and immunoradiometric assay compared. The negative and positive slopes reflect the competitive and non-competitive nature of the respective assays.

Advantages of Immunoradiometric Assays

The immunoradiometric assays carried the promise of greatly improved precision, kinetics, specificity and sensitivity over radioimmunoassays. Since both of the antibodies must be in excess with respect to the antigen, the assay precision is, to a large extent, independent of the precision of pipetting these reagents, and very good precision may be obtained with normal pipetting practices. However, there is still a need for precise pipetting of the test serum. Because of the use of excess reagents, the assay is also less dependent upon antibody avidity than is RIA, and the kinetics of the assay are faster than those of RIA. Increased specificity is obtained by using antisera of two different epitopic specificities in the assay. In order to be recognized and quantitated, the antigen must possess both epitopes. (This also imposes a limitation on the assay, however. It can be applied only to antigens which can be bound by two antibodies simultaneously, i.e. essentially only proteins and other macromolecules.) The increased sensitivity is again derived from the use of excess reagents. By using both antibodies in excess, if the analyte exists in the test solution, it should be possible to trap it and detect it. The only limiting factor to sensitivity is the specific radioactivity of the labelled antibody solution, which must be very high in order that only *labelled* antibodies bind to the trapped antigen. It is theoretically possible to quantitate a single molecule of analyte using this type of assay, providing that a labelled antibody of sufficiently high specific radioactivity is used. In practice this may not be achieved in immuno*radio*metric assays, because of the constant deterioration of the label. However, using non-radioactive labels, such sensitivities are at least theoretically possible. In contrast, such sensitivities can never be possible in RIA. Since RIA depends on saturation of the antibody, assays optimized for greatest sensitivity must use very low concentrations of antibody; this imposes limitations on the equilibrium constant for the assay, and the precision of gamma counting (since the concentration of bound label will also be low). These limitations cannot be overcome, no matter how good the label, and the theoretical limit of sensitivity of such assays has been estimated at 1×10^{-14} mol/l.

Disadvantages of Immunoradiometric Assays

The IRMA system demonstrated few serious disadvantages that were not already seen in RIA, most of which were associated with the use of radioisotopes.

The procedure for purifying, radioiodinating and storing the antibody requires the preparation of specific immunoadsorbent, using relatively large amounts of antigens such as pituitary hormones, which may be difficult to obtain in sufficient quantities.

Some of these difficulties have been overcome by

the use of monoclonal antibody technology. The preparation of immunoadsorbents for the purification, labelling and storage of antiserum is expensive in time and antigen. The availability of a plentiful supply of specific monoclonal antibodies has obviated much of the requirement for such procedures. Radiolabelled specific antibodies may be prepared frequently without attachment to immunoadsorbent, using antibodies which require little or no prior purification. Standard radioiodination methods such as the chloramine-T method may be used. Since the labelled antibodies may be prepared at frequent intervals, the problems associated with the deterioration of the reagents are considerably reduced.

The 'high-dose hook effect', where high concentrations of analyte may lead to a paradoxical fall in binding levels instead of an increase, is seen in most immunoradiometric assays (*see* Fig. 3). To date, no entirely satisfactory explanation has been forthcoming for this phenomenon, although it has been postulated that it may be due to binding of antigen to sites with low binding affinity, and its subsequent loss on washing. The effect may be reduced by the addition of both antibodies to the serum simultaneously, rather than in two separate incubations. This in turn is dependent on the antibody populations used in the assay. Single incubation IRMA methods may only be employed when two specific antibody populations are used for extraction and labelling (i.e. antibodies which react with discrete, unrelated epitopes). Monoclonal antibodies represent such separate populations. Alternatively, affinity-purified polyclonal antibodies may be used. If mixed population antiserum is used, extensive blocking of epitopes may occur, and considerable reduction of sensitivity and specificity may result. The point at which the hook effect occurs varies considerably from assay to assay, and must be determined for any IRMA. Where necessary, samples with expected high values must be diluted for assay. The effect has greater significance in assays where extremely high levels may be encountered (e.g. ferritin, prolactin), than in those where the possible range of levels is more restricted (e.g. TSH).

Applications

Despite their inherent advantages, the full potential of immunoradiometric assays could not initially be realized due to the practical difficulties of producing antiserum of sufficient purity and specificity, the restrictions on the production of high specific activity radioactive labels, and the damaging effects of the radiation on the antibodies. However, more recently, IRMA methods have become popular because, although ultimate sensitivity and specificity may not be reached, the assays are still superior to many of the radioimmunoassays for the same substances. Monoclonal antibody technology has also made the development of IRMA methods more viable commercially. In some cases, the increased sensitivity and specificity afforded by such assays has been invaluable. In the case of TSH, an increase in sensitivity of 10- to 50-fold has been achieved, together with reduced interference from other pituitary hormones and related molecules. Many laboratories have been tempted to use TSH as the main test of thyroid function, since it may now be used to detect and monitor thyrotoxicosis as well as hypothyroidism. In other cases, the advantages of immunometric assays are not so clear-cut: ferritin, for instance, may be quantitated perfectly adequately using radioimmunoassay. There is no requirement for extra sensitivity or specificity in this case (although the enhanced precision of the method could be seen as an advantage).

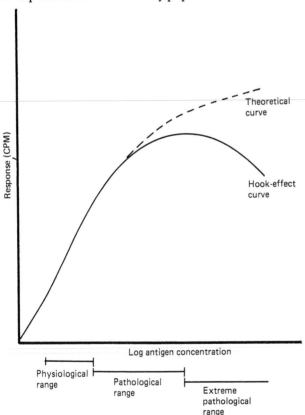

Fig. 3 Immunoradiometric assay standard curve extended beyond normal assay limits to demonstrate the high-dose hook effect. Samples which might be expected to give results beyond the 'hook' must be assayed at a dilution sufficient to bring the result within the reliable part of the curve.

ALTERNATIVE LABELS

The application of non-isotopic labels to immunoassays (together with the development of monoclonal antibody technology previously discussed) fuelled the revival of interest in assays based on labelled antibody. An overview of the use of some enzyme and luminescent labels is given here, and is covered in more detail in later chapters.

Nomenclature

Radioactive isotopes are now by no means the only labels used in immunometric assays, and immuno-radiometric assays have been supplemented by Immuno-enzymo-metric assays, Immuno-Fluoro-Metric Assays (IFMA), Enzyme-Linked Immuno-Sorbent Assays (ELISA) etc., depending on the label attached to the antibody. The generic name of immunometric assays may be applied to all these variations. A clear distinction should be made here between the immunometric assays using enzyme or fluorescent labels (immunoenzymometric or immunofluorometric assays), and enzyme- or fluoro-immunoassays. Although the distinction may initially appear pedantic, the terminology differentiates between non-competitive and competitive assays: because of the limitations of molecular size on the former group, haptens such as thyroid hormones, steroids and drugs cannot be measured using it, and must be measured using the latter type of assay, which is analogous to radioimmunoassay, i.e. it is a *competitive* assay, using enzyme or fluorescence tagged *antigen* as label. Although the use of non-isotopic labels affords longer shelf life for the assays, and is to be encouraged for environmental and safety reasons, it must be recognized that hapten assays using non-isotopic labels are unlikely to show improved sensitivity, precision or specificity.

Enzyme Labels

Many enzymes have been used as labels. Undoubtedly the most popular are horseradish peroxidase and alkaline phosphatase. Suitable enzymes should be readily obtainable, relatively inexpensive, and give good colour development. Several methods have been described for the conjugation of enzymes to antibodies. In general they are simple and give acceptable specific activities, but some are wasteful of enzyme.

In order to increase sensitivity, reaction-rate measurement, and substrate–enzyme systems yielding fluorescent or bioluminescent end-points have been used. (These should not be confused with fluorescent or bioluminescent *labels*.)

Luminescent Labels

Fluorescent. Antibodies labelled with fluorescent compounds (e.g. Fluorescein and Rhodamine compounds) have been used in microscopy-based immunofluorescence procedures for some time. Such uses are not inconsistent with the term immunometric assay, although they are not quantitative, and are assessed subjectively. Precision is reasonable only with skilled interpretation. Antibodies labelled with these fluorescent compounds are not very useful in *chemical* immunofluorometric assays, mainly because of background fluorescence from serum factors and, more particularly, plastic materials.

The success of IFMA methods has been largely due to the introduction of antibody–lanthanide chelate conjugates, and time-resolved fluorimetry. Assays based on this principle are almost exclusively commercially produced, because of the complexities of the label and the procedures required for end-point determination. Time-resolved fluorimetry depends upon the long fluorescence decay times (10–1000 µs) of the lanthanide chelate compared to those of interfering fluorescences (1–20 µs). The fluorimetric response to a flash of light is measured between 400 and 800 µs after excitation. This end-point determination is entirely dependent on specific, dedicated instrumentation which is sophisticated in both the fluorescence measurement and data processing.

Chemiluminescent/bioluminescent. Few immunometric assays have been reported which use chemiluminescent or bioluminescent labels. Enzyme labels which yield chemiluminescent or bioluminescent products have been employed, but these are immunoenzymometric assays or enzyme immunoassays.

A family of immunochemiluminometric assays has been established on the basis of antibodies labelled with acridinium ester. Oxidation of the label gives a flash of light which may be detected in a luminometer.

Applications

Immunometric assays are becoming relatively common in the clinical biochemistry laboratory, and are now used to quantitate a variety of analytes. The example of TSH has been cited above. This hormone may now be assayed using radio-, enzyme-, fluorescent-, or chemiluminescent-labelled immunometric systems, all of which yield excellent results. Non-isotopic assays are also available for other pituitary hormones, tumour markers and many other analytes. The method has also been modified to enable the detection of antibodies to various diseases. In this form of the assay, antigen is immobilized on a solid matrix, and reacted with the test serum. A labelled antiserum specific for the species immunoglobulin is then added, to detect any antibodies reacting with the immobilized antigen. The ELISA system in particular has found wide acceptance in this area, and in-house and commercial methods are available for the detection of antibodies to most infectious diseases, human and animal. Quantitation of such antibodies has proved to be a major problem. The assay is a measure of antibody avidity as well as concentration, and titration curves (the responses from serially diluted test serum samples) from different individuals are not parallel from individual to individual (*see* Fig. 4). Hence it is not possible to use a standard curve derived from either any one individual or a pool of serum samples as a standard preparation.

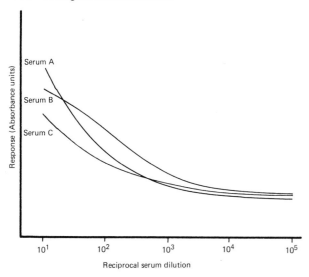

Fig. 4 Typical ELISA response curves from serial dilution of three samples with the same antibody haemagglutination titre. The non-parallelism of the curves reflects the differing avidities of the antibody populations detected by the assay.

Despite attempts to produce ELISA data which reflect the avidity as well as the concentration of the antibody, ELISA methods for antibodies tend to be qualitative or at best semi-quantitative. Complementary ELISA systems for disease antigens are also available, and are similar in principle to those for molecular analytes.

Solid Phases

Solid phase matrices are considered in detail in later chapters. A wide variety of materials has been used for the immobilization of the first antibody (or antigen in the case of assays for antibodies). The most widely accepted medium for immunoenzymometric assays (enzyme linked immunosorbent assays or ELISA) and immunofluorometric assays is the microtitre plate. The antibody is coated onto the surface of the wells of these plates. The microtitre plate was first used widely in assays developed for use in undeveloped countries where instrumentation was not available, and where a visible end point, together with a very robust assay system were essential. Although it has been widely accepted as the matrix of choice for ELISA, its adoption may be due to convention and fashion as much as efficacy. The wells are difficult to label for sample identification and require care in production, preparation and handling for best precision; special instrumentation is necessary for reading the end points.

Particulate solid phases such as cellulose powder and agarose derivatives are not suitable for enzyme-based systems where colour change is to be monitored in the tube, or for fluorescent labelled assays. They have, however, been used extensively in immunoradiometric assays. The major advantages of particulate matrices are the greatly increased surface area available compared with polystyrene tubes or wells, and their suitability for covalent coupling of antibody or antigen.

Immobilization Methods

Immobilization of antibodies or antigens on solid phases may be achieved by simple physical adsorption or covalent bonding with such agents as cyanogen bromide. Covalent coupling is better suited to cellulose and agarose derivatives than unmodified polystyrene, since the latter has no chemical groupings on which covalent bonding may be based. Prior chemical modification of polystyrene (e.g. nitration) tends to reduce its transparency, making it unsuitable for use in media such as microtitre plates when through-the-well readers are to be used. However, covalent bonding onto such carriers as chemically modified plastic beads is practical.

Treatments to increase the extent of physical adsorption to polystyrene have been tried (e.g. radiation, glutaraldehyde), with varying degrees of success. The use of glutaraldehyde is somewhat illogical, since this substance does not react with polystyrene. Glutaraldehyde links proteins through adjacent ε-amino groups. Thus, if any glutaraldehyde adsorbs physically to the polystyrene, its only effect is to cross-link proteins within its vicinity, which will not necessarily ensure higher levels of binding and may alter the presentation of the substance to its complementary antibody or antigen.

DEVELOPMENT OF IMMUNOMETRIC ASSAYS

Many manufacturers of diagnostic immunoassay kits within the clinical biochemistry field are concentrating their efforts on the use of non-isotopic labels, and will often supply the equipment necessary for the detection of the label. Some aspects of immunometric assays have been protected by patents. Most manufacturers now supply kits for both protein and hapten assays, with assays based on non-competitive and competitive principles respectively.

It is becoming clear in the area of clinical biochemistry that immunometric assays are not in general as amenable to in-house development within district hospital laboratories as are radioimmunoassays, although some manufacturers are making some components available. Monoclonal antibodies, where they are necessary to complete the assay system, may be difficult to obtain and this may impose severe limitations on many laboratories. Additionally, the production of large, stable and reproducible batches of immobilized antibody, especially using polystyrene as immobilization matrix, may also be a problem. The immobilization process is inherently wasteful of antiserum, since only a small proportion of added antibody (generally about 10%) is adsorbed onto plastic. Consequently this reagent may be prohibitively expensive for in-house development. Covalent bonding of antibody to solid phase is less wasteful, but is not generally applicable to polystyrene, and is more suitable for particulate solid phases such as cellulose, etc.

In contrast to assays for antigens, the ELISA system for antibodies is relatively easy to develop in-house, providing that facilities exist for the preparation of antigen.

FUTURE DEVELOPMENTS

The future for immunometric assays appears to be promising. Developments have included amplification of the enzyme-generated signal by use of the cyclical NAD/NADH system to give enhanced sensitivity and assays for two or more analytes within the same tube or well by the use of different labels (in both enzyme- and fluorescence-based systems). Automation of the assays is also under continuing development.

Simplification of the ELISA system has been investigated by some manufacturers, and has resulted for instance in pregnancy tests using 'dip-stick' techniques which detect relatively low levels of hCG, and which are suitable for direct use by the public.

Perhaps one of the most exciting potential applications of the immunometric assay system is the development of biosensor devices. Enzyme labels may be used to generate electron flow instead of a colour. This flow may be detected electronically, and specific immuno-reagents may be immobilized on membranes which may be incorporated into such electronic devices. In this way biosensors specific for particular analytes (chemical antigen, disease antigen or antibody) may be developed. Cooperation with the rapidly advancing electronics industry may allow the miniaturization of the entire assembly.

It is clear that immunometric assays will be a major factor in the development of clinical biochemistry and microbiology in the next decade, with an increasing trend towards simplification for the user, and non-laboratory testing.

REFERENCES

1. Miles L. E. M., Hales C. N. (1968). Labelled antibodies and immunological assay systems. *Nature*; **219**: 186 (Letter).
2. Addison G. M., Hales C. N. (1971). The immunoradiometric assay. In *Radioimmunoassay Methods* (Kirkham K. E., Hunter W. M., eds) pp. 447–61 and 481–7. Edinburgh: Churchill Livingstone.
3. Addison G. M., Hales C. N. (1971) Two-site assay for human growth hormone. *Horm. Metab. Res*; **3**: 59–60.

FURTHER READING

Hales C. N., Woodhead J. S. (1980). Labelled antibodies and their use in the immunoradiometric assay. In *Methods In Enzymology* (van Vunakis H., Langone J. J., eds). Vol. 70, pp. 334–55. New York: Academic Press.

Voller A., Bidwell D. E., Bartlett A. (1976). Enzyme immunoassays in diagnostic medicine. *Bull. WHO*; **53**: 55.

Voller A., Bidwell D. E., Bartlett A. (1979). *The Enzyme-Linked Immunosorbent Assay (ELISA). A Guide With Abstracts of Microplate Applications*. Guernsey: Dynatech.

Voller A., Bidwell D. (eds) (1981). *Immunoassays For The Eighties*. Proc. Conf. 1980. London. Lancaster: MTP. (Particularly Ekins R. Merits and disadvantages of different labels and methods of immunoassay, pp. 5–16).

Van Vunakis H., Langone J. J. (eds) (1981). *Methods in Enzymology*, Vol. 73, *Immunochemical Techniques*. Part B. New York: Academic Press.

Van Vunakis H., Langone J. J. (eds) (1982) *Methods in Enzymology*. Vol. 84, Part D, *Selected Immunoassays*. New York: Academic Press.

Van Vunakis H., Langone J. J. (eds) (1983) *Methods in Enzymology*, Vol. 92, Part E: *Monoclonal Antibodies and General Immunoassay Methods*. New York: Academic Press.

Van Vunakis H., Langone J. J. (eds) (1986). *Methods in Enzymology*, Vol. 121, Part I: *Hybridoma Technology and Monoclonal Antibodies*. New York: Academic Press.

Woodhead J. S., Addison G. M., Hales C. N. (1974). The immunoradiometric assay and related techniques. *Br. Med. Bull*; **30**: 44.

33. Enzyme Immunoassay
R. Hubbard and Barry J. Gould

INTRODUCTION

Since the initial studies by Yalow and Berson in 1959, radioimmunoassay (RIA) has developed into an extremely versatile analytical technique. It has been used in clinical laboratories to quantitate a wide variety of compounds. The specificity is dependent upon the antibodies and the sensitivity on both the antibodies and the radiolabel.

However, radioisotopes do have their drawbacks.

The preparation of the radiolabelled antigen involves real risks, which are cumulative. Even when these are prepared commercially the product shows batch-to-batch variation and, generally has a half-life limited to two months. Their toxic nature necessitates the application of strict regulatory control and their measurement requires the use of specialized, sophisticated and hence expensive equipment. The necessity for a separation step has prevented the development of simple automated analyses.

The disadvantages of radiolabels encouraged the search for alternatives, and of these, the use of enzyme-labelled reagents has been established since 1971 and has allowed the development of a diverse range of assay protocols. The more general advantage of enzyme labels, as compared to radio-labels, is their improved shelf-life. Enzyme labels may often be stored under sterile conditions for more than a year at 4°C or at room temperature when freeze-dried. Radiation hazards are obviously avoided.

PRINCIPLES OF ENZYME IMMUNOASSAY

We use the term enzyme immunoassay (EIA) to apply to all immunoassays where the activity of an enzyme is measured to determine the analyte. EIA is generally subdivided into heterogeneous (separation required) assays and homogeneous (separation free) assays. In heterogeneous assays the activity of the enzyme is not affected by the analyte. In homogeneous assays a separation step is not required since the analyte affects enzyme activity. There are two basic types of heterogeneous EIA, the classic competitive EIA, and the immunoenzymometric or sandwich assays. The principles of these various systems are considered below, together with their advantages and disadvantages.

Competitive EIA

This type of assay is analogous to the classical RIA. The assay contains three components, limited and constant quantities of both enzyme-labelled antigen and of antibody specific for the antigen. Also a variable amount of antigen for calibration purposes or unknown amounts of antigen in the test sample (Fig. 1). Since the number of antibody-binding sites is less than the total of unlabelled and labelled antigen molecules, there is competition for the fixed number of antibody-binding sites. The greater the quantity of unlabelled antigen present, the lower will be the quantity of enzyme-labelled antigen molecules that combine with antibody.

After separation of the unbound and antibody-bound enzyme-labelled antigen, the enzyme activity in the bound fraction is measured. The use of varying amounts of antigen is necessary for a calibration curve to be drawn and this allows the unknown amounts of antigen to be determined.

This type of EIA requires a separation step. The simplest way of doing this is to have the antibody

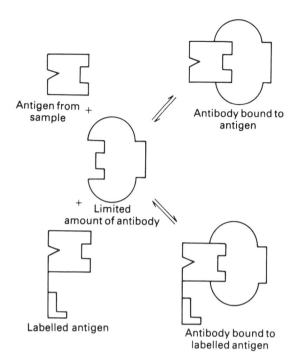

Fig. 1 Classical competitive EIA for antigen. All components are mixed and incubated. Isolation of antibody-bound enzyme-labelled antigen is necessary before measurement of enzyme activity. (Reprinted with permission, from Blake and Gould (1984) *Analyst*; **109**: 533.)

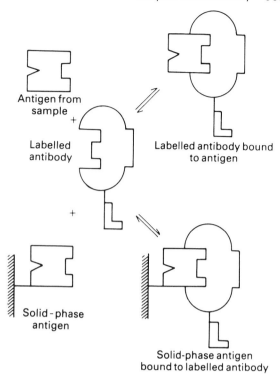

Fig. 2 Competitive EIA for antigen using solid-phase antigen. Enzyme-labelled antibody reacts specifically with antigen in the sample and is then added to excess of solid-phase antigen. After washing, the enzyme label still attached to the solid phase is measured. (Reprinted with permission, from Blake and Gould (1984) *Analyst*; **109**: 533.)

adsorbed to a solid phase which allows for easy washing of the antibody-bound enzyme-labelled antigen complex prior to determination of enzyme activity. This particular type of EIA has no inherent advantage over RIA unless the substitution of the radiolabel is desired either on grounds of safety, or on availability of appropriate equipment. Competitive EIA is the method of choice for small haptens if a sensitive assay (e.g. picogram quantities of hormones) is required. Such assays have a sensitivity comparable with RIA although it is important to use a different chemical link between the hapten–enzyme conjugate and the hapten–protein conjugate used to raise the antiserum.

An alternative assay for antigens depends on competition between a fixed amount of solid-phase antigen and antigen in the sample for a limited amount of specific enzyme labelled antibody (Fig. 2). These assays are also called inhibition assays because the amount of enzyme that will be bound to the solid phase decreases with increasing concentration of the antigen in the sample to be measured. This type of assay can also be used to measure haptens, although the attachment of hapten to the solid phase is not always easy. The sensitivity is at least as good as that achieved with RIA.

Immunoenzymometric Assays

Although competitive assays were used in early EIA there has subsequently been a progressive increase in the use of non-competitive or immunoenzymometric assays. These assays, which are also sometimes referred to as sandwich assays, capture assays or two-site assays rely on the presence of excess reagent. In consequence competition is no longer involved and the final amount of bound enzyme label that is measured is proportional to the concentration of analyte. These assays all use solid-phase reagent, either an antibody or antigen, which allows for easy separation and washing between stages. Because of this, these assays are frequently called 'Enzyme-linked immunosorbent assays' (ELISA) but this term can also include the competitive EIA for which the principles are quite different.

A simple immunoenzymometric assay for antigen is illustrated in Fig. 3. The excess of solid-phase antibody is first incubated with the sample antigens. After washing, the enzyme-labelled antibody is added, and after a further washing stage the enzyme activity retained is measured.

These methods have been widely used in detecting infectious diseases. The use of stable reagents, often combined with simple visual assessment of the test results of up to 100 samples at a time, have made them very suitable for tests on blood bank specimens and for epidemiological surveys. The tests have fre-

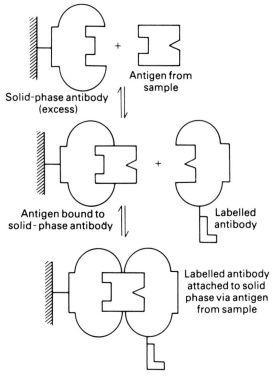

Fig. 3 Immunoenzymometric assay for antigen. Antigen in the sample is mixed with excess solid-phase antibody. After washing of the solid phase, enzyme-labelled antibody which is specific for another site on the antigen is added. The enzyme label which remains bound after washing is measured. (Reprinted with permission, from Blake and Gould (1984) *Analyst*; **109**: 533.)

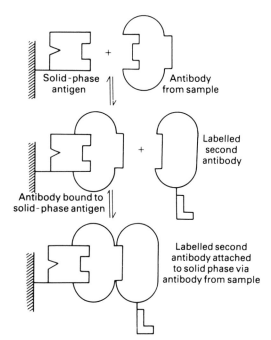

Fig. 4 Immunoenzymometric assay for antibody. Antibody in the sample is mixed with excess solid-phase antigen. After washing of the solid phase, enzyme-labelled second antibody is added. Bound enzyme activity is measured after washing. (Reprinted with permission, from Blake and Gould (1984) *Analyst*; **109**: 533.)

quently been used in the field without the need for complex equipment.

In this type of assay the analyte must be large enough to have at least two reactive antigenic sites a fact that generally excludes its use for haptens. With polyclonal antibodies the same antiserum can be used to coat the surface of the solid phase and in the formation of the enzyme-labelled antibody. An alternative is to use two different monoclonal antibodies. This eliminates one incubation step since both the sample and enzyme-labelled monoclonal antibody can be added at the same time to the solid-phase, which has previously been coated with the second monoclonal antibody. These 'one-step' assays have high specificity, since two antigenic sites are involved, and can be both quick and convenient.

Another important application of immunoenzymometric assays is in the measurement of antibody (Fig. 4). In this case a solid-phase antigen is required to bind initially with antibody in the sample. After washing, the bound antibody is normally detected after the addition of an enzyme-labelled species-specific anti-immunoglobulin and by measurement of enzyme activity.

In the detection of immunoglobulin M class antibodies, false positives may occur in the presence of IgG antibody and IgM anti-IgG rheumatoid factor, and false negatives may be found when competition occurs between IgM and high levels of IgG antibody. These problems can be overcome if a solid-phase anti-IgM is used to capture IgM. Then the specific IgM is detected by the addition of the appropriate antigen which is finally visualized using an enzyme-labelled antibody specific for the antigen.

This type of assay for IgM requires an additional step to the simple immunoenzymometric assay given earlier. However it achieves the purpose of improved assay specificity. Several other variants of immunoenzymometric methodology include additional steps for convenience. These allow the use of general commercially produced enzyme-labelled reagents in the final step and thus make it unnecessary for the user-laboratory to make their own enzyme-labelled reagents. These reagents include enzyme-labelled species-specific antiserum, and enzyme-labelled protein A. It is essential to avoid non-specific binding of these labels.

The rapid growth of immunometric assays has been shown to have a sound theoretical basis. Among the potential advantages of this type of assay design are

1. that the affinity of the antibody is generally less important than in a competitive assay, since more is used,
2. that the precision of antibody pipetting is now generally of minor consequence,
3. a shortening of the assay incubation times.

These advantages should lead to more rapid, rugged and reliable assays with improved sensitivity and specificity, due to the normal two-site assay design. The obvious disadvantage is the increased cost, particularly in terms of amounts of antibodies used.

To take full advantage of the potential of immunoassays, extremely low levels of non-specific binding must be attained. It is also necessary to use labels with a higher specific activity than that of commonly used isotopes. The use of enzymes with a high turnover number is one approach but for optimum sensitivity this will probably have to be enhanced by improved detection facilities which measure fluorescent products, radiolabelled products or chemiluminescence.

Homogeneous EIA

The Enzyme Multiplied Immunoassay Technique (EMIT©; Syva, Maidenhead, UK) is the most widely used homogeneous enzyme immunoassay system. The principle of this type of assay is shown in Fig. 5. The technique is dependent on a change in specific

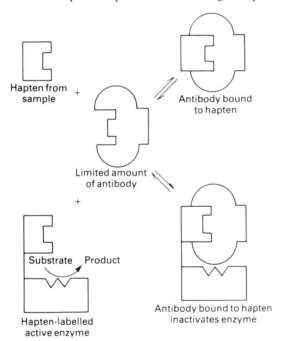

Fig. 5 Principle of the EMIT system of homogeneous EIA. Hapten-labelled enzyme is enzymically active but combination with hapten-specific antibody causes marked inhibition of enzyme activity. The relative amounts of free hapten and hapten-labelled enzyme determine the final measured enzyme activity. (Reprinted with permission, from Blake and Gould (1984) *Analyst*; **109**: 533.)

enzyme activity when enzyme-labelled antigen binds to antibody. The assay contains limited amounts of specific antibody and hapten-labelled enzyme. Normally, in the absence of hapten, enzyme activity is virtually abolished by the binding of antibody.

However in the presence of increasing concentrations of free hapten, required to produce the standard curve, or hapten in the test sample, enzyme activity is increased.

This form of the assay has been widely used for haptens and is most commonly used to assay therapeutic drugs and drugs of abuse. The two most commonly used enzymes are glucose-6-phosphate dehydrogenase and malate dehydrogenase. Hapten conjugates of these enzymes are usually inhibited by up to about 80% by excess of antibody to the hapten, probably as a result of a conformational change. In contrast, when thyroxine is conjugated to malate dehydrogenase, there is a substantial inhibition of enzyme activity which can be partially reversed by the binding of thyroxine antibodies. This phenomenon has been used to develop an homogeneous EIA for thyroxine.

EMIT was originally applied only to small molecules but the system has now been developed so that it can measure proteins. The enzyme used was a protein–β–galactosidase conjugate and the normal substrate *o*-nitrophenylgalactoside was converted into a macromolecular form by attachment to a dextran carrier. On addition of protein-specific IgG the enzyme activity was inhibited by up to 95% due to steric exclusion of the substrate.

The major advantage of the EMIT system is that it is easily automated and then produces rapid results at picomole levels of drug. The commercially available 'kit' method has been adapted for use with continuous-flow systems, automated reaction-rate analysers and centrifugal analysers.

Homogeneous Enzyme-Based Immunoassay

A potential disadvantage of the EMIT system is that the hapten–enzyme complex may not produce a reversible effect on binding to antibody. For this to occur the ligand must be bound close to the active site of the enzyme or to amino acids involved in essential conformational changes. At present the certainty of such reactions occurring cannot be predicted for virtually any enzyme. However, other molecules such as substrates, enzyme cofactors and inhibitors are known to interact directly with the active sites of enzymes. If these small molecules are labelled with hapten, it is more certain that the binding of antibody will interfere with their normal combination with enzyme. Also, since the enzyme is not involved in the chemical reactions, a wider range of reaction conditions may be used.

Enzyme substrates have been used as immunoassay labels. However, since the hapten and hapten-labelled substrate are involved in competition, only small amounts of hapten-labelled substrates can be used, thus preventing the normal amplification due to enzyme catalysis. In order to achieve an adequate sensitivity of micromolar concentrations a fluorescent product is formed as illustrated in Fig. 6. This

SELECTION OF ANTISERUM: MONOCLONAL OR POLYCLONAL ANTIBODIES

Antibody preparations can be exquisitely sensitive and specific reagents. They have been applied in many areas of chemistry, biochemistry, physiology, microbiology and medicine. There are two main types of antibody sample, monoclonal and polyclonal. Monoclonal antibodies are pure, highly specific reagents, available in unlimited quantities, which give excellent reproducibility. Polyclonal antibodies are produced by the immunization of an animal. The isolation of serum from that animal gives polyclonal antibodies which always contain a mixture of antibodies directed against a variety of immunogens. It is possible to purify them partially but due to their great similarity in structure and properties, it is normally impossible to obtain a pure antibody in this way. Both types of antibody can be labelled with radiolabels, fluorescent labels, chemiluminescent labels or enzyme labels, and can be used to detect, to localize, and quantitatively to measure chemical, biochemical, microbiological or cellular material.

Monoclonal Antibodies—Advantages and Disadvantages in EIA

Monoclonal antibodies have several important advantages over polyclonal (conventional) antiserum, notably in quality control and in their ability to react with only one antigenic determinant. Since they are one molecular species they give reproducible results with respect to specificity and to antigen binding. Monoclonal antibodies are standard reagents having identical specificity and constant physical and chemical properties. Another advantage of monoclonals is that an impure immunogen can be used to generate monoclonal antibodies against its components even if this component is only present in small quantity.

There are some limitations to the use of monoclonal antibodies. They are expensive to produce and to characterize; hybridoma technology is time consuming, requires special expertise and is generally less available. Occasionally monoclonal antibodies show some instability problems on the solid phase and it is important that plates should be stored at 4°C rather than at room temperature. The storage of monoclonal antibodies or enzyme-labelled monoclonal antibodies in general does not create a problem but on occasion it has been found necessary to store them at high concentrations rather than at high dilution. A monoclonal antibody is produced against a single antigenic determinant and cannot distinguish between a group of different molecules all bearing the same chemical determinant which it recognizes—this is a genuine cross-reaction. A conventional antiserum, on the other hand, containing antibodies to all the determinants on the antigen, may be used as a 'fingerprint' identification for that antigen. Thus complete genuine cross-reactions can occur for monoclonal antibodies and may cause problems where an immunoassay is being used to assay one molecular species amongst several very similar molecular entities. The specificity of a polyclonal antiserum should be well characterized before it is used. A monoclonal antibody normally has obvious advantages in terms of greater specificity. Nevertheless, there could be a problem with a monoclonal antibody when there is (a) heterogeneity of the antigen, (b) a labile antigenic determinant, and (c) a chance occurrence of a similar antigenic determinant on an unrelated molecule. A monoclonal antibody may be of high or low affinity; either may be advantageous or disadvantageous, dependent on the application concerned. For example, in most immunoassay procedures a high affinity antibody is desirable, whilst for immunopurification (affinity chromatography) using a bound antibody, or for a reusable immunobiosensor, a low affinity antibody is preferable. The cost of continued production of a monoclonal antibody is beginning to match that of producing conventional antiserum and before long their reproducibility will lead to their predominance.

Polyclonal Antibodies (Conventional Antiserum) in EIA

Conventional antiserum is cheaper and quicker to produce, and may contain many different antibodies and irrelevant immunoglobulin in addition to other serum proteins. Polyclonal antibodies usually bind to the antigenic determinants of all the components of the immunogen. The antiserum consists of a typical mixture of all the classes and subclasses of antibody and the physical properties of the antiserum are an average. The antiserum can never be reproduced exactly. Cross-reactions observed may not be genuine. Nevertheless, a purified sample of conventional antiserum may be specific for the material of interest and be suitable for the application concerned.

Choice of Antibody

In assays where the antibody is absorbed to the solid phase, monoclonal antibodies, polyclonal antibodies, IgG fractions and $F(ab')_2$ fractions have been used. When serum is to be used then it is essential that it should be used at a sufficiently high dilution to eliminate non-specific factors. It is important to ensure quality control in each batch of a polyclonal antiserum.

Use of Monoclonal Antibodies in Enzyme Immunoassay

The use of monoclonal antibodies in association with enzyme immunoassay has now been very widely used, not only in clinical applications but also in veterinary medicine, horticulture, agriculture, the food industry, environmental health, and forensic science. Their use is largely because of their advantage with respect to specificity. An international meeting on immunoenzymatic techniques highlighted some interesting applications of monoclonal antibodies in enzyme immunoassay. Among the many applications described were:

1. the localization and detection of specific cell types and subpopulations using enzyme-labelled monoclonal antibodies;
2. quantitative analysis of a wide range of molecules including hormones, drugs, HLA antigens, using highly specific and reproducible antibodies;
3. the detection of a number of microbial antigens, especially those for viral diagnosis.

Recently, monoclonal antibodies have been used in sensitive solid-phase enzyme immunoassays for human immune interferon, for the determination of IgM, IgA and IgG rheumatoid factors, for the detection of E.coli heat-stable enterotoxins, and for two-site sandwich enzyme immunoassays for human α-fetoprotein and chorionic gonadotrophin. The technique of enzyme immunoassay utilizing the specificity of monoclonal antibodies is being increasingly used in the determination of a vast range of antigens.

THE ANTIGEN

Many types of antigen, e.g. molecular, cellular and microbial, have been used in enzyme immunoassays. It is not always possible to predict which antigen preparations will be most suitable. In certain systems crude antigens will be quite suitable whilst in others highly purified materials are needed. Insoluble and soluble antigens, including whole cells, have been used quite satisfactorily, although insoluble antigens tend to adsorb less uniformily. An insoluble antigen may sometimes be solubilized by adjusting the pH of the coating buffer. Sometimes it is difficult or impossible to achieve adequate adsorption of the antigen onto the plate but there are various ways of aiding the adsorption of the antigen (see below).

THE SOLID PHASE

A wide range of solid-phase materials has been used for enzyme immunoassays including cellulose, polyacrylamide, agarose, polystyrene and polyvinylchloride to which the antigen or antibody is adsorbed or covalently bound. When selecting a solid phase, it is advantageous to choose one that is specifically marketed for enzyme immunoassay. The most common materials are polystyrene and polyvinylchloride microtitration plates. These two plate-types show wide variation in adsorption properties. Polystyrene plates bind a wide range of antigens, whilst polyvinyl-chloride plates are suitable for binding antibodies. Polyvinylchloride plates are flexible and have the advantage that they can be cut up easily; unlike the rigid polystyrene plates. Irradiated polystyrene plates adsorb more antigen or antibody than non-irradiated plates whilst polyvinylchloride plates have similar adsorption properties to irradiated polystyrene plates. Polystyrene or polyvinylchloride strips of 8 or 12 microtitration wells are available (Dynatech, Flow Laboratories). It is also possible to use cuvettes, beads or tubes, but whichever solid phase is selected there could be variation within the same batch and from batch to batch. Standard positive controls should always be used in enzyme immunoassays.

It is also important to realize that antibodies and antigens bind to plastic in particular orientations, i.e. specific regions of the molecules bind and produce a limited number of orientations and stereochemistry of that molecule.

Adsorption onto the Solid Phase and Coating Conditions

Heterogeneous enzyme immunoassay requires a separation stage. This is usually achieved by the use of solid surfaces which are coated with antibody, antigen or hapten and are disposable. Normally the required protein or hapten conjugated to protein is allowed to adsorb onto the solid surface which is usually negatively charged. The extent and rate of adsorption of the protein are dependent on the nature of the protein, its concentration, the time, pH and temperature of incubation. The adsorption of a monolayer of protein probably occurs by hydrophobic interactions but if an excess of protein is used protein–protein interactions occur and material is more easily lost. This adsorption process is simple and convenient but it has been claimed that under certain conditions adsorbed antibodies may undergo denaturation or loss of adsorbed protein may occur either during washing or when other proteins plus non-ionic detergents are added to prevent non-specific adsorption of other reagents. Both the sensitivity and the reproducibility of the solid-phase enzyme immunoassay technique can be limited by these effects. Sometimes it is also difficult to bind a protein to plastic and covalent binding to the surface has been claimed to overcome these problems, most commonly by the use of glutaraldehyde or a carbodiimide. Occasionally a particular monoclonal antibody may lose activity once bound to the plastic; plates coated with anti-mouse immunoglobulin have been used to solve this problem in addition to saving on quantity of monoclonal antibody used.

A variety of treatments have been applied to the solid phase in order to improve the adsorption characteristics. The solid phase has been treated with hydrochloric acid, glutaraldehyde, ethanol or poly-L-lysine. The binding of viral antigens and of polysaccharide antigens has been successfully increased by using poly-L-lysine, whereas protamine sulphate has been similarly used to increase the adsorption of DNA.

The adsorption to the solid phase is a passive process and the choice of coating conditions must be carefully chosen to avoid subsequent loss of material. This can occur at higher concentrations of the coating antigen or antibody. Therefore, the highest suitable dilution of the antigen or antibody should be selected from the preliminary results for use in the assay. If this is not done, poor assay reproducibility and reduced assay sensitivity will be a problem. For most proteins coating concentrations of $1-10\,\mu g/ml$ are about adequate.

Adsorption of most proteins takes between 2 and 6 hours. The time required varies according to the stability of the different antigens or antibody preparations and the temperature used for coating. For non-protein antigens, longer incubation periods are required. The length of incubation is also dependent on the concentration of the solutions being adsorbed. Different buffers have been used in the coating process, and of these, phosphate-buffered saline and carbonate/bicarbonate buffer, pH 9.6, are perhaps the most common.

It is often necessary to block any free binding sites on the solid phase and this is normally done by adding a protein of low molecular weight such as albumin, gelatin or casein, either to the buffer at the same time as coating, or to the diluent once the plate is coated.

Washing the Solid Phase

The solid phase may be washed manually or automatically. Although microtitration plates, cuvettes and tubes can be washed manually, this is often tedious since the number of washes required ranges from three to nine. A variety of automatic washers is available for microtitration plates (Flow, Dynatech, Ilacon), for cuvettes (Gilford) and for beads (Pentawash). It is essential to ensure that the washing process is fully adequate so that all excess reagents are completely removed. Again, failure to do this will lead to a poor assay sensitivity or reproducibility. The most common wash buffers which are used include phosphate-buffered saline plus $0.05-0.1\%$ Tween 20 at different pH values. The washing and diluent buffers are normally the same throughout the assay with the exception of the coating and substrate buffers.

EXPRESSION OF RESULTS

Results can be read either spectrophotometrically (including fluorescence) or visually. Different types of reader are available and the widest selection of these are available for microtitration plates. Some readers have a single theme and are semi-automatic, that is the plate must be moved manually and the results written down (Dynatech and Flow micro-ELISA readers). The fully automatic types, with dual-beam facilities have the option of a computer attachment (Dynatech and Flow) and plates may be read very rapidly (30 s).

If the results are read visually then clearly the presence or absence of colour represents a positive or negative result. The results can be expressed as an absorbance value where values greater than a certain absorbance value are positive and those less than that are negative. They may also be expressed as a ratio or an endpoint titre, or be compared with those from a standard curve and the results expressed as a specific unit. It is essential to carry out regular quality control checks on all the reagents used in a solid-phase system and this will serve to guarantee the accuracy and reproducibility of the results.

PREPARATION OF ENZYME LABELS

It is usually possible to produce enzyme-labelled monoclonal or polyclonal antibodies without undue difficulty. A monoclonal antibody is an individual molecule and may be unstable under certain conditions. Monoclonal antibodies are easily purified for labelling and provide clean reagents giving low backgrounds. It is significant that in solid-phase sandwich enzyme immunoassays better results are often obtained with enzyme-labelled $F(ab')_2$ fragments than with whole antibodies labelled with the same enzyme. This is almost certainly due to the fact that whole antibodies cause steric hindrance in a manner such that adjacent antigenic determinants cannot be detected by additional labelled antibodies.

The preparation of enzyme-labelled antibodies and antigens involves the utilization of crosslinking reactions which should produce a good yield of the conjugate with minimum alteration to the activity of the enzyme and antibody or antigen. Because of the chemical nature of antibodies, enzymes and protein antigens, the reagents used for modifying proteins or for polypeptide synthesis can also be used to prepare antibody–enzyme or antigen–enzyme conjugates. The formation of such conjugates involves the use of the nucleophilic functional groups of the amino acids which are present; the functional groups most commonly used include the amino group of lysine and the thiol group of cysteine. Other groups used less frequently are the imidazole group of histidine, the guanidino group of arginine, the carboxyl groups of glutamic and aspartic acids, the hydroxyl groups of serine and threonine, the thioether bond of methionine, and the phenolic ring of tyrosine. A whole range of methods for labelling antigens and antibodies with enzymes has been published. These include coupling reagents such as glutaraldehyde, sodium periodate, water-soluble carbodiimides, diisocyanates, difluorodinitrophenylsulphone, cyanuric chloride, diazonium salts, p-benzoquinone, and N,N'-o-phenylenedimaleimide. Different coupling procedures have been compared and reviewed by Avrameas (see 'Further Reading List'). All the above methods involve producing a covalent linkage between the enzyme and the antibody or antigen. The most common methods are described below.

Glutaraldehyde Method

Glutaraldehyde is a bifunctional aldehyde and the use of this reagent is based on the fact that it cross-links the free amino groups of lysyl residues in proteins. When glutaraldehyde is added to a mixture of an enzyme and an antibody it is possible to produce not only the conjugate but also dimers of the antibody and dimers of the enzyme (see Fig. 9). The reaction

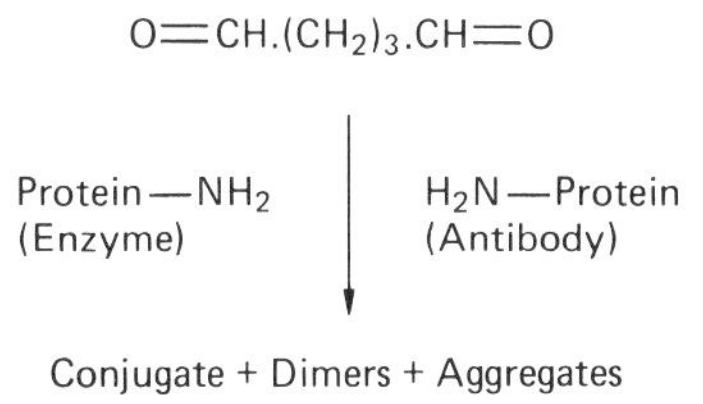

$$O=CH.(CH_2)_3.CH=O$$

Protein—NH$_2$ H$_2$N—Protein
(Enzyme)   (Antibody)

Conjugate + Dimers + Aggregates

Fig. 9 Conjugation of an antibody to an enzyme by the glutaraldehyde method. The antibody–enzyme conjugate is produced in addition to dimers and aggregates of the antibody and enzyme.

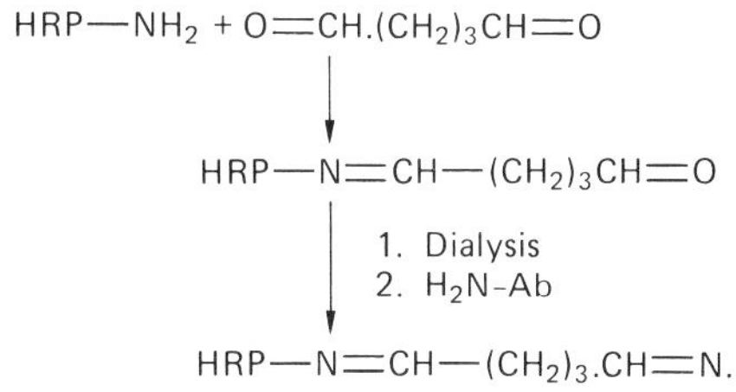

$$HRP—NH_2 + O=CH.(CH_2)_3CH=O$$

$$HRP—N=CH—(CH_2)_3CH=O$$

1. Dialysis
2. H$_2$N–Ab

$$HRP—N=CH—(CH_2)_3.CH=N. Ab$$

Fig. 10 The two-step glutaraldehyde method. The enzyme often used is horseradish peroxidase and this is first treated with glutaraldehyde. Excess aldehyde is removed and the activated enzyme is then reacted with the antibody.

is difficult to control and there is often loss of immunological and enzymic activity. Some of the problems are overcome by the use of the two-step glutaraldehyde method. Peroxidase is the enzyme normally used, as it possesses few free amino groups (see Fig. 10). The enzyme is first treated with glutaraldehyde and the excess aldehyde removed by dialysis. The activated enzyme is then allowed to react with the antibody. Enzyme polymers are still formed but it is possible to obtain a conjugate containing an enzyme:antibody molar ratio of approximately 1:1 by removing the larger enzyme protein complexes when the second stage of the reaction is carried out during molecular sieve chromatography.

The glutaraldehyde method, although it appears to have a number of disadvantages in terms of dimers, aggregates, loss of immunological and enzymic activity, nevertheless often appears to be satisfactory.

Periodate Method

This is a common method for peroxidase enzyme which only has one or two lysine residues available for reaction. However, it also has a number of carbohydrate chains on its surface which may be readily oxidized by sodium periodate (NaIO$_4$) to yield aldehyde groups. These can then react with the ε-amino groups of the antibody in a Schiff's base reaction. The Schiff's base is finally reduced with sodium borohydride to give a stable product and active aldehyde groups are converted into alcohols (see Fig. 11).

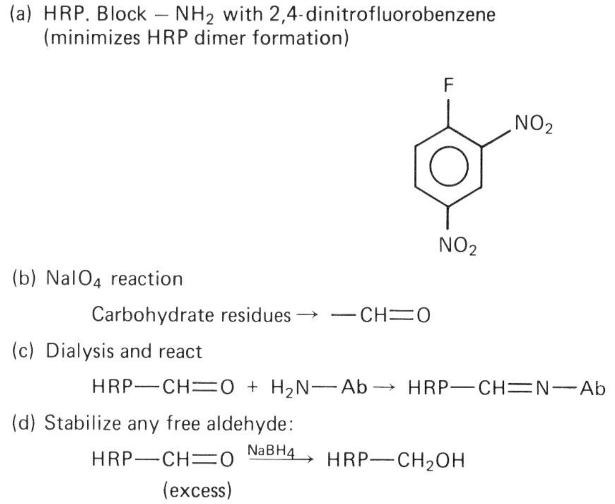

(a) HRP. Block — NH$_2$ with 2,4-dinitrofluorobenzene
    (minimizes HRP dimer formation)

(b) NaIO$_4$ reaction
    Carbohydrate residues → —CH=O

(c) Dialysis and react
    HRP—CH=O + H$_2$N—Ab → HRP—CH=N—Ab

(d) Stabilize any free aldehyde:
    HRP—CH=O $\xrightarrow{NaBH_4}$ HRP—CH$_2$OH
        (excess)

Fig. 11 The periodate method. Free amino groups on horseradish peroxidase are first blocked to reduce dimer formation. Carbohydrate residues are converted into aldehyde and are allowed to react with antibody. The product and residual free aldehyde groups are finally stabilized by reduction.

The use of 2,4-dinitrofluorobenzene to reduce dimer formation is effective to some extent but the reaction still produces over 30% of the peroxidase dimer. Other procedures at a higher pH of 9·5 for the conjugation yield lower quantities of dimer (5%). This second procedure avoids the need to use reagents to block the amino groups. The periodate method has now been extended to utilize glucose oxidase and alkaline phosphatase.

Diisocyanate Methods

Diisocyanates such as toluene diisocyanate (TDIC) are capable of crosslinking antibodies to enzymes via the ε-amino groups of lysine residues. The reaction occurs by addition across the isocyanate residues to give substituted ureas but of course leads to the formation of antibody dimers, enzyme dimers and produces aggregates. The method also has the disadvantage that isocyanates in general are very toxic.

Dimaleimide Method

Maleimide groups react under mild conditions fairly rapidly with thiol groups. The reagent most com-

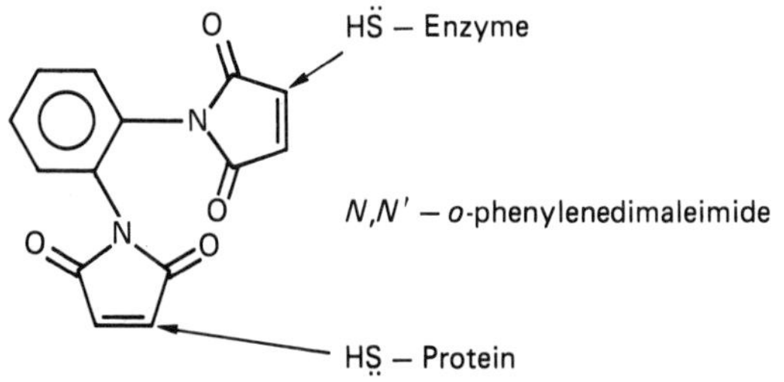

Fig. 12 The dimaleimide method. The nucleophilic reaction of protein or enzyme thiol groups with maleimide double bonds requires very mild conditions and has been utilized to produce conjugates with minimum loss of enzyme activity. This method is only applicable where both enzyme and protein have free thiol groups.

monly used is N,N'-o-phenylenedimaleimide. This has been used for the preparation of a number of conjugates especially with β-galactosidase as this enzyme contains a number of free thiol groups (see Fig. 12). The excess maleimide is removed by gel filtration and typically it is possible to get 50% of β-galactosidase conjugated with a loss of only 5% activity of the enzyme. This method is potentially applicable to all proteins that contain thiol groups. If need be these can be introduced by reaction with 4-methylmercaptobutyrimidate or by a limited reduction of a disulphide bond using 2-mercaptoethylamine. N,N'-o-Oxydimethylenedimaleimide has been utilized to conjugate antibodies with peroxidase, glucose oxidase, β-galactosidase, and penicillinase with high retention of enzyme activity.

Maleimide Ester Method

This method uses m-maleimidobenzoyl-N-hydroxysuccinimide ester (MBS) which reacts at one site with the amino groups of the antibody. Excess of MBS is removed and in a second-stage reaction the thiol groups of the enzyme are reacted with the ester (Fig. 13). Self-polymerization is prevented since anti-

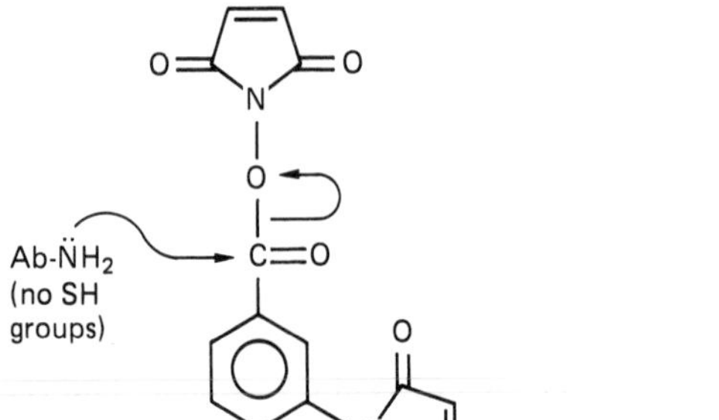

Fig. 13 The m-maleimidobenzoyl-N-hydroxysuccinimide ester (MBS) method. The free amino groups of the antibody first react at the carbonyl site of MBS whilst in the second stage, thiol groups of the enzyme bind to the maleimide double bond. Self-polymerization is prevented by the use of the hetero-bifunctional reagent.

bodies lack thiol groups and a hetero-bifunctional reagent is being used. The reaction to produce the conjugate can be performed in dioxan at pH 7. The solution of antibody in phosphate-buffered saline, pH 7, is added and then passed down a column of Sephadex-200 taking the antibody fractions. The antibody ester conjugate is then reacted finally with the enzyme. Very little loss of enzyme activity or immune reactivity of the individual components occurs in this method. The use of the hetero-bifunctional crosslinking reagent gives a superior linking procedure and a superior conjugate product.

Purification of Enzyme–Antibody Conjugates

Ezyme–antibody conjugates are proteins, and have been purified by a wide variety of techniques including salt fractionation, gel filtration, density gradient centrifugation and affinity chromatography.

In all the conjugation methods the enzyme loses some activity and the antibodies lose some immunoreactivity. The final activity is influenced by the number of enzyme molecules bound to each antibody molecule whereas the immunoreactivity is significantly reduced in polymerized conjugates. There are usually monomeric and polymeric forms of the enzyme and antibody present and they should be removed because they serve to increase the background and decrease the sensitivity of the resulting assay.

Molecular sieve chromatography can be utilized to remove a species of high relative molecular mass. Affinity chromatography generally gives a purer conjugate and is also a more rapid procedure; however, if affinity chromatographic materials are unavailable, it is possible to remove complexes from unbound molecules continuously by allowing the coupling reaction to take place during molecular sieve chromatography. This produces an enzyme–antibody conjugate free from large complexes and the enzyme.

Non-covalent Linkage Between Enzyme and Antibody

Recently, enzyme immunoassay procedures have been developed which are based on the non-covalent, but exceptionally strong interaction of avidin with biotin. Protocols have been produced for the quantitation of both antigens and antibodies. In one method, biotin-labelled antibody, biotin-labelled enzyme and native unlabelled avidin were used to quantitate an antigen. The antigen is allowed to react with the corresponding immobilized antibody, washed and then incubated with an added biotin-labelled antibody. It is washed again to remove excess, and then avidin is added. After further incubation and washing, a biotin-labelled enzyme is added. Measurement of the enzyme associated with the immobilized phase is made. The basis of such assays lies in the fact that avidin possesses four active sites, not all of which are engaged in the interaction with the biotin-labelled antibody. The remaining active sites may then act as acceptors for the biotin-labelled enzyme which is added to the system.

In a second procedure, biotin-labelled antibody and enzyme-labelled avidin are utilized. The biotin-labelled antibody is allowed to react with the antigen previously bound to antibody and, after washing, the enzyme-labelled avidin is added. Following further incubation and washing the enzyme associated with the antigen is quantitated.

The procedures present the advantage of sequential addition of the reagents, therefore the avidin, the antibody and the enzyme label can be introduced independently at chosen concentrations, and in this way a substantial increase in sensitivity of enzyme immunoassays may be achieved.

HAPTEN–ENZYME CONJUGATES

There is a large variety of chemical methods of crosslinking to form hapten–enzyme conjugates and most of these are similar to those used for the preparation of hapten–protein immunogens (see Chapter 31). The reactions used depend on the nature of the hapten, the number of hapten molecules which need to be linked to enzyme, the nature of the bridge, and the site of the bridge, compared to the hapten–protein preparation. If at all possible a different site and crosslinking method should be used, as this avoids interaction between the antibody and the bridge between the hapten and enzyme. This interaction can lead to a decrease in assay sensitivity by as much as 200 times. It is generally advisable to incorporate a spacing group of four to six atoms between the enzyme and hapten so that steric effects on the interaction between antibody and hapten are reduced. The attachment site between hapten and enzyme should be chosen carefully, since this affects the assay specificity.

The enzyme–hapten conjugate must be purified with care as this reduces the sensitivity of enzyme immunoassay. Free enzymes may cause high background signals while the unconjugated hapten will dilute out the enzyme-labelled form. The removal of unconjugated enzyme is not easy but can usually be achieved by affinity chromatography whereas haptens with low relative molecular mass can be readily removed by methods such as dialysis or gel filtration.

Mixed Anhydride Method

Mixed anhydrides of acids are produced at low temperatures and in inert organic solvents, and are then slowly added to the cooled enzyme solution. The protein lysyl and tyrosyl residues react under these conditions. This method has been used with many steroid haptens, morphine and methotrexate. A 10- to 20-fold excess of mixed anhydride is usually needed and the yields are generally fairly low, around 20–30%.

Carbodiimide Method

The carbodiimides contain a reactive N=C=N grouping which readily reacts with amino groups on an enzyme. The water-soluble carbodiimides, 1-ethyl-3-(3-dimethyl-aminopropyl)carbodiimide and 1-cyclohexyl-3-(2-morpholino-4-ethyl) carbodiimide have been used to couple a number of steroid haptens to enzymes. The reaction is carried out at pH 5·5–6·0, and leads to addition of the amino groups of the enzyme across the C=N. One major problem with the carbodiimide method is that intra- and intermolecular crosslinking of enzymes occurs in the reaction.

Periodate Method

Dialdehydes are generated when carbohydrate residues are cleaved with periodate and these can be coupled to amines. This approach should be widely applicable since any amino-containing hapten can be conjugated with a glycoprotein after cleavage with periodate. Nevertheless, the result of coupling certain haptens with enzymes is not efficient.

m-Maleimidobenzoic Acid N-hydroxysuccinimide Ester (MBSE)

MBSE is a heterobifunctional reagent which has been used in a two-stage process to couple haptens to β-galactosidase which contains several free thiol residues. β-Galactosidase has also been conjugated with penicillin and gentamicin using N-(3-maleimidopropionylglycyloxy) succinimide. Using these two reagents, one to produce the enzyme label, and one to produce the immunogen incorporating different bridging groups improves the sensitivity of the resulting enzyme immunoassay. N-(γ-maleimidobutyryloxy) succinimide has been used as a crosslinking agent and has led to the production of several very sensitive enzyme immunoassays. The conjugates mentioned in this section retain very high enzyme activity and immunoreactivity.

Bifunctional Imidates

β-Galactosidase conjugates have been produced using a bifunctional imidate, dimethyl adipimidate which reacts with amino groups under alkaline conditions. The reaction is carried out in two stages, first the imidate and the hapten are reacted under anhydrous conditions, and then they are allowed to react with the enzyme in aqueous solution.

EVALUATION OF THE CURRENT STATUS OF ENZYME LABELS

The main benefits of the use of enzymes as labels in immunoassay have been the development of a wide range of homogeneous immunoassays and the enthusiastic search for improved immunoenzymometric assays.

The homogeneous assays were originally restricted to the assay of haptens in quite high concentrations. However, progress has been made towards measuring large antigens by a range of simple techniques. Many of these assays can be easily automated and are then able to give results in a few minutes. There has always been the worry that these assays would be adversely affected by the presence of interfering substances in biological fluids. In general this has not been a major problem and its possibility is best reduced by developing more sensitive assays so that only small quantities of biological fluid are needed. This problem should not affect the immunometric assays because of the many washing stages that are required.

Another problem with enzyme labels is that their assay may be imprecise when compared to radiolabels. This problem is reduced by using reliable automated equipment for homogeneous assays where rate measurements are required and including the relevant set of standards. In the case of the immunoenzymometric assays the problem is partly overcome because of the batchwise approach to assays. Thus variations in temperature, in particular, affect all the samples in a batch, including the standards.

A potential bonus of homogeneous assays is the development of simple dipstick tests. These have been developed based on the SLFIA, PGLIA, and the 'enzyme-channelling immunoassay'. These allow complicated tests to be performed with good precision and limited equipment, usually a reflectance photometer is required to measure the endpoint. In one case only a scale is needed to measure peak heights.

The preparation of enzyme labels may lead to a range of polymers, only some of which contain both enzyme and antibody. This means that for the most sensitive assays it is necessary to purify the enzyme labels, preferably by affinity methods. In many cases it is possible to include an extra step in an immunoenzymometric assay so as to use a commercially prepared general enzyme label. This extra step obviously takes additional time but may mean that no chemical synthesis is needed. However, for the most sensitive assays the commercially available reagents generally require further purification. It is worth noting that homogeneous assays nearly always use commercially prepared reagents whereas immunoenzymometric assays are simpler for the individual to set up, although they may require the preparation of specific reagents.

This individual approach to immunoenzymometric assay has encouraged the development of three types of assay. Simple qualitative assays, where the development of a coloured product has been of great benefit in large screening surveys. Second, quantitative assays to replace radioimmunoassay when there is a need to avoid radiation hazards or because the equipment necessary for radioactive counting is not available. Thirdly, there are the very sensitive assays

which are only possible using immunometric techniques. These require reliable and precise methodology coupled with large signal amplification. This is generally not possible using straightforward enzyme assays but requires the combined techniques discussed above.

Another advantage of enzymic endpoints is the relevant ease of measuring two analytes in the same sample, although it has yet to be thoroughly exploited.

Properly designed enzyme immunoassays give comparable results to radioimmunoassays in terms of sensitivity, precision, specificity and accuracy. Indeed, the sensitivity can be significantly greater. In addition, the advantages of enzyme immunoassay include stable reagents, low cost, simple equipment and safety.

Solid-phase EIA systems provide sensitive, rapid and inexpensive methods which are particularly suitable for screening large numbers of samples. They are becoming more widely and routinely utilized in laboratories and are replacing some of the more established techniques.

FURTHER READING

Avrameas S., Druet P., Masseyeff R., Feldmann G. (eds.) (1983). *Immunoenzymatic Techniques, Proceedings of the Second International Symposium on Immunoenzymatic Techniques.* Amsterdam, New York, Oxford: Elsevier Science Publishers.

Blake C., Al-Bassam M. N., Gould B. J., Marks V., Bridges J. W., Riley C. (1982). Simultaneous enzyme immunoassay of two thyroid hormones. *Clin. Chem*; **28**: 1469.

Blake C., Gould B. J. (1984). Use of enzymes in immunoassay techniques: A review. *Analyst*; **109**: 533.

Ekins R. P. (1985). Current concepts and future developments. In *Alternative Immunoassays* (Collins W. P., ed.) Chichester, New York, Brisbane, Toronto, Singapore: Wiley.

Engvall E., Perlmann P. (1971). Enzyme-linked immunosorbent assay (ELISA). Quantitative assay for immunoglobulin G. *Immunochemistry*; **8**: 871.

Harris C. C., Yolken R. H., Krokan H., Hsu I C. (1979). Ultrasensitive enzymatic radioimmunoassay: application to detection of cholera toxin and rotavirus. *Proc. Natl. Acad. Sci. USA*; **76**: 5336.

Hubbard R., Wiseman A. (1983). Enzyme immunoassay and the use of monoclonal antibodies. *Trends in Analytical Chemistry*; **2** (7) 7.

Ishikawa E., Imagawa M., Yoshitake S., Niitsu Y., Urushizaki I., Inada M., Imura H., Kanazawa R., Tachibana S., Nakazawa N., Ogawa H. (1982). Major factors limiting sensitivity of sandwich enzyme immunoassay for ferritin, immunoglobulin E and thyroid-stimulating hormone. *Ann. Clin. Biochem*; **19**: 379.

Johannsson A., Stanley C. J., Self C. H. (1985). A fast highly sensitive colorimetric enzyme immunoassay system demonstrating benefits of enzyme amplification in clinical chemistry. *Clin. Chim. Acta*; **148**: 119.

Kemeny D. M., Challacombe S. J. (1986). Advances in ELISA and other solid-phase immunoassays. *Immunology Today*; **7**: 67.

Litman D. J., Lee R. H., Jeong H. J., Tom H. K., Stiso S. N., Sizto N. C., Ullman E. F. (1983). An internally referenced test strip immunoassay for morphine. *Clin. Chem*, **29**: 1598.

Morris D. L., Ellis P. B., Carrico R. J., Yeager F. M., Schroeder H. R., Albarella J. P., Boguslaski R. C. (1981). Flavin adenine dinucleotide as a label in homogeneous colorimetric immunoassays. *Anal. Chem*; **53**: 658.

Ngo T. T., Carrico R. J., Boguslaski R. C., Burd J. F. (1981). Homogeneous substrate-labelled fluorescent immunoassay for IgG in human serum, *J. Immunol. Meth*, **42**: 93.

O'Sullivan M. J. (1984). Enzyme immunoassay. In *Practical Immunoassay: the State of the Art* (Butt W. R. ed.) New York and Basel: Marcel Dekker.

Shalev A., Greenberg A. H., McAlpine P. J. (1980). Detection of attograms of antigens by a high sensitivity enzyme-linked immunosorbent assay (HS-ELISA) using a fluorogenic substrate. *J. Immunol. Meth*; **38**: 125.

Shimizu S. Y., Kabakoff D. S., Sevier E. D. (1985). Monoclonal antibodies in immunoenzymetric assays, In *Enzyme-mediated Immunoassay* (Ngo T. T., Lenhoff H. M., eds) New York and London: Plenum Press.

Van Weeman B. K., Schuurs A. H. W. M. (1975). The influence of heterologous combinations of antiserum and enzyme-labelled estrogen on the characteristics of estrogen enzyme-immunoassays. *Immunochemistry*; **12**: 667.

Voller A., Bartlett A., Bidwell D. E. (1978). Enzyme immunoassay with special reference to ELISA techniques. *J. Clin. Pathol*, **31**: 507.

Voller A., Bidwell D. E. (1980). *The Enzyme Linked Immunosorbent Assay*, Vol. 2. *A review of recent developments*. Guernsey: Microsystems.

Zuk R. F., Ginsberg V. K., Houts T., Rabbie J., Merrick H., Ullman E. F., Fisher M. M., Sizto C. C., Stiso S. N., Litman D. J. (1985). Enzyme immunochromatography—a quantitative immunoassay requiring no instrumentation. *Clin. Chem*; **31**: 1144.

34. Non-isotopic Immunoassays: Luminescence and Fluorescence

G. Wynne Aherne

INTRODUCTION

For over 20 years, radioimmunoassay (RIA) methods have been widely used in clinical chemistry for the measurement of many hormones, proteins and drugs. The principles of RIA have been described in Chapter 31. Whilst laboratories will continue to use RIAs for many years to come, there is a tendency to replace them with non-isotopic immunoassays. The favourable characteristics of RIA, e.g. exquisite sensitivity, specificity, precision and high sample-handling capacity have to be weighed against the disadvantages of the use of radioisotopically labelled antigens. The high cost and instability of radio-labelled antigens coupled to the increasing legislative problems encountered with their use and disposal has led to the development of non-isotopic assays.

In theory, and often in practice, non-isotopic immunoassays retain all the major advantages of RIA, i.e. sensitivity and specificity, since these are to a large extent dictated by the quality of the antiserum or antibody used. Non-isotopic assays are often simpler to perform than RIA and offer similar advantages of high sample throughput and small sample volumes. In RIA, because the signal from the radioisotope cannot be modified, a separation step to distinguish antibody-bound label from free label is essential and automation of complete assays has presented some difficulties.

A number of alternatives to radioactive tracers have been investigated but enzymes have been the most widely used non-isotopic labels,[1] and are discussed separately in this volume. Over the last few years the advantages of fluorescent and luminescent labels in immunoassay have been recognized and such assays, whether developed within individual laboratories or produced commercially, are now a feature of many immunoassay laboratories.

Non-isotopic labels, if they are to replace radioactivity as the end point in immunoassays, should be relatively stable, easy to prepare, inexpensive and should not be associated with potential risks to health. They should retain the potential of sensitivity and their measurement should not be subject to interference from sample components. Equipment for measuring the end point of the assay should be readily available and be able to accommodate the numbers of samples that immunoassay laboratories are used to handling. Such equipment (mostly developed along with commercial immuno-reagents) has become available over the last few years, opening the way for greater acceptance of luminescent and fluorescent assays in routine as opposed to research and development laboratories.

LUMINESCENT LABELS IN IMMUNOASSAY

Both bioluminescent and chemiluminescent molecules have been used to label reagents for use in immunoassays. Three types of assay can be defined.

Bioluminescent Immunoassay

In this type of assay the antigen or antibody is labelled with a bioluminescent reagent such as luciferin or luciferase (obtained from the firefly or bacteria). Alternatively, molecules can be labelled with a cofactor (e.g. NAD or ATP) which is involved in or linked to the luciferase/luciferin reaction.

The firefly luciferase reaction can be depicted by:

$$\text{Luciferin} + O_2 + \text{ATP} \xrightarrow{\text{luciferase}} \text{oxyluciferin} + \text{AMP} + CO_2 \, PP_i + \text{LIGHT}$$

and the bacterial luciferase reaction by:

$$\text{substrate} + \text{NAD} \xrightarrow{\text{dehydrogenase}} \text{NADH} + \text{products}$$

$$\text{NADH} \xrightarrow{\text{oxidoreductase}} \text{NAD} + \text{FMNH}_2$$

$$\text{FMNH}_2 + O_2 + \text{long-chain aldehyde} \xrightarrow{\text{luciferase}} \text{FMN} + \text{RCO}_2\text{H} + \text{LIGHT}$$

As examples, the firefly luciferase reaction was used as label in an assay for methotrexate,[2] and the bacterial system using NAD-labelled reagents has been used for the measurement of steroids.[3]

The availability and stability of highly purified bioluminescence reagents may be a problem for their widespread use in immunoassays but these could be outweighed by the stability and the high quantum yield of light emission.

Chemiluminescent Immunoassay

In this type of assay the antigen or antibody is labelled with a chemiluminescent molecule which upon oxidation emits light. Light emission occurs extremely rapidly (0–10s) allowing high sample throughout but necessitating the carefully timed addition of oxidant and strict standardization of oxidation requirements. Because of the rapid signal generation, the oxidizing reagent must be added directly to the sample once it is in place in the measuring chamber. One disadvantage of such chemiluminescent end points is that the light emission cannot be read again at a later time.

Since each labelled molecule can react to give a signal the potential sensitivity of chemiluminescent labels is higher than for radioactivity. In spite of low

quantum efficiencies, luminescent molecules can be detected at very low levels ($<10^{-18}$ mol), but it must be remembered that immunoassay sensitivity is primarily determined by the antibody used and increased sensitivity will not necessarily be achieved by using a chemiluminescence endpoint. The measurement of chemiluminescence can be affected by quenching of the light output by coloured or fluorescent compounds. Luminescence is theoretically read against a background of zero, although impure reagents and water can cause high levels of background luminescence.

Luminol and Isoluminol Based Immunoassays. Luminol and isoluminol have been widely used in immunoassay for labelling both antigens and antibodies. The oxidation of luminol under basic conditions requires the presence of a catalyst, e.g. microperoxidase or other haem-containing protein and hydrogen peroxide (Fig. 1). If luminol is coupled to antigens

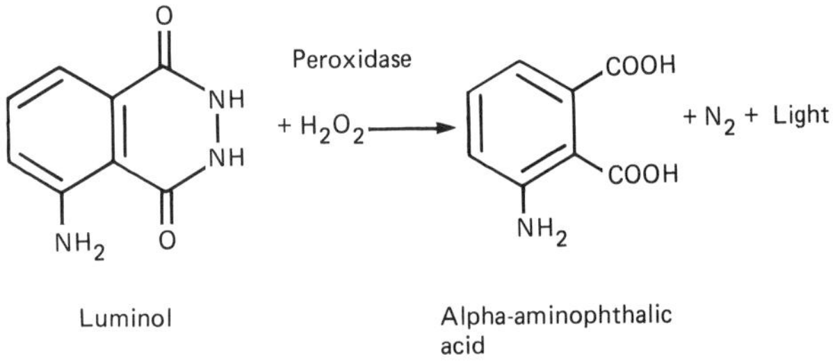

Fig. 1 The oxidation of luminol by peroxidase.

or antibodies via the aromatic amino group the quantum yield of light is drastically reduced. Isoluminol, although only 10% as efficient as luminol, has been extensively used for preparing conjugates, since reaction of the more favourable amino group does not reduce quantum efficiency significantly. Several derivatives of isoluminol, e.g. ABE1 (N- (4-amino butyl)-N-ethyl isoluminol), are available and are easily coupled to antigens and antibodies using chemical methods already familiar to the immunoassayist.

Luminol or isoluminol labels can be used in any type of immunoassay as a direct alternative to a radiolabel, such assays having similar characteristics to the corresponding RIA. These include separation assays using dextran-coated charcoal[4] or antibody precipitation,[5] and solid-phase assays using coated tubes or beads.[6] Immunometric assays[6] have also been developed with luminol labels. The use of a 'Universal Reagent', e.g. isoluminol-labelled second antibody, has been advocated for hapten assays in which an antigen–conjugate is used to coat the solid phase.[7,8] However, problems are encountered with this type of assay when the conjugate used for coating the solid phase is similar to that used to produce the antiserum. Homogeneous (non-separation) assays which depend on enhancement of light output when labelled ligand is bound by antibody have been reported.[9] Although easy to carry out, this type of assay is subject to interference from sample components.

One major disadvantage of the use of luminol-based labels is the necessity for a period of incubation in NaOH (1–5M) following phase separation and prior to light initiation. This incubation not only provides the alkaline pH required for the light reaction but enhances the amount of light produced by dissociating the antibody-bound complexes. Each assay system requires optimization of this incubation step in terms in NaOH concentration, time and temperature. This limitation has been overcome by the use of acridinium ester labels and enhanced luminescence.

Acridinium Ester-based Assays. Acridinium esters[10] have been used as labels for immunoassay with several advantages over luminol-type molecules. The mechanism of the chemiluminescent reaction is represented in Fig. 2.

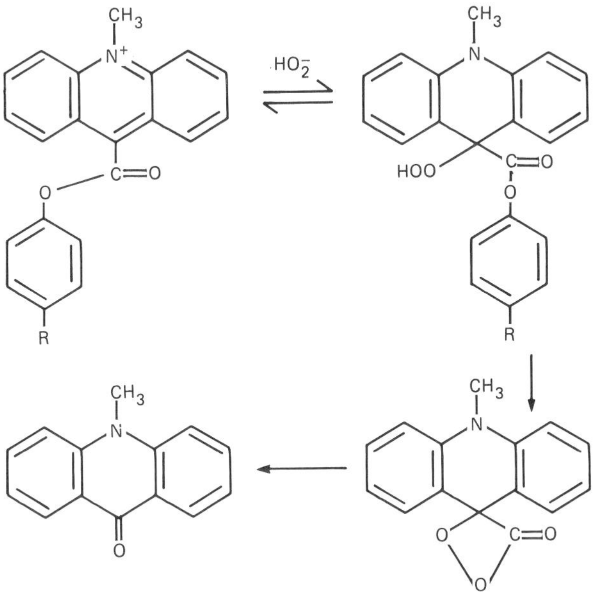

Fig. 2 The mechanism of a chemiluminescent reaction.

In contrast to luminol, light is produced in the presence of dilute alkaline hydrogen peroxide, in the absence of catalyst and without the need of an incubation step. During the reaction, the chemiluminescent moiety is liberated from the antigen or antibody prior to release of light, minimizing quenching and without the need for long incubations in strong alkali.

The usual time course of the acridinium ester light reaction is very rapid (1–5s) but this can be varied from seconds to hours by manipulation of reagent concentrations, etc. As with luminol there is no opportunity to re-read samples. Another advantage of the use of acridinium esters is the ease with which

reagents can be labelled using an activated N-succinimidyl ester form of the compound. Mild conditions can be used to couple this to proteins and haptens thereby minimizing immunological damage.

Acridinium esters have been used to develop extremely sensitive two-site immunometric assays for a number of proteins, e.g. AFP,[11] human TSH,[12] and labelled antibodies and magnetic separation have been used for haptens, e.g. thyroxine.[13] The use of acridinium esters in immunoassays forms the basis of commercially available kits and equipment (e.g. Magic® Lite, Ciba Corning).

Chemiluminescent Enzyme Immunoassay (Enhanced Luminescence)

In this type of assay the immunological reagent is labelled with an enzyme, i.e. horseradish peroxidase, and this is quantitated at the end of the assay using luminol/isoluminol as a substrate in the presence of hydrogen peroxide. Normally, the quantum yield of light from this enzyme-catalysed reaction is low resulting in insensitivity of measurement. The light output of the reaction can be considerably increased (1000–1500 times) by the addition of an enhancer. The first report of enhanced luminescence used firefly luciferin as an enhancer[14] but other chemicals, e.g. 6-hydroxybenzothiazoles[15] and substituted phenols, can also be used. The light produced in enhanced reactions is not only intense, with an improved signal-to-noise ratio, but is produced over a relatively long period of time (20–30 min). The mechanisms of the enhanced reaction are not completely understood but are thought to involve acceleration of rate limiting steps involved in the conversion of luminol.[16]

These characteristics of enhanced luminescence mean that the endpoint of immunoassays can be initiated by the addition of one reagent (containing luminol/isoluminol, enhancer and hydrogen peroxide). The reagent can be added outside the measuring instrument and the samples can be re-read within the time span of 20–30 min. This type of luminescent reaction has been exploited in the Amerlite® immunoassay system (Amersham International plc) and a wide range of analytes can now be measured. Perhaps more importantly, many enzyme immunoassays, e.g. ELISA methods, already use horseradish peroxidase labels with colorimetric end points and these can be readily converted into luminescent assays, with potentially greater sensitivity, now that luminescent plate readers are commercially available (e.g. Dynatech).

The prolonged light emission by enhanced luminescent reactions has also been used to obtain semi-quantitative permanent results using high-speed polaroid films.[17] Camera luminometers (now commercially available) will facilitate the development of rapid screening immunoassays for both laboratory and field use.

FLUORESCENT LABELS IN IMMUNOASSAY

Several types of fluorescent molecules have been used as labels in immunoassay. Labelled reactants have proved extremely stable and are inexpensive to produce. The assay endpoint can be measured rapidly using equipment which is available in most laboratories.

The specific activity of fluorescent labels is potentially very high since for each labelled moiety many detectable events can be identified. However, in practice the sensitivity of fluorescent assays has been disappointingly low because of interferences from biological samples. These include light-scattering effects, caused by lipids and other macromolecules, and inner filter effects caused by light absorption by chromophores such as haemoglobin. Quenching of fluorescence can be caused by a number of factors including binding to proteins such as albumin and specific antibodies. The low sensitivity, though, is mainly due to the presence of endogenous fluorescent compounds in biological samples. The presence of bilirubin for example causes a high background fluorescence in the same region as the commonly used fluorescent probes. The low sensitivity achieved for most fluoroimmunoassays has meant that the most successful assays have been for the measurement of haptens and drugs for which a high degree of sensitivity is not normally required.

Fluorescent labels should ideally retain much of the quantum efficiency of the fluorophore and retain the immunoreactivity of the antigen or antibody upon conjugation. Commonly used fluorescent labels include fluorescein, rhodamine, umbelliferones and rare earth chelates. Fluorescent labels can directly replace the corresponding radiolabel in RIA and, following separation, fluorescence can be measured in either the bound or the free fraction. Solid-phase assays have been widely applied to fluoroimmunoassays as the washing steps involved can minimize background fluorescence although some plastics can contribute to both background and scattering effects. The use of magnetized particles for phase separation has also been used extensively in fluoroimmunoassays[18] since, when the particles have been sedimented at the bottom of the tube, the fluorescence can be measured directly in the supernatant.

Non-separation Fluoroimmunoassays

In contrast to RIA, and to a lesser extent luminoimmunoassays, fluoroimmunoassays (FIA) have provided the means of achieving several types of non-separation or homogeneous assay which have been exploited commercially.

Quenching Fluoroimmunoassay. The fluorescence of a labelled antigen can be quenched as a result of binding to a specific antibody. Antibodies vary in their quenching abilities and the degree of quenching can be related to the amount of antigen bound by specific antibody. The assays are rapid and simple to perform. Direct quenching assays[19] apply only to the measurement of haptens and indirect quenching techniques are needed for the assay of proteins. This type of assay[20,21] depends on the steric hindrance of the specific antibody in an antibody-labelled antigen complex preventing the attachment of a quenching antibody, e.g. anti-fluorescein.

If antigen and antibody are labelled with different fluorophores, e.g. fluoroscein and rhodamine it is possible to develop a quenching assay in which rhodamine absorbs the emitted light from excited fluorescein when antigen–antibody complexes are formed.[22] These assays are analogous to energy transfer assays which utilize reagents labelled with a fluorescent label and a luminescent label.[23]

Release FIA (substrate-labelled FIA). The substrate-labelled fluoroimmunoassay is a homogeneous type of assay in which a non-fluorescent probe, β-galactosyl-umbelliferone, is used to label the antigen (usually a hapten). The label is not fluorescent until, under the action of an enzyme, β-galactosidase, it is hydrolysed to its fluorescent product.[24] When the label is antibody-bound, enzymatic hydrolysis is prevented and there is no release of fluorescence. Therefore, when unlabelled antigen competes with the label for antibody binding there is an increase in fluorescence proportional to the amount of unlabelled antigen present. This assay system forms the basis of the Ames TDA® immunoassay kits for therapeutic drug monitoring which are simple to use, accurate and reliable in routine use.[25]

Polarization FIA. Hapten assays based on the application of fluorescence polarization[26] form the basis of the Abbot TDX® system. In this homogeneous type of assay, antigen labelled with a fluorophore is excited with polarized light and the extent of polarization of the emitted light is measured. Small labelled molecules, with fast random rotation, exhibit a low signal whilst antibody-bound label, with increased size and reduced random rotation, exhibit an enhanced signal. These assays are quick and simple to perform but are applicable only to small molecules ($<20\,000$ mol. wt). The level of sensitivity is low but the assay system is admirably suited to therapeutic drug monitoring.

Time-Resolved Fluoroimmunoassays

Homogeneous fluoroimmunoassay methods offer speed, simplicity and precision of end-point measurement but have been limited by low sensitivity compared with RIA. The main reason for this limited sensitivity is the high background fluorescence associated with components of biological samples. The recent use of time-resolved fluorescence measurement and labels with a long fluorescent decay time have overcome this limitation.

The fluorescence of commonly used fluorophores, such as fluoroscein, decay at a similar rate to the fluorescence of proteins (<10 ns) whereas the decay time of some lanthanide chelates is several orders of magnitude longer (10^3–10^6 ns). By using time-resolved fluorometric measurements it is possible to measure the signal from the chelate after the background fluorescence has decayed. Increased sensitivity is also achieved because the lanthanide chelates have a large Stokes' shift which together with the very sharp emission peak, reduces the background signal arising from non-specific fluorescence and light scattering. Europium chelates have been most thoroughly investigated in the context of immunoassay.[27]

The characteristics of europium fluorescence are dependent on the ligands which chelate the ion and on its physical environment. For immunoassay the ion has to be strongly bound to either the antigen or the antibody and EDTA derivatives, e.g. amino-phenyl-EDTA and isothiocyanate-phenyl-EDTA, have been used. Following the labelling procedures, the europium ions are in a non-fluorescent form and at the end of the assay an 'enhancement solution' is added (containing β-deketone, trioctylphosphine and Triton X-100 at pH 3·2) to dissociate the europium ion from the labelled moiety and to chelate it in a highly fluorescent form.

These principles have now been successfully applied to a range of analytes[28,29] and immunoassay kits and the appropriate instrumentation are commercially available (Delfia®, Pharmacia-LKB). The assays have a wide dynamic range and a high degree of sensitivity. The labels are stable and biochemically inert, and, with very short measurement times, sample throughput is high.

SUMMARY

Both chemiluminescent and fluorescent labels have been successfully used to develop reliable, robust immunoassays which perform as well as or even better than those which utilize radio-labels. RIA techniques will continue to be widely used for some years to come but it is inevitable that there will be an increasing movement to the use of non-isotopic assays. Commercially available reagents and equipment for a range of analytes will ensure that these non-isotopic assay techniques find a place within the clinical biochemistry laboratory. However, complete acceptance of such methods will depend upon the ease with which individual laboratories can adapt their own assays and reagents to the new technologies.

REFERENCES

1. Voller A., Bartlett A., Bidwell D. E. (1978). Enzyme immunoassays with special reference to ELISA techniques. *J. Clin. Pathol*; **96:** 507–20.

2. Wannlund J., Azari J., Levine L., De Luca M. (1980). A bioluminescent immunoassay for methotrexate at the subpicomole level. *Biochem. Biophys. Res. Commun*; **96:** 440–6.

3. Hughes J., Short F., James V. H. T. (1984). Synthesis of a novel bioluminescent conjugate of progesterone for immunoassay. In *Analytical Applications of Bioluminescence and Chemiluminescence* (Kricka L., Stanley P. E., Thorpe G. H. G., Whitehead T. eds), pp. 269–72. New York; Academic Press.

4. Pazzagli M., Kim J. B., Messeri G., *et al*. (1981). Luminescent immunoassay (LIA) of cortisol. 2. Development and validation of the immunoassay monitored by chemiluminescence. *J. Steroid Biochem*; **14:** 1181–7.

5. Pratt J. J., Woldring M. G., Villerius L. (1978). Chemiluminescence—linked immunoassay. *J. Immunol. Methods*; **21:** 179–84.

6. Barnard G. J., Kim J. B., Brockelbank J. L., *et al.* (1984). Measurement of choriogonadotropin by chemiluminescence immunoassay and immunochemiluminometric assay: 1. Use of isoluminol derivatives. *Clin. Chem*; **30:** 538–41.

7. Wood W. G., Fricke H., von Klitzing L., Strasburger C. J., Scriba P. C. (1982). Solid phase antigen luminescence immunoassays (SPALT) for the determination of insulin, insulin antibodies and gentamicin levels in human serum. *J. Clin. Chem. Clin. Biochem*; **20:** 825–31.

8. Hardcastle A., Aherne G. W., Marks V. (1987). A solid phase luminescent immunoassay for methotrexate. In *Bioluminescence and Chemiluminescence. New Perspectives* (Scholmerich J., Andreesen R., Kapp A., Ernst M., Woods W. G., eds) pp. 317–20. Chichester; Wiley.

9. Kohen F., Passagli M., Kim J. B., *et al.* (1979). An assay procedure for plasma progesterone based on antibody enhanced chemiluminescence. *FEBS Lett*: **104:** 201–5.

10. McCapra F., Tutt D. E., Topping R. M. (1977). Assay method utilizing chemiluminescence. *Br. Pat.* 1, 461, 877.

11. Weeks I., Campbell A. K., Woodhead J. S. (1983). Two-site immunochemiluminometric assay for human α_1-fetoprotein. *Clin. Chem*; **29:** 1480–3.

12. Weeks I., Sturgess M., Siddle K., Jones M. K., Woodhead J. S. (1984). A high sensitivity immunochemiluminometric assay for human thyrotrophin. *Clin. Endocrinol*; **20:** 489–95.

13. Sturgess M. L., Weeks I., Mpoku C. N., Laing I., Woodhead J. S. (1986). Chemiluminescent labelled-antibody assay for thyroxin in serum with magnetic separation of the solid phase. *Clin. Chem*; **32:** 532–5.

14. Whitehead T. P., Thorpe G. H. G., Carter T. J. N., Groucutt C., Kricka L. J. (1983). Enhanced luminescence procedure for sensitive determination of peroxidase-labelled conjugates in immunoassay. *Nature*; **305:** 158–9.

15. Thorpe G. H. G., Kricka L. J., Gillespie E., Moseley S., *et al.* (1985). Enhancement of the horse radish peroxidase-catalysed chemiluminescent oxidation of cyclic diacyl hydrazides by 6-hydroxybenzothiazoles. *Anal. Biochem*; **145:** 96–100

16. Thorpe G. H. G., Kricka L. J. (1987). Enhanced chemiluminescent assays for horseradish peroxidase: characteristics and applications. In *Bioluminescence and chemiluminescence. New Perspectives.* (Scholmerich

J., Andreesen R., Kapp A., Ernst M., Woods W. G., eds). pp. 199–208. Chichester: Wiley.

17. Thorpe G. H. G., Kricka L. J., Moseley S. B., Whitehead T. P. (1985). Phenols as enhancers of the chemiluminescent horseradish peroxidase—luminol—hydrogen peroxide reaction: Applications in luminescence-monitored enzyme immunoassays. *Clin. Chem*; **31**: 1335–41.

18. Pourfarzaneh M., White W., Landon J., Smith D. S. (1980). Direct determination of cortisol in serum by fluoroimmunoassay with magnetisable solid-phase. *Clin. Chem*; **26**: 730–3.

19. Broughton A., Frazier M. (1978). A quenching fluoroimmunoassay for the aminoglycoside netilmicin. *Clin. Chem*; **24**: 1033.

20. Nargessi R. D., Landon J., Smith D. S. (1979). Use of antibodies against the label in non-separation non-isotopic immunoassay: 'indirect quenching' fluoroimmunoassay of proteins. *J. Immunol. Methods*; **26**: 307–13.

21. Zuk R. F., Rowley G. L., Ullman E. F. (1979). Fluorescence protection immunoassay: a new homogenous assay technique. *Clin. Chem*; **25**: 1554–60.

22. Ullman E. F., Schwarzberg M., Rubenstein K. E. (1976). Fluorescent excitation transfer immunoassay. A general method for determination of antigens. *J. Biol. Chem*; **251**: 4172–8.

23. Campbell A. K., Roberts P. A., Patel A. (1985). Chemiluminescence energy transfer: a technique for homogenous immunoassay. In *Alternative Immunoassays* (Collins, W. P. ed.). pp. 153–83. Chichester: Wiley.

24. Burd J. F., Wong R. C., Feeney J. E. *et al*. (1977). Homogenous reactant-labelled fluorescent immunoassay for therapeutic drugs exemplified by gentamicin determination in human serum. *Clin. Chem*; **23**: 1402–8.

25. Davis S. J., Marks V. (1983). Measurement of serum theophylline concentrations using a modified Ames TDA® System. *Ther. Drug Monit*; **5**: 479–84.

26. Watson R. A. A., Landon J., Shaw E. J., Smith D. S. (1976). Polarization fluoroimmunoassay for gentamicin. *Clin. Chim. Acta*; **73**: 51–5.

27. Hemmila I., Dakabu S., Mutkala, V.-M., *et al*. (1984). Europium as a label in time-resolved immuno-fluorometric assays. *Anal. Biochem*; **137**: 335–43.

28. Pettersson K., Siitari H., Hemmila I., Soini E. *et al*. (1983). Time-resolved fluoroimmunoassay of human choriogonadotropin. *Clin. Chem*; **29**: 60–4.

29. Suonpaa M. U., Lavi J. T., Hemmila I. A., Lovgren T. N. (1985). A new sensitive assay of human alpha-fetoprotein using time-resolved fluorescence and monoclonal antibodies. *Clin. Chim. Acta*; **145**, 341–9.

FURTHER READING

The following symposia are recommended for those wishing to obtain further details.

Collins W. P., ed. (1985). *Alternative Immunoassays*. Chichester: Wiley.

Collins W. P., ed. (1988). *Complementary Immunoassays*. Chichester: Wiley.

Kricka L. J., Stanley P. E., Thorpe G. H. G., Whitehead T. P., eds (1984). *Analytical Applications of Bioluminescence and Chemiluminescence*. New York: Academic Press.

Scholmerich J., Andreesen R., Kapp A., Ernst M., Woods W. G., eds (1987) *Bioluminescence and Chemiluminescence. New Perspectives*. Chichester: Wiley.

35. Techniques in Automation

J. G. H. Cook and Bernard F. Rocks

INTRODUCTION

The tremendous technological developments which have taken place in recent years have led to the production of small automatic analysers which, although sophisticated in design, are simple and reliable enough to be used by inexperienced staff at the bedside. This has encouraged some eminent clinical biochemists to express the view that the days of the large multichannel analyser are over. This view is not shared by the manufacturers who continue to invest considerable sums of money in the development of large capacity machines of increasing sophistication. Nor is the view shared by the directors of the larger commercial laboratories whose survival depends on cost effectiveness; it is not unknown for several large-capacity analysers to be housed under the same roof. Large multichannel analysers still remain as the workhorse in the UK National Health Service enabling hospital laboratories to cope with ever-increasing workloads without a proportional increase in staff.

In spite of the improvements in machine design which have taken place over the last decade the term 'automation' to describe the mechanization of analy-

tical techniques is still largely a misnomer. Only relatively few modern instruments can boast the automatic feedback control necessary to qualify as being truly automated. However, the term 'automation' is so well entrenched in the vocabulary of biochemists that it and the word mechanization will be used synonymously in this chapter.

As well as the technological developments which have taken place in recent years there has been a simultaneous evolution of reagent systems and analytical techniques which have had a beneficial influence on machine design.

It is worthwhile showing a breakdown of the events necessary for a classical manual biochemical assay, to highlight later the differences in emphasis placed by manufacturers on the different steps of the analytical sequence.

Preliminaries
1. Collection of blood from the patient and transfer into a sample container.
2. Sample reception in the laboratory.
3. Separation of plasma or serum from the whole blood sample.

Assay
1. Precise measurement and transfer of a volume of sample, standard or blank into separate precipitation tubes.
2. Measurement and addition of a volume of one or more protein precipitants.
3. Mixing.
4. Centrifugation or filtration.
5. Measurement and transfer of volumes of protein-free supernatant or filtrate into a reaction vessel.
6. Measurement and transfer of volumes of one or more reagents into the reaction vessel.
7. Mixing.
8. Incubation.
9. Transfer of the solution into a measuring instrument (usually an absorption photometer) and measuring the end-product (usually by absorbance).
10. Calculation of numerical values.

Perhaps the greatest obstruction to the uninterrupted automation of the classical biochemical assay was the protein-removal step. Until Leonard Skeggs, achieved this by dialysis in his ingenious continuous flow system no one else had succeeded.[1] In recent years the development of methods which tolerate the presence of protein have removed this obstacle. With the greater analytical freedom permitted by these assays and the incorporation of microprocessors and computers (for process control as well as calculation) a wide range of analysers has been developed.

TYPES OF AUTOMATIC MACHINES

We have divided the various types of clinical analyser into two general classes, flow-based analysers and

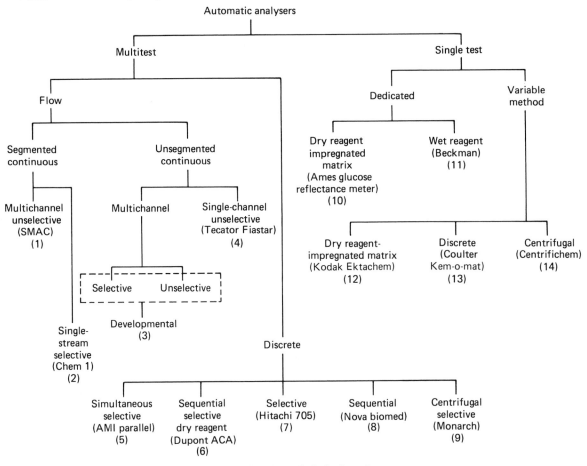

Fig. 1 Classification of clinical analysers.

discrete analysers. These two main categories are then divided into subclasses according to the mode of operation (Fig. 1). In flow analysers samples are determined from a flowing stream; any necessary operations, such as reagent addition and dialysis, are carried out 'on line' prior to the measurement of the reaction products. Samples travel sequentially along the pipeline and determinations are made using flow-through detector cells. In discrete analysers samples are placed in individual vessels for the duration of the chemical reaction. Sample dilution, reagent addition and mixing are performed on each sample at different locations within the analyser. Each treated sample is then presented in sequence to the sensing device. In one large subgroup of discrete analysers this is achieved by centrifugal force.

Flow Analysers

There are two superficially similar approaches to the use of flowing streams in chemical analysis but the two methods are based on entirely different principles. In segmented flow analysis the stream is segmented with air bubbles the purpose of which is to minimize the dispersion of the sample as it is carried through the system. Conversely, in non-segmented flow analysis—more usually referred to as flow injection analysis—the dispersion of the sample bolus is actually encouraged and manipulated for analytical purposes.

When a dilute aqueous solution flows through a tube under laminar flow conditions, frictional forces between the tube wall and the flowing stream cause layers of liquid close to the tube wall to move slower than liquid travelling nearer the centre of the tube. (Note that turbulent flow is unlikely in a steadily flowing stream at flow rates less than 50 ml/min in tubes with internal diameters greater than 0·5 mm.) The drag between the layers of moving liquid establishes a longitudinal parabolic velocity profile (Fig. 2). Under these conditions liquid in contact with the tube surface is practically stationary and the velocity of centrally placed molecules is twice the mean velocity of the liquid. A sample introduced into the stream would then soon be dispersed as illustrated in Fig. 3. In the early days of flow analysis this flow-induced dispersion was considered a nuisance. Typically, tube bores were greater than 2 mm and several metres long. Under these conditions sampling frequency was low since the resulting broad peaks took a long time to pass through the detector. These early non-segmented flow systems, although used by industry for process control purposes, were of little use to the hospital biochemist since reagent consumption was high and throughput was low.

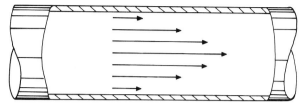

Fig. 2 Velocity profile of water flowing through a tube.

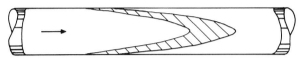

Fig. 3 Sample slug dispersion caused by laminar flow.

Air-segmented Flow Analysis. The first major advance in laboratory automation was made by Skeggs who inserted air bubbles into the flowing stream.[1] The purpose of stream segmentation was to destroy the laminar flow (Fig. 4). Samples can be serially introduced into a segmented reagent stream and transported relatively long distances without carryover becoming significant. Although the thin film of liquid between the bubbles and the tube wall still contributes to carryover, most of the carryover occurs in the non-segmented portions of the manifold and such portions should be shortened or eliminated whenever possible.

A typical arrangement of an early single channel air-segmented continuous-flow analyser is illustrated in Fig. 5. The technique was commercially exploited by Technicon and has since gone through several generations of refinement. Early air-segmented systems (Technicon AutoAnalyzers) were modular in

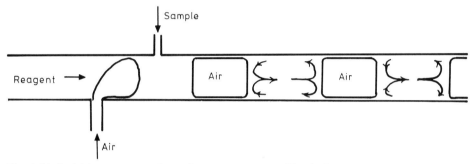

Fig. 4 Air bubble segmentation of reagent stream. The bubbles destroy laminar flow and encourage intraslug mixing. The sample is spread over many segments of reagent.

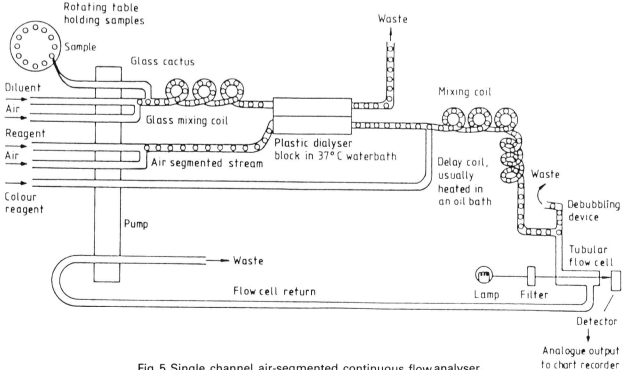

Fig. 5 Single channel air-segmented continuous flow analyser.

design, consisting of an auto-sampler, proportionating pump, dialyser, mixing coils, flow-through measuring device (usually a photometer) and a strip chart recorder. Although recent more-sophisticated multichannel designs are no longer modular the principle of operation is essentially the same. Samples are placed in plastic cups held in holes on a circular tray which is indexed round at preset intervals. A probe connected by plastic (usually polyvinyl chloride) tubing to the proportionating pump is dipped serially into successive samples. The volume of sample aspirated is determined by the adjustable dwell time of the probe and by pumping rate. Between samples the probe resides in a wash solution. During the transfer it aspirates air. The internal diameters of the different pump tubes determine the relative flow rates of sample, reagent and air. The pumping technique makes use of the peristaltic action produced by a series of stainless-steel rollers passing along an array of parallel pliable pump tubes (Fig. 6). The

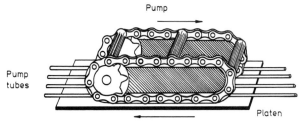

Fig. 6 AutoAnalyzer proportioning pump. (Reprinted from reference 10 with permission from CRC Press Inc.)

rollers are arranged on a continuous chain belt drive, and occlude the manifold pump tubes as they press them against a spring-loaded metal plate (the platen). The solution in front of an advancing roller is forced forward while solution behind the roller is drawn forward by the vacuum created as the roller advances. Near the end of the platen the roller lifts off the tubes but back flow is limited as subsequent rollers begin to press on the tubes and maintain the motion of the streams. However, some pulsing is apparent. The plastic pump tubes, all of which have the same wall thickness, are available in a range of internal diameter sizes. Therefore, although the linear velocity of the solution in each individual pump tube will be the same the volume pumped in a fixed time will be proportional to the square of the internal radius. By judicious choice of manifold tubes a wide range of sample to reagent ratios is possible. The manifold may be seen as replacing the use of different sizes of pipettes in manual methods. Streams can be merged by connecting the pump tubing to glass connecting pieces called cacti, and T-shaped pieces may be used for stream splitting. At least one of the manifold tubes is used to pump air into the system. As the air enters the reagent stream it forms bubbles and the sample stream is introduced into this segmented reagent stream. As already described the

function of the air bubbles is to minimize intersample mixing. Complete intrasegment mixing of reagent and sample is achieved by passing the stream through multi-turn glass coils mounted so that the coil axis is horizontal.

Efficient mixing is dependent on the regular segmentation of the stream by air bubbles in the proportion of 1 volume of air to about 2 volumes of liquid. As a segment of fluid held between two air bubbles passes around one turn of the coil the outer part of each slug travels faster than the inner so that stability of the segment breaks down and mixing occurs. Also as a segment passes around one turn of the coil, which lies in the vertical plane, the segment is inverted and mixing enhanced. The number of inversions depends on the number of turns in the coil. Some mixing coils are jacketed to allow a stream of cold water to flow past the outside of the coil to cool its contents.

When continuous-flow analysis was first introduced many of the reagents of that time worked only in the absence of protein. Most manual estimations required that the proteins were removed before addition of reagent to the protein-free solution. This was usually achieved by adding a protein precipitant (e.g. trichloroacetic acid). After centrifugation the supernatant fluid could be pipetted off and the reagent added to it. This widely used method of protein separation was difficult to automate. Skegg's solution to the problem was to use a continuous-flow dialysis module.

The dialyser consists of two plates into which mirror-image grooves have been cut. When the plates are placed together the grooves form a circular channel. A semipermeable membrane (e.g. cellophane) is placed between the plates dividing the groove in half. The segmented stream containing the serum sample moves along one side of the membrane while a second recipient stream is pumped in the same direction and at the same rate along the other side of the membrane. Molecules of low molecular weight can pass through the membrane into the recipient stream, whereas high-molecular-weight molecules (e.g. proteins) remain in the donor stream and flow to waste. For those reactions that require a heating step the recipient stream, plus any additional reagents is passed through a thermostatically controlled coil held at the required temperature. The reaction time can be regulated by choosing a coil of the appropriate length. For most determinations an absorption photometer fitted with a flow-through cuvette serves as the measuring device. For sodium and potassium assays the detector is often a flame emission photometer or more recently ion-selective electrodes have been used. Fluorimetry finds application in the analysis of a small number of substances which, because of their low concentration, are not readily measured by absorption photometry; these include catecholamines, corticosteroids, oestrogens, triglycerides and certain drugs.

With first-generation AutoAnalyzers it was necessary to debubble the stream before it entered the colorimeter. This was to avoid the large signal caused by light scatter as bubbles move through the flow cell. For absorbance assays it was convenient to pass the signal from the detector through a logarithmic converter and to plot the resulting negative signals as a series of peaks on a strip-chart recorder. Provided that Beers Law is obeyed the absorbance signal (peak height) is proportional to analyte concentration (see Chapter 9). A series of standards or calibrators were used to construct, manually, a graph of peak heights against concentration. The test peak heights were measured and by comparison with the calibration graph the test values were assigned.

Multichannel machines of this type first became available during the 1960s. The sample stream from a single sampler was split so that it fed several channels. The various colorimeters shared a common light source and the output from each detector was registered sequentially on a single recorder. This arrangement requires that the signal peak plateau from a particular channel coincides with the period during which the channel output is being recorded. Phasing coils of different lengths are used to achieve this. The recorder trace is a series of horizontal lines crossing the scales of precalibrated chart paper appropriate to the assays being carried out. A demerit of this approach is that the slowest test determines the speed at which the analyser can operate. The most widely used of this type was the Technicon Corporation's SMA 12/60, a 12-channel analyser which operated at 60 samples per hour. For many years such multichannel analysers were the mainstay of the majority of hospital laboratories and although the SMA 12/60 is now out of production large numbers are still in use.

The present generation of air-segmented continuous-flow multichannel analysers use computers and miniaturization of flow channels to produce results more rapidly and with less operator intervention. The most sophisticated of these is the Sequential Multiple Analyser plus Computer (SMAC), again manufactured by Technicon. The sampler accommodates 19 racks each holding eight tubes. The racks can easily be added or removed, except for the rack actually being sampled. While the sample is being aspirated the sample identification is read by an optical scanner from a bar-coded card placed in front of the sample tube. About 0·5 ml is sampled for 20 separate analyses. The air introduction system consists of two pinch bars whose motion is synchronized with the pump rollers. Air at a specified pressure is introduced against one of the bars which occludes the tube. The volume of air is kept under pressure by the latter pinch bar which then compresses the tube. The forward bar is then released and the pressurized air expands and enters the flowing stream of reagent. Ninety reactant segments are formed per minute. The analytical cartridge contains all the necessary components including mixing coils, heating

blocks and dialysers. The mixing coil and connecting tubing both have an internal diameter of 1 mm (compared with 1·6 mm on the SMA 12/60 and 2 mm or larger diameter on first generation analysers) and the length of tubing is kept as short as possible. To this end the flow cell is positioned very close to the analytical cartridge. Additionally, air bubbles are not physically removed before the stream enters the cuvette but are electronically filtered out by computer recognition of the large light scatter caused by the air bubbles. The miniaturization of the analytical conduits and the electronic 'debubbling' produces less carryover, and better cuvette washout characteristics, enabling faster sample throughput.

The SMAC has only one visible and one UV radiation source. Light is transmitted to and from the flow cells by total internal reflection through a fibre-optic system. The flow cells have internal diameters of between 0·5 and 1·0 mm and are 7 to 12 mm in length. The light beams pass through the cells and are returned by fibre-optics to either a single UV or visible detector. The radiation is filtered and by means of slots in a rapidly rotating wheel the light from each channel is presented in sequence to the appropriate photomultiplier. The scanning occurs at a rate of four scans of each channel per second. In this way the computer builds up the entire test curve for each channel and compares the curve shape to the pattern expected for that particular chemistry. When curve quality does not meet preselected criteria, the computer flags the result for review. Recalibration is performed whenever the computer recognizes the need, producing an analyser with an element of feedback much more like true automation than the simple mechanization of the early systems. Malfunction of any channel is notified by an audible alarm and a visual error signal. Sodium and potassium are determined using continuous-flow ion-selective electrodes instead of flame photometry.

Patients' details and test requests are entered via a keyboard/visual display unit attached to the computer. Although the machine is fitted with two chart recorders they are intended for trouble shooting on individual channels and not for routine analytical purposes. Test results are presented in a printed format. The usual SMAC configuration is as a 20-channel analyser operating at a speed of 150 samples per hour.

Because in a multichannel air-segmented analyser all samples must follow the same path through the various tubes it is not possible to make these systems discretionary. The SMAC, for example, carries out all 20 analyses on all samples regardless of which tests are requested. The printer can, however, be instructed to report only the requested tests. Another disadvantage is that because of the compressibility of the bubbles these machines take a long time to settle down after being switched on. For this reason unless they are already running they are not suitable for emergency use. In practice these analysers are left running continuously throughout the working day; they continually pump reagent even when samples are not being analysed. In the present economic situation this inefficient use of reagent is no longer acceptable and these rather wasteful machines have fallen from favour.

As mentioned above the major source of carryover in air-segmented flowing streams is the presence of an annular liquid film on the inside wall of the tubing through which the liquid segments move. This slower-moving ring of residual fluid is responsible for the 'leakage' between liquid segments. The liquid film, however, also provides the sliding surface upon which the air bubbles flow. It might be thought that the use of tubing made from a non-wettable material, for example Teflon, might reduce carryover since a film would not form on the tube wall. This is indeed the case but in these circumstances there is a tendency for the air bubbles to break up and disrupt the regular pattern of segmentation. Introducing an inert fluorocarbon fluid into the Teflon tube allows the conduit walls to be wetted and hence air bubbles to flow smoothly over the thin film of liquid. The water immiscible fluorocarbon liquid also prevents aqueous solutions from leaking past the air bubbles, hence carryover is drastically reduced.[2] This feature is used in the latest type of air-segmented analyser.

Operation of the Chem-1 system (Technicon), introduced in 1985, is based on the formation of test 'capsules' consisting of a liquid segment containing the sample combined with the first reagent and separated from a segment of second reagent by a small air bubble. Each chemistry 'capsule' is separated from the next test 'capsule' by two larger inter-test air bubbles and a wash segment of a buffer solution (Fig. 7a). A simplified illustration of the flow channel

is shown in Fig. 8. Sample ($1\,\mu l$), reagent one ($7\,\mu l$), air and reagent two ($7\,\mu l$) are aspirated into the system through a common Teflon probe. A diaphragm pump is used to draw in the $1\,\mu l$ volume of serum. The probe functions as a calibrated volumetric pipette. Light-emitting diodes and optical sensors are located along its length. As the meniscus of the various segments pass the appropriate sensor a series of stop valves are activated to control air and liquid volumes. During the sampling phase fluorocarbon fluid is pumped around the outside of the probe. Additionally, the sample and reagent surfaces are coated with a film of fluorocarbon liquid. Therefore as the probe aspirates either sample or reagent the fluorocarbon film on the inside wall of the probe is renewed. The sample is thoroughly mixed with the first reagent by passage through a multi-contorted tube. The intact segments then pass through the first of a series of in-line detectors. The absorbance of each of the segments is measured and used for blanking purposes.

The reaction of the two separate segments of each test 'capsule' is initiated by increasing the internal diameter of the Teflon tube from $1\cdot0\,mm$ to $1\cdot9\,mm$. As a result of this change in tube diameter, the small intra-test air bubble floats to the top of the stream and no longer occludes the tube. The two liquid segments then merge into a larger ($15\,\mu l$) reaction segment (Fig. 7b). This segment is homogeneously mixed by passing it through another multi-contorted coil. It then passes through a series of eight additional detectors arrayed along its path. These detectors are spaced so that the initial reaction reading is taken 30s after the sample has been mixed and further readings are taken at intervals of 30, 30, 30, 90, 90, 90

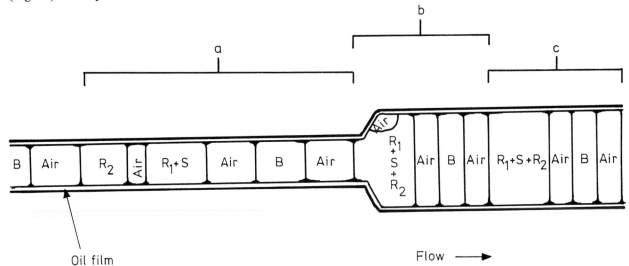

Fig. 7 Mixing of reagent and sample segments by widening the flow channel. A series of 'test packages' are formed consisting of two liquid segments separated by a small air bubble. The 'test packages' are separated from each other by two larger air bubbles and a buffer wash segment. a. Segments flowing through the narrow part of the tube. The first reagent (R_1) and the sample (S) have already been mixed and are separated from the second 'starter' reagent (R_2) by a small air bubble. b. When the tube widens the small air bubble floats to the top and $R_1 + S$ and R_2 are combined. The next large air bubble will collect the small air bubble and the process will be repeated. c. The mixed reagent segments flow towards the detectors.

and 90s. The total time for a sample to pass through the system is about 15 min.

Light from a single tungsten–halogen light source is passed through a rotating filter wheel containing eight filters and distributed to each of the detectors via quartz optical fibres. The light then passes through the tube and is monitored by individual silicon photodiodes. In addition to end-point chemistries the row of detectors allow 8-point kinetic measurements to be made. When necessary polychromatic and nephelometric determinations are also possible.

This improved method of limiting longitudinal dispersion is so successful that each test capsule can contain different reagents allowing the same channel to be used for a variety of different chemistries. The Chem-1 has a refrigerated reagent turntable capable of holding up to 32 different reagent cassettes. The instrument can be programmed to carry out any combination of available chemistries on each sample. Test 'capsules' pass through the reaction tube at a constant rate of 720 per hour regardless of chemistry selection. The sample throughput will of course depend on the average test per sample ratio. If say eight colorimetric assays are requested on each specimen then the rate of analysis will be 90 samples per hour. A parallel channel fitted with ion-selective electrodes is used to determine sodium, potassium and bicarbonate at a maximum rate of up to 360 samples per hour. This dual channel multitest air-segmented analyser uses much less reagent than the multichannel type but the relatively slow sample throughput restricts its use to the small to medium size laboratory.

Non-segmented Flow Analysis. In recent years a better understanding of the flow-induced dispersive process has led to a new approach to flow-based analysis. In non-segmented flow analysis, dispersion of sample and reagent slugs are controlled and used to produce analytical results rapidly and with minimal reagent consumption. Initially a syringe was used to inject a sample into a flowing (non-segmented) stream of reagent and the technique became known as flow-injection analysis (FIA). To date no manufacturer has produced an FIA machine designed specifically for the hospital laboratory but clinical biochemists have experimented with improvised equipment and it would appear that the technique has great potential.[3] For this reason we will outline the essential features of this new technique.

The simplest form of flow-injection analyser is illustrated in Fig. 9a. A precisely metered volume of sample is introduced into a stream of reagent moving under conditions of laminar flow. As the sample slug is swept through the narrow bore reactor tube it progressively disperses into the reagent. At the appropriate distance downstream a flow-through detector monitors the products of reaction. When necessary, additional reagents may be added by using convergent streams.

Soon after injection the slug will take up the shape of a hollow bullet, gradually elongating as it traverses the system (Fig. 3, p. 531). The interface between the slug and the carrier solution rapidly increases the mixing of sample and carrier solution results predominantly from radial molecular diffusion across the interface. Radial diffusion also limits the length of the slug tail since molecules will encounter faster moving carrier solution when they diffuse away from the tube wall. Likewise molecules at the tip of the slug head will encounter slower moving carrier when they diffuse from a central position. This type of diffusion-induced dispersion has a moderating effect on the longitudinal dispersion caused by carrier flow.

The degree of dispersion (dilution) of the slug is affected by sample size, tube bore and tube length. For analytical purposes the peak height is usually

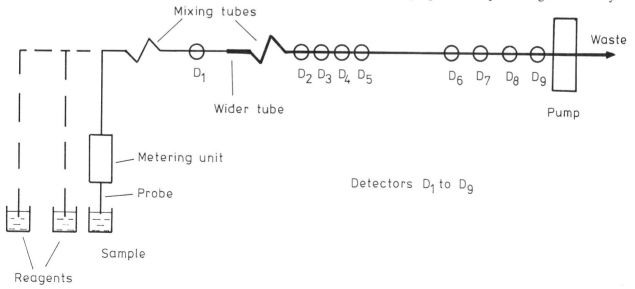

Fig. 8 Chem-1 flow channel.

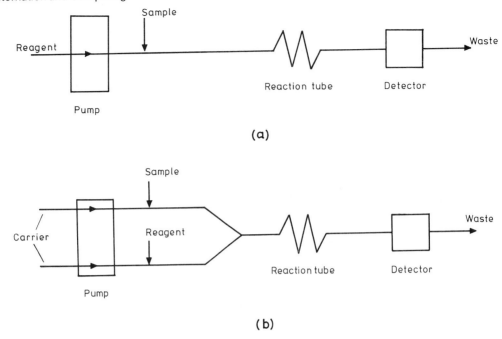

Fig. 9 a. Flow-injection analyser. b. Merging zone flow-injection analyser.

measured and a convenient method of comparing the effect of different conditions on dispersion is to inject dye solution into the system and to measure the resulting peak height. The greater the dispersion of the dye the smaller will be its peak height. Defined in this way dispersion is proportional to (1) the square of the tube radius, (2) the square root of the tube length, and inversely proportional to the sample size (provided the sample is small relative to the total volume of the system). Flow rates used in FIA are usually between 1 and 4 ml/min and over this range flow-rate has no significant effect on dispersion.

In order to maximize sample throughput the tube dimensions are kept as small as is practically possible. Reaction tubes (Teflon) are typically about 50 cm long with an internal diameter of 0·5 mm. Dispersion is best varied by adjusting the injected volume. Sample introduction is usually achieved by means of a mechanized injection valve fed from an autosampler. Both slider valves and rotary valves have been used; a variable length valve 'loop' is necessary to allow different volumes to be injected.

When rapid reactions are involved sample throughput is typically between 150 and 300 per hour. The system processes one sample at a time and the analytical readout (peak height) is available seconds after sample injection. With chemistries involving slow reactions when the reaction zone reaches the cuvette the flow is stopped and the initial rate of reaction is computed as a rate of change in absorbance. The accurate placement of a section of a stream in the cuvette can only be achieved with non-segmented systems. If the stream contained bubbles this would be impossible because the compressible gas bubbles would cause some movement of the stream even after the pump had been halted. In this mode of operation sample throughput is reduced to about 120 assays per hour. Another advantage of the bubble free approach is that 'start up' and 'close down' is rapid, typically 30s.

As described above reagent consumption is between 1 and 3 ml per analytical cycle. However, the sample reacts only with reagent in its immediate vicinity. The bulk of the reagent does not take part in the reaction but serves merely as a sample carrier. A more efficient use of reagent is obtained by using the technique of merging zones. In this technique a double-injection valve is used to inject slugs of sample and reagent simultaneously into independent, inert carrier streams (Fig. 9b). The carrier streams are synchronized so that the reagent and sample slugs merge at a confluence point before reaching the detector. Distilled water, or dilute buffer or detergent solution may be used as carrier in both streams; hence reagent consumption may be very low. For example, Mindegaard[4] used merging zones to determine serum albumin with bromocresol green reagent. Sample volume was 8 μl, reagent volume 15 μl and throughput 300 assays per hour.

One reason why manufacturers have been slow to develop clinical analysers based on FIA is that injection valves waste sample. Although the injected volume might only be, say, 2 μl a much larger volume of sample must be drawn through the valve and connecting tubes to remove the residue of the previous contents. Also, when subjected to large daily workloads valves wear and frequently develop leaks. It was to overcome these and other disadvantages associated with valves that Riley et al.[5] developed an alternative method of sample introduction. This valveless

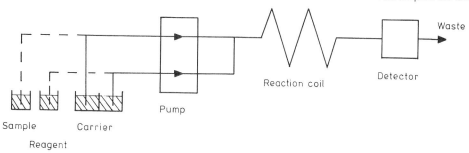

Fig. 10 Controlled-dispersion flow analyser. The probes which are attached to a small transfer arm normally rest in a trough of carrier solution (demineralized water). During the sampling phase the pump is halted, so that air does not enter the system, and the probes transferred to the sample and reagent cups. The broken line represents probe movements. Small volumes of sample and reagent are aspirated into the probes and they are then returned to the carrier trough. The lengths of the connecting tubes are arranged so that when the pump restarts the sample and reagent zones merge before being swept to the detector.

system, which is referred to as controlled-dispersion analysis, is illustrated in Fig. 10. Sample and reagent probes are attached to an arm that can transfer them to and fro between a trough containing distilled water, where the probes normally rest, and the sample and reagent cups. The peristaltic pump is driven by a computer-controlled stepping motor, this allows very precise metering of sample and reagent volumes. After sampling the pump is halted while the probes are returned to the carrier solution and the pump restarted. The sample and reagent slugs travel through the system, merging at a T-piece before reaching the detector.

Systems employing non-segmented flowing streams are quicker to start up and close down, and produce results more rapidly than air-segmented systems. However, the non-segmented approach is less well suited to analytical methods requiring long incubations. The use of several parallel holding coils into which samples can be diverted and held for a fixed period of time before being pumped to the detector may overcome this limitation.[6]

Discrete Analysers

The majority of commercially available analysers fall into this broad category. We shall not attempt to describe all of the available analysers or to describe any one instrument in detail except where an instrument is unique enough to merit special description. Instead a discussion of the underlying principles will be presented.

The adjective discrete, in this context, implies that individual samples are contained in separate vessels during the period of chemical reaction. These machines allow manual methods to be replicated by means of a series of automatic operations. In most analysers of this type both sample and reagent solutions are metered into reaction vessels, test tubes or specially designed cuvette cells. Some systems, however, employ cells containing prepacked quantities of the necessary reagents. In these analysers it is necessary to add only the sample and diluent if required.

Single-channel Single-chemistry Analysers. The basic configuration of an early discrete analyser is illustrated in Fig. 11. This is a single-channel single-chemistry analyser. Specimens for analysis are placed in a circular tray by the operator. A measured volume is aspirated by a sampler-diluter probe and the sample turntable advances by one position. The sampler-diluter dispenses the sample followed by a measured volume of diluent into the reaction vessel situated in a thermostatted reaction rotor. The reaction rotor indexes around at constant predetermined intervals. At appropriate positions reagents are added to each reaction vessel as they pass beneath the reagent dispensers. The reagent is often added as a jet, the kinetic energy of which is used to mix the solution. Other methods of mixing include the use of small rotating paddles, mechanical agitation of the tubes, and the use of a stream of air bubbles blown through the solution. Further around the perimeter of the reaction rotor, the distance determines the reaction time, the detector (usually a colorimeter) is situated. In older machines the reaction mixture is aspirated from the reaction tube into a colorimeter fitted with a flow-through cuvette. The reaction solution rests in the colorimeter for several seconds to allow any bubbles to clear before the absorbance is measured, after which the solution is discharged to waste. A disadvantage of this approach is that reaction rates cannot be continuously monitored as the reaction vessels move around the system. In some analysers the tubes then pass through a laundry station where they are washed, dried and passed onwards to be used again. A commonly used system will be described in more detail later in this chapter. Other machines discard the tubes after use.

Analysers of this type are used to assay batches of samples sequentially for a single analyte at a time.

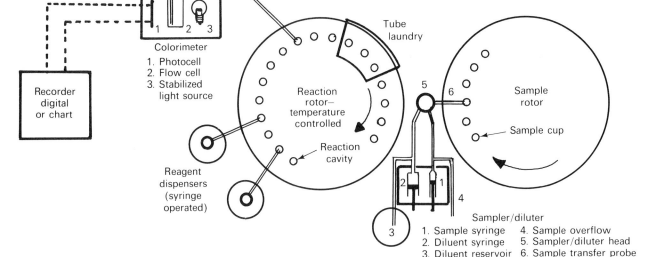

Fig. 11 Single-channel single-chemistry discrete analyser.

By changing the reagents, colorimeter filter and dispenser volumes different chemistries can be performed. Several of these simple chemistry units can be combined to form a multichannel instrument. When this type of multichannel analyser was first introduced in the early 1970s lack of computing power meant that they were not selective. That is they performed their complete battery of tests on every sample regardless of how many determinations were requested.

This first generation of discrete analysers processed samples in batches and once a batch had been scheduled for assay and details entered into the instrument it was inconvenient to interrupt the work pattern with an urgent specimen. Specifically to meet this need so called 'stat' analysers were developed to carry out a single analysis on demand. In these small analysers all measurements are made in a single reaction cell and only one sample is assayed at a time. Sample and reagents are pipetted or pumped into the reaction cell, mixed and at the appropriate time the reaction products are measured. The cell contents are then pumped to waste and the cell flushed with fresh reagent in preparation for another analytical cycle. Usually the sample is manually injected into the reaction area by means of a special pipette or syringe. Sometimes the measuring device will employ potentiometry rather than colorimetry. Analysers for the determination of glucose, bilirubin, creatinine, urea, sodium, potassium and blood gases are currently available. Because these analysers have few moving parts they are relatively inexpensive to purchase and are potentially reliable. Another attribute is that, since each sample is analysed in an identical environment, precision should be good. The main disadvantage is that throughput is low, typically one sample per minute, since it is controlled by the speed at which the reaction cell can be cycled between specimens. Mechanized sample introduction has also been used. The Beckman Astra combines either four or eight of this type of unit to form a small multichannel analyser in which the sampler mechanism, which travels on a track at the front of the instrument, dispenses sample into the appropriate unit.

Single-channel Multi-chemistry Analysers. In more recent years developments in microprocessor technology together with more sophisticated engineering has enabled the design of single-unit selective, multichemistry analysers. This is a rapidly developing area of laboratory automation and at least a dozen analysers of this type have been introduced onto the UK market during the past 5 years. We expect this trend to continue.

A typical arrangement is shown in Fig. 12. The analyser has three major components. A sample tray, a refrigerated tray in which reagent containers are

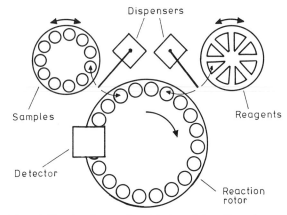

Fig. 12 Single-channel multi-chemistry discrete analyser.

placed and a temperature-controlled reaction rotor in which the reaction cells are held (typically, the sample carousel would hold about 40 sample cups, reagent tray 20 different reagents, and the reaction tray 100 cells). A machine-readable label is attached to the sample container so that the instrument can identify the sample and pair the results with specimen details entered previously by the operator and held in the computer. Because of this system samples can be entered anywhere on the sample turntable at any time.

A sipper probe (described later) attached to a transfer arm is used to aspirate sample and to introduce it with diluent into the reaction tube. Similarly appropriate reagent is then added to the reaction cell as it passes under the reagent probe. The use of this method allows the same probe to be used with all reagents without the need to purge the dispenser between reagents. To minimize contamination of one reagent by another various methods have been used to wash the outside surface of the probe between different reagent additions. The simplest method involves a water wash while another method involves the use of an immiscible fluorocarbon liquid to provide a barrier between the reagent and the probe, thus avoiding cross contamination.

Many recently introduced analysers use transparent reaction tubes or specially designed cells that also serve as colorimeter cuvettes. In these instruments the absorbance reading is taken as the cuvette is indexed through the measuring unit. In order to obtain several readings during the course of a reaction several different approaches have been employed. A series of colorimeters placed at intervals around the perimeter of the reaction rotor may be used.

A more elegant approach involves rotating the reaction rotor through 360° plus one position every time a sample is added. In this way each reaction cell passes through a single colorimeter many times during an assay. In the Dacos (Coulter Electronics Inc.) rather than the tubes rotating through the light beam the light beam is made to rotate through the reaction cuvettes. In each of these cases readings, which are usually taken at several wavelengths either by means of a rapidly rotating filter wheel or by use of a diode array detector (Fig. 13), are subjected to sophisticated data-processing algorithms. These frequent readings permit the calculation of reaction rates as well as end-points and the observations at several wavelengths enable blank values to be subtracted.

Samples can be processed in batches or continuously and most instruments have a facility for giving priority to urgent specimens. The machines which analyse samples serially have a special position close to the sample rotor reserved for the location of urgent specimens. If this dedicated 'stat' position is occupied during a run the system will complete the analysis of any sample that is underway, then immediately

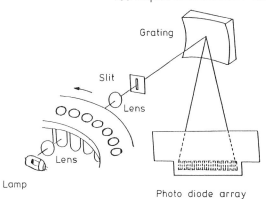

Fig. 13 Combined holographic grating and diode array detector. The detector used in the Genesis 21 measures up to 15 wavelengths at once. (Diagram courtesy of Allied IL.)

proceed with the urgent sample before assaying the remaining routine samples. Many of this new generation of analysers, however, enable the user to process specimens in any order, regardless of the sequence in which they are placed in the sample tray. Tests may also be performed in any selected order. This capability is often referred to by American manufacturers as 'random access'. This facility offers greater flexibility to sample handling. Preference can be given to urgent samples through a keyboard command and some analysers can automatically optimize the workflow to achieve the fastest throughput of collated patient reports. After the final absorbance measurement the reaction cells may be laundered *in situ* for further use or they may be discarded and replaced by fresh cuvettes. Sodium and potassium determinations are performed by means of an ion-selective electrode module, often sold as an 'optional extra' and operating in parallel with the colorimetric assays. Unfortunately, the short life span of some of the electrode systems has blemished their reputation.

The basic analyser geometry can vary from that shown in Fig. 12. For example, the reagent rotor can be placed concentrically within the sample holder. The inner ring holding the reagent containers while the outer ring holds the sample cups. The Japanese-manufactured Genesis 21 (Fig. 14) uses racks to hold both sample and reagent containers. The racks are automatically moved so that the probe assemblies can aspirate from the appropriate cups. There are also other arrangements.

Analysers are easily 'programmed' via a keyboard and a visual display unit is incorporated for operator guidance. Microprocessors control all functions from mechanical movement to evaluation of results, reporting and quality control statistics. If required the analyser can accept patient details from and download results to a central laboratory computer, commonly via an RS232C interface. The menu of available tests amenable for inclusion on these analysers is constantly increasing. Several manufacturers

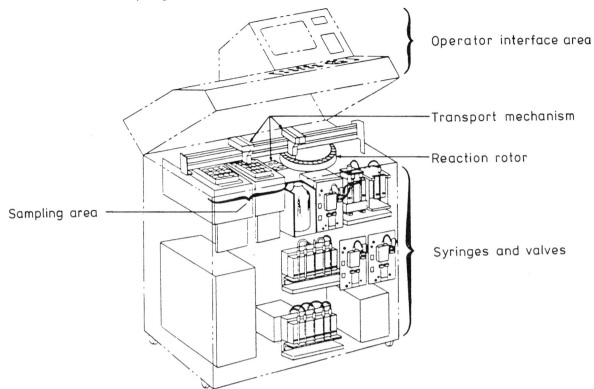

Operator interface area

Transport mechanism

Reaction rotor

Sampling area

Syringes and valves

Fig. 14 Working areas of the Genesis 21; a typical modern discrete analyser. (Diagram courtesy of Allied IL.)

now offer a selection from more than 50 different assays. These include, in addition to the most frequently requested tests, determinations of therapeutic drugs and thyroid function tests. Other attractive features of these single-channel machines is that they require little daily maintenance and can be left in a 24-hour ready state.

The processing rate of these systems varies between 100 and 1200 determinations per hour, depending on the choice of analyser. However, the sample throughput is often disappointingly low particularly when the test per sample ratio is high. Therefore, this type of machine is best suited to small or medium-sized laboratories or as a complementary instrument in the larger hospital facility.

It is common for these analysers to be fitted with the type of sample holder that requires the plasma to be manually removed from the primary collection tube into a small plastic cup. No doubt this simplifies the design of the autosampler system but decanting specimens can lead to potentially serious mix ups. The remedy is for the manufacturer to fit samplers, similar to those used on certain multichannel machines, which are capable of holding the tube into which the blood specimen has been collected.

Multichannel Analysers. To cope with the high workload of the largest hospital laboratories high capacity analysers are required. This need is best met by selective multichannel analysers such as the Parallel manufactured by American Monitor International (AMI)

or the Clinicon Prisma. These machines have the facility to run many different chemistries simultaneously. For example, the Parallel operates at 240 samples per hour and can carry out up to 30 determinations on each sample, and is thus capable of producing a maximum of 7200 test results per hour. Within-run analysis time is about 12 minutes using sample volumes of 3–50 µl with an average reagent consumption of 1 ml per assay.

There have been several different approaches to the mechanically complex problem of tube transport in multichannel machines. A bank of single-chemistry analytical units can be fed samples via a conveyor belt. As the samples pass each dedicated chemistry module, the unit can take an aliquot of sample for analysis. The now obsolete Vickers M-300 was of this general type.

Another approach is to integrate all the chemistry channels within a single unit; one way of achieving this is illustrated by Fig. 15. The specimen tubes are placed on a conveyor that indexes them past a bank of sampler-diluter pipettes, each pipette being dedicated to a particular assay. A bar-code reader deciphers the code attached to the sample tube and finds from the database which tests have been scheduled, accordingly the pipettes transfer an aliquot of the sample into an adjacent reaction tube held in a long rack. The racks which are situated in a thermostatted water bath are transported through the system by a chain drive. Placed above the tube racks at appropriate positions are a series of reagent dispensers,

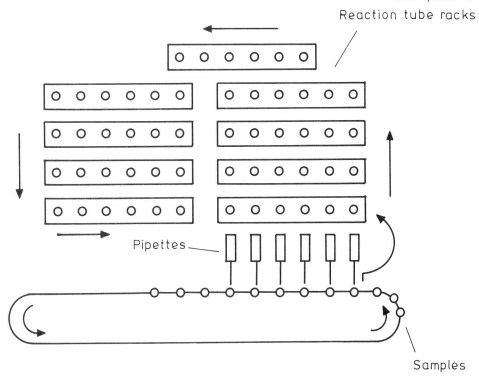

Fig. 15 Tube transport in a multi-channel analyser.

mixers and colorimeters (not shown in the figure). As the racks progress through the analyser they encounter a laundry area where the reaction tubes are washed, dried and moved back to the sampling station for another specimen.

These large computer-controlled machines have all the utilities of the single-channel analysers plus a greater capacity for storing patient results. On the negative side the capital cost of such equipment is likely to exceed £200 000 and the huge number of moving parts makes these machines prone to mechanical breakdown. Startup time is relatively long and, contrary to the claims by the manufacturers, they are in practice generally unsuitable for 'out-of-hours' use.

Centrifugal Analysers. The technique of centrifugal analysis was invented by Anderson in the late 1960s.[7] Originally it was devised to carry out identical analyses very quickly on various cell fractions isolated by zonal centrifugation but with some modification it has found a place in the clinical laboratory. The central feature of the machine is a rotor which is usually constructed of transparent plastic, glass or teflon. The rotor forms a transfer disc in which are machined a number of radially arranged cavities connected by channels as shown in Fig. 16.

In most of the original models there were 15 such channels carrying samples, standards and reagents but later machines with 30- and 42-place rotors were developed. Each channel contains two or more wells into which the sample and reagent are pipetted. The wells are so arranged that samples and reagents remain in their separate compartments until the rotor is mounted in the machine and rotated rapidly. Samples and reagents are then transferred centrifugally and almost instantaneously into outer chambers, where after rapid mixing, the change in absorbance of the solution is measured. This is achieved by means of a light source and photomultiplier mounted in such a way that the light beam passes vertically through the cuvette chambers as they rotate. In the original models, signals from the photomultiplier were displayed on an oscilloscope the sweep circuit of which was synchronized with the rotor through a photoelectric sensor mounted close to the rotor edge.

In the first generation of centrifugal analysers sample and reagent were introduced off-line into the transfer disc. Because each series of radially arranged depressions is concerned with the assay of only one sample and because there is no lateral interconnection, tests remain discrete. The design of the sample diluter and reagent dispenser in this generation was such that they operated only as intermittent batch analysers.

After radial transfer of reagents from the inner pockets to the peripheral cuvettes in the Centrifichem C400, mixing is effected by applying vacuum at the centre of the rotor and by drawing air back through drainage siphons contained in each cuvette. Mixing in the IL Multistat III with its disposable 20-place acrylic rotor was achieved by an abrupt stop in rotation which caused the back and forth movement of a tidal wave of sample and reagent in each separate radial channel. The time taken for the assay of a batch of tests once loaded into the rotor is very short,

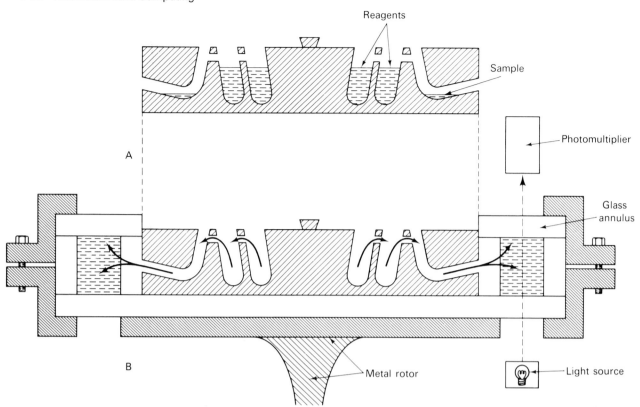

Fig. 16 Section through rotor of a centrifugal analyser. A. Transfer disc with unmixed sample. B. Transfer disc in cuvette rotor after centrifugation to mix sample and reagents.

ranging from just a few seconds to a few minutes. However, the rate-limiting step in the whole system is in the sample and reagent loading which is usually around 240 samples per hour.

The advantage of offline systems is that several sampler diluters can be used to load the transfer discs at the same time thus increasing the analytical throughput. The disadvantage, of course, is the need for the operator to set up the diluter and when the operation is complete transfer the disc.

In more recent years there have been developments in the design of centrifugal analysers which are of benefit to the user and provide a greater degree of flexibility. The Cobas Bio system (Roche Products Ltd) is designed so that its disposable acrylic rotor is charged with standards, sample and reagents *in situ*. The operator simply has to position the loaded sample ring, the standard and reagent rack and the analysis rotor, press the button which sets the parameters for the required test and actuate the rotate button. The results are automatically printed out on completion of the batch of assays.

The rotor is specially constructed of a transparent acrylic plastic. It has 30 positions each with two wells, one for the sample with a maximum capacity of 80 μl and the other for reagent with a maximum capacity of 370 μl. During centrifugation the rotor speed is 2500 rev./min and the sample and reagent pass rapidly over a baffle into the adjoining optical

cuvette. Mixing is achieved by rapid speed variation of the rotor which imparts a juddering motion. It is possible to add a second 'start' reagent; in certain tests the rotor is programmed to stop, allowing the second reagent to be introduced into the sample well. On restarting this reagent is mixed with the previous sample and reagent mixture and the reaction initiated.

Optical measurements are made with the rotor speed at 1000 rev./min with pulsed light from a xenon source passing radially through the length of the cuvette, through a grating monochromator (wavelength range 285–750 nm) and reflected onto a semiconductor photodiode, light detector. Longitudinal measurement through the reaction cuvette has certain advantages: (1) the absorbance is not influenced by evaporation of the reaction mixture; (2) the result is independent of small variation in reagent or diluent volume; (3) the calculation depends only on the volume and concentration of sample used.

Further tests may be carried out on the same samples simply by changing the standard and reagent rack and pressing the appropriate test button followed by the start button. If there are any samples not requiring a second test these will be excluded if the tube is not pushed fully home into the sample ring during loading. It is not necessary to have a full rotor of tests to initiate a reaction. Providing the rotor is left *in situ* the machine can be successively programmed to process small numbers of different tests until all spaces on the reaction rotor are used.

A logical development of the Cobas Bio system is the Cobas Fara. The design of this analyser allows complete flexibility of operation in batch, selective or stat mode. The machine will accept up to 150 patient samples in sealed sample cups, loaded in parallel rows in special test tube racks. As many as 50 reagents may be handled with free selection of reagent combinations. There is a level detector for both sample and reagents. Stat samples may be analysed at any time.

In addition to a colorimeter similar to that described for the Cobas Bio analyser there are options for fluorimetry and nephelometry. If any of these additional options is chosen provision is made for the automatic switch-over from one measurement mode to the other as the assay demands it. In addition to colorimetric and fluorimetric assays the option is available for the simultaneous measurement of sodium and potassium using ion-specific electrodes (ISE) with autocalibration. A range of working temperature options is available. By means of a built-in cooling device it is possible to select temperatures between 25 and 40°C.

The versatility of this instrument is due mainly to its central control unit which provides simple one-key access to routine and stat programmes. There is capacity for storing up to 100 different test programmes. In addition there is continuous access to information programmes for patient data, including collated patient reports. From the operational point of view there are user-selectable calibration modes, built in quality-control programmes, manual data input, diagnostic programmes and a facility for the continuous monitoring and control of sample and reagent consumption.

An even greater versatility is seen in the IL Monarch analyser which was introduced in 1985. In this instrument an ISE assembly for the measurement of sodium, potassium and chloride operates side by side with an analytical system working on the centrifugal principle. A combination of powerful software and robotics controls the automatic transfer of disposable 40 place acrylic rotors from a supply stack to a loading station and thence to an analysis station and finally, on completion of the assays, to a discard stack. The loading of a rotor and the analysis in the previously loaded one, are simultaneous operations so that an analysis rate of up to 600 tests per hour is possible.

The work may be scheduled:

1. in a time-optimized mode to give results in the fastest possible time by means of a test-load organizer
2. according to 'patient priority' in random access mode
3. in a stat mode for immediate results.

Detection may be by fluorescence, absorbance, light scatter and potentiometry (with the ISEs).

The system provides a programmable menu of 100 tests with random access to any of 23 reagents loaded at any one time. Reagents for the centrifugal assays are loaded onto a 20-place removeable circular tray. Each reagent is enclosed in a wedge-shaped container which is bar coded for machine identification. The seals protecting the opening to each reagent container are easily penetrated by the reagent probe and reseal automatically when the probe is withdrawn. The reagent tray is free to rotate so that the appropriate reagent (identified by its bar code) may be brought rapidly into the sampling position for each different assay.

Sample volumes are typically 2 to 20 µl for the centrifugal assays and 30 µl for the ISEs and reagent volumes are between 150 and 200 µl. As with some other centrifugal analysers Monarch can be used for enzyme-immunoassay and fluoroimmunoassay as well as routine colorimetric chemistries, special proteins and therapeutic drugs.

On the whole centrifugal analysers do not have the versatility of modern discrete analysers and are best reserved for kinetic reactions where it is advantageous to make the first absorbance measurement as near as possible to zero time. However, the features of the Fara and Monarch which permit stat sample handling and random access make them more competitive.

A novel approach to centrifugal analysis was described by Schultz et al.[8] This is the Vision System of Abbott Laboratories. It is a desk-top analyser which uses disposable test packs, injection moulded from acrylic or polystyrene. A top is sealed onto the test pack so that within its body are multiple cavities joined by a labyrinth of passages. Within each pack is a sealed polypropylene cup which contains the concentrated reagent and diluent, specially partitioned. The reagent cup is free to move within the test pack.

For use, the pack requires the introduction of 40–80 µl of whole blood into an opening on its cover. This may be achieved directly from the punctured surface of the skin by touching the capillary opening in the pack against the blood droplet.

Calibration of the instrument is carried out in a separate calibration run; two drops of calibrant, instead of blood, are introduced into the pack which is then positioned in the analyser and the calibrate button actuated. Up to three different assays may be calibrated simultaneously. Once calibrated the machine may be loaded with any number or type of test pack up to a maximum of ten. Packs are available for the measurement of enzyme activity and the concentrations of electrolytes and other analytes, each is labelled with the assay name and a unique bar-coded test pack number. Results are printed out in less than 10 min. Controls are treated in the same way as blood samples and, unlike calibrators, can be run at the same time.

The centrifuge is self balancing so that test packs may be randomly loaded. Each test pack position has an aluminium disc with a mechanism which allows a secondary rotation of the pack through 90°. When the start button is pressed the developing centrifugal force causes the reagent cup to move downwards within the pack. The lid is peeled from the cup and the reagent and diluent empty into the reagent measuring chamber. As this is happening the blood sample fills a cell-separating chamber from which excess sample passes into primary and secondary chambers. The optical detection of sample in the secondary chamber indicates that there is sufficient for analysis.

The first test pack rotation now takes place and the mixture of reagent and diluent moves to a mixing chamber. At the same time separated plasma moves to a delay chamber and the primary sample overflow chamber empties. As the pack returns to its upright position the reagent moves into an optical cuvette chamber in the pack and the plasma into a measuring chamber of capacity 4 μl. At this stage a reagent blank reading is taken to determine its suitability.

With a second rotational cycle of the test pack sample and reagent are mixed. On returning to the upright position again the absorbance of the reaction mixture is measured to check for the presence of haemoglobin, lipaemia or bilirubin. After this measurement the reaction is incubated and the absorbances measured for kinetic and end-point assays.

Fluidics in Discrete Analysis. In all automatic analysers the sample is introduced unmeasured in a disposable plastic tube or cup. The sample container is loaded onto a mechanical device which offers each sample in turn, usually for a fixed period, to a narrow tubular probe which aspirates a precise volume for analysis. The sampling device is usually used in conjunction with a diluter so that the measurement and transfer of the sample is followed by the addition of a volume of diluent. Probably the most precise device so far developed for the purpose of sampling and dilution is the two-syringe dilutor. This has appeared in various forms but the basic principles remain as shown in Fig. 17. The 'sipper' probe, which is usually made from narrow small-bore Teflon tubing, is dipped into the specimen and the piston of the sample syringe is withdrawn, aspirating the required volume of sample into the probe. Simultaneously the diluent syringe aspirates the required volume of diluent. The probe is then transferred to the reaction tube and the motorized rotary valve turned clockwise through 90° connecting the diluent syringe to the probe. Both syringe pistons are then pushed in. By this means not only is the sample diluted but the diluent, which is usually deionized water, serves to wash the inside of the probe. Carryover on the outside of the probe is minimized if the probe just touches the liquid surface of the diluted sample, otherwise a droplet may remain hanging on the tip of the probe when it is withdrawn. Hence, probes are often fitted with a fluid level sensor, which limits the immersion depth of the sampling tip to

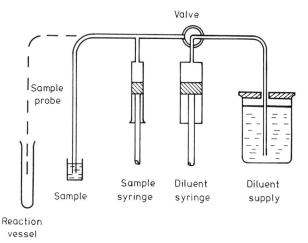

Fig. 17 Two-syringe 'sipper' probe. The broken line represents probe movements.

about 2 mm. In some analysers the outside of the probe is washed by running water between samples. For precise working the syringes must be kept free of air bubbles. To this end it is best if the diluent is deaerated before use and that the syringes are arranged vertically with their exits at the top. The syringes may be driven pneumatically; when they are pushed between adjustable stops, or mechanically. Stepping motors are particularly appropriate. The length of time that the motor drives in one direction is proportional to the distance that an attached piston syringe will move. The positioning of these motors is extremely accurate (because the motor is wired so that the armature will stop only in specific positions when the current is shut off) and their starting and stopping positions are easily adjusted via the software. To withdraw a designated volume of liquid, power is applied to the motor for the appropriate length of time.

In single-chemistry units and in multichannel analysers where each channel is dedicated to a particular chemistry the reagent can be added by means of a syringe drawing and discharging through non-return valves, by peristaltic pumping or from pressurized reagent reservoirs. When pressurized reservoirs are used a constant pressure is applied to the reservoir and reagent discharge is regulated by microprocessor-controlled electromagnetic valves. The volume of reagent added is determined by the pressure, the dimensions of the connecting tube, and the time over which the reagent is allowed to flow. If the pressure is kept constant the volume of reagent added to the reaction tube is proportional to the time during which the valve is open.

Discrete Analysers with Dry Reagents. Some discrete analysers employ dry reagents packaged in quantities sufficient for a single assay. Essentially these fall into two main groups:

1. Those in which the reagents are automatically

reconstituted with a volume of solvent (usually water) at the start of the analytical sequence.

2. Those which require only the addition of the sample, either neat or diluted, to provide the necessary liquid to dissolve the reagents and initiate the reaction.

In the latter, the reagents are usually layered onto the fibres of a matrix of cellulose or other fibrous material (e.g. the Ames Seralyzer or BCL Reflotron) or incorporated into one or more layers of a multi-layer package (e.g. Kodak Ektachem). Instruments using this approach have been described in Chapter 17 of this book so only the first category will be discussed here.

Although these are classified as discrete analysers it is worth considering them as a separate group since they are designed to be used by personnel with little or no formal laboratory training. The user is required only to separate the plasma, introduce it into the appropriate container, place it onto the machine, select and load the reagents and press a button.

Perhaps the most familiar analyser in this group is the Dupont ACA which was introduced into the UK market more than a decade ago. The concept upon which it is based was revolutionary and outstandingly different from any other developments taking place at the time. It was introduced with a limited range of chemistries and with less than perfect performance but the main reason for its lack of popularity in this country is the high cost of the reagent packs and the lack of user-freedom to add new methods or modify old.

As the years have passed so the reliability of the system has improved and the range of available assays increased to nearly 50. In addition to the large free-standing model there is also a smaller bench-top model (the ACA SX). The main feature of the ACA system is the analytical test pack (Fig. 18) which consists of a transparent plastic disposable pouch which

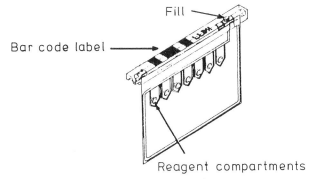

Fig. 18 ACA test pack.

contains seven sealed compartments, one or more of which contains precisely measured quantities of dried reagents necessary for the required assay. Each pouch is fixed to a rigid header through which the sample and diluent are introduced. The header is marked with the test identity in both operator- and machine-readable form.

To operate this machine the patient's sample is introduced into a cup on a plastic 'header' similar in dimension to the pack headers. Each sample cup is given a patient identification number. The sample carrier followed by the different packs for the required tests (in any order) are loaded onto a tramway and with the press of a button the analytical sequence is initiated. The appropriate volumes of sample and diluent are determined from the optical recognition of the binary code on the headers of each test pack and are automatically added to the packs.

The test packs serve as flexible cuvettes which are carried by a transport belt, first to a breaker/mixer where reagent compartments 1, 2, 3 and 4 are broken open and the contents mixed with the sample and diluent by oscillation. Next the pack is transported to a delay station where the sample is incubated and after a second breaker/mixer, which breaks and mixes the reagents in pockets 5, 6 and 7, the reaction progresses to completion. The pack finally passes to a photometer where the plastic pouch is compressed into a precise optical cell and the absorbance of the reaction mixture measured at a number of specific wavelengths generated by interference filters. The computer calculates the appropriate analytical results which are printed out under the patient's code number on a permanent record card by an alphanumeric thermal printer.

With this system the first test takes 7.5 minutes and subsequent results are produced every 77 seconds regardless of the tests ordered. Stat samples can be given priority at any time. The machine is always on standby and requires no start-up or shut-down operations. Although a very slow analyser these features make it most suitable for emergency use.

In 1985 Eppendorf introduced into the UK their 'Easy' analyser which works on a similar principle. With this analyser the dry reagents (Diagnostica Merck) are provided in rigid clear plastic vessels which also act as optical measuring cuvettes. The patient's sample which is identified by a bar-code label is inserted into a metal rack with the bar-coded test cuvettes. The action of loading this rack into the analyser is sufficient to initiate the analytical process.

Even more recent is the Paramax Analytical system (American Dade, American Hospital Supply) which has not yet reached the UK market. This is a multi-channel analyser in which disposable reaction cuvettes are supplied in reels of 2100. These form a continuous cuvette track into which reagent tablets are dispensed from a carousel which can accommodate 32 reagent tablet dispensers. The carousel rotates under microprocessor control to bring the correct tablets to the dispensing point. A diluent and liquid reagent dispenser adds the correct volume of liquid for tablet solution. The reaction cuvette is maintained at a temperature of 37°C in a water bath and the tablets totally dissolve by exposure to high efficiency ultrasound for 45 s. The quality of the reagent solution thus prepared is checked by on-line colorimeters prior to the addition of the sample.

Samples in bar-coded tubes are loaded onto a carousel with a capacity for up to 96 tubes. From this Loading Carousel sample tubes are passed on to a Transfer Carousel which feeds patients' samples into the system to allow maximum throughput. At the same time the patient's sample is adjusted to a height which brings the meniscus to a level for proper aspiration with minimum carryover and a bar-code reading is taken. In the transfer rotor are special priority access stations for urgent samples.

The sampler is capable of aspirating from 2 to 20 μl of patient's sample every 5 s. To prevent contamination and carryover the sample probe is flushed with diluent. Each patient's sample is also dispensed into a cuvette without reagent and monitored for icterus, lipaemia and haemolysis. This provides a sample blank.

There are eight photometric read stations connected by eight guides to a single light source. The stations are located in positions appropriate for the different methods used and for either end-point or kinetic determinations. The Paramax analyser has the capacity to provide more than 600 patients' results per hour with a range of 32 different tests. Like the other machines in this group it is ideal for emergency use with 24-hour accessibility and stat capacity. The cuvettes are automatically sealed before disposal.

Table 1 lists selected details for many of the analysers presently on sale in the UK. Only those instruments capable of producing more than 100 results per hour on any analyte have been included. The information was largely abstracted from a survey of large analysers prepared in July 1985 on behalf of the North West Thames Regional Biochemistry Sub-Committee.[9] Full information was not available on some of the newer instruments and for those not yet launched in the UK. For up-to-date information the reader should contact the manufacturer or their agents.

PRACTICAL CONSIDERATIONS

Cleaning Automatic Analytical Systems

All automatic analytical systems, whether they use the continuous flow or discrete principle must have some means of removing the residue of the previous reaction mixture so that it does not interfere with subsequent assays. As well as chemical cleaning it is also important to ensure freedom from contamination from potentially infectious material. Some companies, understandably, will not allow their engineering staff to service instruments which have not been disinfected in a manner which eliminates the possibility of infection by HIV or hepatitis B viruses (*see* DHSS circular HN(87)22, 'Decontamination of health care equipment'). Laundering and disinfection of analysers has been achieved in a variety of ways.

Cleaning Continuous Flow Analysers.

Reactions in continuous-flow analysers develop as successive samples, mixed with reagents, progress along the same length of tubing. In the period between sampling, the reagents only are drawn into the flow-line and as they progress along it, they help to remove traces of the previous reaction mixture and so reduce contamination. In the early models of the Technicon sampler no provision was made for washing the sample line with water between samples. As a result of this severe sample carryover was experienced with some methods and it became the practice to alternate sample and water cups thus doubling the time required for a batch of tests. To correct this the sampler was redesigned to allow a water wash between successive samples.

At the end of each batch of tests it is important to clean both sample and reagent lines by pumping distilled water through the system. It is also sometimes necessary to use detergent solutions or solutions of sodium hypochlorite or chromic acid to remove material which has been deposited on the walls of the transmission tubing. Complete replacement of the entire manifold tubing becomes necessary when contamination is not removed by this treatment. When this is the case the new manifold should be thoroughly flushed with a solution of wetting agent to ensure a good bubble pattern from the start. The use of freshly prepared sodium hypochlorite solution containing 2500 ppm available chlorine is suitable for disinfecting after processing samples from AIDS or hepatitis B patients.

Cleaning Discrete Analysers.

Some discrete analytical systems avoid the interaction of successive reaction mixtures by using disposable reaction vessels (e.g. in the Technicon RA 1000). Some, now obsolete, analysers required an off-line laundering of the tubes after removal from the rotor or left *in situ*, with the whole rotor being transferred to a separate laundry unit. Most modern discrete analysers arrange for laundry of tubes to take place automatically between one assay and the next. This is achieved by first aspirating the dregs of the reaction mixture remaining after colorimetry and then cleaning each tube by the alternate injection and aspiration of deionized water. This arrangement does not on its own prevent water droplets adhering to the walls of the reaction cavities in sufficient volume to cause significant dilution errors. In the early stages of development of the now-obsolete Vickers M-300 analyser consideration was given to overcoming this problem by injecting a volatile water-miscible solvent followed by an air jet but it was realized that this could influence temperature control. The problem was overcome by means of an additional tube terminating in an elongated bullet-shaped tip of Teflon machined to fit the reaction cavity fairly closely. Vacuum was applied to a hole drilled down the centre of the tip. As the tip passed down the reaction cavity the vacuum created a strong

TABLE 1

COMPARATIVE DETAILS OF CHEMICAL ANALYSERS

Instrument	Type (see Fig. 1)	Basic cost exc. VAT £	Sample tray capacity	Max. no. tests available at one time	Sample volumes (μl) for U + E	Sample volumes (μl) for LFT	Samples assayed per hour for U + E	Samples assayed per hour for LFT	Time for U + E from startup, standby	Calibration frequency
Abbott VP Super	7	21 000	32	6	No U + E	44	No U + E	44	No U + E	Every run
Allied IL Genesis 21	7	50 000	50	21	82	132	30	25	13·5 min	8–24 h
Allied IL Monarch	9	68 000	38	23	47	61	60	55	6 min	2 h–5 day
AMI Parallel	5	203 500	150	30	75	135	240	240	—	Daily
AMI Perspective	10	97 500	40	64	98	84	120	100	<10 min	Daily
Baker Encore	7	49 500	96	6	No U + E	117	No U + E	57	No U + E	Each 30 tests
BCL Hitachi 705	7	52 000	40	19	130	78	45	26	30 min	Varies
BCL Hitachi 737	7	129 000	60	23	44	47	75	151	1 h	Daily
BDH Eppendorf ERIS	7	69 500	100	23	84	91	100	59	35 min	Each batch
BDH Eppendorf EPOS	7	33 500	200	1	No U + E	88	No U + E	39	No U + E	Daily
BDH Eppendorf EXTRA	13	180 000	200	43	84	91	200	118	35 min	Daily
BDH Eppendorf EASY	7	—	9	—	—	—	15	8	0 min	See ERIS
BDH Eppendorf EXSEL	7 + 13	140 000	300	24	84	88	100	50	35 min	8 h
Beckman RIIC ASTRA	5	34 000	38	23	110	144	65	98	7 min	Each batch
Chemlab System 4	1	25 000	80	4	N/A	N/A	N/A	N/A	75 min	Each batch
Chemlab Chemilyser	5	45 000	80	6	50	N/A	120	N/A	60 min	Daily
Clinicon Prisma II	13	179 000	220	35	300	50	300	65	25 min	Each batch
Coulter Kemomat 2	13	16 400	32	1	182	49	50	32	No U + E	Each 32 tests
Coulter Dacos	6	104 180	64	28	No U + E	62	No U + E	54	32 min	Varies
Dade Paramax	7	—	102	32	No U + E	62	No U + E	720	No U + E	30 days
Dupont Dimension 380	7	—	60	37	128	145	200	100	3 min	3 mths
Dupont Dimension 760	7	—	120	37	128	145	400	200	3 min	3 mths
Dupont Dimension 1140	13	—	180	37	128	145	600	300	3 min	3 mths
Gilford 400E		27 500	60	1	No U + E	220	No U + E	<20	15 min	Varies
Greiner G-400		50 000	30	28	150	135	42	37	24 min	2–3 mth
Hilger Chemispek	1	45 000	60	16	175	200	120	120	No U + E	Monthly
Hilger Saitron CLP	8	68 000	150	20	No U + E	190	No U + E	120	16 min	Each batch
Hilger Saitron CLS 4/30	7	—	40	32	—	—	81	57	25 min	
Kone Progress	7	45 000	84	27	180	50	30	21	12 min	>2 h
Nova Biomed 1 + 1	8	10 170	40	Na/K	N/A	N/A	N/A	N/A	No U + E	Auto Cal
Nova Biomed 4 + 4	8	17 890	40	Na/K/Cl/Bicarb	N/A	N/A	N/A	N/A	No U + E	Auto Cal
Nova Biomed 5 + 5	8	14 700	40	Na/K/Cl	N/A	N/A	N/A	N/A	No U + E	Auto Cal
Roche Cobas FARA	9	45 000	150	50	85	78	45	28	1 min	Varies
Roche Cobas MIRA	7	27 000	90	30	85	108	45	19	1 min	Varies
Technicon SMAII	1	118 000	40	18	1200	1200	90	90	25 min	10 min
Technicon SMACII	1	165 000	144	23	450	1200	150	150	35 min	96 samples
Technicon SRA 2000	1 + 7	215 000	174	35	450	450	150	150	20 min	see SMACII
Technicon RA 1000	7	47 000	30	15	35	90	60	34	0 min	2 wk ISE 4 h
Technicon RA2X	7	110 000	60	27	35	90	120	69	<5 min	2 wk ISE 4 h
Technicon Chem 1	2	160 000	288	35	13	7	240	103	3·5 min	2 wk ISE 4 h
Ultrolab Altaire	7	56 500	150	16	No U + E	103	No U + E	—	No U + E	Daily

Footnotes: U + E = sodium, potassium, chloride, bicarbonate, urea, and creatinine.
LFT = bilirubin, total protein, albumin, alkaline phosphatase and 3 other enzymes.
— = No data available.
N/A = Not applicable.

current of air in the narrow annulus around the 'bullet'. This caused the water droplets to precede the 'bullet' down the walls and finally to be aspirated through the central hole in the vacuum tube and to waste. This highly efficient method of drying the reaction tubes, invented and later published by Riley,[10] is seen in several currently marketed discrete analysers.

This arrangement does not eliminate inter-sample contamination in the flow-cell of the colorimeter but this can be minimized by careful design to avoid sharp angles in which residual solution can be trapped and suitable shaping to encourage drainage between samples. The system should also be arranged so that about four cell volumes of the reaction solution are rinsed through the cell before its absorbance is measured.

Recommendations for sterilizing automatic analysers after the assay of infectious samples vary with the manufacturer. It is the policy in some health districts to allow the assay of samples from AIDS victims only by means of automatic analysers. The wide, often alarmist, publicity given to the increasing incidence and the high mortality associated with this disease have urged some manufacturers to take precipitate action in providing protocols for machine sterilization. There are several agents which have been recommended for this purpose but some seem to affect the behaviour of assays, giving rise to higher coefficients of variation. For instance, Totacide recommended by AMI, appears to interfere with the measurement of albumin using bromocresol green reagent and possibly also with AST, cholesterol and protein assay. The use of sodium hypochlorite as described for continuous-flow analysers overcomes these problems.

As well as influencing the performance of certain assays, sterilization protocols can also be so time consuming as to bring about the need to alter work schedules. It takes up to 50 min to complete the wash and disinfection cycles at the end of each day on the AMI Parallel analyser.

Cleaning Centrifugal Analysers. In those centrifugal analysers which do not employ disposable rotors the transfer disc is usually cleaned *in situ* by the introduction of deionized water, methanol or other solvents into the rotor cavities and subsequent centrifugation.

Chemical Methods in Automatic Analysis

One of the main aims in the development of an automatic analytical system should be to ensure its overall simplicity. As the requirements increase (e.g. high speed, mechanical transfer, *in situ* protein removal, automatic drift correction, tests selection and *in situ* laundering) this becomes more difficult to achieve. However, if the interdependency of machine and chemistry is recognized from the start a blend of ana-lytical and mechanical compromise may go a long way towards simplifying the system. This section deals with the interrelationship of machine and method and illustrates cases where a slight modification to an assay has saved mechanical complication and also the converse where mechanization has allowed the simplification of a method.

The different approaches in handling serum or plasma protein, mentioned earlier in the chapter, illustrates both these aspects. The Technicon Auto-Analyzer was invented at a time when most conventional analytical methods required the preliminary removal of protein. Dialysis was used to achieve this without interrupting analytical continuity. Inefficient though this method is, it has not been surpassed in simplicity and reliability in any automatic analytical system. Thus with the inclusion of an extra functional entity a system has been provided which makes possible the assay of a wide range of substances without major alteration of the original chemistry methods.

On the other hand the rapid development of work-simplified techniques arising from the discovery of new and often more specific reagents, has led to the realization that protein removal is no longer essential for the accurate and reproducible assay of a wide range of substances in the body fluids. This has been of vital importance in the fundamental design of all modern high-speed, discrete analysers.

Improvement of Fluid Flow. In both continuous-flow and discrete analysers the addition to one of the reagents of a small amount of surfactant improves the flow characteristics of the reaction solution (in the case of the discrete analyser through the flow cell of the colorimeter). It is important that these agents are not used in excess since frothing can result which decreases the accuracy of colorimetry. A final concentration in the reaction mixture of about 0·02% v/v is sufficient for most purposes.

Reduction of Specific Gravity of Reagents. With reagents of high specific gravity there may not only be mixing problems but also problems with filling the colorimeter flow cell. A reaction mixture of high specific gravity makes fine control difficult, so that errors arise from improper filling of the cell. For example, such a reagent combination is found in the bilirubin method of Ichida and Nobuoka[11] which employs concentrated urea-benzoate solution as the accelerator and alkaline potassium sodium tartrate (Fehling's II) solution for the formation of azobilirubin blue complex. The efficiency of filling the colorimeter cuvette in this case, is improved first by changing to a less concentrated accelerator of caffeine–sodium benzoate and still further by using sodium hydroxide instead of Fehlings II solution. The omission of potassium sodium tartrate from the alkalinizing reagent in no way reduces the accuracy of this method.

Beneficial Effects of Mechanization on Chemical Methods. One of the main advantages of an automatic analytical system is the precise timing of the operational sequence which ensures that every sample is identically processed at every stage of the reaction. The implications of this, when adapting or devising methods for machines are not always fully appreciated. They are:

1. Some reagents, used in manual methods to ensure the precise termination of the reaction become unnecessary. The bilirubin method once more provides an example. Some workers use a sodium ascorbate reagent which probably prevents the continued development of azo-pigments in alkaline solution[12] which, with anything but strict timing, would lead to differences in relative absorbance. With precise timing of the reaction it has been found unnecessary to use the reagent.
2. Methods dependent on the measurement of reaction rate may be employed. These have the following advantages:
    a. It is often possible to measure absorbance well before colour development is complete thus shortening assay time;
    b. Relative and not absolute measurements are made so that with a constant source of interference, e.g. slight opalescence, in the reaction mixture no blank is necessary.
    c. The measurement of individual components of a mixture of substances with closely related chemical properties may be made without first separating them. Such measurements may be achieved in substances whose rate constants differ by a factor of 10 or more.

As well as the advantages of kinetic methods Malmstadt, Delaney and Cordos[13] also mention limitations:

1. The half-time of the reaction must be greater than the mixing time of the system. At the other extreme very slow reactions, with half-times greater than a few hours, are not suitable for routine kinetic analysis.
2. The precision of the measurement depends on good reproducibility for all experimental conditions such as temperature, pH, ionic strength, composition of the reagents and even the size and shape of the reaction vessels.

Reaction-rate Measurements. It is true to say that the growth of interest in the application of kinetic methods for routine biochemical analysis has been made practicable by the development of instruments for improving the precision of measurement. The greatest developments have undoubtedly taken place in the field of enzyme assay but in more recent years the advantages of the kinetic approach have been shown to apply just as much to other areas of analytical biochemistry. For example the measurement of creatinine in the presence of protein, using the Jaffé reaction, is made possible only by the use of reaction-rate measurements.[14] Furthermore, by the judicious choice of reaction conditions and measurement period the influence of some, if not all interfering substances can be overcome.

In recent years, with the much greater use of computers for process control in automatic analysers, a more detailed monitoring of the analytical process is possible. The result is that multiple, very closely spaced and accurately timed absorbance measurements can be achieved in kinetic assays. Thus what was once only a two-point assay becomes multipoint and errors in the determination of slope sometimes encountered with say chance bubbles in the colorimeter or very rapid consumption of the substrate due to high enzyme activity are minimized.

Effect of Reagents on Machine Components. As little as a decade ago the most widely used methods for cholesterol assay employed the use of Lieberman–Burchard reagent or some modification of it. This reagent consists of a mixture of acetic anhydride and concentrated sulphuric acid which, of course, is highly corrosive and presents problems in both discrete and continuous flow analysis. The problems associated with the use of this reagent led to the development of an alternative method involving the enzymatic oxidation of cholesterol to Δ4-cholestanone and hydrogen peroxide.[15] This is now widely used as the method of choice for both manual and automatic assay of cholesterol.

The use of alkaline picrate solution for the measurement of creatinine in body fluids is not without potential hazard. On contact with metals such as copper and iron it forms complexes which may explode on percussion. It is possible that this reagent too will be replaced by enzyme systems although the development in this field has been very slow. First mentioned in the 1930s it has taken until the mid 1980s for a commercial kit to appear on the market. Produced by Boehringer Mannheim, the kit, which incorporates creatininase, creatinase, sarcosine oxidase and peroxidase, is not easy to apply to automatic analysers. It is also costly when compared with the traditional Jaffé reagent. The alternative system which employs creatinine desmidase and leads to the production of N-methylhydantoin and ammonia may be simpler to adapt for machine use but production of the enzyme appears to be more difficult.

Factors Governing Assay Sequence. In some of the earlier analysers little attention was paid to the effect of carryover. Even in the Vickers M300 the effect of certain of the diluents on the sample was noticeable. For instance carryover of phosphate buffer diluent, even though of small proportion, was sufficient to cause the elevation of inorganic phosphate concentration if this assay was downstream of any channel employing phosphate buffer as diluent. As a result of this type of contamination analytes such as sodium, potassium, calcium and phosphate were always measured early in the test profile. Manufacturers of modern analysers pay much closer attention to the avoidance of this type of carryover on sample and diluent probes. The most common approach being to insert a rinse station between sample and reagent vessels.

Even in some modern analysers, however, the organization of test patterns cannot be neglected, although more from an economic than from an analytical standpoint. The design of the AMI Parallel analyser is such that in advance of the first sample for the assay of a particular analyte reagent lines are flushed through twice to ensure that fresh reagent is used for the analysis. If there is a break in sequence or even if there is a random scatter of samples requiring a particular test two reagent purges will always precede the delivery for the actual assay. In certain assays, particularly for the measurement of enzyme activity this can be very costly; in the case of spaced, random samples the cost will be three times that for sequential batches of the same test. Careful planning of test sequences should be made and samples for the less-frequently requested tests should be grouped.

Sensitivity and Specificity of Reaction. The measurement of certain constituents of serum or plasma may be rendered inaccurate by the presence of substances which interfere with the reaction and these may be of endogenous or exogenous origin. It is often possible by careful selection of reagents or reaction conditions to correct such errors and to improve the specificity of the assay. An example of this is seen in the kinetic method for the determination of creatinine (*see* under 'Reaction-Rate Measurements'). Sometimes, however, the interference is not the result of chemical side-reactions but is due to the presence of a coloured material in the plasma which absorbs at the same wavelength as that chosen for the assay. A common source of this colorimetric interference is free oxyhaemoglobin in the plasma. This arises from the haemolysis of erythrocytes in the blood sample and causes absorbance in more than one region of the spectrum (i.e. between 400 nm and 448 nm and around 540 nm and 578 nm). Interference of this type can usually be corrected by means of sample blanks which use the same volume of serum or plasma as the test but are treated with the reagents, or modified reagents, in a way which prevents the colour reaction. Subtraction of the blank from the test absorbance therefore corrects for the presence of the interfering colour.

In automatic analysis the need for a sample blank means the use of a channel which might otherwise be occupied by an additional assay. Thus the possible range of tests is reduced and the cost per test increased. The dialyser in continuous-flow systems affords some protection against interference from coloured compounds of large molecular weight, such as haemoglobin but in discrete systems there is no such protection so the following alternatives must be considered:

1. Sample monitoring for the presence of interfering chromophores and the rejection of samples which contain them;
2. Choice of a method with a coloured product the absorption maximum of which is in a different spectral region from the interfering substances;
3. Provision of facilities for blank correction;
4. Measurement of the absorbance of the interfering substance and application of an appropriate correction factor for each of the affected methods.

A serum or plasma monitor is now provided in some instruments. In the Vickers machine the purpose of the plasma monitor was to detect and reject those samples which showed excessive haemolysis, lipaemia or icterus. With the increased computer capacity of modern machines such as the AMI Parallel analyser it has been possible to incorporate a plasma monitor and with so-called 'Math' factors automatically 'correct' for the influence of the interfering substances in the final calculation.

PURCHASING AN AUTOMATIC ANALYSER

The purchase of a new automatic analyser is a major event in any laboratory. The choice is wide and the mechanical principles adopted by the different manufacturers to meet the analytical requirements are varied (Fig. 1, p. 530). The life expectancy of an analyser may be up to ten years, sometimes more. The cost is almost always high and in the present climate of financial stringency the competition for capital is intense. Against this background there is a clear need to reduce to a minimum the risk of making the wrong choice. It is also essential to prepare a strong case-of-need if one is to succeed in obtaining funds from limited financial resources.

Justification for Purchasing an Automatic Analyser

The need for an automatic analyser arises from an increase in laboratory workload to a point where the staff are no longer able to meet demands with the existing equipment during a normal working day. In laboratories already equipped with an automatic analyser replacement may become necessary for a variety of reasons: (1) that analytical demand has increased to the point where it exceeds the capacity of the present analyser; (2) that machine breakdown is unacceptably frequent and repair costs high; (3) that the present analyser is of a (outmoded) design that is uneconomical in the use of sample and reagents; (4)

that the results are frequently of an unacceptably low quality (as demonstrated by quality control records) resulting in the frequent necessity to repeat batches of tests.

Choice of Analyser

DHSS evaluation reports in the UK, and similar reports by other independent bodies, can be of help in making a choice between instruments which have been on the market for some time. Unfortunately the pace of introduction of new analysers is so fast that it outstrips the capacity of the evaluators to provide up-to-date reports. If one is to take advantage of the latest choice in analysers it is necessary either to carry out one's own evaluation or to make personal contact with a user to discuss his or her experiences. Many manufacturers will now loan models of even the medium-sized analysers to allow user familiarization and evaluation before committing themselves to its purchase. With larger analysers where temporary installation is too costly manufacturers are usually happy to arrange visits to existing sites where the machine is in use. User-evaluation will be discussed later in this chapter.

Capacity of the Analyser

The capacity of an analyser is usually expressed in terms of the number and range of tests which may be performed in a specified period of time. It is a simple matter to calculate the average workload in the same terms and make a shortlist of those analysers with a large enough capacity. Bearing in mind that the life expectancy of an automatic analyser is around ten years it is important to extrapolate the trends in workload for a decade and incorporate this into calculations for determining the size required.

It is important at this stage to recognize the difference between those analysers which are described as handling say 300 tests per hour and those described as handling 300 samples per hour. In the former, the various assays are measured sequentially through the same colorimeter. The frequency of measurement is usually expressed in terms of a batch of the same, relatively simple, end-point assays. Kinetic enzyme measurements or assay changes can significantly reduce the achievable analysis rate. In the case of samples per hour, assays for all the different analytes are often measured simultaneously in several colorimeters and the rate of analysis is unaffected by the complexity of the assays.

In a situation where the capacity of a large analyser is too great, even when taking into account future developments, the possibility of using the alternative of two medium-sized analysers should be considered. Although ergonomically not as satisfactory as a single faster analyser it could be a cheaper approach and because of the low risk of simultaneous breakdown there will be a partial back-up facility.

Performance Specifications

Size of Sample and Reagent Volumes. Most modern analysers require only a few microlitres of sample and reagents. This enables samples from small children and adults to be processed economically on the same analyser, thus overcoming the need for a separate ultramicro, paediatric service, so simplifying quality control. Until recently economy of reagent was not possible using continuous-flow instruments but the introduction of the Chem-1 system (Technicon) and the use of merging zones in non-segmented streams should remove this disadvantage.

Analytical Flexibility. With some instruments it is not possible for the user to employ home-made reagents, to introduce new assays or even to modify existing ones; analysers such as the Dupont ACA or the BDH Eppendorf Easy are dependent on dry reagents supplied by the manufacturer in special bar-coded reaction packs. In such cases the availability, cost and quality of the assays is entirely in the hands of the manufacturer and outside user control.

Similar limitations apply to those analysers which rely on special disposable components for their operation, e.g. the reaction rotor for the IL centrifugal analysers. Although the user is free to modify the manufacturers assay protocols or introduce new ones the analyser will not function without these unique disposables. In spite of the fact that these features are convenient and labour saving for the user it should be remembered that a failure in supply of the reagent packs or plastic components means that the machine is totally inoperable. Furthermore, they are not without significant revenue consequences which can be increased by the manufacturer at any time. Also the possibility that a manufacturer might withdraw availability of an essential disposable item cannot, unfortunately, be totally discounted.

Facility for Processing Urgent Samples

Many discrete analysers are designed to allow the operator to insert urgent samples for preferential treatment during a routine analytical sequence. A stand-by facility is also commonly available which allows the analyser to be used with negligible delay after a period of non-use. These facilities allow urgent work to be done in the same way as routine thus reducing the need to staff a separate emergency laboratory and also ensuring the continuity of results. It is not easy to arrange stat handling with conventional continuous-flow analysers and stand-by can only be achieved with considerable wastage of reagents.

Machine Dimensions

Apart from all other considerations it is important not to overlook the size, weight and shape of the machine. Not only must the analyser be small enough to fit into the available laboratory space but there must be sufficient all round clearance to permit unhindered routine maintenance. For bench-standing models there must be sufficient free bench space to allow activities such as the temporary parking of samples during loading.

It is also worth remembering that some analysers, even in the medium-capacity range are too wide to pass through the standard door, too long to manoeuvre round a tight corner, or too heavy to be transported in a lift. It may even exceed the weight-bearing capacity of the floor. These problems can be very expensive to overcome so careful pre-planning should go into the siting and installation of the analyser.

Operator Instruction and Engineering Courses

The more complex the analyser the greater the need for user training. Suitable training courses should be available for a sufficient number of staff at no extra cost to the purchaser. It is also of value to negotiate with the manufacturer a rather more advanced course to allow first-line engineering problems to be solved and rectified without calling on the services of the company's engineers. Although a maintenance contract may have been negotiated with the firm the response time of the engineer can be unacceptably long. Informed self help reduces the chance of excessive machine down-time for trivial reasons. Furthermore, maintenance contracts can add significantly to the revenue consequences of installing a particular analyser. The annual cost of comprehensive maintenance cover is approximately 10% of the purchase price of the analyser. There are usually reduced scales for less complete cover, therefore certain amounts of in-house engineering can save considerably in maintenance costs.

Installation

The cost of installing an automatic analyser can be very high and the arrangements complex. With some of the large, computer-controlled analysers it may be necessary to provide a clean 30 amp, 3-phase power supply, a large-capacity deionizing plant for water, piped gases for flame photometry, air conditioning and perhaps even acoustic tiles to reduce noise levels.

It is not always apparent from the manufacturers' literature that extra items of equipment are essential before the analyser can function and that the preparations for installation can be extensive and time consuming. It is important to check the requirements carefully preferably having a site meeting with the installation engineers. The supplier should be asked to include all the extras (even the provision of services up to the required standard) in the purchase price of the analyser; this could save months of local negotiation.

Different problems arise in the case of large-analyser replacement. It may seem ideal to provide a completely new set of services for the new analyser so that the old one may be used for the routine work until the installation and evaluation of the new one is complete. However, even if space is not limiting the cost of this approach could be very high compared with reusing the existing services. To arrange this may require a transition period of some weeks during which time the requests for biochemistry services must be met. This may be achieved in a variety of ways each involving local arrangements for temporary clinical restraint in demand for tests together with either:

1. The loan of an intermediate capacity analyser requiring no special installation facilities. It may be possible to negotiate the free loan of such an instrument if manufactured by the same company as the one to be purchased.
2. The temporary transfer of non-urgent work to a local laboratory, with the provision of technical help for transport and sample and reagent preparation.

User Evaluation and Acceptance

Following the installation of an automatic analyser it is important, before formal acceptance, to determine whether the achievable standard of analytical performance meets that claimed by the manufacturer. There are numerous published protocols for evaluation of clinical analysers; many of these have been discussed by Westgard.[16] For the most part, however, these schemes are too ponderous and time consuming for use in acceptance trials.

The detail of the acceptance trial will vary with the size and complexity of the machine. Often, with the larger analysers, groups of would-be purchasers and representatives from the government health service are asked to agree acceptable standards of precision for each analyte and a test protocol is drawn up. The design of the protocol should be such that it tests precision, linearity and carry-over over the physiological and pathological ranges of all the analytes and allows correlation with chosen reference methods.

In general terms the machine should first be standardized according to the manufacturer's instructions and then a series of well-mixed, low, medium and high analyte pools assayed in patterns from which precision, linearity and carry-over may be calculated. The number of tests required will depend on the capacity of the analyser and should not be less than one complete rotor of samples (in the case of the AMI Parallel analyser this is 151). This should be repeated on at least three occasions and only if the agreed performance is achieved on all three should the machine be accepted. Standardization material, control samples and reagents during the acceptance trial should be supplied by the manufacturer.

Standardization and Quality Control

It has become the tradition to standardize an automatic analyser at least once a day and sometimes even before each run. Additional quality control checks are then carried out within run by the introduction of machine-identifiable control material placed at intervals within each batch. It is advantageous, when controls are used, to have some means of displaying the results during the run, to identify drift or significant changes in precision in time to take immediate action. Many instruments will permit only off-line calculation of quality control data so that no within-run correction is possible. Most manufacturers recognize the high cost of standardization and control materials and some (e.g. Kodak Ektachem, Dupont ACA) taking advantage of advances in material sciences, analytical techniques, electronics and computer sciences have developed systems in which the need for standardization has been reliably reduced to a frequency of 3 months or less. The revenue savings brought about by the reduction in use of standardization materials and controls, together with an improved reliability of the intermittent assay of urgent samples must be weighed against the high cost of the individual reagent packages. There is little doubt that with the increased stability and decreased drift of modern colorimeters the whole question of standardization and control is in need of review.

Print-out of Results

An aspect of analyser operation which can easily be overlooked in the decision-making process is the form of output of the results, and yet this may not be compatible with existing laboratory reports. The format of the output of some analysers is so rigid as to require pre-printed paper. Others, although accepting standard computer paper, allow no flexibility in the way the results may be presented. This can be a great drawback necessitating a modification to the structure of the patient's notes. Manufacturers are often unsympathetic to this problem and sometimes object to changing software to allow print-out format to user specification. If this is considered important the available options should be determined before deciding to purchase.

Staff Involvement

It would be a mistake to arrange the purchase of an analyser without discussing the options with the biochemistry staff. There is, however, a tendency for some laboratory workers to favour only those instruments which work on principles with which they are familiar, an attitude, which if allowed to prevail, will almost certainly impede progress towards the use of analysers employing new technology. The popularity of conventional continuous-flow systems marketed almost exclusively by Technicon is almost entirely due to their early dominance in the field of automation in clinical biochemistry. Only recently has this firm acknowledged the greater flexibility of discrete analysers by introducing the RA 1000 series to be used in conjunction with the SMAC, with its fixed test profiles. The new generation of flow analysers will doubtless allow operator discretion in the choice of tests but as yet they are relatively untried. If uninformed prejudice is to be overcome it is important to arrange an educational programme to highlight the advantages and disadvantages of the different options.

CONCLUDING REMARKS AND FUTURE DEVELOPMENTS

The needs of laboratories vary enormously and the universal clinical chemistry analyser has not yet been produced. In the large laboratories the majority of specimens requiring multi-component analyses are most efficiently processed using a large selective multichannel machine. These machines are inflexible, expensive and because of their mechanical complexity require frequent attention by a skilled operator. The high-capacity analysers that are currently available were all designed at least 10 years ago and the introduction of state-of-the-art technology into this area is urgently required. Perhaps, a future generation of multichannel machines could be based on the use of non-segmented flowing streams and merging zone techniques.

In recent years the instrument manufacturers have concentrated their efforts on lower capacity units where sales potential is greater. The resulting competition in this lucrative sector of the market has produced an excellent choice of up-to-date small- to medium-sized analysers. Extensive use of microprocessors has reduced operator time and the required skill level. These developments have been complimented by advances in reagent formulation. Thus in some instances an instrument can be calibrated and the calibration retained for many weeks. The recent advent of the discrete analyser capable of taking frequent readings during the course of a reaction will no doubt speed the decline of the centrifugal analyser. The menu of tests available for implementation on discrete analysers will continue to grow.

The trend away from the use of radioactive labels in immunoassay is likely to continue and there is a need for more sensitive homogeneous methods of detecting the antigen–antibody complex. The use of lanthanide chelates and time-resolved fluorimetry looks promising but as yet no easily automated method has been developed.

The concept of management budgeting is currently being discussed in the UK National Health Service. If this is implemented, laboratory directors will become even more cost conscious and the cost benefit of all new equipment will be increasingly scrutinized. Under the proposed scheme physicians will be charged a fee for each laboratory request and the laboratory will have to generate its own resources by selling its services to the clinicians. This environment will produce a desire for machines with low capital and running costs, albeit at some loss of precision and accuracy. After the introduction of management budgeting a laboratory can expect an immediate decline in the number of requests, but we expect the decrease in workload to be short lived. In the long run workloads will continue to increase. However, the increasing work will almost certainly have to be accommodated by increased automation and not by large increases in staff numbers (staff salaries are by far the largest laboratory expenditure).

Dry reagent chemistry has advanced rapidly during the past decade and it might reasonably be expected that broader applications will emerge in the years ahead. So far this technology has had little impact on laboratory automation but management budgeting may cause some clinicians to investigate its possibilities.

An area of high manual activity still devoid of automation is the sample reception and preparation room. Here specimens are booked in, centrifuged, split and a laboratory sample number—usually via a bar-code label—is fitted. Developments in this area could make a useful contribution to laboratory efficiency. In order to minimize sample handling all automatic analysers should be able to receive the tube into which the sample was collected and also to read the sample identification number.

A further reduction in tedious manual work could be achieved if more analysers could process whole blood instead of plasma. It would then be logical to include in the test repertoire, the measurement of haemoglobin concentration and the determination of the numbers of red and white cells. As, in the UK, these tests are usually considered to be the province of the haematologist such a machine may not find much favour, but in some other countries, where haematology and biochemistry are considered a single discipline, the view may be different.

The commonly employed optical methods are obviously unsuitable for direct determinations on whole blood samples. Electrochemical methods have proved useful for a few analytes but a more generally applicable selective technique would be desirable. The slow trend towards the use of whole blood will continue particularly in those appliances sold specifically to deal with urgent specimens.

REFERENCES

1. Skeggs L. T. (1957). An automated method for colorimetric analysis. *Am. J. Clin. Pathol*; **28**: 311.
2. Cassaday M., Diebler H., Herron R., Pelavin M., Svenjak D., Viastelica D. (1985). Capsule chemistry technology for high speed clinical chemistry analysers. *Clin. Chem*; **31**: 1453.
3. Riley C., Rocks B. F., and Sherwood R. A. (1984). Flow injection analysis in clinical chemistry. *Talanta*; **108**: 879.
4. Mindegaard J. (1979). Flow multi-injection analysis—a system for the analysis of highly concentrated samples without prior dilution. *Anal. Chim. Acta*; **104**: 185.
5. Riley C., Aslett L. H., Rocks B. F., Sherwood R. A., Watson J. D. McK., Morgon J. (1983). Controlled dispersion analysis: Flow injection analysis without injection. *Clin. Chem*; **29**: 332.
6. Rocks B. F., Sherwood R. A. (1986). The use of holding coils to facilitate long incubations in unsegmented flow analysis. *Anal. Chim. Acta*; **179**: 225.
7. Anderson N. G. (1969). Analytical techniques for cell fractions XIII. A multiple-cuvette rotor for a new microanalytical system. *Anal. Biochem*; **28**: 545.
8. Schultz S. G., Holen J. T., Donohue J. P., Francoeur T. A. (1985). Two-dimensional centrifugation for desk top clinical chemistry. *Clin. Chem*; **31**: 1457.
9. Fyffe J. A. (1985). A review of large biochemistry analysers. *Commun. Lab. Med*; **1**: 118.
10. Riley C. (1984). The design of automated analysis machines. *Crit. Rev. Biomed. Eng*; **10**: 27.
11. Ichida T., Nobuoka M. (1968). Ultramicro method for the determination of total and direct bilirubin in serum by modified alkaline azobilirubin blue reaction. *Clin. Chim. Acta*; **19**: 249.
12. With T. K. (1968). *Bile Pigments*. p. 64. London: Academic Press.
13. Malmstadt H. V., Delaney C. J., Cordos E. A. (1972). Reaction-rate methods of chemical analysis. *Crit. Rev. Anal. Chem*; **2**: 559.
14. Cook J. G. H. (1971). Creatinine assay in the presence of protein. *Clin. Chim. Acta*; **32**: 485.
15. Richmond W. (1972). The development of an enzymatic technique for the assay of cholesterol in biological fluids. *Scand. J. Clin. Lab. Invest*; suppl. 126: abstract 325.
16. Westgard J. O. (1981). Precision and accuracy: concepts and assessment by method evaluation testing. *Crit. Rev. Clin. Lab. Sci*; **18**: 283.

36. The Use of Computers in Laboratories

André De Bats

INTRODUCTION

For over twenty years, scientists have had held out to them the promise of revolutionary developments in laboratory practice following the installation of what have disrespectfully been described as 'all-singing, all-dancing' computer systems. When these promises were made in the early 1960s, there was a need to distinguish between the terms mechanization, automation and the use of computers. This was due, in part, to the limitations of technology and the types of computers available at that time. However, with the development of today's discretionary analysers together with the newer instruments designed to operate nearer the patient, I attempt here to examine the effectiveness of computers in laboratory medicine in the light of current knowledge.

This chapter also attempts to consider the future of computerization in clinical biochemistry by the evidence presented in the commercial environment since, because of its size, the commercial market is where the major developments are taking place.

HISTORICAL

To answer the question as to why the computer was invented, the reply must be because it had to be.

The pressures of World War II led to research into many areas including night bombing, attempting to shoot at targets that could not be seen, calculating the speed and direction of enemy movements, and much more. The events that led up to the invention of the computer are briefly described below.

1642 Blaise Pascal. Blaise Pascal developed a mechanical calculating aid using gears, wheels and dials.

Pascal was the son of a Tax Superintendent in Paris. His father had the tedious task of manually calculating tax returns and to ease this burden, Blaise, at the age of 18, invented his calculator. Basically, it consisted of a number of wheels, each of which was divided into 10 segments and a carryover lever. An example of this today is a mileometer trip meter.

1694 Gottfried Wilhelm von Leibnitz. The limitation of Blaise Pascal's calculator was that it treated multiplication as repeated addition. It was therefore a logical progression to mechanize the multiplication process. This was done first by von Leibnitz. He was 25 years old when he began work on a machine which could perform the four basic functions of arithmetic, addition, subtraction, multiplication and division. Von Leibnitz took 23 years to complete his machine, which was designed for both scientific and commercial arithmetic. Unfortunately, because of the limited technology of the day, the components could not be cut with sufficient precision and the machine proved to be of limited accuracy.

Von Leibnitz, being a philosopher as well as a mathematician, anticipated the use of binary arithmetic in computer design. He saw binary arithmetic as the image of creation. God is represented as 1 and nothing (the void) as 0. The beauty and scepticism of von Leibnitz's binary arithmetic is said to have converted the Emperor of China to the belief in a god who could draw all beings from the void.

1791 Charles Babbage. It was left to the genius of Charles Babbage to design a machine, which was to be the forerunner of the electronic computer.

Charles Babbage was born in 1791 in Totnes, Devon, the son of a wealthy banker. He was educated privately at home until he went to study mathematics at Cambridge. In 1828 he was awarded the Lucasian chair of Mathematics, which he held for 11 years without giving a single lecture.

The difference engine. The idea for this machine came to Babbage whilst he was mulling over some tables in his room at the Analytical Society. It was based on an entirely new principle—the levels of difference for particular formulae:

taking the formula $y = x^2 + 3x + 1$
when $x = 0$ $y = 1$
$x = 1$ $y = 5$
$x = 2$ $y = 11$
$x = 3$ $y = 19$ etc.

Babbage noticed that between consecutive values for y, there was a first level of difference, i.e. 4, 6, 8, etc., and between these values there was a second level of difference which was a constant, i.e. 2 (Table 1). The interesting point Babbage made was that by adding together the previous value for y with the previous values in the 1st and 2nd difference columns, then the next value of y was obtained.

i.e.   Taking the value of y for $x = 2$ as 11, in the above example then the value of y for $x = 3$ is $11 + 6 + 2 = 19$
$y = 19$

TABLE 1
DIFFERENCE TABLE FOR $y = x^2 + 3x + 1$

x	y	First difference in y	Second difference in y
0	1	–	–
1	5	4	2
2	11	6	2
3	19	8	2

The first difference engine was abandoned due to lack of funds; his personal fortune was lost.

The second difference engine was conceived to compute tables from a formula with six levels of difference and produce results to 21 places. It also failed, because it was too ambitious. As late as 1934, it was regarded as a major achievement to compute six orders of difference to 13 places.

1840 Analytical engine. During 1840, Babbage went to Turin and presented a paper on the Analytical Engine. It was intended to be completely automatic and capable of performing the basic arithmetic functions for any mathematical problem at a speed of 60 additions a minute.

The Analytical Engine was to consist of five parts

A *store* to hold integers.

An *arithmetic* unit which Babbage called the 'mill'.

A *control* unit for ensuring that the machine performed the desired functions.

An *input* device to pass into the machine both integers and instructions as to which arithmetic operation to perform.

An *output* device to display the results obtained from the calculations.

Charles Babbage died in 1871. His concept of a 'computer' remained but an idea. Some 75 years later, an article by Comrie[1] appeared in *Nature* entitled 'Babbage's dream comes true'. The paper describes the Harvard Mk 1 computer designed by Howard Aiken, who was quoted as saying 'if Babbage had lived 75 years later I would have been out of a job'.

Harvard Mk 1. In 1937, Howard A. Aiken, using a technique already developed for punched cards,

began work in collaboration with the International Business Machines Corporation (IBM) on the design of a fully automatic calculating machine to solve complex differential equations. Seven years later the Harvard Mk 1 was produced and donated to Harvard University where it was initially used for classified work for the US Navy. The Mk 1 was complex in design; physically the machine measured 51 feet in length and 8 feet in height. It was said to contain 0.75 million parts and in construction to have used 500 miles of wire. This was the birth of the digital computer.

The innovation of very high speed vacuum tube switching devices led to the first all-electronic computer, the Electronic Numerical Integrator and Calculator (ENIAC) (1946). Before the completion of ENIAC, a significant event occurred. This was the publication of a paper entitled 'Theory and Techniques of Electronic Digital Computers' by John von Neumann, a consultant to the ENIAC project. Von Neumann's most significant concept was that of the 'stored program'. This embodied the concept that a sequence of instructions might be held in the store of a computer, for the purpose of directing the flow of operations and that these instructions themselves may be altered and manipulated in much the same way as data. EDVAC, the Electronic Discrete Automatic Computer was to be such a machine.

EDVAC. This computer made use of acoustic delay lines, consisting of tanks of mercury in which the trains of pulses representing data circulated and recirculated until required to be operated upon by the arithmetic unit. Both instructions and integers to be used for calculation were stored in the memory unit.

There were a number of engineering difficulties with EDVAC, which was in part due to the departure from the project of two key figures, Eckert and Manchly, who left to form their own manufacturing company.

1947 EDSAC. The Electronic Delay Storage Automatic Calculator was produced in 1947 by a British team under the leadership of Maurice Wilkes, who had spent some time with the EDVAC team in the United States of America. The machine executed its first program in May 1949, and with this function the forerunner of digital computers as they are produced today had arrived.

Computer Generations. There is no clear cut pattern of development after EDSAC had emerged. The following framework clarifies the development of computers until today

1940–1952	1st Generation systems—based on Vacuum tube devices —EDVAC, EDSAC
1952–1964	2nd Generation systems—Magnetic drum or magnetic core storage and transistors instead of vacuum tubes

1964–present 3rd/4th Generation systems—Integrated circuits, multi-programming, multi-users.

The distinction between 3rd and 4th generation systems has been a hotly debated point. Those manufacturers who based their new product lines on integrated circuitry claim this to be the dividing line, whereas others who developed multi-programming and multi-sharing contend this to be the dividing line.

In general, prior to 1968 the development was mainly hardware based. Since 1968 the generations have been extended to include both the hardware and software components of the complete system.

The Development of 5th Generation Systems. Already at the beginning of the 1960s there was growing interest in the development of electronic 'tools' for non-numeric data processing. However, due to financial constraints, the construction of specialized hardware was terminated. Attention was then drawn to the development of special software for the hardware which existed at the time. A major breakthrough was the creation of LISP by J. McCarthy,[2] an early high-level language designed for non-numeric data processing. Further development of LISP has led to the creation of 'super' high level languages designed for knowledge manipulation. These form the basis of the 'expert' systems now being developed.

SOFTWARE

Of the two major components of a laboratory computer system, the software and the hardware, it is the software that enables the system to perform as a laboratory computer rather than as one to be used in, say, a business environment. It is the software more than the hardware, which is tailored to the user's needs and makes one laboratory's system different from that of another. Also, it should be said, that problems with the software are usually found responsible for failures of the system to perform as required.

The software is usually constructed at several different levels:

1. At the most fundamental level is the 'bootstrapping' function which is usually built into the hardware and which responds immediately on switching on the system, often by loading the operating system from a storage device, such as a magnetic disc or tape. This is the initial phase of 'booting up' the system.
2. The operating system is that part of the software which controls the passage of information between the various parts of the system, such as keyboards, VDUs, printers, on-line instruments and the data-processing unit(s). It is also responsible for providing the framework for the efficient storage of data and program files on storage devices, and for loading such files into processor memory available to the user.

Many modern operating systems, of which three of the most currently popular are OS2, Pick and UNIX, additionally provide a wide range of facilities for sophisticated manipulation of files, for text editing, for programming, for graphical or textual presentation of data and for mathematical computation.

Most of these facilities are routines that programmers have written to assist them in their own work and have been thought useful enough to retain in the system for the benefit of other users. In earlier days, however, operating systems provided the bare minimum and users were able to communicate with the system only through the programming language provided.

3. Programming languages are described as low level or high level, depending on how close they are to the binary code understood by the computer, or how similar they are to everyday language.

In order for high level languages to be understood by the computer processor they must be translated into binary code. This can be done either by translating the written program as a whole, and using the compiled program to instruct the computer (compiled languages) or translating one high level instruction at a time, which is then acted upon in sequence by the computer (interpreted languages). Compiled languages have the benefit of speed.

In the UK in the 1960s and 1970s, the languages mainly used were BASIC, FORTRAN, or COBOL, or a language idiosyncratic to the particular hardware. These languages were not ideal for hospital laboratory purposes and have been largely replaced by others more suitable including the Pascal family of languages of which the current favourite is probably the 'C' language. With the advent of artificial intelligence and expert systems, languages that are more suitable for these purposes may become more popular.

4. Much faster in execution, but more difficult to write, is assembler code, which addresses the processor functions more directly than the high level languages.
5. In earlier times, at least in the UK, laboratory personnel were largely responsible for writing the programs that were most successfully used in biochemistry departments, and the programming language was an important interface between the laboratory and the computer. Procedures for inputting patients' details and tests required; for taking in results of tests and assigning them to the correct patient's file; for formatting and printing reports; and for storing these data in a form that it could be quickly recalled; all these functions were frequently written from

scratch by laboratory programmers. The resulting complex of program and data files are referred to as the application software.

It is evident that such programs and data files are interdependent. For example, results-input programs may take in results from analysers or keyboard, call up a validation program so that the result can be accepted, call up a tests file so that the result is assigned to the right test, and call up a patients' file to assign that result to the correct patient. In the 1970s similar interconnected routines were being developed, on a much larger scale, for business and commercial purposes, and it became clear that much programming effort was being wasted in writing individual programs and connecting them together to form workable systems.

As a result, the concept was introduced of producing an interconnected framework of programs which would enable programmers or even end-users to develop complex data-handling facilities, suitable for their own individual purposes, without the necessity of starting each application from scratch. The idea of a 'database' system was therefore developed and in recent years databases have become the foundation on which laboratory systems have been built.

It is quite possible to use a laboratory computer system without coming into direct contact with any of the areas of software described above, and it is certainly no longer necessary for laboratory personnel to be involved in writing programs, although history would indicate that it may be difficult to stop them. In order to get the best out of a laboratory system, however, it is advisable for some personnel to have a working knowledge of the database and its facilities. For this reason this subject will now be covered in more detail.

INTRODUCTION TO DATABASES

The Evolution of Databases

The term database became current in the early 1960s. Prior to that time the computer world talked about files of data and data sets. However, before the third generation of computers (1965) most files were handled in a serial manner (Fig. 1). The physical data structure was essentially the same as the logical file structure. The physical file structure is embedded in the applications programs. If the data structure or storage device is changed, the application program must be re-written, re-compiled and re-tested.

Some random access files were used at this stage, permitting the user to access any record at random instead of scanning the entire file. The means of addressing these files had to be coded into the program.

The next stage (Fig. 2) acknowledged the changing nature of files and their storage devices and

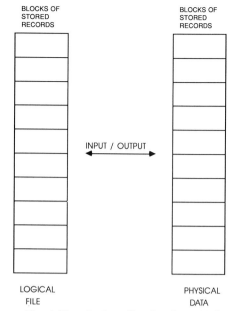

Fig. 1 Simple data files (early 1960s).

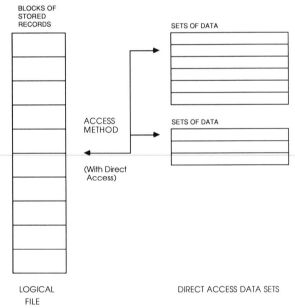

Fig. 2 File access (late 1960s).

attempted to insulate the application from the effects of hardware changes. The software allows change of the physical data layout without changing the logical view of the data. Data structures are usually serial, indexed sequential or simple direct address.

In general, if a laboratory purchases a commercial system, the exact structure of the database—whether it is network, hierarchical or relationally based—would seem superfluous, provided of course that the system performs the tasks placed upon it in an efficient manner and is capable of evolution. Indeed many manufacturers of pathology systems use a number of different structures within the database, dependent on the requirements placed upon the database. A knowledge of the limitations of each database structure will, however, provide the biochemist with added insight to enable selection of a system knowing something of the limitations resulting from its design.

Structures and Manipulations

A database may be defined as a collection of inter-related data stored together, without harmful or unnecessary redundancy (*see* below), in order to serve multiple applications. The various items that comprise the data are stored in a manner which enables them to be independent of programs which use the data. A common and controlled approach is used in adding new data and in modifying and retrieving existing data within the database.

It would seem appropriate here to define some of the terms used in describing the items of a database.

Record A group of related fields of information treated as a unit by an application program, i.e. a patient's record.
File A set of similarly constructed records.
Set A set is a named collection of record types. As such, it establishes the characteristics of an arbitrary number of occurrences of the named set.
Field/Data Item The smallest unit of data that has meaning in describing information.
Logical File A file as perceived by an application program. It may be in a completely different form from that in which it is stored on the storage units.
Physical File A file in which the data items exist in reality. Data is often converted by software from the form in which it is physically stored, to a form in which a user or programmer perceives it.

The intention of a database is that the same collection of data should be available to as many applications as possible, and permit the retrieval and continuous modification of the data needed for the control of operations. It should be possible to search the database to obtain answers to specific queries or to produce long-term information for managing and planning the laboratory. The database may serve several different departments, cutting across all disciplines.

Redundancy. In many databases, data items are stored redundantly; that is they are stored more than once in different parts of the database. However, controlled duplication in a database can be very efficient and those databases with no redundancy can be slow and tedious, because of the time required to search and access the database. There is a trade-off between non-redundancy and other desirable criteria, so the use of controlled redundancy or minimal redundancy is generally accepted.

Uncontrolled redundancy can have several disadvantages. First, there is the added cost of sorting multiple copies. Second, a much more serious aspect is that multiple operations are necessary to update at least some of the redundant copies. Third, because the different copies of the data may be in different stages of updating, the system may give inconsistent information.

Relationships Between Data Items. When a single set of data items serves a variety of applications, different application programs perceive different relationships between the items of data. A database used for many applications may have multiple interconnections between the data. In this environment, the control of accuracy, privacy and security of the data is much more difficult than when simple interconnected files are stored.

On some systems, a reason for using database techniques is to permit users to employ the data in a way which cannot be precisely anticipated by the system designers. One of the advantages of 'Management Information Systems' is that laboratory managers may ask unanticipated questions of their computer system. Instead of being organized into application-oriented files, which must always be addressed in the same way, the data is organized so that it can be addressed in a variety of different ways and can be used to answer a diversity of queries.

As commercial data processing evolved, it became clear that it was desirable to isolate the application programs not only from changes in the file hardware and the effects of increasing file size, but also from additions to the data that is stored, i.e. new fields, new relationships. Development of database software attempted to accomplish this and recognized that a database is continually evolving and will be used for new applications. As multiple logical files can be derived from the same data (Fig. 3), so this same data may be accessed in different ways, by applications with different requirements. The next stage (Fig. 4), which is the current situation, utilizes the concept of the independence of logical and physical data. Logical data independence means that the overall logical structure of the data may be changed, without changing the applications programs. Physical data independence means that the physical layout and organization of the data may be changed, without changing either the overall logical structure of the data, or the applications programs.

The central block in Fig. 4 is extremely important in modern database design and is a conceptual view of the data as a whole. It is sometimes referred to as a *model* of the data or a *conceptual model*. It should be designed to be as stable as possible and to be able to grow to incorporate more data types.

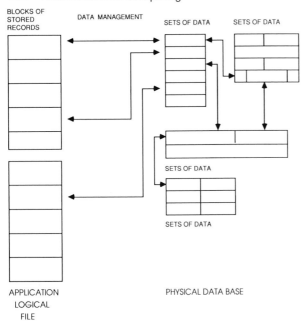

BLOCKS OF STORED RECORDS · DATA MANAGEMENT · SETS OF DATA · SETS OF DATA · SETS OF DATA · SETS OF DATA · APPLICATION LOGICAL FILE · PHYSICAL DATA BASE

Fig. 3 Early database system (early 1970s).

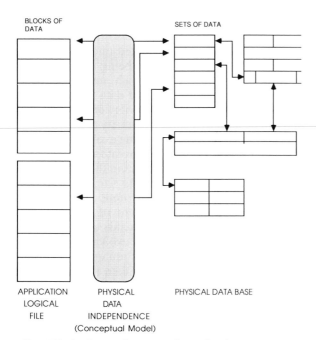

BLOCKS OF DATA · SETS OF DATA · APPLICATION LOGICAL FILE · PHYSICAL DATA INDEPENDENCE (Conceptual Model) · PHYSICAL DATA BASE

Fig. 4 Today's requirements for a database system.

The Objectives of Database Organization

The principles of database organization have been studied at great length by many bodies, who have issued reports on the requirements for database management systems.[3,4] Some characteristics required of a database system are shown in Table 2.

Three types of structures will be discussed to demonstrate the difference between the types of structures that are found in database relationships.

TABLE 2
CHARACTERISTICS REQUIRED OF A DATABASE SYSTEM

1. Ability to represent the inherent nature of the data.
2. High level of performance.
3. Low level of cost.
4. Minimal redundancy.
5. Fast and flexible search capability.
6. High level of data integrity.
7. Database security and privacy
    data should be protected from physical damage
    data should be reconstructable after incidents
    data should be auditable
    data should be tamper proof
    use of database should be positively identified
    the system should establish that user's actions are authorized
    the system should ensure that user's actions are monitored
8. Ability to update database for future requirements.
9. System should be able to be tuned to user's requirements.
10. Frequently used data should be accessed quickly and conveniently.
11. Ability to support a high level of query or report generation languages.

From Computer Data-Base Organization[5]

Hierarchical Databases

Hierarchical, in the context illustrated here, means a tree-structured database. Unfortunately additional terminology has to be introduced, but it will be kept to a minimum. The physical representation of these databases is described elsewhere.[5]

Figure 5 represents a tree structure. A tree is composed of a hierarchy of elements called *nodes*. The uppermost level of the hierarchy has only one node, called a *root*. With the exception of the root, every node has one node related to it at a higher level, and this is called the parent. No node can have more than one parent. Each element can have one or more elements related to it at a lower level. These are called children. Trees such as shown in Fig. 5 are used in both logical and physical data descriptions. In physical data organizations, they are used to describe sets of pointers and relations between

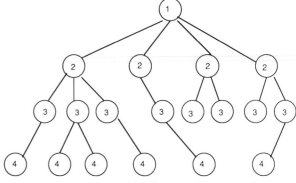

Fig. 5 A tree structure. No element has more than one parent.

entries in indices. Trees are usually drawn upside down with the *root* at the top and the *leaves* at the bottom.

To bring this into clinical biochemistry terms: Level 1, the patient identification record (PID); Level 2, active requests for that patient; Level 3, tests associated with those requests, Level 4, results and comments associated with those tests.

Network Based Databases

If a child in a data relationship has more than one parent, the relationship cannot be described as a tree or hierarchical structure. Instead it is described as a *network* or *plex structure* (Fig. 6). The term network

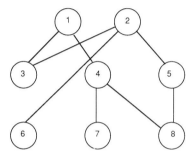

Fig. 6 Example of a plex structure (network). One or more nodes have multiple parents.

is used here to imply a CODASYL database structure.[3] Ever since this structure was proposed in the late 1960s it has been subject to *de facto* standardization.[3] As with a tree structure, a plex structure may be described in terms of children and parents, and drawn in such a way that the children are lower than the parents.

In many plex structures showing the relationships between record types or data aggregate types, the mapping between parents and children is similar to that in a tree. The parent-to-child mapping is complex and the child-to-parent mapping is simple, i.e. a child has one or two parents, whereas a parent may have many children.

Figure 7 shows a simplex plex structure with parent-to-child relationships. This model is found to be most useful when repeated and predictable transactions are executed against a large database, with the constraint that the execution must be fast. In this case it is advantageous that there is a direct link between certain nodes, rather than just a complicated link as in a hierarchical structure.

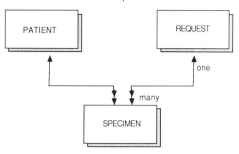

Fig. 7 A schema depicting a simple plex structure.[6] A patient may have many specimens, whereas the specimen is from one patient.

Relational Databases

It is possible to avoid the entanglements that build up in tree and plex structures, when additional items of data are added, or when different forms of query are requested by the users. This is a technique known as normalization,[6] which has been designed and much advocated by Codd.[7]

A way of describing data was advocated that:

1. Can be understood by users with no training in programming.
2. Makes it possible to add new data items, records and associations.
3. Permits the maximum flexibility in handling unanticipated uses of data or spontaneous enquiries at terminals.

The computer enthusiasts of normalization have a vocabulary of their own and often have a tendency to express simple terms in a complex form.

Table 3 shows what is referred to as a *relation*. A database constructed using relations is referred to as a relational database. The relational approach is taken from the mathematical theory of relations and the vocabulary is taken from this branch of mathematics. Hence operations on data may be described with precision.

The relation or table is a set of *tuples*, where a tuple can be regarded as a number of sets of data. If there are n tuples (i.e. the table has n columns), the relation is said to be of degree n. Relations of degree 2 are called binary, degree 3 called tertiary and so on.

A set of values of one item, i.e. one column in a relation (Hospital no. in Table 3) is referred to as a domain.

TABLE 3

Laboratory number	Surname	Forename	Sex	Hospital no.	Hospital	Ward
1234	Smith	John	M	678908	Any	1
1463	Jones	Alf	M	134678	Any	2
1643	Brown	Michael	M	167348	Any	1
1786	Robinson	Belinda	F	134867	Any	3

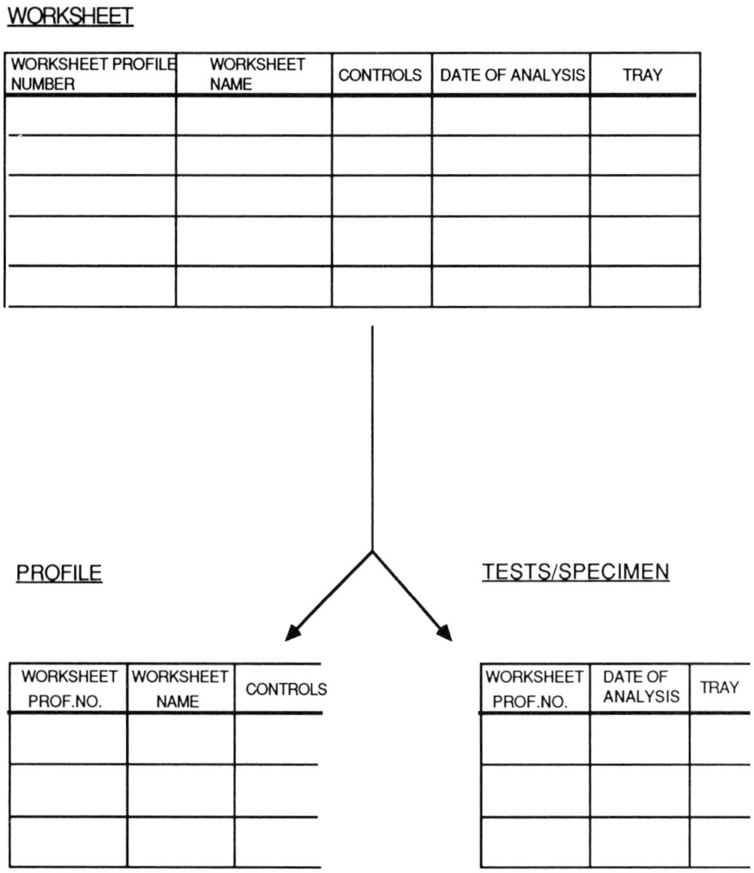

WORKSHEET

WORKSHEET PROFILE NUMBER	WORKSHEET NAME	CONTROLS	DATE OF ANALYSIS	TRAY

PROFILE

WORKSHEET PROF.NO.	WORKSHEET NAME	CONTROLS

TESTS/SPECIMEN

WORKSHEET PROF.NO.	DATE OF ANALYSIS	TRAY

Fig. 8 Taken from Rappoport.[9]

Repeating groups. A file which is 'flat' except for a repeating group can be normalized by removing the repeating group into a separate table or flat file. The new file or relation thus formed is given a separate name (e.g. 'Tests per specimen' in Fig. 8).

Keys. Each tuple must have a key with which it can be identified. The tuple may be identifiable by means of one attribute, i.e. Worksheet Profile No. in Fig. 8. However, more than one attribute may be necessary to identify the tuple. No one attribute is sufficient to identify a 'tests/specimen' tuple in Fig. 8. Therefore a key would consist of more than one attribute e.g. 'Worksheet Profile No.' and 'Date of Analysis'.

The key should have two main properties:

1. It must provide unique identification.
2. No attribute in the key can be discarded without destroying the property of unique identification.

HARDWARE

It is beyond the scope of this chapter to cover the subject of the technology of electronic data-processing hardware; the interested reader can refer to the many excellent books, both general texts and those specific to particular processors and applications, that are readily available in book shops.

By and large, the computer equipment now available to the laboratory for processing its data is well able to carry out the desired functions efficiently and with adequate speed. This applies both to the central processing unit (whether comprising a large mainframe system, a medium-sized minicomputer, or a number of inter-connected microcomputers) and to peripheral devices such as VDU/keyboard terminals, storage devices, printers, bar-code readers, etc. There is no great difficulty in obtaining equipment from the many reputable hardware manufacturers that will do the job adequately. But it is essential that the workload expected of it, both current and projected, is properly assessed, and that equipment is chosen which is appropriate to the task required and is capable, in terms for example of memory size, speed and robustness, of meeting the necessary requirements[6].

There have been great advances in the available hardware over the past decade, particularly in the speed of the microprocessors, in the amount of processor memory, and in the availability of on-line data-storage devices, such as the Winchester disc drives. Recent advances in hardware technology, such as the video disc, and even better microprocessor chips will soon bring even greater computing power to clinical laboratories.

Despite this great advance in hardware technology, the implementation of laboratory systems has not developed as much as it should, partly because of limitations in suitable software, as discussed earlier, and partly because of poor application of networking and interfacing procedures. Because of the importance of this aspect of the subject, networking will now be discussed.

NETWORKS AND CLINICAL COMPUTING

A most desirable feature for computing in clinical laboratories is that the laboratory computer should be connected to another computer, e.g. Patient Administration System (PAS), to allow interchange of information. Because of costs and practicalities, the laboratory system may be designed to maintain an index of patients, which amounts to a sub-set to that contained in the PAS computer. In some cases it is not a proper sub-set and some discrepancies may be present between the two indices.

Within a hospital there will probably be a number of computers, each dedicated to its own particular function (e.g. clinical biochemistry, x-ray, appointments, accident/emergency and personnel). These computers will contain items of data that exist on other machines, with the same problem of discrepancies. Clearly there is a need for the data used by all the computers to be consistent and therefore they need to be interconnected in some way.

The most flexible type of interconnection is known as a 'Local Area Network (LAN). There are various types of LAN that can be purchased and some are already in use in a hospital environment.[8]

The successful transfer of information from one computer to another may be achieved in three functional blocks:

1. The hardware level—responsible for physical connection and transfer protocol.
2. The software level—responsible for the link to the LAN, ensuring a reliable transmission of data.
3. The applications level—responsible for whether applications or service programs are initiated.

All these levels together make up a LAN.

A LAN may be one of several distinct types:

1. Star Network
2. Ring Network
3. CSMA/CD Network
4. Token passing

Star Network

Historically the star configuration was the first, with a central host computer surrounded by terminals (Fig. 9). The trend then moved to remote job-entry satellites, which were themselves star networks. The

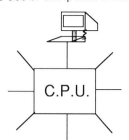

Fig. 9 Star network.

drawbacks of these LANs were the cabling required for large sites and the potentially critical elements such as the central controller.

Ring Network

A ring network usually consists of a simple coaxial cable run around the site (Fig. 10). Each computer/

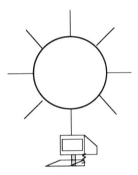

Fig. 10 Ring network.

instrument/terminal is connected to the ring via a station or node. When a data package is sent by the node, it has a destination 'address' attached to it. The data package passes around the ring until the destination node removes the package from the ring.

For the safe and efficient operation of the ring, a number of additional items of hardware are necessary: (a) a central controller which provides the timing and power for the nodes and can monitor traffic; (b) repeater nodes which 'boost' the data package around the ring. The main problem with ring networks is that they have poor resilience under cable faults.

CSMA/CD Networks

These networks are generically known as Carrier Sensing Multiple Access with Collision Detection (i.e. two people picking up the telephone at the same time) or Ethernet. These LANS (Fig. 11) allow multiple access and a contention scheme is necessary to detect collisions when under high load. The very nature of contention allowed on Ethernet, which permits collisions to take place, dictates that the user of such a system is allowed a probability that a colli-

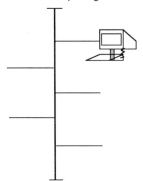

Fig. 11 CSMA/CD network.

sion will take place on each occasion he attempts to transfer information.

This mode of operation is wasteful under heavy loads. Even under moderate loads, the protocols may fail to guarantee access to other users within a given timeframe.

Token Passing

This network can be either on token ring or token bus (Fig. 12). Each of these schemes utilizes the prin-

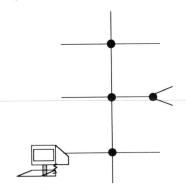

Fig. 12 Token passing.

ciple of an 'Invitation to Transmit' or 'Token' in which an electronic signal is used to synchronize the access of users of the LAN. With co-ordinated access of the media, guaranteed throughput is obtained with either ring or bus structures. After receipt of a token, the holder is allowed to transmit directly to any other user on the network.

In effect, the token-based network combines the advantages of the other protocols without the drawbacks.

COMPUTING IN CLINICAL BIOCHEMISTRY

There are available comprehensive reviews on the early development of computing in clinical biochemistry laboratories, to which the reader requiring a detailed understanding is recommended to refer.[10–13] We examine here the main changes which have occurred in pathology computing to the present day.

The development of computing in pathology may be summarized under three main headings.

1. The early batch-oriented computers.
2. The interactive systems.
3. Further developments of interactive systems.

The Early Batch-oriented Computers

During the 50s and 60s an increased demand was made on the clinical laboratory to perform tests accurately, swiftly and economically. This was the time of the greatest growth in the medical sciences. Due to the paucity of technically trained staff at the time and the increased demands made upon the manually orientated laboratory, there was a gradual introduction into the laboratory of newly invented mechanized devices, leading to the development of (mechanically) automated laboratories.

These 'automated' laboratories were able to deal effectively with the technical performance of the physico-chemical procedures which eventually led to the establishment of a measurable reaction or result. A corollary of this development was the large amount of paper work necessary to document the entire procedure. This activity included the identification of the patient, specimen and test to be performed; the creation of appropriate calibration curves or reference standard values and the establishment of values for quality control procedures. In addition, the results had to be manually transferred to the patient's laboratory report and delivered to the appropriate ward or clinic.

Clearly the two areas which required development at this time were the manual calculation of results and the labour-intensive manual reporting of these results. A small number of eminent and intrepid scientists in the field,[14,15] began to introduce a second phase of automation, namely data processing. Their vision was to merge the two discrete automated systems into a single continuous process.[9]

A number of courageous attempts were made to develop laboratory computer systems often, in the United Kingdom, with the help of the Department of Health & Social Security (DHSS). These computer systems were batch processors which were configured to accept paper tape input and output, with all output printed off-line, at a rate of 10 characters per second, on a Teletype printer.[14,15]

The sequence of operations using these off-line systems is outlined in Fig. 13. Entry to the batch processor was usually via punched tape. The limitations of these early systems were abundantly clear and working practices were altered to keep the number of occasions the computer was accessed during the day to a minimum. The peripheral devices used, i.e. magnetic tape, teletypes and punch readers, were mechanically based and therefore less robust and reliable than the computer itself.[4] These reasons added together meant that early computer processing in cli-

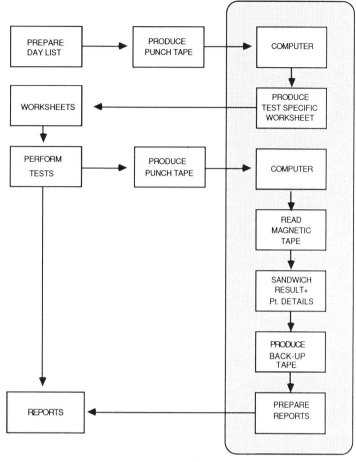

Fig. 13 Data-flow chart for early off-line computerized systems.

nical biochemistry was labour intensive and time consuming.

The Interactive Systems

The early concepts, that laboratory computer systems in use were considered as being data acquisition units, programmed as if arithmetical operations were the most critical problem facing the laboratory were soon proved to be untrue. Advances in the instrumentation resulted in the calculation functions being incorporated into the analyser, therefore producing results in a calculated form. It soon became clear that data management was becoming the more important function for the computer system.

Coincident with the development in computer hardware, the DHSS instituted a project, which became known as the Three Lab Project, which allowed the design of systems which could be operated with confidence by laboratory staff, without the intervention of specially trained computer personnel. The design criteria incorporated a requirement for the individual transactions to be carried out quickly and with little effort, so that the introduction of such a system resulted in the saving of time and effort rather than the reverse.

Two major laboratory systems developed in the UK at this time were the Phoenix[12] and Socrates[13] systems which incorporated several design requirements.

1. Multi-user and multi-tasking facilities.
2. An indexed random access filing system with instantaneous retrieval.
3. A high-level applications language such that laboratory staff are able to understand and maintain the software.
4. Interfaces for handling on-line instruments.

Further Developments of Interactive Systems

With the development of microprocessors, whereby more intelligence is being incorporated into clinical analysers, the requirements of the laboratory computer system have changed. Although the laboratory computer has taken on the role more of a laboratory information management system, there has not been a significant development of computers in the Health Service, similar to that during the 1960s and 1970s.

The reasons for this can be postulated as being—

1. The relatively small size of the NHS market, making systems development uneconomical.

2. The general reduction of development funds of the NHS.
3. The relatively high cost of software compared with the much lower cost of hardware.

Developments in hardware have allowed the Health Service to benefit from:

faster processing speeds
    —faster response
better database design
    —faster response
larger storage capacity
    —winchester disc technology
'fault tolerant' computers
    —dual processors, mirror discs and transaction logging

Developments in software have allowed:

better base search facilities
    —correlations and epidemiological studies
non-numeric result entry
    —free text and word processing
generated results
    —creatinine clearance, etc.
structured results of complex tests
    —TRH test, GTT, etc.
management information
    —workload, other management statistics, normal range assessment
research information
    —clinical, biochemical
query languages
    —for example—provide me with a *list* of *all patients* who are between the *ages* of *60–80* and have a *T4* less than *140 nmol/l* etc.
quality assurance
access to other databases
    —via telecommunication services, etc.
data protection and confidentiality

The development of so called 'expert systems' for pathology systems are still some way off and will be discussed below.

COMPUTERIZING NEEDS NOT PROBLEMS

It is surprising that although each routine clinical biochemistry laboratory is performing essentially the same repertoire of tests, there is a wide variability in the apparent requirements for laboratory computing. It has been suggested that often departmental heads are asking computing systems to sort out departmental procedural problems, rather than optimizing the procedures prior to installing the computer.

There is no doubt that putting a bad, inefficient laboratory system onto a computer can only lead to a bad computer system. It is important to ensure that any project is well thought out and driven by need rather than technology. It is very important therefore

to define the laboratory's real needs and problems. Once these have been defined, the problems must be sorted out in the organization structure, as they exist prior to computerization, before installing the laboratory information management system.

Introducing a computer system into a laboratory will produce considerable changes in the overall operation of the laboratory. It is better to acknowledge and accept these changes rather than attempt to select a system that mimics exactly the laboratory's previous working practices. However, it is essential that the requirement of good laboratory practice and good laboratory management still apply and are not jeopardized.

There is also a little confusion in the terminology used between the computer supplier/laboratory interface. This is the definition of the terms, features and benefits. Unfortunately many features of a computer system are presented as benefits. This confusion of terms must be clearly understood by the negotiating body so that the right laboratory information management system is installed.

The Oxford Dictionary defines a *feature* as *a distinctive or characteristic part of a thing, part that arrests attention* and a *benefit* as *an advantage*. Table 4 shows a brief list of the features incorporated by a hypothetical computer system.

TABLE 4
FEATURES OF LABORATORY COMPUTER SYSTEMS

Interactive on-line test requesting.
Logging receipt of samples/requests into day book.
Automatic creation of worksheets.
On-line data organization.
On-line quality control.
Flagging unusual findings.
Graphical reports for dynamic tests.
Aid with interpretation of results—indication of normality.
Electronic transmission of reports to satellite laboratories.
Speed with telephone enquiries.
Storage of results occupying less space.

EXPERT SYSTEMS AND ARTIFICIAL INTELLIGENCE

The term 'expert systems' has a futuristic and sometimes sinister connotation but there are a number of projects being implemented in the commercial and Health Service environments, although these are decidedly modest in scope.

The level of interest that has been generated by the Alvey and Esprit (European Strategic Programme for Research and Development in Information Technology) programmes and the Japanese fifth generation computer program, has led to expectations of highly sophisticated systems which, in the commercial world, purport to replace human experts!

Over the past 15 years, research interest and expertise in applying knowledge-based systems to clinical practice has expanded rapidly in the United States.

A number of expert systems were being developed in the 1970s (CASNET, MYCIN and DIGITALIS ADVISOR etc.) which explored ways of representing and manipulating expert knowledge in medical science.

The way a clinician arrives at a diagnosis can be proposed as being:

1. Initial information is obtained from the patient —patient database
2. This is matched to clinical knowledge (body in health state versus body in disease state) —knowledge database
3. Diagnosis achieved through deterministic reasoning

In the field of medicine and health care it is, of course, impossible to reduce human knowledge and experience to a system of rules that involve strict implication. Expert systems provide a modification of the strength of an inference in their rules in the form of so-called certainty factors.

In Shortliffe's MYCIN which was developed at Stanford University, rules are in the form

Rule 91　IF the patient has abdominal pain AND the pain is maximal in the Right Iliac Fossa AND there is rebound tenderness THEN the patient may have appendicitis.

This type of rule expresses an association between simple elements but rarely includes the relationships of true cause and effect. They may be considered as rules of thumb or *heuristic*. These rules are further extended to introduce the concept of uncertainty, by noting a level of probability associated with the conclusion, i.e. *likely* (0.9), which expresses the uncertainty associated with this inference.

Early programs for control of the knowledge base were written in one of the few high logic programming languages designed for knowledge manipulation. Several early systems were developed in LISP[2] which has more recently been standardized as COMMON LISP PROLOG which is a development from COMMON LISP and is more frequently used in systems associated with medicine.

Inference. In operation, the inference system may respond to a user enquiry, a consultation system or be activated by fresh terms of data. The control program may itself contain the strategies for manipulating a knowledge base or these may exist separately as a distinct set of rules.

One of the main characteristics of the control program, which is central to the concept of expert systems, is its ability to provide the user with an explanation of how it obtained its conclusions (when required). A scientist may thus validate the computer's statement by examining the knowledge base and the inference procedures used to reach it.

Early in the development of expert systems used in medical science, it became clear that control programs could be dissociated from any one particular area of knowledge. Independent control programs formulated into knowledge bases of different subject areas (*domains*) could be fitted. EMYCIN, derived from the MYCIN system, was the first of the expert system 'shells' to be used for domains outside the initial area in which it had been developed (Table 5).

TABLE 5
SOME EXPERT SYSTEMS USED IN MEDICINE

System	Expert function	Author	Publisher
MYCIN	Diagnosis and treatment of bacterial infection	Shortcliffe	Stanford
EMYCIN	Expert system shell of MYCIN	Shortcliffe	Stanford
NEOMYCIN	A teaching version of MYCIN	Clancy	Stanford
DIALOG INTERNIST I—II	Diagnosis of disorders in internal medicine	Pople	Pittsburgh
DIGITALIS ADVISOR	Advisor for digitalis therapy	Swartout	MIT
PUFF	Interpretation of pulmonary function data	Aikins	Stanford
ABEL	Solution of problems in acid–base balance	Szolovits	MIT

The Knowledge Base

Construction of any knowledge base is always the bottle-neck in any expert system. Knowledge acquisition can be obtained by a number of people from domain experts either by direct interview or discussion. Accumulating the knowledge base is a slow and tedious process and is usually followed by the equally laborious task of encoding the acquired knowledge into the chosen representation system. Very few functional examples have so far been published, and their clinical acceptability is remarkably low.

EXPERT SYSTEMS IN PATHOLOGY—THE FUTURE

Domain Experts. The careful selection of subject areas which are relatively contention free and where there is full co-operation and agreement of domain experts is clearly the first stage for the successful implementation of any medical expert system.

Natural Language. Most scientists are instinctively addicted to natural language. However, the task of instructing a computer to understand a natural language is a hard one because of the inherent imprecision and ambiguity of language.

The process usually deals with analysing three

general components: syntax, semantics and pragmatics. Syntactic analysis separates the natural language sentence into its constituent parts. This separation aids in the nearly simultaneous semantic analysis in which the internal representation for the meaning of the entire sentence is constructed.

Pragmatic analysis goes one step beyond this by considering the *intent* of the speaker—not just a literal translation of the words used.

Knowledge Representation. For efficient problem solving, a knowledge base must hold both shorthand, heuristic rules and deeper casual knowledge. Clearly more research will be needed into the languages and systems to achieve efficient knowledge representation.

Knowledge Manipulation. Time-dependent data and uncertainty parameters need to be built into more knowledge bases, e.g. the pharmokinetics of drug therapy.

The Experts' Expert. Immense effort is required to develop systems which will provide even modest expert inferences in a limited domain. The near future should see acceptable systems which can provide sensible information to clinicians about specialist topics and the development of knowledge acquisition across a range of related disciplines leading to the subsequent representation of this data with the minimum of ambiguity.

When these developments are achieved in parallel with advances in hardware and software tools, medical sciences should see a further major leap forward in computing.

REFERENCES

1. Comrie L. J. (1946). Babbage's dream comes true. *Nature*; **158**: 567–8.
2. McCarthy J., Brayton R., Edwards D., Fox P. A., Hodes L., Luckham D., Maling K., Park D., Russell S. (1960). *LISP 1 Programmers' Manual*; Cambridge, Ma: MIT Press.
3. CODASYL Systems Committee (1971). *Feature Analysis of Generalized Database Management Systems; Technical Report*. New York: Assoc. for Computing Machinery.
4. CODASYL Programming Languages Committee (1971). *Database Task Group Report*. New York: Assoc. for Computing Machinery.
5. Martin J. (1977). *Computer Data-base Organization*. New Jersey: Prentice Hall.
6. Hirst A. D. (1983). Systems analysis of a laboratory. In *A Guide to Data Processing in Clinical Laboratories*. (de Bats A., O'Meara J. eds) pp. 10–25. Epsom: PRC Associates.
7. Codd E. F. (1970). A relational model of data for large shared data banks. *Comm. ACM*; **13**: 377–87.
8. Stokes A. V. (1984). The implementation of an Ethernet in West Lambeth Health Authority. *Proc. Networks*; **84**: 651–61.
9. Rappoport A. E. (1969). *J. Clin. Pathol*; **22**, Suppl 3: 125–6.
10. Whitehead T. P. ed. (1969). *Symposium: Automation and Data Processing in Pathology. J. Clin. Pathol*; **22**, Suppl 3.
11. Flynn F. V. (1978). Computers in clinical chemistry. In *Recent Advances in Clinical Biochemistry*; **1**: 255–79.
12. Abson J., Prail A., Wootton I. D. P. (1977). Data processing in pathology laboratories: the Phoenix system. *Ann. Clin. Biochem*; **14**: 307–29.
13. Flynn F. V., Ball S. G. (1982). Comprehensive computerised data management in a chemical pathology laboratory with SOCRATES. *Med. Inform*; **7**: 275–305.
14. Wootton I. D. P. (1969). Computer processing of biochemical information without going on-line. *J. Clin. Pathol*; **22**, Suppl 3: 101–6.
15. Flynn F. V. (1969). Problems and benefits of using a computer for laboratory data processing. *J. Clin. Pathol*; **22**, Suppl 3: 62–73.

INDEX